Fifth Edition

Ebersole and Hess'

Gerontological Nursing & Healthy Aging

Theris A. Touhy, DNP, CNS, DPNAP
Emeritus Professor
Christine E. Lynn College of Nursing
Florida Atlantic University
Boca Raton, Florida

Kathleen Jett, PhD, GNP-BC
Clinical Care Coordinator
Gerontological Nurse Practitioner, Board Certified
Oak Hammock at the University of Florida
Division of Geriatric Medicine
Department of Aging and Geriatric Research
University of Florida College of Medicine
Gainesville, Florida

ELSEVIER

ELSEVIER

3251 Riverport Lane
St. Louis, Missouri 63043

EBERSOLE AND HESS' GERONTOLOGICAL NURSING & HEALTHY AGING, FIFTH EDITION ISBN: 978-0-323-40167-8

Notices

Knowledge and best practice in this field are constantly changing. As new research and experience broaden our understanding, changes in research methods, professional practices, or medical treatment may become necessary.

Practitioners and researchers must always rely on their own experience and knowledge in evaluating and using any information, methods, compounds, or experiments described herein. In using such information or methods they should be mindful of their own safety and the safety of others, including parties for whom they have a professional responsibility.

With respect to any drug or pharmaceutical products identified, readers are advised to check the most current information provided (i) on procedures featured or (ii) by the manufacturer of each product to be administered, to verify the recommended dose or formula, the method and duration of administration, and contraindications. It is the responsibility of practitioners, relying on their own experience and knowledge of their patients, to make diagnoses, to determine dosages and the best treatment for each individual patient, and to take all appropriate safety precautions.

To the fullest extent of the law, neither the Publisher nor the authors, contributors, or editors, assume any liability for any injury and/or damage to persons or property as a matter of products liability, negligence or otherwise, or from any use or operation of any methods, products, instructions, or ideas contained in the material herein.

Previous editions copyrighted 2014, 2010, 2005, and 2001.

Library of Congress Cataloging-in-Publication Data

Names: Touhy, Theris A., author. | Jett, Kathleen Freudenberger, author.
Title: Ebersole and Hess' gerontological nursing & healthy aging / Theris A. Touhy, Kathleen Jett.
Other titles: Ebersole and Hess' gerontological nursing & healthy aging | Ebersole and Hess' gerontological nursing and healthy aging | Gerontological nursing & healthy aging
Description: Fifth edition. | St. Louis, Missouri : Elsevier, [2018] | Includes bibliographical references and index.
Identifiers: LCCN 2016040080 | ISBN 9780323401678 (hardcover)
Subjects: | MESH: Geriatric Nursing | Aged | Aging | Holistic Nursing | Health Promotion
Classification: LCC RC954 | NLM WY 152 | DDC 618.97/0231—dc23 LC record available at https://lccn.loc.gov/2016040080

Senior Content Strategist: Sandy Clark
Content Development Manager: Billie Sharp
Associate Content Development Specialist: Laurel Shea
Publishing Services Manager: Jeff Patterson
Book Production Specialist: Carol O'Connell
Design Direction: Maggie Reid

Printed in China

Last digit is the print number: 9 8 7 6 5 4 3 2 1

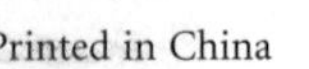

To my beautiful grandchildren, Colin, Molly, and Auden Touhy.
Being your Gramma TT makes growing older the best time of my life and I love you.

To my sons and daughters-in-law, thanks for surrounding me with love and family.

To my husband, just thanks for loving me for 49 years even though it's not always easy!

To all the students who read this book. I hope each of you will improve the journey toward healthy aging through your competence and compassion.

To all of my students who have embraced gerontological nursing as their specialty and are improving the lives of older people through their practice and teaching.

To the older people I have been privileged to nurse, and their caregivers, thanks for making the words in this book a reality for the elders you care for and for teaching me how to be a gerontological nurse.

Theris Touhy

To my husband, Steve, and our wonderful children and grandchildren, who never cease to remind me that the best parts of life are in the adventures we share.

To Dr. Michael Johnson, who is a never-ending guide in pathfinding through chaos.

And to the persons around me who teach me both the challenges and opportunities of aging with grace and dignity.

Kathleen Jett

REVIEWERS AND EVOLVE WRITERS

REVIEWERS

Janet E. Bitzan, PhD, RN
Clinical Professor Emeritus
College of Nursing
University of Wisconsin–Milwaukee
Milwaukee, Wisconsin

Mariann Harding, PhD, RN, CNE
Associate Professor of Nursing
College of Nursing
Kent State University–Tuscarawas
New Philadelphia, Ohio

Cheryl A. Lehman, PhD, RN, CNS-BC, RN-BC, CRRN
Owner, Independent Consultant
Lehman Consulting LLC
Boerne, Texas

Arlene H. Morris, EdD, MSN, RN
Professor of Nursing
School of Nursing
Auburn University–Montgomery
Montgomery, Alabama

Margo L. Thompson, EdD, RN, CNE, BSN, MA, MSN
Associate Graduate Faculty, Department of Nursing
University of Central Missouri
Warrensburg, Missouri

EVOLVE WRITERS

Dia Campbell-Detrixhe, PhD, MSN, BSN
Associate Professor of Nursing
Kramer School of Nursing
Oklahoma City University
Oklahoma City, Oklahoma

Mariann Harding, PhD, RN, CNE
Associate Professor of Nursing
College of Nursing
Kent State University–Tuscarawas
New Philadelphia, Ohio

Anne Van Landingham, RN, BSN, MSN
Instructor, Medical Career Magnet
Orange Technical College–OCPS
Apopka High School
Apopka, Florida

Sharon Wexler, PhD, RN, FNGNA
Associate Professor
ABSN Program Director
Pace University
College of Health Professions Lienhard School of Nursing
New York, New York

PREFACE

This text is intended to tell the story of both health and the health challenges we face as we age. A holistic approach, addressing body, mind, and spirit along a continuum of wellness, and grounded in caring and respect for the person, provides the framework for the text. It is designed to provide nurses, faculty, and students with the key information needed to promote heathy aging. We draw on the most current evidence-based information whenever it is available. As in the fourth edition, this edition provides content consistent with the *Recommended Baccalaureate Competencies and Curricular Guidelines for the Nursing Care of Older Adults* developed by the AACN in collaboration with the John A. Hartford Foundation Institute for Geriatric Nursing at New York University.

We have written this to be used in all courses to provide more expansive coverage than can be found in the several paragraphs of aging applications usually found at the end of many texts. In this way it is highly complementary to any other text and provides more thorough information in care of older adults. It is intended to serve the needs of the undergraduate student in both associate and bachelor's degree programs. For faculty considering a text for use in master's and doctoral programs, we refer you to our sister text, *Toward Healthy Aging*.

The chapters have been reorganized and modified to facilitate student learning. Content has been totally updated, and new chapters have been added on metabolic and neurological disorders, gerontological nursing across the continuum, and caregiving. The goals set forth by the U.S. document *Healthy People 2020* are highlighted whenever there are applications to aging.

We have divided the chapters into five sections that build on one another. Section 1, **Foundations of Healthy Aging**, presents key elements that provide the background—in other words, context—to all other sections. In Section 2, **Foundations of Gerontological Nursing**, the focus is on the nurse with the presumption that all of us provide gerontological care. By 2020, up to 75% of nurses' time will be spent with older adults, and every older person should expect care provided by nurses with competence in gerontological nursing. Section 3, **Fundamentals of Caring**, provides in-depth coverage of areas that may affect functional abilities as we age and presents nursing and interprofessional interventions to enhance wellness, maintain optimal function, and prevent unnecessary disability. Section 4, **Promoting Health in Chronic Illness**, will appear at first glance to be short discussions of a number of disease processes. The disease processes selected are those that commonly develop as we age, but in no case have they been determined to be "normal changes with aging." The content is pointedly directed at how these health problems interact with the normal changes with aging and what the nurse can do to promote healthy aging in the presence of the condition. Finally, Section 5, **Caring for Elders and Their Caregivers**, addresses the added circumstances of living, dying, and aging within one's social sphere and issues that affect older adults and their families/significant others, be they traditional nuclear families, extended families, or fictive (affective) groups of persons.

The text is organized for optimal student learning experiences. Each chapter begins with the phenomenological consideration of the lived experience of an elder. The chapters end with key concepts, learning activities, and discussion questions to stimulate further educational growth. For readers who wish to seek additional information, resources are provided at http://evolve.elsevier.com/Touhy/gerontological.

Gerontological nurses have always assumed a leadership role in improving care for elders and promoting healthy aging. Since the first edition of this text, there has been an explosion, not only of persons in later life, but also of knowledge, research, interest, and resources in gerontological nursing. Today, the expectation is that all nurses will be prepared to care for the growing number of diverse older adults all over the globe and have the knowledge and skills to promote healthy aging for people of all ages. We can look forward to the coming years when aging in health will be the norm, and we hope this text will provide the knowledge nurses need to play a key role in making this happen.

ANCILLARIES

Ancillaries are available at http://evolve.elsevier.com/Touhy/gerontological.

For Instructors

- **TEACH for Nurses Lesson Plans:** Detailed listing of resources available to instructors for each book chapter include learning objectives; key terms; student and instructor resources; suggested classroom activities; answers to Critical Thinking Activities in the book; and clinical activities that can be used for classroom discussion, projects, and further study. Also included is an outline of nursing curriculum standards for each chapter that includes QSEN, Concepts, and BSN Essentials, and a unique Case Study for each book chapter.

- **PowerPoint Presentations:** Lecture slides to accompany each chapter (approximately 750 slides total)
- **Test Bank:** Approximately 500 questions in the latest NCLEX® examination format
- **Image Collection:** Over 75 illustrations and photos that can be used in a presentation or as visual aids

For Students

- **NCLEX®-Style Review Questions:** Questions organized by chapter for additional help in preparing for the NCLEX® examination
- **Case Studies:** Accompanying select chapters, these provide short case studies with questions to help students see content put into practical use

ACKNOWLEDGMENTS

We would like to thank Priscilla Ebersole and Patricia Hess, the creators of the first edition of this book, for their trust in providing us the opportunity to continue their legacies as we share their beautiful words and passion for gerontological nursing. We hope that our work honors them and the specialty we all love. It has been a real privilege for us to be a part of the work of two gerontological nurses from whom we have learned to care.

We would also like to thank the people at Elsevier who helped produce this book, including Sandy Clark, Billie Sharp, Laurel Shea, and Carol O'Connell.

Theris A. Touhy
Kathleen Jett

CONTENTS

SECTION 1 Foundations of Healthy Aging

1 **Introduction to Healthy Aging,** 1
Kathleen Jett
The Years Ahead, 2
How Old Is Old?, 3
Moving Toward Healthy Aging, 6

2 **Cross-Cultural Caring and Aging,** 11
Kathleen Jett
Culture, 12
Diversity, 12
Health Disparities and Inequities, 13
Cultural Knowledge, 15
Integrating Concepts, 20

3 **Biological Theories of Aging and Age-Related Physical Changes,** 22
Kathleen Jett
Biological Theories of Aging, 22
Physical Changes That Accompany Aging, 26

4 **Psychosocial, Spiritual, and Cognitive Aspects of Aging,** 40
Theris A. Touhy
Psychosocial Theories of Aging, 41
Spirituality and Aging, 46
Adult Cognition, 48
Learning in Later Life, 51

SECTION 2 Foundations of Gerontological Nursing

5 **Gerontological Nursing and Promotion of Healthy Aging,** 55
Theris A. Touhy
Care of Older Adults: A Nursing Imperative, 55
History of Gerontological Nursing, 56
Gerontological Nursing Education, 58
Organizations Devoted to Gerontology Research and Practice, 58
Research on Aging, 59
Gerontological Nursing Roles, 60

6 **Gerontological Nursing Across the Continuum of Care,** 66
Theris A. Touhy
Community Care, 67
Skilled Nursing Facilities (Nursing Homes), 69
Long-Term Care and the U.S. Health Care System, 70
Quality of Care in Skilled Nursing Facilities, 71
Transitions Across the Continuum, 74

7 **Economic and Legal Issues,** 79
Kathleen Jett
Late Life Income, 79
Health Care Insurance Plans in Later Life, 81
Legal Issues in Gerontological Nursing, 88

SECTION 3 Fundamentals of Caring

8 **Assessment and Documentation for Optimal Care,** 92
Kathleen Jett
The Assessment Process, 93
The Health History, 94
Physical Assessment, 96
Assessment of Mental Status, 99
Functional Assessment, 102
Comprehensive Geriatric Assessments, 103
Documentation for Quality Care, 105

9 **Safe Medication Use,** 110
Kathleen Jett
Pharmacokinetics, 111
Pharmacodynamics, 114
Chronopharmacology, 114
Medication-Related Problems and Older Adults, 115
Psychoactive Medications, 120

10 **Nutrition,** 130
Theris A. Touhy
Nutrition, 130
Obesity (Overnutrition), 133
Malnutrition (Undernutrition), 133
Factors Affecting Fulfillment of Nutritional Needs, 134

11 **Hydration and Oral Care,** 145
Theris A. Touhy
Hydration Management, 145
Dehydration, 145
Oral Health, 148

12 **Elimination,** 154
Theris A. Touhy
Urinary Incontinence, 155
Urinary Tract Infections, 163
Bowel Elimination, 163

Accidental Bowel Leakage/Fecal Incontinence, 167
13 **Rest, Sleep, and Activity,** 170
Theris A. Touhy
Rest and Sleep, 170
Activity, 178
14 **Promoting Healthy Skin,** 185
Theris A. Touhy
Skin, 186
Common Skin Problems, 186
Skin Cancers, 190
Pressure Injuries, 192
15 **Falls and Fall Risk Reduction,** 201
Theris A. Touhy
Falls, 201
Restraints and Side Rails, 212
16 **Promoting Safety,** 217
Theris A. Touhy
Home Safety, 217
Vulnerability to Environmental Temperatures, 217
Vulnerability to Natural Disasters, 221
Transportation Safety, 221
Emerging Technologies to Enhance Safety of Older Adults, 223
Elder-Friendly Communities, 225

SECTION 4 Promoting Health in Chronic Illness

17 **Living With Chronic Illness,** 228
Kathleen Jett
Acute Illness, 229
Chronic Illness, 229
Theoretical Frameworks for Chronic Illness, 231
18 **Pain and Comfort,** 236
Kathleen Jett
Acute and Chronic Pain, 237
Barriers to Providing Comfort for Those in Pain, 238
19 **Diseases Affecting Vision and Hearing,** 249
Theris A. Touhy
Visual Impairment, 249
Diseases and Disorders of the Eye, 250
Hearing Impairment, 258
Interventions to Enhance Hearing, 259
Tinnitus, 262
20 **Metabolic Disorders,** 265
Kathleen Jett
Thyroid Disease, 265
Diabetes, 267
21 **Bone and Joint Problems,** 276
Kathleen Jett
Musculoskeletal System, 276
Osteoporosis, 277
The Arthritides, 279
22 **Cardiovascular and Respiratory Disorders,** 286
Kathleen Jett
Cardiovascular Disease, 286
Respiratory Disorders, 291
23 **Neurological Disorders,** 297
Kathleen Jett
Cerebrovascular Disease, 298
Neurodegenerative Disorders, 301
Communication and Persons With Neurological Disorders, 305
24 **Mental Health,** 309
Theris A. Touhy
Mental Health, 309
Factors Influencing Mental Health Care, 310
Mental Health Disorders, 313
Schizophrenia, 317
Psychotic Symptoms in Older Adults, 318
Bipolar Disorder, 320
Depression, 321
Suicide, 326
Substance Use Disorders, 328

SECTION 5 Caring for Elders and Their Caregivers

25 **Care of Individuals With Neurocognitive Disorders,** 336
Theris A. Touhy
Neurocognitive Disorder: Delirium, 336
Care of Individuals With Mild and Major Neurocognitive Disorders, 342
Communication, 344
Behavior Concerns and Nursing Models of Care, 346
Providing Care for Activities of Daily Living, 351
Wandering, 353
Nutrition, 353
Nursing Roles in the Care of Persons With Dementia, 354
26 **Relationships, Roles, and Transitions,** 360
Theris A. Touhy
Later Life Transitions, 360
Relationships in Later Life, 363
Families, 364
Intimacy, 369
Sexuality, 370
Sexual Health, 371

Sexual Dysfunction, 373
Alternative Sexual Lifestyles: Lesbian, Gay, Bisexual, and Transgender, 375
Intimacy and Chronic Illness, 376
Intimacy and Sexuality in Long-Term Care Facilities, 376
Intimacy, Sexuality, and Dementia, 379
HIV/AIDS and Older Adults, 379

27 Caregiving, 386
Theris A. Touhy
Caregiving, 386
Elder Mistreatment, 392

28 Loss, Death, and Palliative Care, 397
Kathleen Jett
Grief Work, 398
Dying, Death, and Palliative Care, 404
Dying and the Nurse, 407
Decision-Making at the End of Life, 410

Index, 415

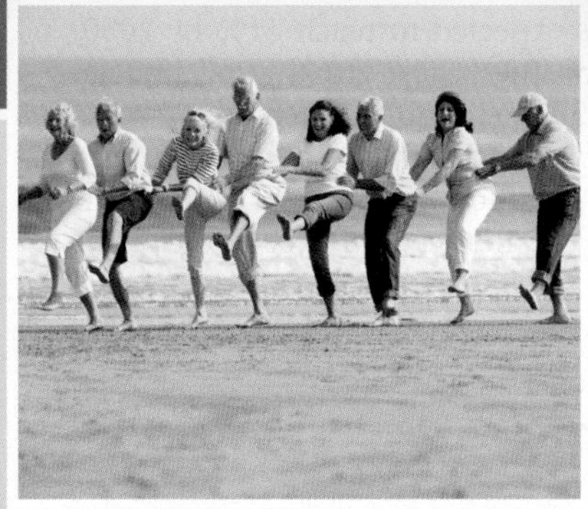

1

Introduction to Healthy Aging

Kathleen Jett

evolve.elsevier.com/Touhy/gerontological

LEARNING OBJECTIVES

Upon completion of this chapter, the reader will be able to:

- Identify at least three factors that influence the aging experience.
- Define health and wellness within the context of aging and chronic illness.
- Describe the trends seen in global aging today.

THE LIVED EXPERIENCE

I believe a human life is like a river, meandering through its course, rushing through rapids, flowing placidly over the plains, twisting and turning through countless bends until it spends itself. It is the same river; yet it looks very different from one place to another. So it is with our lives; circumstances vary from one time to another in the course of a life but there is also value to living.

Georgia, age 80

Caring for older adults gives us a unique opportunity to influence their quality of life in so many ways.

Nursing student, age 19

Aging is part of the life course. Caring for persons who are aging is a practice that touches nurses in all settings: from pediatrics involving grandparents and great-grandparents; to the residents of skilled nursing facilities and their spouses, partners, and children; to nurses providing relief support in countries outside of their own. Holroyd and colleagues (2009) have estimated that "by 2020, up to 75% of nurses' time will be spent with older adults" (p. 374). The core knowledge associated with gerontological nursing affects all of the profession and is not limited to any one subgroup of nurses (Young, 2003).

Gerontological nurses can help shape a world in which persons can thrive and grow old, not merely survive. They have unique opportunities to facilitate wellness in those who are recipients of care. As we move forward in the twenty-first century, the manner in which nurses respond to our aging society will determine our character because we are no greater than the health of the country and the world in which we live. This chapter provides an introduction to how the nurse can help facilitate some level of health for persons in later life regardless of where they are on the continuum between complete well-being and the final moments of life.

THE YEARS AHEAD

As we look to the future, the world's population will soon include more persons older than 60 years than ever before (Fig. 1.1). In the United States the percentage of persons at least 65 years old has increased from 9% to 12% since 1994 and is expected to reach 21% by 2050, making this population the fastest growing of any age group (Fig. 1.2). By 2020 the number of persons 60 years of age and older worldwide outnumbered those younger than 5 years of age, at 2 billion; up from 900 million in 2015 (WHO, 2015a). The majority of those older than

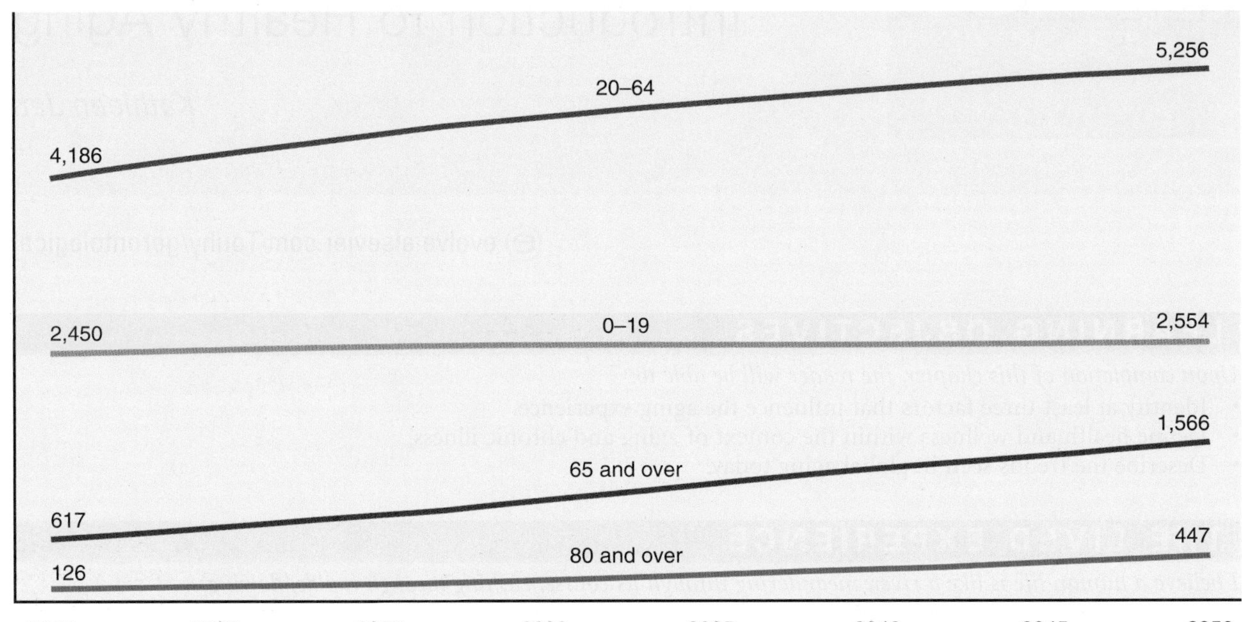

FIGURE 1.1 Percent change in world population by age: 2015 to 2050. (Redrawn from He W, Goodkind D, Kowal P: U.S. Census Bureau, International Population Reports, P95/16-1. *An aging world: 2015,* Washington, DC, 2016, U.S. Government Publishing Office.)

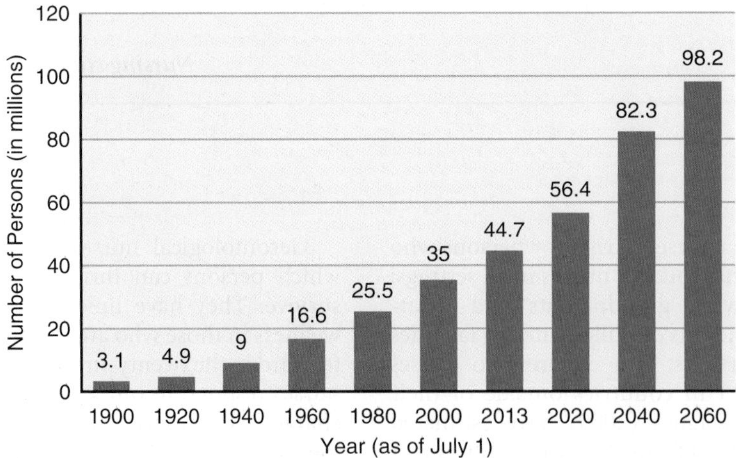

FIGURE 1.2 Number of persons 65+: 1900–2060. (Redrawn from U.S. Department of Health and Human Services: *Administration on aging, future growth.* Available at http://www.aoa.acl.gov/Aging_Statistics/Profile/2014/4.aspx. Retrieved April 2016. Data from U.S. Census Bureau, Population Estimates and Projections.)

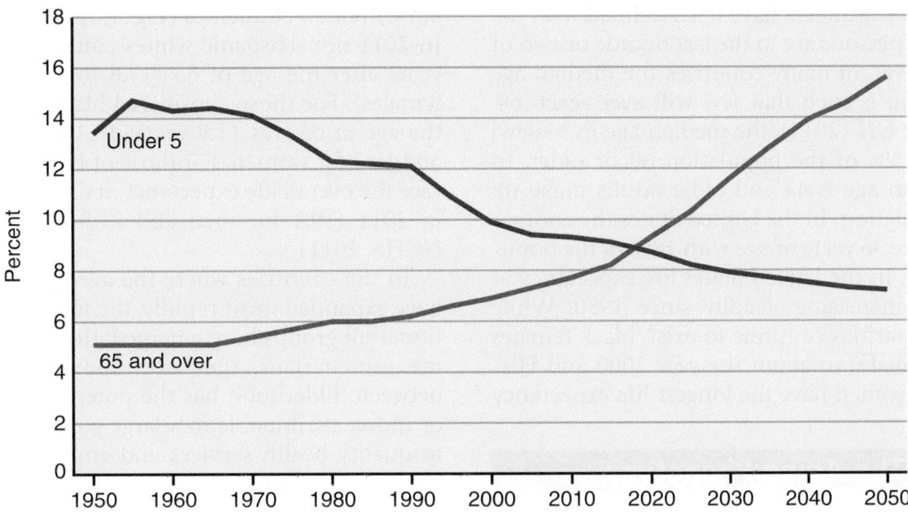

FIGURE 1.3 Average annual percent growth of older population in developed and developing countries: 1950 to 2050. (Redrawn from He W, Goodkind D, Kowal P: U.S. Census Bureau, International Population Reports, P95/16-1. *An aging world: 2015,* Washington, DC, 2016, U.S. Government Publishing Office.)

60 (about 66%) live in less developed areas in the world, with this percentage expected to grow to 80% by the year 2050 (WHO, 2015a) (Fig. 1.3). The majority of those in this exploding population are women (United Nations [UN], 2014).

This population growth will change the face of aging as we know it and present many challenges today and in our future. Although healthy aging is now an achievable goal for many in developed and developing regions, it is still only a distant vision for many living in less developed areas of the world, where lives are shortened by persistent communicable diseases, inadequate sanitation, and lack of both nutritious food and health care. It is essential that nurses across the globe have the knowledge and skills to help people of all ages achieve the highest level of wellness possible. Some questions must be asked. How can global conditions change for those who are struggling? How can the years of elderhood be maximized and enriched to the extent possible, regardless of the conditions in which one lives?

HOW OLD IS OLD?

Each culture has its own definition of when one is recognized as "old." A range of terms is used to refer to those considered old, including elderly, senior citizens, elders, granny, older adult, tribal elder, or "na" among the !Kung San of Botswana (Rosenberg, 1990). In some cultures elderhood is defined in functional terms—when one is no longer able to perform one's usual activities (Jett, 2003). For example, while "na" was an honorific title, among this same group, those who had become functionally impaired were called "da kum kum" or "old to the point of helplessness." Social aging is often determined by changes in roles, such as retirement from one's usual occupation, appointment as a wise woman/man of the community, or at the birth of a grandchild. Transitions may be marked by special rituals, such as birthday and retirement parties, invitations to join groups such as the American Association of Retired Persons (AARP, 2014), the qualification for "senior discounts" (Box 1.1), or recognition of special honor. Aging is defined in both biological and chronological terms. Biological aging is described in Chapter 3.

Chronological Aging

In most developed and developing areas of the world, chronological late life is recognized as beginning sometime between the ages 50 and 65, with the World Health Organization using the age of 60 in their discussions (WHO, 2016a). In 1935, with the establishment of a national retirement system (Social Security), the time when one became "old" was set at 65 in the United States. In the 2000s this age is creeping toward 70 when one becomes eligible for pensions and other monetary benefits based on age.

These arbitrary numbers have been defined with the expectation that persons are in the last decade or two of their lives; however, in many countries the median age of the population is such that few will ever reach 60. According to the UN (2013), the median age in Malawi is 17 with only 5% of the population 60 or older. In Japan the median age is 44 and older adults make up 29% of the population. In the United States the comparable numbers are 36 years of age with 18% of the population at least 60. In the United States life expectancy at birth has been increasing steadily since 1980. While racial/ethnic disparities continue to exist, black females overtook white males in about the year 2000 and Hispanic men and women have the longest life expectancy at birth of all ethnicities (Fig. 1.4) (CDC/NCHS, 2013). In 2011 non-Hispanic whites could expect to live 19.1 years after the age of 65 (17.8 for males and 20.3 for females). For those considered black, life expectancy at the age of 65 was 17.9 years; 16.1 more years for men and 19.2 for women. For those of Hispanic origin of any race the overall life expectancy at 65 was 20.7 more years in 2011 (19.1 for men and 21.8 for women) (CDC/NCHS, 2011).

BOX 1.1 The Aging Phenotype

A few years ago I stopped coloring my hair, which is almost completely silver now. It was quite a surprise to me the first time the very young clerk in the booth at the movie theater assumed I was 65 and automatically gave me the "senior discount." My husband's hair is only fading to a dull brown. When he goes to the theater alone they tentatively ask, "Do you have any discounts?"

Kathleen, age 60

In the countries where the average life expectancies have expanded most rapidly, the following four generational subgroups have emerged: the super-centenarians, the centenarians, the baby boomers, and those in-between. Elderhood has the potential to span 40 years or more, attributable in a large part to increased access to quality health services and emphasis on improving the health of the public.

The Super-Centenarians

The super-centenarians are those who live until at least 110 years of age (Box 1.2). This elite group emerged in the 1960s as those first documented to have lived so long. The Gerontology Research Group has an ongoing study and keeps a running tabulation of validated super-centenarians; they refer to this list as "Table E." After the

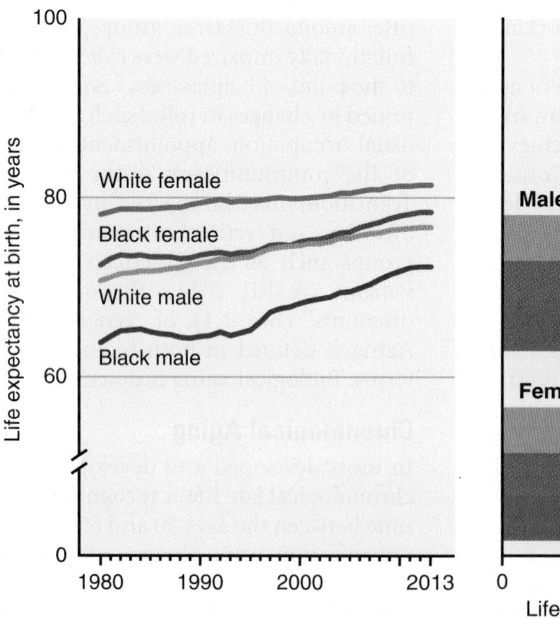

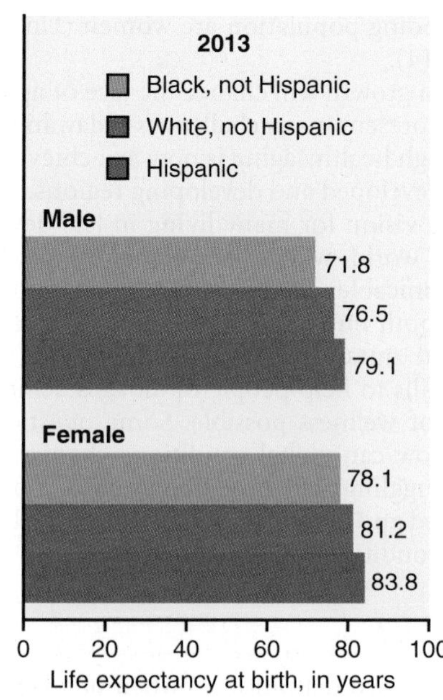

FIGURE 1.4 Life expectancy at birth: United States, 1980–2013. (Redrawn from National Center for Health Statistics: *Health, United States, 2014,* Hyattsville, MD, 2015. Data from the National Vital Statistics System. Available at http://www.cdc.gov/nchs/data/hus/hus14.pdf. Retrieved June 2016.)

BOX 1.2 Super-Centenarian Extraordinaire: Jeanne Louise Calment

Jeanne Louise Calment died in France at age 122. At that time she was believed to be the longest-lived person in the world. She outlived her husband, her daughter, her only grandson, and her lawyer. Her husband died in 1942, just 4 years before their 50th anniversary. Her daughter died in 1936 and her grandson in 1963. She was 4 years old when the Eiffel tower was built and reportedly once sold art supplies to Vincent Van Gogh. She not only lived a long life but also approached life with vigor. Madame Calment took up fencing at 85 and was still riding a bike at 107. She smoked until she was 117 and ate a lifelong diet rich in olive oil. Her longevity remains a mystery to experts and researchers.

From Dollemore D: *Aging under the microscope: A biological quest*, Bethesda, MD, 2006, National Institute of Aging, National Institutes of Health, Publication #02-2756.

TABLE 1.1 Global Flu Pandemics

Year(s)	Historical Name
1918	The Spanish flu; Le Grippe (H1N1)
1957–1960	Asian flu (H2N2)
1968–1969	Hong Kong flu (H3N2)
2009–2010	H1N1 (Swine flu)

death of 116-year-old Susannah Mushatt Jones in May of 2016, Emma Morano has replaced her, born slightly after Mrs. Jones in November 1899. The majority of long-lived persons presently live or have lived in Japan (Gerontology Research Group, 2015).

As teens or young adults the super-centenarians of today survived the influenza pandemic of 1918 to 1919, which killed an estimated 50 million people or one fifth of the world's population. In 1 year the life expectancy in the United States dropped by 10 to 12 years (National Archives, n.d.). Those alive today have also survived the three subsequent global epidemics, four pandemic flu threats (Table 1.1), and outbreaks of cholera, typhoid, and polio.

A study of 32 super-centenarians in the United States found that "A surprisingly substantial portion of these individuals were still functionally independent or required minimal assistance" (Schoenhofen et al., 2006, p. 1237). Most functioned independently until after age 100, with no signs of frailty until about the age of 105. They were found to be remarkably homogeneous. None had Parkinson's disease, only 25% had ever had cancer, and stroke and cardiovascular disease were rare if they occurred at all. Few had been diagnosed with dementia. A study of super-centenarians in Japan corroborated these findings. It is theorized that these unusual persons have survived this long for "rare and unpredictable" reasons (Willcox et al., 2008). Biologically and sociologically they are comparable to each other. Scientists report that contributing factors include improvements in sociopolitical conditions, medical care, and quality of life (Vacante et al., 2012). While the number of super-centenarians alive today is small, it is predicted to grow as the centenarians behind them live longer and healthier (Robine and Vaupel, 2001).

The Centenarians

Centenarians today are between 100 and 109 years of age, the majority of whom are between 100 and 104 years old (Meyer, 2012). Smallpox has been a threat to centenarians until about 1980 when it was essentially eradicated globally (WHO, 2016b). Many centenarians had all or most of the "childhood" diseases, such as measles, mumps, chickenpox, and whooping cough; some survivors of today also had polio as children.

The percentage of those older than 100 years of age is rising more rapidly than the total population in many countries. However, several countries have a higher percentage of centenarians per 10,000 persons in their population (Fig. 1.5).

In the United States, 53,364 persons were at least 100 in 2010, a 66% increase from 1980 (U.S. Census Bureau, 2010). The UN estimates that a worldwide population of less than one-half million centenarians in 2013 will grow to more than 3 million by 2050. Among centenarians, women are between four and five times more numerous than men (UN, 2013). Based on the U.S. Census report of 2010, centenarians were overwhelmingly white women living in urban areas of the Southern states (AOA, 2014). For the first time in history, parents and their children and grandchildren may all belong to this same "generation."

Those In-Between

There is also a unique cohort born in the 30 years between 1915 and 1945, that is, between those referred to as the baby boomers and the centenarians. This age group includes some of the last survivors of the Holocaust. Many fought in World War II.

Polio infection was a major fear for this cohort and for some of these individuals, either they or their friends were affected. A vaccine was not available in the United States until 1955, providing the most benefits to the youngest of the "in-betweeners" (CDC, 2014). Many had friends and loved ones who died of the AIDS epidemic before treatment was available. Penicillin, first discovered in 1928 by Alexander Fleming, became usable in humans in the 1940s and likely has prevented

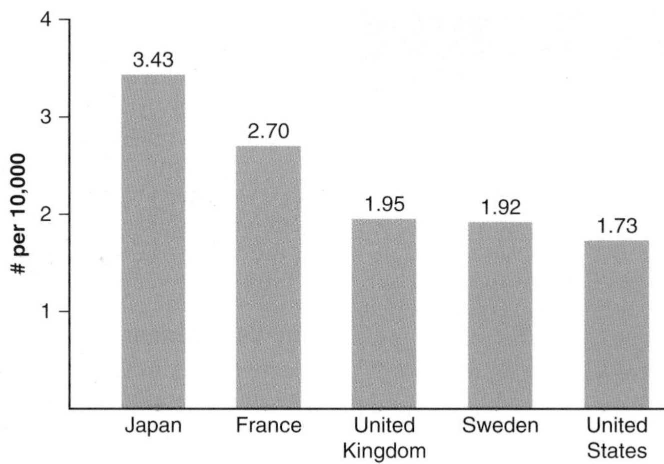

FIGURE 1.5 Number of persons older than 100 per 10,000 persons in the population (select countries). (Data from Meyer J: *Centenarians: 2010, 2012*. 2010 Census special reports C2010SR-03. Available at https://www.census.gov/prod/cen2010/reports/c2010sr-03.pdf. Accessed April 2016.)

much infection-related mortality from then to the present time.

The number of persons between the ages of 70 and 99 is growing at an exponential rate as the boomers begin to join their ranks. At this time the population in the United States of those 85+ years of age is expected to more than double between 2013 and 2060—from 6 million to 14.6 million. There is also a growing racial and ethnic heterogeneity among older adults. The number of persons of color has increased from 6.3 million in 2003 to 9.5 million in 2013 and is projected to increase to 21.1 million by 2030, a rate far exceeding their white, non-Hispanic counterparts. Between 2013 and 2030 the number of white non-Hispanic elders is expected to increase by 50% compared to 123% from other groups (AOA, 2014). Those who self-identify as Hispanic comprise the group growing older at a particularly rapid rate (U.S. Census Bureau, 2014).

The "Baby Boomers"

The youngest of the "older generation" are referred to as "baby boomers" or "boomers." They were born sometime between approximately 1946 and 1964 depending on how they are defined by any one country. In the United States the first to become baby boomers turned 64 in 2010; the last will do so 21 years later in 2031. More babies were born in the United States in 1946, the year after the end of WWII, than any other year—3.4 million or 20% more than in 1945. These numbers increased every year until they tapered off in 1964. In just 18 years, 76.4 million babies had been born (*History*, 1996–2013). Each day another 11,000 "boomers" turn 50 years old (AHA, 2007).

Although the super-centenarians and centenarians may not have received the immunizations as they became available, they became a standard of care from 1960 on, when the eldest boomer was 13 years of age. The ability to produce the potent antibiotic penicillin and those to follow has been significantly influential in the survival of this cohort into 2017. The baby boomers of today have better access to medication and other treatment regimens than previous cohorts. Although they have high rates of chronic conditions, especially obesity, diabetes, arthritis, heart disease, and dementia, today's baby boomers will nevertheless live longer with these chronic diseases than any of their predecessors. It is hoped that the social emphasis today on healthier lifestyles will go far to help persons reach higher levels of wellness, but for this group, the challenges are many.

MOVING TOWARD HEALTHY AGING

From a perspective of Western medicine, health was long considered the absence of physical or psychiatric illness. It was measured in terms of the presence of accepted "norms," such as a specific range of blood pressure readings and results of laboratory testing, and the absence of established signs and symptoms of illness.

When any of the parameters negatively affected the ability of the individual to function independently, debility was assumed. The measurement of a population's health status was usually inferred almost entirely from morbidity and mortality statistics: how long we live, what illness we have, and how many people die from a specific illness. The numbers provided information about illness and death but the quality of life and wellness of the population could not be inferred. The data do not reflect the lives of persons with functional limitations, their ability to contribute to the community, or their self-esteem.

Although there had been efforts for many years to recognize that health meant more than the absence of disease, a national effort was not organized in the United States until 1979. At that time initial national goals were set and described in the document *The Surgeon General's Report on Health and Disease Prevention* (U.S. Department of Health and Human Services [USDHHS], 2015a). This has been updated every 10 years with the most current document referred to as *Healthy People 2020* (USDHHS, 2015b). Many new topical areas that are especially important to the promotion of health while aging have been added to the newest version. Among these are goals related to quality of life and wellness while aging and the preparation of health care professionals to provide the highest quality care to adults as they age (USDHHS, 2015c). The importance of social well-being as a part of physical and mental health was recognized by the World Health Organization (WHO) in 1949 with the continuation of on-going support voiced in the global forums on aging (WHO, 2015b).

The strong emergence of the holistic health movement has resulted in even broader definitions of health and wellness. Wellness involves one's whole being—physical, emotional, mental, and spiritual—all of which are vital components (Fig. 1.6). In a classic work, Dunn (1961) defined the holistic approach to health as "an integrated method of functioning which is oriented toward maximizing the potential of which the individual is capable within the environment where he is functioning." Wellness involves achieving a balance between one's internal and external environment and one's emotional, spiritual, social, cultural, and physical processes.

This holistic paradigm has reshaped how health is viewed and revolutionized the way health care and health are perceived. Wellness is a state of being and feeling that one strives to achieve through effective health practices. Instead of snapshots in time during a person's illness, a state of wellness can be uniquely defined anywhere along the continuum of health. Age and illness influence the ease at which one moves along the continuum but do not define the individual.

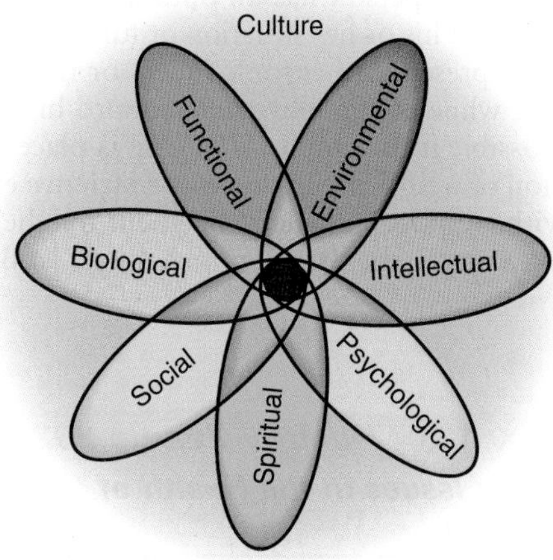

FIGURE 1.6 Flower model.

An individual must work hard to achieve wellness. In working toward wellness, an individual may reach plateaus in his or her ascension to higher-level wellness. Even for those with chronic illnesses, regression from an illness or acute event or crisis can be a potential stimulus for growth and a return to moving along the wellness continuum (see Chapter 17).

Consistent with Dunn (1961), health in later life is often thought of in terms of functional ability (i.e., the ability to do what is important to a given person) rather than the absence of disease. This may mean the person's ability to live independently or the ability to enjoy great-grandchildren when they visit at the nursing home, but it is always individually determined. Well-being for those older than 60 years of age is strongly related to functional status but is affected also by socioeconomic factors, degree of social interaction, marital status, and aspects of one's living situation and environment.

For the first time, older adults are identified as a priority area, with the specific goal to improve their health, function, and quality of life (USDHHS, 2015c). The importance of this is triggered by the recognition of the growth of the baby boomer generation and the number of chronic conditions they are and will be facing. Improving the health of persons with diabetes (see Chapter 20), arthritis (see Chapter 21), congestive heart failure (see Chapter 22), and dementia (see Chapter 23) will be the foci in the years to come as well as an emphasis on the use of clinical preventive services (USDHHS, 2015b).

Approaching aging from a holistic viewpoint of health emphasizes strengths, resilience, resources, and capabilities rather than focusing on existing pathological conditions. A wellness perspective is based on the belief that every person has an optimal level of health independent of his or her situation or functional ability. Even in the presence of chronic illness or multiple disabilities or while dying, movement toward higher wellness is possible if the emphasis of care is placed on the promotion of well-being in the least restrictive environment, with support and encouragement for the person to find meaning in the situation, whatever it is (Box 1.3).

BOX 1.3 *Healthy People 2020*

Emerging Issues in the Health of Older Adults

- Coordinate care.
- Help older adults manage their own care.
- Establish quality measures.
- Identify minimum levels of training for people who care for older adults.
- Research and analyze appropriate training to equip providers with the tools they need to meet the needs of older adults.

From U.S. Department of Health and Human Services: *Healthy People 2020. Topics and objectives: older adults.* Available at http://www.healthypeople.gov/2020/topicsobjectives2020/overview.aspx?topicid=31. Accessed October 2015.

❖ IMPLICATIONS FOR GERONTOLOGICAL NURSING AND HEALTHY AGING

As life expectancy increases how will we define aging? How will these definitions, as well as the meaning and the perception of aging, change as the health and wellness of individuals, communities, and nations improve? How will nursing roles and responsibilities change? How can we promote wellness in those who have a much greater chance of living into their 100s?

It is the responsibility of the nurse to assist elders to achieve the highest level of wellness in relation to whatever situation exists. The nurse can, through knowledge and affirmation, empower, enhance, and support the person's movement toward the highest level of wellness possible. The nurse assesses and can help explore the underlying situation that may be interfering with the achievement of wellness, and work with the person and significant others to develop affirming and appropriate plans of care. The nurse can utilize the resources available, such as *Healthy People 2020* and the *Clinical Preventive Services Guidelines,* to maximize the potential for health (Table 1.2). The nurse and the elder collaboratively implement interventions to achieve individual goals and evaluate their effectiveness. The goals of the nurse are to care and comfort always, to cure sometimes, and to prevent that which can be prevented.

TABLE 1.2 Example of Interventions to Promote Wellness

Preventive Service	Wellness and Person-Oriented Intervention
Promoting influenza, pneumococcal, and streptococcal immunizations	Consider new approaches to community outreach, such as home visits, neighbor-to-neighbor campaigns. Develop effective reminder systems.
Breast cancer screening	Develop effective reminder systems. Provide one-to-one education and counseling. Reduce structural barriers, such as transportation difficulties.
Colorectal screening	Develop effective reminder systems. Reduce structural barriers, such as transportation difficulties.
Vaginal and cervical cancer screening	Help women determine eligibility and appropriateness.
Diabetes screening	Help identify people at risk.
Diabetes self-management training	Encourage participation to help the person achieve glycemic goals.
Hearing and balance exams	Offer exams for those with identified problems. For those with impairments, work with them to obtain care.
Shingles vaccination	Promote public education regarding the importance of this. Engage in policy activism to promote insurance coverage.
HIV screening	Encourage open conversations to include discussions of "safe sex" and the importance of screening.
Prostate screening (PSA and DRE)	Stay informed about current status and recommendations about these screening exams.

KEY CONCEPTS

- Gerontological nursing is an opportunity to make a significant difference in the lives of older adults.
- The meaning of aging is influenced by many factors.
- Nurses have a responsibility to contribute to the nation's goals of increasing the quality of life lived and to reduce health disparities.
- Individual persons become more unique the longer they live. Thus one must be cautious in attributing any specific characteristics of older adults to "old age."
- All persons, regardless of age or life and/or health situation, can be helped to achieve a higher level of wellness, which is uniquely and personally defined.
- Gerontological nurses have key roles in the provision of the highest quality of care to older adults in a wide range of settings and situations.

ACTIVITIES AND DISCUSSION QUESTIONS

1. Discuss the ways in which elders contribute to society today.
2. Interview an older person, and ask how he or she has changed since 25 years of age.
3. Discuss health and wellness with your peers. Develop a definition of aging.
4. Explain wellness in the context of chronic illness.
5. Discuss how you seek wellness in your own life.
6. Discuss what you can do to enhance the quality of life for the persons to whom you provide care.
7. Draw a picture of yourself at 80 years of age. Compare your drawing to those of others who have done the same and discuss the implications of the representation.
8. Discuss how older adults are portrayed in popular TV shows, commercials, and movies.

REFERENCES

AARP (American Association of Retired Persons): *Member advantages* (2014). Available at http://discounts.aarp.org/memberbenefits. Accessed October 15, 2015.

AHA (American Hospital Association): *When I'm 64: How boomers will change the face of heath care*, 2007, American Hospital Association. Available at http://www.aha.org/content/00-10/070508-boomerreport.pdf. Accessed October 15, 2015.

AOA (Administration on Aging): *Profile of older Americans* (2014). Available at http://www.aoa.acl.gov/Aging_Statistics/Profile/index.aspx. Accessed October 15, 2015.

CDC (Centers for Disease Control and Prevention): *Polio disease: Questions and answers* (2014). Available at http://www.cdc.gov/vaccines/vpd-vac/polio/dis-faqs.htm. Accessed October 15, 2015.

CDC/National Center for Health Statistics (NCHS), Administration on Aging, Agency for Healthcare Research and Quality and Centers for Medicare and Medicaid Services: *Enhancing use of clinical services among older adults*, Washington, DC, 2011, AARP.

CDC/NCHS: *Health, United States*, 2013. See list of table available at http://www.cdc.gov/nchs/hus/contents2013.htm#017. Accessed October 15, 2015.

Dunn HL: *High-level wellness*, Arlington, VA, 1961, Beatty.

Gerontology Research Group: *Validated living supercentenarians* (2015). Available at http://www.grg.org/Adams/TableE.html. Accessed October 15, 2015.

History: Baby boomers, 1996–2013. Available at http://www.history.com/topics/baby-boomers. Accessed October 15, 2015.

Holroyd A, Dahlke S, Fehr C, et al: Attitudes toward aging: Implications for a caring profession, *J Nurs Educ* 48(7):374–380, 2009.

Jett KF: The meaning of aging and the celebration of years, *Geriatr Nurs* 24(4):209–293, 2003.

Meyer J: *Centenarians: 2010*, 2010 Census special reports C2010SR-03, 2012.

National Archives: *The deadly virus: The influenza epidemic of 1918* (n.d.). Available at http://www.archives.gov/exhibits/influenza-epidemic/index.html. Accessed October 15, 2015.

Robine J, Vaupel JW: Supercentenarians: Slower aging individuals or senile elderly? *Exp Gerontol* 36(4–6):915–930, 2001.

Rosenberg H: Complaint discourse, aging, and caregiving among the !Kung Sun of Botswana. In Sokolovsky J, editor: *The cultural context of aging: A worldwide perspective*, New York, 1990, Bergin and Garvey, pp 19–42.

Schoenhofen EA, Wyszynski DF, Andersen S, et al: Characteristics of 32 supercentenarians, *JAGS* 54:1237–1240, 2006.

UN: *Profiles of ageing 2013* (2013). Available at http://www.un.org/en/development/desa/population/publications/dataset/urban/profilesOfAgeing2013.shtml. Accessed October 15, 2015.

UN: *Concise report on the world population statistics in 2014* (2014). Available at http://www.un.org/en/development/desa/population/publications/pdf/trends/Concise%20Report%20on%20the%20World%20Population%20Situation%202014/en.pdf. Accessed October 15, 2015.

U.S. Census Bureau: *Population estimates and projections, 2010 census special reports* (2010). Available at http://www.aoa.gov/aging_statistics/profile/2012/3.aspx. *Note: per citation the information is a compilation of multiple sources.*

U.S. Census Bureau: *Future growth* (2014). Available at http://www.aoa.acl.gov/Aging_Statistics/Profile/2014/4.aspx. Accessed October 15, 2015. *Note: per citation the information is a compilation of multiple sources.*

USDHHS (U.S. Department of Health and Human Services): *History and development of* Healthy People (2015a). Available at http://www.healthypeople.gov/2020/about/History-and-Development-of-Healthy-People. Accessed October 15, 2015.

USDHHS: *Healthy People 2020* (2015b). Available at http://www.healthypeople.gov/. Accessed October 15, 2015.

USDHHS: *Healthy People 2020: Older adults* (2015c). Available at http://www.healthypeople.gov/2020/

topicsobjectives2020/overview.aspx?topicid=31. Accessed October 15, 2015.

Vacante M, D'Agata V, Motta M, et al: Centenarians and supercentenarians: A black swan. Emerging social, medical and surgical problems, *BMC Surg* 12(Suppl 1):S36, 2012.

WHO: *Media Centre: Ageing and health* (2015a). Available at http://www.who.int/mediacentre/factsheets/fs404/en. Accessed July 28, 2016.

WHO: *Report on the 2nd WHO global forum on innovations for ageing populations: imagine tomorrow.* (2015b). Available at http://www.who.int/topics/smallpox/en. Accessed July 28, 2016.

WHO: *Definition of an older or elderly person* (2016a). Available at http://www.who.int/healthinfo/survey/ageingdefnolder/en. Accessed October 15, 2015.

WHO: *Smallpox* (2016b). Available at http://www.who.int/topics/smallpox/en/. Accessed July 28, 2016.

Willcox BJ, Willcox DC, Ferrucci L: Secrets of healthy aging and longevity from exceptional survivors around the globe: Lessons from octogenarians to supercentenarians, *J Gerontol A Biol Sci Med Sci* 63(11):1201–1208, 2008.

Young H: Challenges and solutions for an aging society, *Online J Issues Nurs* 8:1, 2003.

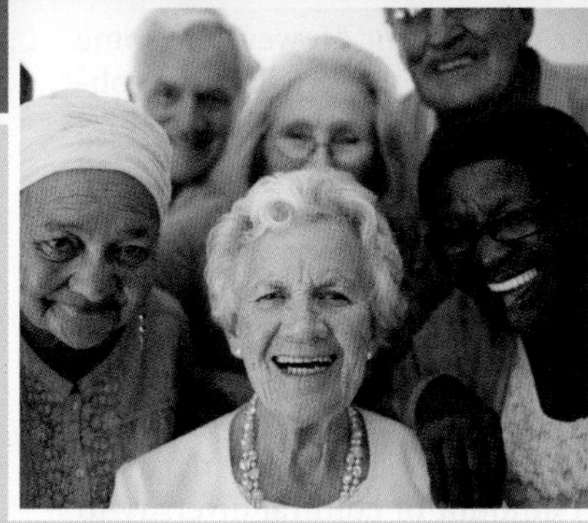

2

Cross-Cultural Caring and Aging

Kathleen Jett

evolve.elsevier.com/Touhy/gerontological

LEARNING OBJECTIVES

Upon completion of this chapter, the reader will be able to:

- Compare and contrast factors influencing health outcomes for vulnerable populations.
- Identify nursing care interventions appropriate for the increasingly diverse population of elders.
- Formulate a plan of care incorporating sensitive interventions to facilitate improved outcomes in cross-cultural nursing situations.

THE LIVED EXPERIENCE

I feel so out of place here. If my children weren't so busy, I suppose I could live with them, but they seemed relieved when this retirement home would accept me. I wonder if they knew I was the only Chinese person in this place. A sweet young Chinese student tried to talk with me, but she only spoke Mandarin and I speak Cantonese. She had never lived in China. I want so much to talk to someone my age that lived in China and speaks my language.

Shin, a 75-year-old woman

I thought all old people were the same. I am very surprised that they are not!

Helen, an 18-year-old nursing student

As the number and diversity of persons of all ages grows it has become mandatory for nurses to provide culturally proficient care to persons with different life experiences and perspectives, values and beliefs, styles of communication, and ages.

Providing skillful cross-cultural care is especially important in gerontological nursing because of the numbers of elders immigrating—to the United States and other countries. Many others have spent their lives in self-contained, homogeneous communities and have not become accustomed to the larger culture of their adopted countries. Instead, they are now faced with confronting unfamiliar health care approaches when they receive the specialized care needed for the treatment of acute and chronic conditions that are more prevalent with aging. This situation is likely to result in cultural conflict in the health care setting and a high risk for poor outcomes.

This chapter provides an overview of culture and aging, as well as strategies that gerontological nurses can use to best respond to the changing face of aging (see Chapter 1). In doing so, the nurse promotes healthy aging and helps reduce health inequities. These strategies include the skills needed to work with a person who is different from the nurse to find a way to identify and achieve goals for healthy aging. It is moving from cultural destructiveness to proficiency in the care of older adults.

CULTURE

Culture is most often referred to in terms of the shared and learned values, beliefs, expectations, and behaviors of a group of people. Culture guides thinking and decision-making, and beliefs about aging, health and health-seeking, illness, treatment, and prevention (Jett, 2003; Spector, 2012).

Cultural values extend into the delivery of health care any time the "seeker" and "giver" meet. The giver determines the problems that are recognized, the treatments that are appropriate, and the way seekers are expected to respond. Many of the oldest adults in the United States today grew up during a period when paternalism was the primary principle from which health care was delivered. That is, the patient assumed that the physician would make the best decision for him or her, one that "he" would make for his own child. Persons in many cultures across the globe and subcultures within the United States continue to view the health care encounter from this perspective to a great extent. However, in some cultures the seekers decide if they agree with the problems identified, if they will accept the "prescription," and if they will act on it.

DIVERSITY

Extending the idea of culture is that of *cultural diversity* or simply the existence of more than one group with differing values and perspectives. Morin (2013) describes the extent of diversity in the world, identifying those countries with the least amount of cultural diversity to those with the most. In Argentina, 97% of the citizens are white (of European descent) and are Roman Catholic. At the other end of the spectrum are many of the countries on the African continent. For example, the 37 different tribal groups in Togo speak 39 different languages and share little in common other than geography. Canada is the only "Western" country in the top 20 in terms of diversity (Morin, 2013).

The United States ranks near the middle (Fig. 2.1). Diversity in the United Stated usually refers to the seven major ethnoracial groups: black/African American,

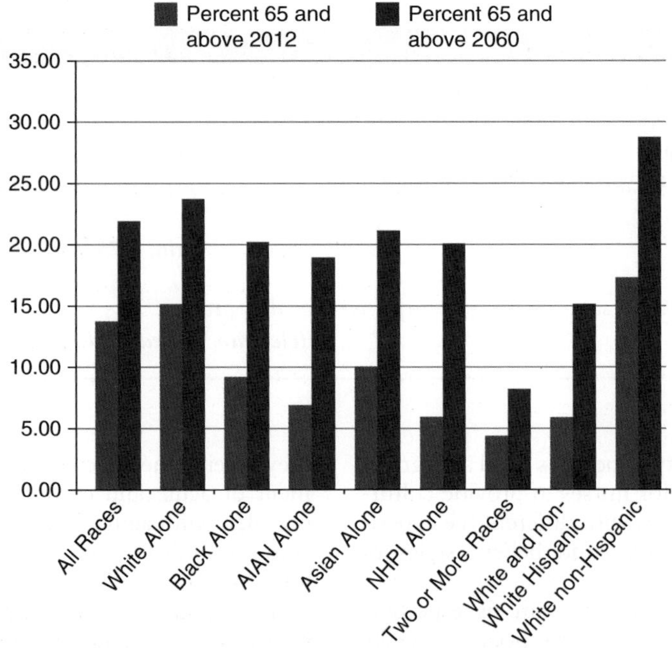

FIGURE 2.1 Anticipated percentage in growth of distribution of race and ethnic groups of persons 65 and older in the United States, 2012 to 2060. *AIAN,* American Indian/Alaska Native; *NHPI,* Native Hawaiian/Pacific Islander. (From Touhy TA, Jett K: *Ebersole and Hess' toward healthy aging,* ed 9, St Louis, 2016, Elsevier. Data from U.S. Census: *2012 National population projections,* 2013. Available at http://www.census.gov/population/projections/data/national/2012.html. Accessed March 2014.)

Asian American, Native Hawaiian/Pacific Islander, American Indian/Alaskan Native, white (of European descent), multiracial, and the ethnic group who self-identify as Hispanic or Latino, regardless of race (Office of Minority Health [OMH], 2015). The categories of "mixed race" and "middle Eastern" may appear in a future U.S. census. Of note: The most accurate use of the term "African American" is technically limited to the descendants of the more than 4 million people who were transported to the United States against their will between 1619 and 1860 (Spector, 2012). It does not apply to individuals who have more recently migrated from the African continent.

It is important to recognize that within any one group, culturally similar or disparate, there is diversity of other kinds, most notably that of gender, education, power, and status. These factors, in particular, greatly influence the delivery and receipt of health care in many, if not all, places in the world.

HEALTH DISPARITIES AND INEQUITIES

The terms *health inequities* and *health disparities* are often used interchangeably. Although they are somewhat different, both have implications for health care outcomes. Health inequities most often relate to differences as a result of distribution of wealth and their effect on health outcomes. One of the most dramatic examples is the 37-year discrepancy in life expectancy between the impoverished nation of Malawi and the high-income country of Japan (see Chapter 1). It is always important to note that health inequities are not limited to those between countries. In London the life expectancy of men ranges from 88 years of age to 71 years of age, depending on neighborhood, from the most affluent to the least, respectively (World Health Organization [WHO], 2011).

The term *health disparity* refers to differences in health outcomes between groups. It is usually discussed in terms of the excess burden of illness in one group compared with another. Most often the latter hold the majority of the power and influence in a culture, including control of the resources, such as health care.

In any country where older adults are marginalized simply because of their age, they are especially vulnerable to health disparities. If the person has other characteristics (e.g., skin color, religion, or sexual orientation) that cause further differentiation between the person and those with power and status, the disparities are amplified (Centers for Disease Control and Prevention [CDC], 2014; Gushulak & MacPherson, 2006; Pan American Health Organization [PAHO]/WHO, 2013; WHO, 2008). Cognitive impairment or sensory or physical disability increases the person's risk even further.

BOX 2.1 Examples of Health Disparities Relevant to Older Adults

African Americans

- Although African American adults are 40% more likely to have hypertension, they are 10% less likely than their non-Hispanic white counterparts to have their blood pressures controlled.
- In 2013 African American men were 20% more likely than non-Hispanic white men to die of heart disease.
- African American women are 60% more likely to have hypertension than their non-Hispanic white counterparts.

From CDC Office of Minority Health Disparities: *Heart disease and African Americans.* Available at http://minorityhealth.hhs.gov/omh/browse.aspx?lvl=4&lvlID=19. Accessed October 2015.

Health inequities refer to the excess burden of illness or the difference between an expected incidence and prevalence and that which actually occurs in excess in a comparison population group. The inequities are often the result of both historical and contemporary injustices. Those found to be especially vulnerable to health disparities and inequities are older adults from ethnically or racially different from the majority population (Box 2.1).

❖ IMPLICATIONS FOR GERONTOLOGICAL NURSING AND HEALTHY AGING

◆ Moving Toward Cultural Proficiency to Improve Health Outcomes

Gerontological nurses can learn to more expertly provide care as they move along a continuum from cultural destructiveness to cultural proficiency (Fig. 2.2). This requires a willingness to become more self-aware, to learn the perspectives of others (i.e., "where they are coming from"), and finally to apply new skills to more effectively support rather than hinder their personal and cultural strengths in achieving healthy outcomes (Box 2.2).

Cultural Destructiveness

Cultural destructiveness is the systematic elimination of the culture of another. Examples include the genocide of the Jews in Eastern Europe and the historical treatment of American Indians and African Americans in the United States. In both Australia (WHO, 2008) and the United States cultural destructiveness occurred with the removal of children to boarding schools where the language, dress, and food of their origins were forbidden

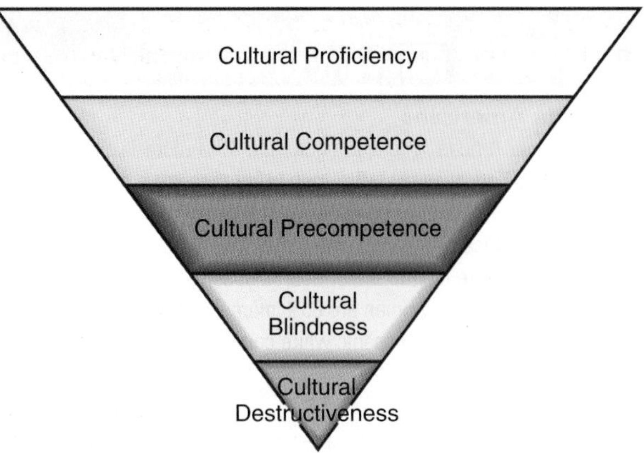

FIGURE 2.2 A model for cross-cultural caring. (From Touhy TA, Jett K: *Ebersole and Hess' toward healthy aging,* ed 9, St Louis, 2016, Elsevier. Adapted from Cross T, Bazron B, Dennis K, et al: *Toward a culturally competent system of care,* vol 1, Washington, DC, 1989, CASSP Technical Assistance Center, Center for Child Health and Mental Health Policy, Georgetown University Child Development Center; Goode TD: *Cultural competence continuum,* Washington, DC, revised 2004, National Center for Cultural Competence, Georgetown University Center for Child and Human Development, University Center for Excellence in Developmental Disabilities; and Lindsey R, Robins K, Terrell R: *Cultural proficiency: A manual for school leaders,* Thousand Oaks, CA, 2003, Corwin Press.)

BOX 2.2 Moving Toward Cultural Proficiency and Healthy Aging

- Become familiar with your own cultural perspectives, including beliefs about disease etiology, treatments, and factors leading to outcomes.
- Examine your personal and professional behavior for signs of bias and the use of negative stereotypes.
- Remain open to viewpoints and behaviors that are different from your expectations.
- Appreciate the inherent worth of all persons from all groups.
- Develop the skill of attending to both nonverbal and verbal communication.
- Develop sensitivity to the clues given by others, indicating the paradigm from which they face health, illness, and aging.
- Learn to negotiate, rather than impose, strategies to promote healthy aging consistent with the beliefs of the persons to whom we provide care.

(Lewis, 2013). American Indian healing ceremonies, performed by tribal elders, were forbidden. Practices referred to as "traditional" or "folk" healing were and continue to be discounted. Suspiciousness of Western medicine is still present among many African American and American Indians, especially those who are in their 80s and 90s today; who may have first- or second-hand knowledge of the cultural destruction to which they and others were subjected (Grandbois et al., 2012) (Box 2.3).

BOX 2.3 Racism in the Boston Naming Test*

During a study to evaluate the cultural applicability of several standard psychological tools sometimes administered by nurses, an 82-year-old African American woman reluctantly agreed to take what is called the Boston Naming Test. This measure of verbal fluency used in the diagnosis of dementia comprises a packet of pictures. The patient is asked to name the pictures. After doing so the volunteer shared, "Did you know that one of the pictures is a hangman's noose? Do you have any idea what that means to a black person to look at that picture!" Indeed, none of the white researchers had noticed this.

*Personal experience of Kathleen Jett.

Cultural Blindness

It is hoped by this point the reader has begun to understand that there are multiple cultures coexisting in countries and continents and that such things as age and other factors affect the health care experience. Yet some people, including health care providers (including nurses), voice that they see the outward differences such as skin color and age but believe that "everyone is the same." In addition, they see no harm in applying negative stereotypes such as "all old people have a little dementia" but are blind to the fact that life experiences, such as being subjected to such stereotyping, prejudice, and historical trauma, can affect an individual's beliefs and behavior. All of these experiences and the failure to recognize them frequently lead to poor health care outcomes by influencing both the pursuit and the receipt of health care by older adults. It is not possible to provide cross-cultural care or reduce health disparities in the context of cultural destructiveness or cultural blindness unless individual and community health belief paradigms, factors such as ageism, poverty and racism, are considered (Feagin & Bennefield, 2014; Williams & Mohammed, 2009). Cultural blindness prevents the nurse from providing sensitive and, more importantly, effective care.

Cultural Precompetence

The development of precompetence begins in the cross-cultural setting with self-awareness of one's personal biases, prejudices, attitudes, and behaviors toward persons different from oneself in age and many other factors. It is becoming aware of one's own ageist attitudes as well as ageism found in the person's world (Box 2.4).

BOX 2.4 Unintentional Ageism in Language and Its Effects

- Use of general labeling terms: sweet old lady, little old lady, geezer.
- Use of terms applied in the health care setting: fossil, bed blocker (debilitated person in the hospital awaiting a bed in a nursing home), GOMER (get out of my emergency room).
- When speaking: exaggerated pitch, demeaning emotional tone, lower quality of speech.
- Consequences of ageism in language: reduced sense of self, lowered self-esteem, lowered sense of self-competence, decreased memory performance.

Adapted from International Longevity Center: *Ageism in America* (2006). Available at http://www.graypanthersmetrodetroit.org/Ageism_In_America_-_ILC_Book_2006.pdf. Accessed October 2015.

BOX 2.5 Unrecognized Privilege and Ethnocentrism

A gerontological nurse responded to a call from an older patient's room. While she was with him, he repeatedly, and without comment, dropped his watch on the floor. She calmly picked it up, handed it back to him, and continued talking. One time an aide walked in the room when the patient dropped the watch. The aide picked it up and handed it back to him just as the nurse had done. The patient immediately started yelling and cursing at the aide for attempting to steal his watch. When telling this story, the nurse thought the whole situation odd, but not too remarkable.

The patient and nurse were white and the aide was black. The nurse did not realize that the behavior of the patient was both ethnocentric and culturally destructive until the nurse learned these concepts while taking a formal class on cross-cultural health care.

For persons whose culture or status places them in a position of power, cultural awareness is realizing that this alone often means special privilege and freedoms (White Privilege Conference, 2015) (Box 2.5). Achieving cultural precompetence requires a willingness to learn how health is viewed by others. It means playing an active role to combat ageism in society and thereby contribute to the reduction of health disparities.

Cultural Competence

The nurse who moves beyond precompetence is able to step outside of one's biases and accept that others bring a different set of values, choices, and even priorities to the health care encounter. The nurse who is able to provide competent cross-cultural care accepts that all persons are unique and deserving of respect and that the older the adult is, the more he or she has experience in dealing with personal health problems. The nurse has some knowledge of other cultures, particularly those she or he is most likely to encounter in the health care setting. This is especially important when the nurse and the elder are of different ages or have different values, backgrounds, and cultures from each other. The acquisition of cross-cultural knowledge takes place in the classroom, at the bedside, and in the community. Cultural knowledge is both what the nurse brings to the caring situation and what the nurse learns from others (Fung, 2013).

Cultural Proficiency

To provide the highest quality of care, it is now expected that the nurse not only demonstrate competence but also strive for cultural proficiency, that which is respectful, compassionate, and relevant (see Fig. 2.2). Cultural proficiency includes putting cultural knowledge to use in assessment, communication, negotiation, and intervention. The culturally proficient nurse is able to move smoothly between two worlds for the promotion of healthy aging and the care of persons. The nurse enters into an unknown conceptual world in which time, space, religion, tradition, and wellness are expressed through a unique language that conveys the perceived nature of the health, illness, and humanity.

Culturally proficient care includes the recognition that there may be factors beyond culture to consider, such as the effects of past and current trauma, social status, and poverty, which can lead to health disparities and inequities. The nurse providing proficient cross-cultural health care is able to work with, and build relationships with, members from a variety of age and cultural groups as a natural part of daily practice. The relationship building results in the ability to communicate effectively, sensitively and effectively assess the individual's health status, formulate mutually acceptable goals, and support interventions that are culturally acceptable, empowering, and possible within the limitations of available resources.

CULTURAL KNOWLEDGE

Cultural knowledge grows as the nurse learns about older adults, their families, their communities, their beliefs, and their expectations of the health care experience. Essential knowledge includes the elder's way of life (ways of thinking, believing, and acting). This knowledge is obtained formally and informally through the individual's professional experience of nursing. It is expected that knowledge will allow the nurse to more appropriately and effectively improve health outcomes (Campinha-Bacote, 2011; Kirmayer, 2012).

Although cultural knowledge is essential, caution must be used with regard to the potential for stereotyping or the application of limited knowledge about one person with specific characteristics to other persons with the same characteristics. The nurse will hear "old people just become more like children…" Stereotyping limits the recognition of the heterogeneity of the group. At the same time, relying on knowledge of a positive stereotype can be useful as a starting point, but it too can be used to limit understanding of the uniqueness of the individual and impose unrealistic expectations. For example, a common stereotype of the African American culture is that the church is a source of support. The nurse's assumption can easily have a negative outcome, such as fewer referrals for formal services support (e.g., home-delivered meals). This stereotype can also be used to start conversations about discharge planning. The non–African American nurse may say to an African American elder, "I understand that the church can sometime serve as source of support in the African American community. Is this one of the resources in your church that is available to you when you return home?" If so, it is necessary to elaborate. "What kinds of help will you be able to receive and for how long?" For example, the nurse may discuss services such as parish nurses or agencies that provide meals. It is important that the nurse uses such an opening to this conversation because the elder may not mention a lack of such resources in order to avoid embarrassment.

Orientation to Family and Self

An important concept in cross-cultural health care is orientation to self and family. Many North Americans, especially those of northern European descent, place great value on independence, that is, personal autonomy and individuality (Fung, 2013). In the classic study, Rathbone-McCune (1982) found that a large group of American elders living in a segregated ("white") senior apartment building went to great lengths and lived with significant discomforts rather than ask for help. To seek or receive help was considered a sign of weakness and dependence, something to be avoided at all costs.

In the United States the cultural expression of autonomy was institutionalized in the passing of the Patient Self-Determination Act of 1990 wherein individuals were recognized as the sole decision-makers regarding their health. Health care providers are now legally bound to restrict access to health care information only to the patient, unless the person provides explicit permission.

This orientation is in sharp contrast to that of a collectivist or interdependent culture, a norm in many parts of the world. In the Latino culture this is referred to as "familism" (Lukwago et al., 2001; Scharlach et al., 2006). Self-identity is drawn from family ties (broadly defined) rather than the individual. The "family" (e.g., extended, tribe, or clan) is of primary importance; decisions are made by the group or designee based on the needs and beliefs of the group rather than those of the individual. Within families, the exchange of help and resources is both expected and commonplace. For example, older adults may care for their grandchildren or great-grandchild in exchange for housing and assistance with their own needs, including health-related decision-making. When a nurse from a culture in which independent decision-making is expected cares for an elder whose dominant value is interdependence or vice versa, the potential for cultural conflict and poor outcomes is great.

Orientation to Time

Orientation to time is often overlooked as a culturally constructed factor influencing the use of health care and preventive practices (Lukwago et al., 2001). Time orientations are culturally described as future, past, or present. Conflicts between the future-oriented Westernized medical care and those with past or present orientations are many. Patients are likely to be labeled as *noncompliant* for failing to keep an appointment or for failing to participate in preventive measures, such as a "turning schedule" for a bed-bound patient to prevent pressure ulcers or immunizations to prevent future infections.

Members of present-oriented cultures are often accused by the media of overusing hospital emergency departments in the United States, when in fact it may be considered the only reasonable option available for today's treatment of today's problems. For older adults who are dependent on others this is particularly salient. If the health care provider (and perhaps the elder as well) believes that future care is adequate, then caregivers must agree with this and make a plan to meet the needs (e.g., transportation). Similarly if the elder and caregivers believe that the problem is urgent and a health care provider does not agree, *or* the mechanics needed for future care (e.g., transportation) are not possible, the use of emergency facilities may be the only option available to them.

Health Beliefs

The diversity of the population has brought the strong potential for a clash of health beliefs. Aging itself further increases the diversity of beliefs because of the lifelong experiences and practices related to illness and treatment of self, family, and others. In most cultures, older adults are likely to treat themselves and others for familiar or chronic conditions in ways they have found successful in the past, practices that are referred to as *domestic medicine,* folk medicine, or folk healing. Folk medicine is, and always has been, based on beliefs regarding the appropriate treatment for the symptoms and presumed diagnoses. Only when self-treatment fails will a person consult with others known to be knowledgeable or experienced with the problem, such as an elder family member, neighbor, community, or indigenous healer known to the community. When this too fails, people may seek help within a formal health care system.

The culture of nursing and health care in the United States is one that advocates what is called the *Western or biomedical model*. The health care providers within this model usually consider it to be superior to all other models, a highly ethnocentric viewpoint. However, many of the world's people have different beliefs, such as those based on *personalistic* (magicoreligious) or *naturalistic* (holistic) models (Table 2.1). Each model includes beliefs and attitudes about disease prevention, disease causation, acceptable treatment, and definitions of health. It is not uncommon for ethnic elders to adhere to beliefs other than the biomedical approach. However, many of us, nurses included, often practice health care based on a combination of models. Nonetheless, nurses who are familiar with the range of health beliefs and realize their importance will be able to provide more sensitive and appropriate care. In the absence of understanding there is great potential for conflict.

❖ IMPLICATIONS FOR GERONTOLOGICAL NURSING AND HEALTHY AGING

Perhaps in cross-cultural gerontological nursing more than any other fields skill is based on mutual respect between the nurse and the elder. It is working "with" the person rather than "on" the person.

Contact between elders and gerontological nurses often begins with assessment. During that process, each has an opportunity to know the other as discussed earlier. Several tools have been developed to accomplish

TABLE 2.1 Comparison of Health Belief Models

Model	Illness Causation	Assessment and Diagnosis	Treatment	Prevention	Health
Western (biomedical)	Invasion of germs or genetic mutation identified as a "disease"	Objective identification of pathogen or process May include consultation with a health practitioner identified as a specialist in the subcategory of disease (e.g., oncologist)	Remove or destroy invading organism; repairing, modifying, or removing affected body part	Avoidance of pathogens, chemicals, activities, and dietary agents known to cause abnormalities	Absence of disease
Personalistic (magicoreligious)	The actions of the supernatural, such as gods, deities, or nonhuman beings (e.g., ghosts, or spirits) A punishment for a breach of rules, breaking a taboo, or displeasing or failing to please the source of power	Consultation with a health practitioner associate specializing in the particular subcategory of practice (e.g., minister, curandero)	Religious practices, such as praying, meditating, fasting, wearing amulets, burning candles, and "laying of the hands"	Making sure that social networks with their fellow humans are in good working order Avoid angering family, friends, neighbors, ancestors, and gods	A blessing or reward of God
Naturalistic (holistic)	Physical, psychological, or spiritual imbalance resulting in disharmony	Consultation with a health practitioner specializing in the specific subcategory of practice (e.g., Chinese physician, herbalist)	Dependent on the particular type of submodel (e.g., hot/cold practices of treating a hot illness with a cold treatment)	Life practices that maintain balance	Balance (e.g., the right amount of exercise, food, sleep)

BOX 2.6 The LEARN Model

L Listen carefully to what the elder is saying. Attend to not just the words but to the nonverbal communication and the meaning behind the stories. Listen to the elder's perception of the situation, the desired goals, and the ideas for treatment.
E Explain your perception of the situation and the problems.
A Acknowledge and discuss both the similarities and the differences between your perceptions and goals and those of the elder.
R Recommend a plan of action that takes both perspectives into account.
N Negotiate a plan that is mutually acceptable.

From Berlin EA, Fowkes WC: A teaching framework for cross-cultural health care: Application in family practice, *West J Med* 139(6):934–938, 1983.

this (e.g., Leininger's Sunrise Model) (Kleinman et al., 1978; Leininger, 2002; Schim et al., 2007; Shen, 2004). However, like the comprehensive assessments described in Chapter 8, a comprehensive "cultural" assessment takes time, often more time than is possible in today's health care setting, and somewhat objectifies the person.

An alternative is that of the LEARN Model, a negotiated plan of care that includes identification of the availability of culturally appropriate and sensitive community resources (Berlin & Fowkes, 1983) (Box 2.6). When using the LEARN Model in goal setting and care plan development with older adults, it is necessary to pay close attention to any sensory limitations that might interfere with communication; for example, hearing aids need to be both functional and used so that beneficial conversations can ensue. When others are directly involved in a person's day-to-day life, they should be present (see Chapter 19). The LEARN Model is easy to use and incorporates the collection of the most useful assessment data needed to construct a focused, problem-oriented care plan. Because it requires an interactive process it has the highest potential for success (i.e., improved outcomes).

◆ L—Listen

Listening as a part of communication includes paying attention to more than just verbal expressions. It includes physical contact, eye contact, the spoken word, and the nonverbal communication behind the words. The nurse listens carefully to the person for his or her perception about the problem at hand, the situational and cultural context, desired goals, and beliefs about treatment.

◆ Physical Contact

In caring for others, especially those in distress, it may seem natural for many nurses to feel that they should touch their patient in some way (such as a hug, a pat on the shoulder, or a touch of the hand) to show that they are listening. However, in the Muslim culture, cross-gender physical contact of any kind may be considered highly inappropriate or even forbidden and care arrangements may need to be modified. Before the nurse makes physical contact with an elder of any culture, he or she should ask the person's permission or follow the person's lead, such as an outstretched hand.

◆ Eye Contact

Eye contact is another highly culturally constructed behavior. In some cultures direct eye contact is believed to be a sign of honesty and trustworthiness. Nursing students in the United States are taught to establish and maintain eye contact when interacting with patients, but this behavior may be misinterpreted by persons from other cultures.

A more traditional American Indian elder may not allow the nurse to make eye contact, moving his or her eyes slowly from the floor to the ceiling and around the room. During a health care encounter in most Asian cultures, direct eye contact is considered disrespectful. To impose eye contact with an elder may be particularly rude. The gerontological nurse can again follow the lead of the elder by being open to eye contact but neither forcing it nor assigning it any inherent value.

◆ Verbal Communication

Respectful communication is vital at all times; it is essential, however, with older adults from cultures in which there are specific age-related norms. For example, in some Asian and Middle Eastern cultures children are expected to speak only when invited to do so by an elder. Respectful communication includes addressing the person in the appropriate manner (using the surname unless otherwise instructed by the elder) and using acceptable body language.

In many cross-cultural health care encounters the providers and the patients do not speak the same language or may not communicate at the fluency needed for the situation; some cultural traditions prevent the elder from speaking directly to the nurse (e.g., cross-gender care). To optimize the opportunity to promote healthy aging, an interpreter may be needed. *The more complex the decision that must be made, the more important the skills of the interpreter are, such as when determining the elder's wishes regarding life-prolonging measures or the family's plan for caregiving* (Box 2.7).

◆ Working With Interpreters

It is ideal to engage persons who are trained medical interpreters and who are of the same age, sex, and social status as the elder. Unfortunately, it is too often

BOX 2.7 When a Professional Interpreter Is Needed

An interpreter is needed any time the nurse and the elder speak different languages, when the elder has limited proficiency in the language used in the health care setting, or when cultural tradition prevents the elder from speaking directly to the nurse. The more complex the decision-making situation, the more important are the interpreter and his or her skills. These circumstances are many, such as when discussions are needed about the treatment plan for a new condition, the options for treatment, advanced care planning, or even preparation for care after discharge from a health care institution. The use of a specially trained interpreter is essential in the setting of lowered levels of health literacy.

necessary to call upon strangers, such as housekeepers or younger relatives, to act as interpreters. When children and grandchildren are asked to act as interpreters, the nurse must realize that the child or the elder may be "editing" comments because of intergenerational boundaries or cultural restrictions about the sharing of certain information (e.g., some information may not be considered appropriate to share between an elder and a child).

◆ E—Explain

Once the nurse has listened carefully and obtained a basis for further discussion (see Box 2.8 for helpful lines of inquiry), he or she explains the medical problem or situation from the context in which the care is being delivered. This portion of the conversation requires utmost tact and gentleness so the nurse does not appear judgmental or exhibit any disrespect for the views and beliefs of the elder. Kleinman's suggestions can be used for both listening and explaining. The nurse explains to the person his or her views about the nature of the illness.

◆ A—Acknowledge

The process of goal setting and the chance of achieving desired outcomes will stop at this point unless there is a mutual acknowledgment of both the similarities and differences between the nurse's perceptions and those of the elder. This acknowledgment forms the basis for the final step of negotiation. For those on either side of the conversation who hold a preconceived cultural belief in the authority of the health care provider, this may be especially difficult. When an informal interpreter is used there is the added risk that he or she edits the conversation in a way that makes a "meeting of the minds" impossible.

BOX 2.8 The Explanatory Model for Culturally Sensitive Assessment

1. How would you describe the problem that has brought you here? *(What do you call your problem; does it have a name?)*
   a. Who is involved in your decision-making about health concerns?
2. How long have you had this problem?
   a. When do you think it started?
   b. What do you think started it?
   c. Do you know anyone else with it?
   d. Tell me what happened to that person when dealing with this problem.
3. What do you think is wrong with you?
   a. How severe is it?
   b. How long do you think it will last?
4. Why do you think this happened to you?
   a. Why has it happened to the involved part?
   b. What do you fear most about your sickness?
5. What are the chief problems your sickness has caused you?
6. What do you think will help clear up this problem? *(What treatment should you receive; what are the most important results you hope to receive?)*
   a. If specific tests and/or medications are listed, ask what they are and do.
7. Apart from me, who else do you think can make you feel better?
   a. Are there therapies that make you feel better that I do not know? *(Maybe in another discipline?)*

Adapted from Kleinman A, Eisenberg L, Good B: Culture, illness, and care: Clinical lessons from anthropologic and cross-cultural research, *Ann Intern Med* 88(2):251–258, 1978.

◆ R—Recommend

With careful and thorough consideration the nurse can now assimilate the aforementioned information, discussion, and knowledge of the person's beliefs and personal experiences with health care and develop a unique, *potential* plan of care. This is presented to the elder and/or to the person(s) designated by the elder to be involved in receiving the information.

◆ N—Negotiate

Finally, cross-cultural skills include the ability to negotiate a plan of action that is mutually acceptable that takes both perspectives into account (Berlin & Fowkes, 1983). In many cases the nurse cannot change the person's belief system. It is difficult, if not impossible, and usually counterproductive. This is particularly true when working with older adults who carry a lifetime of beliefs about prior illness experiences and treatments. The nurse attempts to preserve helpful beliefs and practices, accommodate beliefs that are neither helpful nor harmful, and help persons modify beliefs or practices that are known to be harmful. A sense of caring is conveyed by giving support to the elder's traditional beliefs and practices. At the same time, respectfully explaining concern about potentially harmful practices with the offer of possible alternatives may show the person that the nurse is considering the person's preferences. Unbiased caring can surmount cultural and age differences.

INTEGRATING CONCEPTS

The migration of some elders born outside of the United States or other adopted countries was uneventful. They moved easily with their parents or made conscious decisions to join their child in a new country. Many others suffered horrifically in their home country before the move or during their immigration process, and for many, safety and security were never certain. Several years ago the staff of a nursing home for Jewish residents complained that it was particularly difficult getting some of the residents with dementia to shower. Some were Holocaust survivors. It was some time before the staff realized that as the residents' dementia progressed, they were no longer able to distinguish the difference between a shower for hygiene and the fear of "going to the showers" (i.e., to the gas chamber) in the concentration camps of their youth (Weissman, 2004).

Changes are threatening the historical role of aging in families across the globe. Different degrees of assimilation between generations create a communication gap between the young and older immigrants as they join their families in new countries where the language and customs may be unknown to them. This may cause isolation and estrangement between the oldest and youngest generations (see Chapter 26).

Economic independence and mobility of the younger members of the family are chipping away at the insulation afforded by the community (Jett, 2006). Intergenerational discontinuities created by assimilation produce a communication gap between the young and the old. This may cause isolation and estrangement between the oldest and youngest generations. Members of ethnic and sexual minorities are especially vulnerable in old age (Box 2.9). Nurses can take an active role in facilitating self-actualization by enabling expression of the uniqueness of the individual, by attending to the elder's spiritual and cultural needs, and by taking the lead in optimizing the health and abilities of those who seek our care.

The study of aging is one of the most complex and intriguing opportunities of our day. Realistically, it will be almost impossible to become familiar with the whole range of clinically relevant cultural differences of older adults one may encounter. Attempting to provide care holistically and sensitively is the most challenging opportunity leading to personal growth for both the nurse and the person receiving care.

To skillfully assess and intervene, nurses must develop cultural proficiency through awareness of their own ethnocentricities. They must be acutely sensitive to the cues suggested (e.g., eye contact) to know how best to respond. Promoting healthy aging in cross-cultural settings includes the ability to develop a plan of action that considers the perspective of both the elder/family and the nurse/health care system to negotiate an outcome that is mutually acceptable. Skillful cross-cultural nursing means developing a sense of mutual respect between the nurse and the elder. A sense of caring is conveyed in gestures of personal recognition. It is working "with" the person rather than "on" the person; and in doing so, health disparities and inequities, if they exist, can begin to be reduced and movement toward healthy aging can be facilitated. Unbiased caring can surmount many cultural differences.

BOX 2.9 Where Did the Community Go?

A middle-aged African American woman talked about her community and care of persons with dementia. She said that when she grew up, "it was expected that the neighbor would watch out for you. Like if someone saw you out and about and knew you would get lost they would just take you home again... That just doesn't seem to be happening anymore... we don't even know each other!"

From Jett KF: Mind-loss in the African American community: Dementia as a normal part of aging, *J Aging Stud* 20(1):1–10, 2006.

KEY CONCEPTS

- Population diversity will continue to increase rapidly for many years. This suggests that nurses will be caring for a greater number of persons from a broad range of ethnicities and ages than in the past.
- Nurses can contribute to the reduction of health disparities and inequities by moving toward cultural proficiency.
- Cultural awareness, knowledge, and skills are necessary to move toward cultural proficiency.
- Nurses caring for diverse elders must let go of their own ethnocentrism before they can give effective care.
- Many elders hold health beliefs that are different from those of the biomedical or Western medicine used by most health care professionals in the United States.

- Lack of awareness of the elder's health belief model and time orientation has the potential to produce conflict in the nursing situation regardless of the setting in which it takes place.
- The more complex the communication or decision-making needs in a given situation, the greater the need for skilled interpreter services for persons with limited English proficiency.
- Programs staffed by persons who reflect the ethnic background of the participants and speak their language may be preferred by the elderly.
- The LEARN Model provides a useful framework for working with elders of any ethnicity or background to develop achievable and acceptable goals.

ACTIVITIES AND DISCUSSION QUESTIONS

1. Discuss your personal beliefs regarding health and illness and explain how they fit into the three major classifications of health models. How can this affect culturally competent care for elders who hold differing beliefs?
2. Explain the types of questions that would be helpful in assessing an elder's health problem(s) in a way that is respectful of the person and his or her cultural background and ethnic identity.
3. Propose strategies that would be helpful in planning care for elders from different ethnic backgrounds.
4. Discuss your familial and culturally determined views of aging after speaking to older family members.

REFERENCES

Berlin EA, Fowkes WC: A teaching framework for cross-cultural health care: Application in family practice, *West J Med* 139(6):934–938, 1983.

Campinha-Bacote J: Delivering patient-centered care in the midst of a cultural conflict: The role of cultural competence, *Online J Nurs Issues* 16(2):5, 2011.

Centers for Disease Control and Prevention (CDC): *Minority health*, 2014. Available at http://www.cdc.gov/minorityhealth/. Accessed October 2015.

Feagin J, Bennefield Z: Systematic racism in U.S. healthcare, *Soc Sci Med* 103:7–14, 2014.

Fung HH: Aging in culture, *Gerontologist* 53(3):369–377, 2013.

Grandbois DM, Warne D, Eschiti V: The impact of history and culture on nursing care of Native American elders, *J Gerontol Nurs* 38(10):3–5, 2012.

Gushulak BD, MacPherson DW: The basic principles of migration health: Population mobility and gaps in disease prevalence, *Emerg Themes Epidemiol* 3:1–11, 2006.

Jett KF: The meaning of aging and the celebration of years among rural African American women, *Geriatr Nurs* 24:290–293, 2003.

Jett K: Mind-loss in the African American community: A normal part of aging, *J Aging Stud* 20(1):1–10, 2006.

Kirmayer LJ: Rethinking cultural competence, *Transcult Psychiatry* 49(2):149–164, 2012.

Kleinman A, Eisenberg L, Good B: Culture, illness, and care: Clinical lessons from anthropologic and cross-cultural research, *Ann Intern Med* 88(2):251–258, 1978.

Leininger M: Culture care theory: A major contribution to advance transcultural nursing knowledge and practices, *J Transcult Nurs* 13(2):189–192, 2002.

Lewis JP: The importance of optimism in maintaining healthy aging in rural Alaska, *Qual Health Res* 23(11):1521–1527, 2013.

Lukwago S, Kreuter MW, Bucholtz DC, et al: Development and validation of brief scales to measure collectivism, religiosity, racial pride, and time orientation in urban African American women, *Fam Commun Health* 24:63–71, 2001.

Morin R: *The most (and least) culturally diverse countries in the world*, Pew Research Center, July 18, 2013. Available at http://www.pewresearch.org/fact-tank/2013/07/18/the-most-and-least-culturally-diverse-countries-in-the-world. Accessed October 2015.

Office of Minority Health (OMH): *Racial and ethnic populations*, 2015. http://www.cdc.gov/minorityhealth/populations/remp.html. Accessed October 2015.

Pan American Health Organization (PAHO)/World Health Organization (WHO): *Addressing the causes of disparities in health service and utilization for lesbian, gay, bisexual and trans (LGBT) persons* (WHO ref. no. CD52/18), 2013. Available at http://www.who.int/hiv/pub/populations/lgbt_paper/en. Accessed October 2015.

Rathbone-McCune E: *Isolated elders: Health and social intervention*, Rockville, MD, 1982, Aspen.

Scharlach AE, Kellam R, Ong N, et al: Cultural attitudes and caregiver service use: Lessons from focus groups with racially and ethnically diverse family caregivers, *J Gerontol Soc Work* 47:133–156, 2006.

Schim SN, Doorenbos A, Benkert R, et al: Culturally congruent care: Putting the pieces together, *J Transcult Nurs* 18(2):57–62, 2007.

Shen Z: Cultural competence models in nursing: A selected annotated bibliography, *J Transcult Nurs* 15(4):317–322, 2004.

Spector RE: *Cultural diversity in health and illness*, ed 8, Upper Saddle River, NJ, 2012, Prentice Hall.

Weissman G: *Personal communication*, April 10, 2004.

White Privilege Conference: *What is white privilege?*, 2015. Available at http://www.whiteprivilegeconference.com/white_privilege.html. Accessed October 2015.

Williams DR, Mohammed SA: Discrimination and racial disparities in health: Evidence and needed research, *J Behav Med* 32(1):20–47, 2009.

World Health Organization (WHO): Australia's disturbing health disparities set Aboriginals apart, *Bull World Health Org* 86(4):241–320, 2008.

World Health Organization (WHO): *10 facts on health inequities and their causes*, 2011. Available at http://www.who.int/features/factfiles/health_inequities/en. Accessed 2015.

3

Biological Theories of Aging and Age-Related Physical Changes

Kathleen Jett

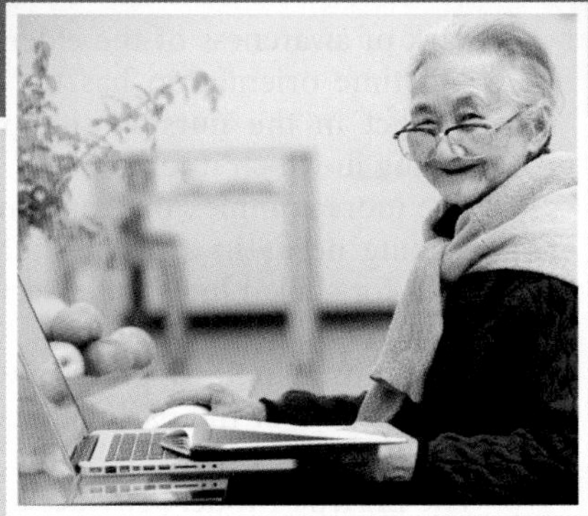

evolve.elsevier.com/Touhy/gerontological

LEARNING OBJECTIVES

Upon completion of this chapter, the reader will be able to:

- Suggest ways in which normal age-related changes are supported or refuted by the major theories of aging.
- Identify the physical changes that are associated with normal aging.
- Begin to differentiate normal age-related changes from those that are potentially pathological.
- Describe at least one age-related change for each body system that has the most potential to impair function.
- Make a plan of care for the older adult that targets prevention and health promotion.

THE LIVED EXPERIENCE

Until I started learning about the science of the aging process I had no idea how complicated it could be. We seem to have learned so much but still have so much more to learn.

Helena, age 20

When I was a young girl Einstein was proposing the molecular theory of matter and we had never heard of DNA or RNA. We only knew of genes in the most rudimentary theoretical sense. Now I hear that scientists believe there is a gene that is controlling my life span. I really hope they find it before I die.

Beatrice, age 72

Theories are attempts to explain phenomena, to give a sense of order, and to provide a framework from which one can interpret and simplify the world (Einstein, 1920). Most theories can be neither proved nor disproved, but they are useful points of reference. The biological theories of aging have helped both scientists and bedside nurses understand the physical changes of aging.

Many apparent age-related changes do not happen to everyone. Others are universal but do not occur at the same chronological age (e.g., menopause). In this chapter several of the current prominent biological theories of aging and some of the major physical changes associated with normal aging are discussed. With this knowledge the nurse can begin to differentiate normal aging from health problems that necessitate treatment, and thereby promote healthy aging.

BIOLOGICAL THEORIES OF AGING

The current biological theories of aging are attempts to explain senescence or changes in the organism leading ultimately to its death (Campisi, 2013). Although there is a growing body of knowledge about the genetics

BOX 3.1 Can We Postpone Aging?

The caloric restriction theory has garnered interest for many years. A significant amount of bench research has been conducted with nonhumans. The results have been conflicting. In a recent report published by the National Institutes of Health, a diet composed of 30% fewer calories than the standard diet in rhesus monkeys did not extend their lives. A restriction to this level would be intolerable to most humans.

Data from NIH: *Can we prevent aging?* (2014). Available at http://www.nia.nih.gov/health/publication/can-we-prevent-aging#calorie. Accessed April 2014.

related to aging, complex questions remain. Are the changes orderly and predictable or random and chaotic? What are the roles of cellular mutation and epigenetics, that is, the effect of the environment? What are the effects of lifestyle choices? Can we extend life (Box 3.1)? The major focus of today's research is on activities at the cellular level.

Today's aging theories have evolved from the groundbreaking work of earlier scientists (Box 3.2). Advancements in technology now allow us to see changes within one of the most basic structures in cells, the mitochondria. Aging changes appear to have negative effects on the functioning and longevity of the organism, be it a yeast cell or a human being. They may result from unchecked damage from atoms or clusters of atoms called "free radicals" (Fig. 3.1), or from genetic mutation, or even from long-term environmental stressors such as pollution and/or those associated with the stress of poverty (Lagouge & Larsson, 2013).

The normal changes of aging are made visible in what is referred to as the "aging phenotype," that is, ways our appearance changes as we accumulate years of life (e.g., sagging skin) (Carnes et al., 2008). Some changes are potentially harmful (e.g., slowed reaction time) and others are harmless (e.g., graying of hair). Just why the changes occur has been of interest to scientists for decades as they have unceasingly searched for the mythical "fountain of youth" (Walston, 2010).

Cellular Functioning and Aging

Survival of an organism depends on successful cellular reproduction. The genetic components of each cell (deoxyribonucleic acid [DNA] and ribonucleic acid [RNA]) serve as templates for ensuring that, theoretically, reproduction results in new cells that are exactly the same as the old cells in form and function. If reproduction was always perfect, the organism would never age. Instead, cells become increasingly complex over time. For example, an infant does not learn to walk until the associated neurons have adequate myelination, that is, until the myelin sheath is thick enough to facilitate smooth and rapid transmission of messages to the brain (Nomellini et al., 2008).

BOX 3.2 The Building Blocks of Contemporary Theories of Aging

The "Biological Clock" Theory

In 1981 Hayflick and Moorhead coined the term "biological clock" (1981). They purported that each cell had a preprogrammed life span; that is, the number of replications was limited and not dependent on other factors. Taken literally, programmed aging means that the age at which cells die in any one person is predetermined and inevitable. Although programmed theories of aging still have many proponents (Goldsmith, 2013), they are being eclipsed by those made possible by advances in cellular research.

Wear-and-Tear Theory

One of the earliest theories of aging is known as "wear-and-tear." This theory states that there are an increasing number of cellular errors during reproduction with aging because of the combination of continued use and trauma. Internal and external stressors increase the number of errors and the speed with which they occur (e.g., in shoulder joints of pitchers or knees of runners). These errors are random and unpredictable.

Cross-Link Theory

Cross-link theory explains aging in terms of the accumulation of errors initiated by the stiffening of proteins within the cell. Proteins "link" with glucose and other sugars in the presence of oxygen and become stiff and thick (Marin-Garcia, 2008). Because collagens are the most plentiful proteins in the body, this is where the cross-linking is most easily seen. Skin that was once smooth, silky, firm, and soft becomes drier and less elastic with age. Although this linking does occur, it is an explanation for many of the changes of aging rather than the "cause" of aging.

Oxidative Stress Theories

Advances in scientific methods have enabled scientists to examine cells at the molecular level, particularly the activity and effect of reactive oxygen species (ROS) and the ways that ROS affect the aging cell. As natural products in the metabolism of oxygen, ROS have an important role in homeostasis. The number of ROS is increased by external factors (such as pollution and cigarette smoke) and by internal factors (such as inflammation) (Dato et al., 2013). If there is a dramatic rise in the level of ROS, significant damage to the cell results, referred to as oxidative stress (Harman, 1956; Murphy,

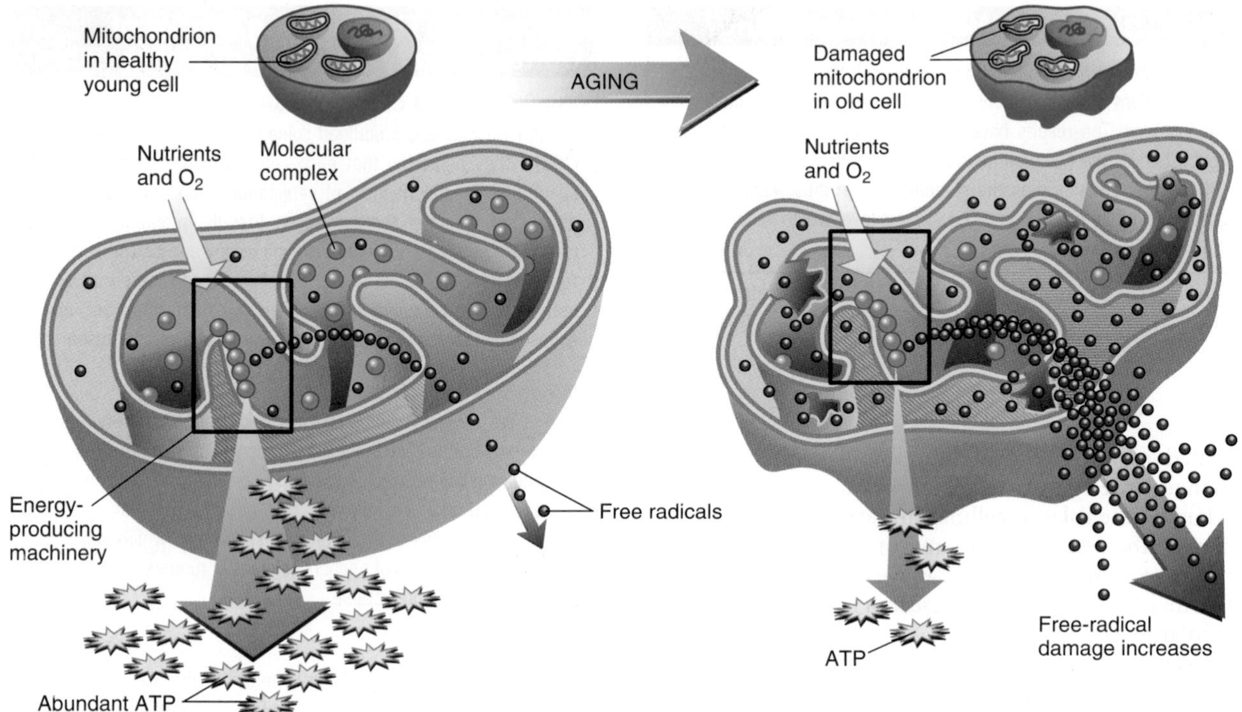

FIGURE 3.1 Mitochondria in young and old cells. *ATP,* Adenosine triphosphate. (From McCance KL, Huether SE: *Pathophysiology: The biologic basis for disease in adults and children,* ed 6, St Louis, 2010, Mosby.)

2009). The damage is seen as an accumulation of errors in reproduction until the cell is no longer able to function (Short et al., 2005). According to oxidation stress theories, the damage appears to be random and unpredictable, varying from one cell to another and from one person to another. Although they are still questioned by some researchers, oxidative stress theories (OST) are among those most studied and widely accepted at this time (Shi et al., 2010). As evidence accumulates, oxidative stress theories of aging have garnered strong support (Goldsmith, 2013; Jang & Van Remmen, 2009; Lagouge & Larsson, 2013).

Free Radical Theory

The "free radical theory of aging" is among the most understood and accepted of the OST (Jang & Van Remmen, 2009; Vine, 2013). Free radicals are natural by-products of cellular activity and are always present in the cell. In youth, naturally occurring vitamins, hormones, enzymes, and antioxidants neutralize the free radicals as needed (Valko et al., 2005). The changes we associate with normal aging and with vulnerability to many of the diseases common in later life have been suggested to develop when the accumulation of damage from free radicals occurs faster than the cells can repair themselves (see Fig. 3.1) (Dato et al., 2013; Grune et al., 2001; Hornsby, 2010).

It is known that exposure to environmental pollutants, especially smog and ozone, pesticides, and radiation, increases the production of free radicals and increases the rate of damage (Abdollahi et al., 2004; Lodovici & Bigagli, 2011). There is also evidence that chronic exposure to discrimination increases evidence of oxidative stress. This may provide some explanation for a number of the disparities in incidence and prevalence of several diseases that are associated with free radicals, such as heart disease (Pashkow, 2011).

For many years it was thought that the consumption of supplemental antioxidants, such as vitamins C and E, could delay or minimize the effects of aging by counteracting the damage caused by free radicals (Box 3.3). However, it is now known that the intake of supplemental antioxidants is deleterious to one's health (National Center for Complementary and Alternative Medicine [NCCAM], 2013). At the same time, diets inclusive of natural antioxidants, such as those high in fruits and

BOX 3.3 Tips for Best Practice

High doses of supplemental antioxidants have been found to be harmful. Some studies have shown that high-dose beta-carotene supplements increase the risk for lung cancer in smokers and high doses of vitamin E increase the risk for stroke. There are also a number of potential and actual drug/supplement interactions; for example, the combination of warfarin and vitamin E increases the risk of bleeding. Check to make sure that the total amount of multivitamin used does not exceed the daily recommended requirement. Encourage people to stay away from those products advertised as "mega-vitamins."

vegetables or a Mediterranean diet rich with red wine and olive oil, are clearly healthful (Dato et al., 2013).

Immunological Theory of Aging

The immune system in the human body is a complex network of cells, tissues, and organs that function separately. Together and separately the network protects the body from invasion by substances such as bacteria and helps regulate our response to internal conditions such as emotional stress.

This theory suggests that aging is a result of an accumulation of damage to the immune system, or immunosenescence. The decreased ability of the cells to counteract inflammation appears to have a broad effect, including the inability of the body to use fever to fight illness (Castelo-Branco & Soveral, 2014; Delves, 2016). The combination of a chronic state of inflammation and an increasing number of ROS in the cells appear to be key factors in the aging process and in the development of many health problems common in later life, such as heart disease (Fulop et al., 2014; Swain & Nikolich-Zugich, 2009).

Aging and DNA

The rapidly growing field of genomics has allowed scientists to examine the DNA (basic hereditary material) within cells. There is growing evidence suggesting that ROS and free radicals alone do not trigger the aging process, but instead lead to mutations in the basic DNA that in turn cause the errors in reproduction noted earlier (Lagouge & Larsson, 2013). While supported by early research, the findings are not yet conclusive.

Telomeres

Perhaps the most promising work in this area is that related to the examination of telomeres, small caps at the tip of each strand of DNA (Fig. 3.2). As long as the enzyme telomerase is present the telomeres can reproduce and therefore the DNA can be replicated

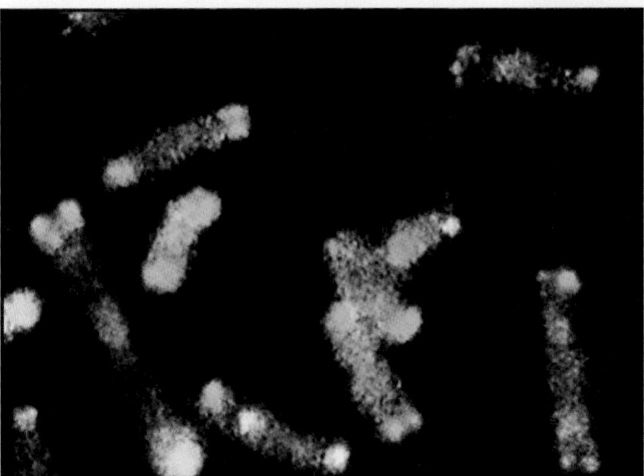

FIGURE 3.2 Chromosomes with telomere caps. (Modified from Jerry Shay and the University of Texas Southwestern Medical Center at Dallas, Office of News and Publications, 5323 Harry Hines Blvd, Dallas, TX 75235.)

BOX 3.4 Telomeres and Aging

Telomere length decreases at a rate of 24.8–27.7 base pairs per year. A number of lifestyle factors can increase the rate of shortening. Smoking one pack of cigarettes a day for 40 years is associated with the loss of 5 additional base pairs or 7.4 years of life. Obesity also causes accelerated telomere shortening resulting in 8.8 years of life lost. Excessive emotional stress results in the release of glucocorticoids by the adrenal glands. They have been shown to reduce levels of antioxidants and thereby increase oxidative and premature shortening of telomeres. Shorter telomeres are suggested as greatly increasing one's vulnerability to early onset of age-related health problems such as heart disease.

From Shammas MA: Telomeres, lifestyle, cancer and aging, *Curr Opin Clin Nutr Metab Care* 14(1):28–34, 2011.

(Cefalu, 2011). The length of the telomere may affect immunity, longevity, and overall health (Box 3.4) (Dehbi et al., 2013). Each telomere appears to have a maximum length before it begins to undergo senescence (aging). Consistent with the findings of Hayflick and Moorhead (1981) (see Box 3.2), the telomere may have its own "biological clock." At the same time, the shortening both results from and is influenced by oxidative stress. Premature shortening can occur, increasing the individual's risk for any number of disease states and a decreased life span (Shammas, 2011). Research related to aging and the reproductive ability of telomeres has become an intriguing area of inquiry, showing great promise to untangling the mysteries of the aging process.

It is apparent that the theories are no longer distinct but together provide clues to the aging process (Viña et al., 2013). The science of aging continues to advance at a rapid pace, fueled in large part by growth in the understanding of genetics. Areas of intense inquiry are the relationship between oxidative stress and the development of diseases in addition to the science of epigenetics, or how genes are influenced by environment, lifestyle, and other factors (Borghini et al., 2013; Brooks-Wilson, 2013; Cefalu, 2011). It is hoped that more research will lead to the discovery of other pathways and key changes in gene expression seen as the aging phenotype and perhaps, more importantly, their association to preventable and treatable illnesses.

It is important for the nurse to understand that the exact cause of aging is unknown; there is considerable variation in the aging process. There is variation not only between persons but also between the systems of any one person. Aging is an entirely unique and individual experience, but at the same time there are also common changes in each physical system of the body as discussed next.

PHYSICAL CHANGES THAT ACCOMPANY AGING

Skin

As the largest, most visible organ of the body, the various layers of the skin mold and model the individual to give much of his or her personal and sexual identity. The skin and hair provide clues to heredity, race, and physical and emotional health (Spector, 2012).

Many age-related changes in the skin are functionally inconsequential, but others have more far-reaching impact with implications for organs throughout the body (Table 3.1). Skin changes occur due to both internal factors (such as genetics) and external factors (such as wind, sun, and pollution) to which skin is especially sensitive. Cigarette smoking causes coarse wrinkles, and the photodamage of the sun is evidenced by rough, leathery texture, itching, and mottled pigmentation. Sun damage in particular increases the risk of skin cancer, common among older adults. Skin changes from aging include dryness, thinning, decreased elasticity, and the development of prominent small blood vessels. Skin tears, purpura (large purple spots), and xerosis (excessive dryness) are common but not normal aspects of physical aging (see Chapter 14). Visible changes of the skin—quality of color, firmness, elasticity, and texture—affirm that one is aging.

TABLE 3.1 Key Aspects of Normal Age-Related Changes With Aging: Skin and Nails

Changes	Effects
Epidermis	
Reduced number of melanocytes	Increased risk for solar damage such as skin cancers
Thinning	Bruises more easily and blood vessels more fragile Tears more easily
Increase time for cell renewal	Increased healing time
Dermis	
Reduced thickness	Pallor, less ability to withstand cooler temperatures
Reduced elastin	Sagging Increased risk for injury
Hypodermis	
Thinning	Reduced ability to modulate environmental temperatures
Reduced sebum production	Reduced ability to produce vitamin D when skin is exposed to sunlight
Nails	
Thickening of the nails	Increased risk for fungal infections

Epidermis

The epidermis is the outer layer of skin and is composed primarily of tough keratinocytes and squamous cells. Melanocytes produce melanin, which gives the skin color. With age, the production of melanin lessens, the epidermis thins, and blood vessels and bruises are much more visible. Cell renewal time increases up to 33% after the age of 50; 30 or more days may be necessary for skin to repair itself after an injury when compared to a younger adult (Gosain & DiPietro, 2004).

If the skin is injured (e.g., a cut or scrape) in a younger adult, the surrounding tissue becomes red (erythematous) almost immediately. This inflammatory response is the first step in the natural healing process. In an older adult, this inflammation may not begin for 48 to 72 hours. A laceration that becomes pink several days after the event may be misinterpreted by as having become "infected," when in reality, it is a sign of the beginning of the healing process. Evidence of a true skin infection in older adults is no different than that in younger adults, namely, odor, increasing redness, and purulent drainage.

The aging skin changes color and texture and is more at risk for the development of cancers. The tone lightens as the number of melanocytes in the epidermis decreases. With a decrease in the amount of protection from ultraviolet rays, the importance of sunscreen and regular "skin check-ups" for early signs of cancer increases (see Chapter 14). However, in some body areas, melanin synthesis increases. Pigmented spots (freckles or nevi) enlarge and can become more numerous in areas exposed to ultraviolet light such as the backs of the hands and the wrists and on the faces of those with lighter skin. Lentigines, also called "age spots" or "liver spots," appear and are completely benign. Thick, uniformly brown, raised lesions with a "stuck on" appearance are usually seborrheic keratosis; this condition is more common in men and is of no clinical significance but may be cosmetically disturbing to the person.

All skin cancers (melanoma, squamous cell, and basal cell) are increasingly common in older adults after a lifetime of sun exposure especially for those with very light skin or who have spent a good deal of their earlier years outdoors (e.g., in an occupation such as farming or in a sport such as tennis) (Skin Cancer Foundation, 2015). Actinic keratosis is a precancerous growth on the skin that can easily be confused with the benign seborrheic keratosis. However, on close examination, a very small red or pink ring can be seen surrounding it. This requires a visit to a dermatology office where it will probably be removed. Skin cancer is never a normal change with aging (see Chapter 14).

Dermis

The dermis, lying beneath the epidermis, is a supportive layer of connective tissue composed of a combination of yellow elastic fibers that provide stretch and recoil and white fibrous collagen fibers that provide strength. It also supports hair follicles, sweat glands, sebaceous glands, nerve fibers, muscle cells, and blood vessels, which provide nourishment to the epidermis.

Many of the visible signs of aging skin are reflections of changes in the dermis. The aging dermis loses about 20% of its thickness (Friedman, 2011). This thinness causes older skin to look more transparent and fragile. Dermal blood vessels are reduced, which accounts for resultant skin pallor and cooler skin temperature. Collagen synthesis decreases, causing the skin to "give" less under stress and tear more easily. Elastin fibers thicken and fragment, leading to loss of stretch and resilience and a "sagging" appearance. Loss of elasticity accentuates jowls and elongated ears and contributes to the formation of a "double" chin. Breasts begin to sag. As will be discussed, the impact of the change in elastin has implications for a number of other systems as well.

Hypodermis: Subcutaneous Layer

The hypodermis is the innermost layer of the skin containing connective tissues, blood vessels, and nerves, but the major component is subcutaneous fat (adipose tissue). The primary purposes of the adipose tissue are to store calories and provide temperature regulation. It also provides shape and form to the body and acts as a shock absorber against trauma. With age, some areas of the hypodermis thin.

Changes in the hypodermis increase the chance for the person to become more sensitive both to cold, because the natural insulation of fat is diminished, and to heat (overheated or hyperthermia), as a result of the reduced efficiency of the eccrine (sweat) glands. Sweat glands are located all over the body and respond to thermostimulation and neurostimulation in response to both internal (e.g., fever, menopausal "hot flashes") and external causes (e.g., increases in environmental temperatures). The younger body's response to heat is to produce moisture or sweat from these glands and thus cool the skin by evaporation. With aging, the glands become fibrotic, and surrounding connective tissue becomes avascular. This leads to a decline in the efficiency of the body to become cool. It is not uncommon for persons to complain of being either too hot or too cold in environments that are comfortable to others.

Sebaceous (oil) glands also atrophy. Sebum, produced by the gland, protects the skin by preventing the evaporation of water from the epidermis; it possesses bactericidal properties and contains a precursor of vitamin D. When the skin is exposed to sunlight, vitamin D is produced and absorbed through the skin. Continuing to produce vitamin D is especially important because of the high incidence of osteoporosis (see Chapter 21). All people need limited exposure to natural ultraviolet (UV) light (with protection); therefore, vitamin D supplementation (800 international units) is recommended, especially for those who are frail or residents of care facilities and have few opportunities to be exposed to the sun. When caring for frail older adults, gerontological nurses can promote healthy aging by helping their patients avoid extremes of temperature, prevent dryness, and prevent exposure to toxic products (see Chapter 16).

Hair and Nails

Hair is part of the integument with biological, psychological, and cosmetic value. It is composed of tightly fused horny cells that arise from the dermal layer of the skin and are colored by melanocytes. Genetics, race, sex, and testosterone and estrogen hormones influence hair texture, color, distribution, and loss in both men and women.

In some persons, their genetic backgrounds related to race produce distinctive hair characteristics, which should be kept in mind when caring for or assessing the person. For example, persons of Asian descent often have sparse facial and body hair and it is dark, silky, and straight. Persons of African descent often have slightly more head and body hair than Asians; however, the hair texture varies widely. It is always fragile, and it ranges from straight to spiraled, and from thin to thick. Persons of European descent have the most head and body hair, with an intermediate texture and form ranging from straight to curly, fine to coarse, and thick to thin and of any color.

Men and women in all racial groups have thinner and less hair as they grow older. Scalp hair loss is prominent in men, beginning as early as the twenties. The hair in the ears, the nose, and the eyebrows of older men increases and stiffens. Women have less pronounced scalp hair loss (Luggen, 2005). The accustomed hair color remains for some, but for most there is a gradual loss of pigmentation (melanin) and it becomes dryer and coarser. Older women develop chin and facial hair attributable to a decreased estrogen to testosterone level ratio. Leg, axillary, and pubic hair lessens and in some instances eventually disappears altogether after menopause. The absence of lower extremity hair can be misinterpreted as a sign of peripheral vascular disease in the older adult, whereas it is a normal change of aging.

Fingernails and toenails become harder and thicker, and more brittle, dull, and opaque with age. They change in shape, becoming at times flat or concave instead of convex. Decreasing amounts of water, calcium, and lipid in the body result in vertical ridges. Reduced blood supply slows nail growth rate. The half-moon (lunula) at the base of the fingernails may entirely disappear; the color of the nails may vary from yellow to gray, although the long-term effect of the widespread use of nail acrylic is not yet known.

The development of fungal infections of the nails (onychomycosis) is quite common but not the result of aging. Fungus invades the space between the layers of the nail, leaving a thick and unsightly appearance. The slowness of growth and the reduced circulation in older nails make treatment very difficult.

Musculoskeletal

A functioning musculoskeletal system is necessary for the body's movement in space, gross responses to environmental forces, and the maintenance of posture. This complex system comprises bones, joints, tendons, ligaments, and muscles.

Although none of the age-related changes to the musculoskeletal system are life-threatening, any of them could affect one's ability to function and therefore one's quality of life (Table 3.2). Some of the changes are visible to others and have the potential to affect the person's self-esteem. As seen with the skin, changes in the musculoskeletal system are influenced by many factors, such as age, sex, race, and environment; signs of musculoskeletal changes begin to become obvious in the forties.

TABLE 3.2 Key Aspects of Normal Age-Related Changes With Aging: Musculoskeletal

Changes	Effects
Dryer ligaments, tendons, and joints	Reduced flexibility
Reduced muscle mass	Reduced strength
Reduced bone mineral density	Increased risk for fractures, spontaneous and traumatic
Reduced body water	Increased risk of dehydration

The musculoskeletal changes that have the most effect on function are related to the ligaments, tendons, and joints; over time these structures become dry, hardened, and less flexible. In joints that had been subjected to trauma earlier in life (injuries or repetitive movement), these changes can be seen earlier and are more severe. If joint space is reduced, arthritis is diagnosed.

Muscle mass can continue to build until the person is in his or her fifties. However, between 40% and 50% of the skeletal muscle mass of a 30-year-old person may be lost by the time the person is in his or her eighties (Brown & McCarthy, 2015; Yu et al., 2014). Disuse of skeletal muscle (sarcopenia) accelerates the loss of strength. The amount of muscle tissue mass decreases (atrophies) whereas levels of adipose tissue increase. The replacement of lean muscle by adipose tissue is most noticeable in men in the area of the waist and in women between the umbilicus and the symphysis pubis.

Stature, Posture, and Body Composition

Changes in stature and posture are two of the more obvious signs of aging and are associated with multiple factors involving skeletal, muscular, subcutaneous, and fat tissue. Vertebral disks become thin as a result of both gravity and dehydration, causing a shortening of the trunk. These changes may begin to be seen as early as the fifties (Crowther-Radulewicz, 2014). The person may have a stooped appearance from kyphosis, a curvature of the cervical vertebrae arising from reduced bone mineral density (BMD). Some loss of BMD in women is associated with the normal age-related lowered

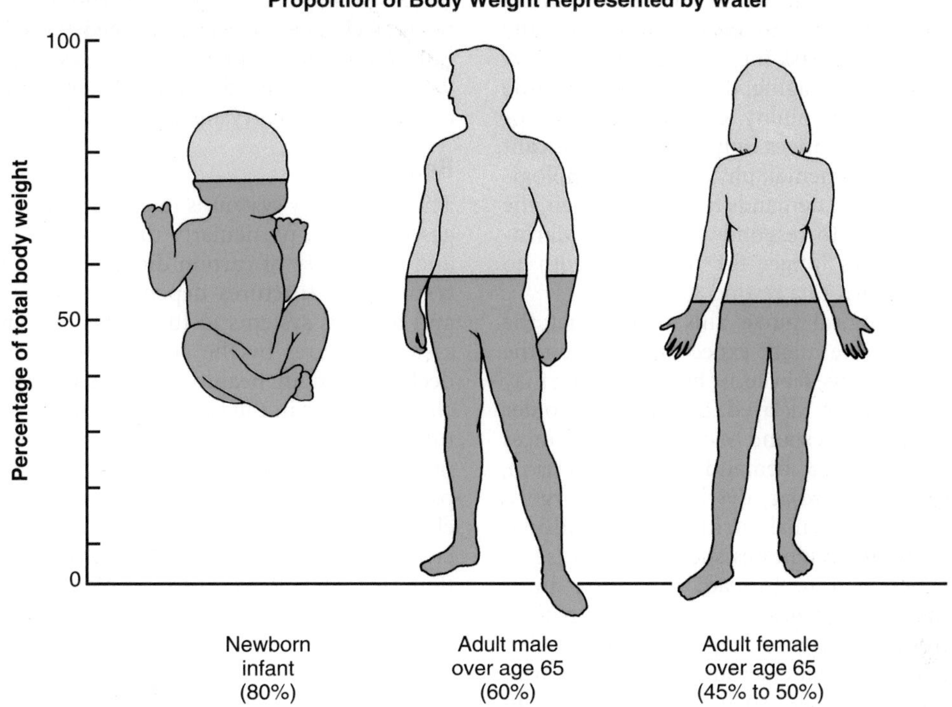

FIGURE 3.3 Changes in body water distribution. (From Thibodeau GA, Patton KT: *Structure and function of the body,* ed 13, St Louis, 2008, Mosby.)

postmenopausal estrogen levels. With the shortened appearance, the bones of the arms and the legs may appear disproportionate in size. If a person's bone mineral density is very low, it is diagnosed as osteoporosis and a loss of 2 to 3 inches in height is not uncommon (see Chapter 21).

From 25 to 75 years of age, the fat content of the body increases by 16%, slowly altering body shape and weight as the amount of lean body mass declines. Age-related loss of body water is significant: 54% to 60% in men; 46% to 52% in women (Kee & Paulanka, 2000). This water loss results in a dramatically increased risk for dehydration (Fig. 3.3).

TABLE 3.3 Key Aspects of Normal Age-Related Changes With Aging: Cardiovascular

Changes	Effects
Stiffening and thickening of the heart tissue	Decreased ability to respond to the need for increased circulation/oxygen Longer time for the heart to return to a resting state after stress
Decreased elasticity of the arterial walls	Increased risk for hypertension Reduced blood flow to some organs (e.g., kidney)

Cardiovascular

The cardiovascular system is responsible for the transport of oxygenated and nutrient-rich blood to the organs and the transport of metabolic waste products to the kidneys and bowels. The most relevant age-related changes in this system are myocardial (heart tissue) and blood vessel stiffening and, in particular, decreased responsiveness to sudden changes in cardiovascular demand (Table 3.3) (Cunningham et al., 2014). Changes in the cardiovascular (CV) system are progressive and cumulative.

Cardiac

The age-related changes of the heart (presbycardia) are structural, electrical, and functional. Although the overall size of the heart remains relatively unchanged in healthy adults, the wall thickens and the shape changes somewhat. Maximum coronary artery blood flow, stroke volume, and cardiac output are decreased, making the person at a much greater risk for heart failure (Strait & Lakatta, 2012). In healthy aging, the changes have little or no effect on the heart's ability to function in day-to-day life. As noted, the changes only become significant when there are environmental, physical, or psychological stresses. With sudden demands for more oxygen, the heart may not be able to respond adequately (Marin-Garcia, 2008). It takes longer for the heart both to accelerate and to return to a resting state.

For the gerontological nurse, this means that the increased heart rate one might expect to see when the person is in pain, anxious, febrile, or hemorrhaging may not be present or will be delayed. Similarly, the older heart may not be able to respond to other circumstances requiring increased cardiac demand, such as infection, anemia, pneumonia, cardiac dysrhythmias, surgery, diarrhea, hypoglycemia, malnutrition, drug-induced illnesses, and noncardiac illnesses such as renal disease and prostatic obstruction. Instead, the nurse must depend on other signs of distress in the older patient and be diligently alert to signs of rapid decompensation both of the previously well elder and of the elder who is already medically fragile, such as those living in nursing homes.

Heart disease is the number one cause of nonaccidental death in the world (WHO, 2015). Often the changes associated with disease are thought to be "normal," but they are not. The nurse promotes healthy aging by providing recommendations for heart-healthy life choices and urging the elder to seek and receive excellent health care (see Chapter 22).

Blood Vessels

Several of the same age-related changes seen in the skin and muscles affect the lining (intima) of the blood vessels, especially the arteries. As in the skin, the most significant change is decreased elasticity limiting the consistent forward movement of blood to the organs. In health, change in blood flow to the coronary arteries and the brain is minimal, but decreased blood flow to other organs, especially the liver and kidneys, has potentially serious implications for medication use (see Chapter 9). When a person already has or develops arteriosclerosis or hypertension, the age-related changes can have serious consequences (see Chapter 22).

Less dramatic changes are found in the veins, although they do stretch and the valves, which keep the blood from flowing backward, become less efficient. This means that lower extremity edema develops more quickly and that the older adult is more at risk for deep vein thrombosis (blood clots or DVTs) because of the increased sluggishness of the venous circulation. The normal changes, when combined with long-standing but unknown weakness of the vessels, may become visible in varicose veins and explain the increased rate of stroke and aneurysms in older adults.

Respiratory

The respiratory system is the vehicle for ventilation and gas exchange, particularly the transfer of oxygen into and the release of carbon dioxide from the blood. The respiratory structures depend on the musculoskeletal and nervous systems to function fully. The respiratory system matures by the age of 20 and then begins to decline, even in healthy individuals. Although subtle changes occur in the lungs, the thoracic cage, the respiratory muscles, and the respiratory centers in the central nervous system, the changes are small and, for the most part, insignificant. The specific changes include loss of elasticity resulting in stiffening of the chest wall, inefficiency in gas exchange, and increased resistance to air flow (Fig. 3.4). Respiratory problems are common but

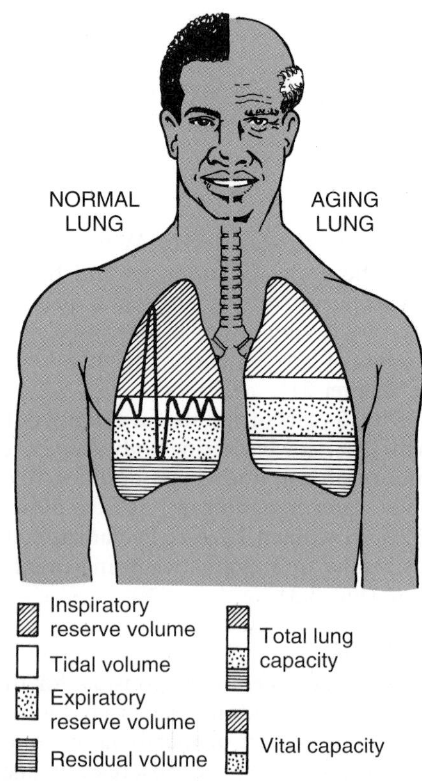

FIGURE 3.4 Changes in lung volumes with aging. (From McCance KL, Huether SE: *Pathophysiology: The biologic basis for disease in adults and children,* ed 7, St Louis, 2014, Mosby.)

almost always the result of past or present exposure to environmental toxins (e.g., pollution, cigarette smoke) rather than a consequence of the aging process (Sheahan & Musialowski, 2001) (see Chapter 22).

Like the cardiovascular system, the biggest change is in the efficiency, in this case, of gas exchange. Under usual conditions, this has little or no effect on the performance of customary life activities. However, a respiratory deficit may become evident when an individual is confronted with a sudden demand for increased oxygen. The body is not as sensitive to low oxygen levels or elevated carbon dioxide levels, each indicating the need to increase the rate of breathing. The changes that occur in the anatomical structures of the chest and altered muscle strength can significantly affect one's ability to cough forcefully enough to quickly expel materials that accumulate in or obstruct airways. In addition, the respiratory cilia (small fibers in the respiratory system) are less effective. Together these place the person at high risk of potentially life-threatening infections and aspiration. In the presence of impairment, such as difficulty swallowing or decreased movement of the esophagus, the risk is even more increased; this is often the case after a person has had a stroke or during end-stage dementia. All of these potential complications make the promotion of health through the prevention of respiratory illnesses in older adults of the highest importance.

Renal

The renal system is responsible for regulating concentrations of water and salts in the body and maintaining the acid/base balance in the blood. Blood is filtered in the nephrons in the kidneys with each beat of the heart. The glomerulus is the key structure that controls the rate of filtering (glomerular filtration rate [GFR]). Among the many changes to the kidneys are those of blood flow, GFR, and the ability to regulate body fluids. As a result of vascular and fixed anatomical and structural changes blood flow through the kidneys decreases by about 10% per decade, from about 1200 mL/min in young adults to about 600 mL/min by 80 years of age, (Macias-Nunez & Cameron, 2005; Wiggins & Patel, 2009). Yet the kidneys lose as many as 50% of the nephrons with little change in the body's ability to regulate body fluids and maintain adequate day-to-day fluid homeostasis.

Age-related changes in the renal system are especially significant because of resultant heightened susceptibility to fluid and electrolyte imbalance and because of structural damage caused by medications and contrast media used in diagnostic tests. Even healthy kidneys have a reduced capacity to respond (renal reserve) to either salt or water load or deficit or even a fever, and therefore older adults are at greater risk for renal insufficiency and failure than healthy younger adults (Choudhury & Levi, 2011).

Whereas plasma creatinine level is constant throughout life, urine creatinine level should decline even in normal aging because of the reduced lean muscle mass. The urine creatinine clearance rate is an important indicator for appropriate drug therapy, reflecting the ability to handle medications passing through and metabolized by the kidneys. Kidney function is measured through the calculation of the creatinine clearance (CrCl) rate as described in Chapter 9.

SAFETY ALERT

Persons with a reduced creatinine clearance rate usually need a reduction in the dosages of their medications to prevent potential toxicity, and caution must be used in the administration of intravenous fluids.

Endocrine

The endocrine system, working in tandem with the neurological system, provides regulation and control of the integration of body activities through the secretion of hormones from glands that can be found throughout the body. As the body ages, most glands shrink and the rate of secretion decreases. However, other than the decrease in estrogen level, leading to menopause, the impact of the changes is not clear.

Pancreas

The endocrine pancreas secretes insulin, glucagon, somatostatin, and pancreatic polypeptides. The secretion of these substances does not appear to decrease to any level of clinical significance. However, there is increased insulin resistance and accelerated aging for those with chronic inflammation and obesity, leading to diabetes mellitus type 2 (Akintola & van Heemst, 2015). Older adults have the highest rate of type 2 diabetes of any age group, with significant variation by ethnicity and region (see Chapter 20). When the pancreas is stressed with sudden concentrations of glucose, blood levels are higher for longer. These temporary levels of increased blood glucose make the diagnosis of diabetes or glucose intolerance difficult.

Thyroid

Slight changes occur in the structure and function of the thyroid gland, which may explain the increased incidence of hypothyroidism in older adults (Brashers et al., 2014). Some atrophy, fibrosis, and inflammation occur.

Although other evidence of change is inconclusive at this time, diminished secretion of thyroid-stimulating hormone (TSH) and thyroxine (T_4) appear to be age-related. Serum T_3 level decreases with age, perhaps as a result of decreased secretion of TSH by the pituitary gland. When thyroid replacement is needed, lower doses are usually effective and higher doses contraindicated. In addition, the therapeutic dose of thyroxine may change over time and monitoring is required (see Chapter 20).

Collective signs, such as a slowed basal metabolic rate, thinning of the hair, and dry skin, are characteristic of hypothyroidism in the young but are normal manifestations in the aged who have no history of thyroid deficiencies, making the recognition of thyroid disturbances difficult (see Chapter 20). The number of persons affected by thyroid disturbances is so low that they cannot be considered normal changes with aging.

Reproductive

The reproductive systems in men and women serve the same physiological purpose—human procreation. Although both aging men and women undergo age-related changes, the changes affect women significantly more than men. Women lose the ability to procreate after the cessation of ovulation (menopause), whereas men remain fertile their entire lives. Regardless of the physical changes, the need for sexual expression remains (see Chapter 26).

Female Reproductive System

As menopause signals the end of the reproductive phase in a woman's life, several other age-related changes occur, particularly in breast tissue and urogenital structures. The testosterone to estrogen ratio changes, with sometimes a significant drop in a woman's relative estrogen level. Older breasts are smaller, pendulous, and less firm. Outwardly, the labia majora and minora become less prominent and pubic hair thins and may disappear altogether. The cervix, uterus, and ovaries slowly atrophy, the latter to the point where they may not be palpable on exam. The vagina shortens, narrows, and loses some of its elasticity, typical of aging muscle and skin. Vaginal walls also lose their ability to lubricate quickly, especially if the woman is not sexually active. More stimulation is needed to achieve orgasm. The vaginal epithelium changes considerably with an increase in pH and increased risk for vaginitis (Tufts et al., 2014). The vaginal changes result in the potential for dyspareunia (painful intercourse), trauma during intercourse, increased susceptibility to infection, and urinary incontinence.

Male Reproductive System

Although men have the ability to produce sperm throughout their lives, they also experience changes in the functioning of the reproductive and the urogenital organs in late life. The changes are usually more subtle and noticed only as they accumulate, beginning when men are in their fifties. The testes atrophy and soften. Although sperm count does not decrease, fertility may be reduced because a higher number of sperm lack motility or because of structural abnormalities such as sclerosis or fibrosis of the seminiferous tubules. Erectile changes are also seen: more stimulation is needed to achieve a full erection, ejaculation is slower and less forceful, and refractory periods (time between erections) are longer (Tufts et al., 2014). As with women, alterations in hormone balances may play a part in the age-related changes in men. Testosterone level is reduced in all men but only rarely to the level at which it would be considered a true deficiency.

By 80 years of age more than 80% of men in the United States are likely to have some degree of prostatic enlargement (Cunningham & Kadmon, 2015). The condition known as benign prostatic hyperplasia (BPH) is so common that some are beginning to call it a normal part of aging. The only time it is considered a problem is when the enlargement compresses the urethra and interferes with bladder emptying. As a result, the man may experience urinary retention leading to repeated urinary tract infections and overflow incontinence. Intervention is pursued only when the symptoms of BPH interfere with the man's quality of life (Kamel & Dornbrand, 2004). In addition to aging, obesity, high glucose levels, and insulin resistance have been found to increase the risk of developing BPH (Chen et al., 2015).

Gastrointestinal

The digestive system includes the gastrointestinal (GI) tract and the accessory organs that aid in digestion. Several age-related changes affect function, with these changes seen as early as the fifties (Doig & Huether, 2014). Additionally, a number of common health problems can have a great effect on the digestive system (Table 3.4).

Mouth

Age-related changes affect both the teeth and the mouth. With the wear and tear of years of use, the teeth eventually lose enamel and dentin and then become more vulnerable to decay (caries). The roots become more brittle and break more easily. The gums recede and are more susceptible to infection and chronic inflammation and may influence cardiac health (National Institute of Dental and Craniofacial Research [NIDCR], 2013).

TABLE 3.4 Key Aspects of Normal Age-Related Changes With Aging: Gastrointestinal

Changes	Effects
Mouth: wear and tear of teeth	Increased risk for decay
Gums recede	Increased risk for oral and cardiac disease
Esophagus: sluggish and erratic movement of muscles	Increase stress to lower end leading to discomfort and increased risk for GERD (gastroesophageal reflux disease)
Stomach: decreased motility, reduced bicarbonate and gastric mucus	Early sensation of fullness, increased risk for pernicious anemia and peptic ulcer disease
Intestines: reduced function of intestinal villi	Reduced ability to adequately absorb nutrients
Liver: reduced blood flow	Increased half-life of fat-soluble medications

Without care, teeth may be lost. Taste buds decline in number, and salivary secretion lessens. A very dry mouth (xerostomia) is common. The nurse ensures the fit and cleanliness of any whole or partial dentures worn.

Even in health, these changes combine to create the potential for decreased pleasure and comfort in eating, which in turn can lead to anorexia and weight loss. A number of medications taken for common health problems can quickly exacerbate potential problems, especially xerostomia. When the gerontological nurse administers medications to older adults or conducts medication education, he or she should warn them about this potential and how to minimize its effects (see Chapter 9).

Esophagus

In youth, food passes quickly through the esophagus to the stomach because of the strong and coordinated contractions of associated muscle and peristalsis. In aging, the contractions increase in frequency but are more disordered, and therefore propulsion is less effective. This is referred to as presbyesophagus. The sluggish emptying of the esophagus may cause the lower end of the esophagus to dilate, creating greater stress in this area and possibly causing digestive discomfort. Pathological processes that are increasingly seen as adults become older include gastroesophageal reflux disease (GERD) and hiatal hernias.

Stomach

Age-related changes in the stomach include decreased gastric motility and volume, and reductions in the secretion of bicarbonate and gastric mucus. Loss of smooth muscle delays emptying time, which may lead to anorexia or weight loss as a result of distention, meal-induced fullness, and the feeling of satiety (Price & Wilson, 2002). It will prolong the amount of time medications stay in the stomach, affecting drug metabolism (see Chapter 9). Gastric atrophy results in insufficient levels of hydrochloric acid and other digestive substances, leading to a decrease in the ability to produce intrinsic factor, the key component needed for the utilization of ingested vitamin B_{12}. Without vitamin B_{12} pernicious anemia develops. The lessening or loss of protective gastric mucus makes the stomach more susceptible to peptic ulcer disease, particularly when nonsteroidal anti-inflammatory drugs such as aspirin and ibuprofen are used.

Intestines

The age-related changes of the small intestine include those noted earlier that involve smooth muscles as well as those related to the gastric villi, the anatomical structures in the intestinal walls where nutrients are absorbed. The villi become broader and shorter and less functional. Nutrient absorption is affected; proteins, fats, minerals (including calcium), vitamins (especially B_{12}), and carbohydrates (especially lactose) are absorbed more slowly and in lesser amounts (Doig & Huether, 2014). Changes in motility, epithelial membranes, vascular perfusion, and gastrointestinal membrane transport may affect absorption of lipids, amino acids, glucose, calcium, and iron.

Peristalsis is slowed with aging and there is a blunted response to rectal filling; the extent of the change should not be such to cause problems with defecation. In other words, constipation is not a normal part of aging. Instead, constipation is more often a side effect of medications, life habits, immobility, inadequate fluid intake, and lack of attention to the gastrocolic reflex (the urge to defecate after eating). The role of the gerontological nurse in addressing elimination needs is presented in Chapter 12 with suggestions on promoting healthy digestion.

Accessory Organs

The accessory organs of the digestive system are the liver and the gallbladder. The liver continues to function throughout life despite a decrease in weight (mass) and blood flow. The blood flow may decrease 30% to 40% by the late nineties (Hall, 2009). The decrease is associated with an increased half-life of fat-soluble medications (see Chapter 9). While slow, liver regeneration is not greatly impaired, and liver function tests remain unaltered with age.

There does not seem to be a specific change in the gallbladder; however, the incidence of gallstones increases (Hall, 2009). This is possibly caused by the increased lipogenic composition of bile from biliary cholesterol. Decreased bile salt synthesis increases the incidence of cholelithiasis and cholecystitis but these are not normal age-related illnesses (Hall, 2009).

Neurological

Contrary to popular belief, the older nervous system, including the brain, is remarkably resilient and changes in cognitive functioning are not a normal part of aging. Although many neurophysiological changes occur with aging, they do not occur in all older persons and do not affect everyone the same way, and therefore cannot be attributed to normal aging. For example, the presence of neurofibrillary tangles is a classic sign of dementia and is found in the brains of all persons with Alzheimer's disease, but they are found also in the brains of persons without dementia. Although it is very difficult to show a true cause and effect of age-related changes in the nervous system, several changes appear to be more common (Table 3.5). Nonetheless neither the patient nor the nurse should accept an assessment of "confusion" without making sure the cause is identified and treated if at all possible.

Central Nervous System

The major changes in the aging nervous system are found in the central nervous system (CNS). With aging, the dendrites appear to be "wearing out," and the number of neurons found in several areas of the brain decreases. The older brain is smaller and weighs less than a younger brain. This change in size is seen primarily in the frontal lobe and diagnosed as "normal age-related atrophy" on computed tomography (CT) scans or magnetic resonance imaging (MRI). Decreased adherence of the dura mater to the skull, increased fibrosis, thickening of the meninges, narrowing of the gyri, widening of the sulcus, and an increase in the subarachnoid space also occur (Sugarman, 2014). These changes are important because of the increased potential damage that can occur following a traumatic brain injury (see Chapter 16).

Subtle changes in cognitive and motor functioning occur in the very old. Mild memory impairments and difficulties with balance may be seen as normal age-related changes in neurodegeneration and neurochemistry (see Chapter 23). The intellectual performance of the older adult without brain dysfunction remains constant; however, the performance of tasks may take longer, which is an indication that central processing is slowed. There are also decreasing levels of the neurotransmitters choline acetylase, serotonin, and catecholamines. Reduced levels of circulating serotonin probably increase the elder's risk for endogenous depression. Other enzymes such as monoamine oxidase (MAO) have increased levels. Redundancy of brain cells may forestall the effects of these changes, but the exact number of cells required for certain functions is unknown.

TABLE 3.5 Key Aspects of Normal Age-Related Changes With Aging: Neurological

Changes	Effects
Central nervous system: reduced number of dendrites, atrophy of brain itself	Decrease in brain weight and size, increased risk for trauma
Slight changes in physiology and chemistry of brain	Mild memory impairments Increased risk for slight balance difficulties
Peripheral nervous system: Significantly reduced vibratory sense in lower extremities Decreased sensory functions at the periphery Decreased proprioception	Greatly increased risk for injury (e.g., from fire or falling)

Peripheral Nervous System

The most important effect of the normal changes in the aging peripheral nervous system is the increased risk for injury. Vibratory sense in the lower extremities may be nonexistent. Somesthetics, or tactile sensitivity, decreases in connection with the loss of nerve endings in the skin. This is most notable in the fingertips, the palms of the hands, and the lower extremities. This decreased sensitivity is translated into delayed reactions to things such as hot surfaces, significantly increasing the risk for burns and the extent of burns should they occur. The presence of a functioning smoke detector is particularly important for healthier and safer aging.

Kinesthetic sense, or proprioception (awareness of one's position in space), is altered because of changes in both the peripheral and the central nervous systems. If one is less aware of body position and has less tactile awareness, the risk for falling is dramatically increased (see Chapter 14). For example, the person may be walking on a flat surface that suddenly becomes uneven. With reduced proprioception, it takes a little longer to realize the surface is uneven and a little longer still to realize that one has tripped (changed position in space). Whereas a younger person would be able to immediately restore his or her body position and prevent a fall, this slight delay may result in a fall in an older adult. Conditions such as arthritis, stroke, some cardiac disorders, or damage to the structures of the inner ear may also affect peripheral and central mechanisms of mobility and exacerbate these changes in proprioception.

Sensory Changes

As we age, we cannot totally escape some loss of smell, sight, sound, and touch. The creative gerontological nurse can make a big difference in the quality of life for the person with sensory changes (see Chapter 19) (Table 3.6).

Eyes and Vision

Changes in vision and eyes begin very early and are both functional and structural. All the changes affect visual acuity and accommodation, that is, the ability to adjust to changes in environmental light.

Presbyopia is an age-related decrease in near vision that begins to become noticeable in midlife. Nearly 95% of adults older than 65 years of age wear glasses for close vision (Burke & Laramie, 2003), and 18% also use a magnifying glass for reading and close work. Although presbyopia is first seen between 45 and 55 years of age, 80% of those older than 65 years of age have fair to adequate far vision past 90 years of age.

TABLE 3.6 Key Aspects of Normal Age-Related Changes With Aging: Sensory

Changes	Effects
Eyes	
Decrease in near vision (presbyopia)	Necessity of wearing reading glasses or using a magnifying glass for close work
Changes to eyelids: sagging, entropion, and ectropion	Reduced vision, excessive tearing, and scratching of cornea
Reduced efficiency of goblet cells	Uncomfortable, drying of eye
Cornea: flatter, thicker, less flexible	Increased far-sightedness
Lens and intraocular: potential thickening and yellowing, reduced flexibility	Need for increased levels of light, decreased depth and color perception
Ears	
Atrophy of cerumen glands	Thicker, dryer cerumen and increased risk for impactions that temporarily reduce hearing
Stiffening of joints within the ear (presbycusis)	Sensorineural hearing loss, permanent

Extraocular. Like the skin elsewhere age-related changes affect both form and function of the extraocular structures. The eyelids lose elasticity, and drooping (senile ptosis) results. In most cases, this only affects appearance. In extreme cases the lids sag far enough to block vision. Spasms of the orbicular muscle may cause the lower lid to turn inward. If it stays this way, it is called entropion. The lower lashes that curl inward irritate and scratch the cornea. Surgery may be needed to prevent permanent injury. Decreases in the orbicular muscle strength may result in ectropion, or an out-turning of the lower lid. Without the integrity of the trough of the lower lid, tears run down the cheek instead of bathing the cornea. This and an inability to close the lid completely lead to excessively dry eyes and the need for artificial tears. The person may need to tape the eyes shut during sleep. Exacerbating this problem, the number of goblet cells that provide mucin (essential for eye lubrication and movement) decreases. A severe deficiency of lubrication is known as "dry eye syndrome."

Ocular. The cornea is the avascular transparent outer surface of the eye globe that refracts (bends) light rays entering the eye through the pupil. With aging, the cornea becomes flatter, less smooth, thicker, and duller in appearance. The result is increased far-sightedness (hyperopia). For the person who was myopic (near-sighted) earlier in life, this change may actually improve vision. Arcus senilis, a gray-white to silver ring or partial ring, may be observed 1 to 2 mm inside the limbus at the juncture of the iris and cornea; it is composed of deposits of calcium and cholesterol salts. It does not appear to have any clinical significance.

The anterior chamber is the space between the cornea and the lens. The edges of the chamber include canals that control the volume and movement of aqueous fluid within the space. With aging, the chamber decreases slightly in size and capacity because of thickening of the lens. Resorption of the intraocular fluid becomes less efficient with age. If the decrease is significant, it can lead to increased intraocular pressure and glaucoma (see Chapter 19) (Huether et al., 2014). Any acute changes in vision or eye pain should be considered medical emergencies and responded to accordingly.

Reduced accommodation and the need for greater levels of lighting are the result of reduced responsiveness of the pupils and changes in the lens. The lens, a small, flexible, biconvex, crystal-like structure just behind the iris, is most responsible for visual acuity; it adjusts the light entering the pupil and focuses it on the retina. Age-related changes in the lens are probably universal and begin in the forties. The origins of these changes are not fully understood, although exposure to ultraviolet rays of the sun contributes to the problem, with cross-linkage of collagen creating a more rigid and thickened lens structure.

Light scattering increases, and color perception decreases. As a result, glare is a problem created not only by sunlight outdoors but also by the reflection of light on any shiny object (Meisami et al., 2007). Eventually, people require three times as much light to see things as they did when they were in their twenties. It is more effective to place high-intensity light on the object or surface to be observed rather than increasing the intensity of the light in the entire room. For example, it would be more effective to focus a light directly on the newspaper a person was reading.

SAFETY ALERT

As a result of age-related changes in vision there is an increased sensitivity to glare. The floor in the care facility may be very clean, but if it is also shiny it could increase the older adult's risk for falling.

Intraocular. The retina, which lines the inside of the eye, has less distinct margins and is duller in appearance than in younger adults. Color clarity diminishes by 25% in the sixth decade and by 59% in the eighth decade, especially that of the blues, the violets, and the greens of the spectrum; light colors such as reds, oranges, and yellows are more easily seen. Some of this difficulty is linked to the yellowing of the lens and impaired transmission of light to the retina. Finally, the number of rods and associated nerves at the periphery of the retina is reduced, resulting in peripheral vision that is not as clear or is absent (Meisami et al., 2007). Arteries in back of the eye may show atherosclerosis and slight narrowing. Veins may show indentations (nicking) as they pass over the arteries if the person has a long history of hypertension but this is not an age-related change in eye structure. As long as these changes are not accompanied by distortion of objects or a significant decrease in vision, they are not clinically significant.

Ears and Hearing

Like the eye, age-related changes affect both the structure and the function of the ear. The appearance of the ear changes, especially in men (Fig. 3.5). The auricle loses flexibility and becomes longer and wider as a result of diminished elasticity. The lobe sags, elongates, and wrinkles. Together, these changes make the ear appear larger. Coarse, wiry, stiff hairs grow at the periphery of the auricle, and the tragus enlarges in men. On otoscopic examination the tympanic membrane appears dull and gray.

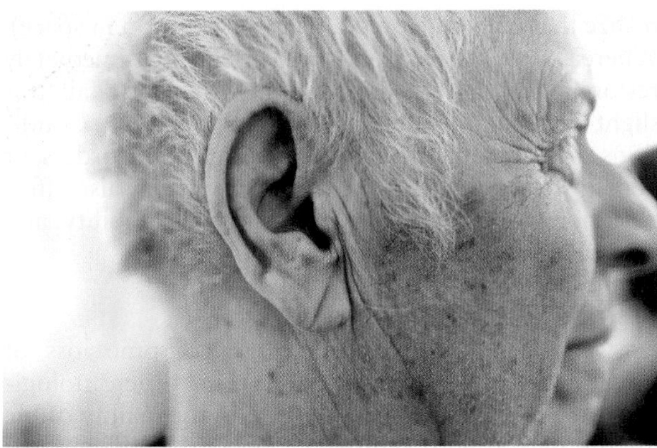

FIGURE 3.5 Ear of a senior adult man. (© iStock.com/themacx.)

The auditory canal narrows through inward collapse. Stiffer and coarser hairs line the canal. Cerumen glands atrophy, causing thicker and dryer wax, which is more difficult to remove. This is a substantial cause of temporary, reversible obstructive hearing loss. The gerontological nurse should be sensitive to this possibility and be skilled at safe cerumen removal. Once the cerumen is removed the associated obstructive hearing loss is restored (see Chapter 19).

Aging can change structures within the ear; for example, the joint between the malleus and the stapes can become calcified, causing reduced vibration of these bones and a mechanical reduction in the amount of sound transmitted to the auditory nerve, in turn impairing transmission of sound waves to the brain. This age-related hearing loss is known as presbycusis and sensorineural (SNL) in origin. The loss develops slowly, and in contrast to obstructive loss, is irreversible.

Presbycusis is primarily the loss of the ability to hear high-frequency sounds such as consonants, the chirping of birds, the rustling of leaves, and whispering. Although the person may be able to eventually decipher what is said if it is within context, this processing takes longer than usual or language is processed incorrectly. It is important to note that with normal age-related hearing loss the person can still hear but may not be able to make sense of the partially heard words, especially in places where there is a great deal of environmental noise such as restaurants. Inaccurate responses too often lead to the incorrect suspicion of dementia or confusion

TABLE 3.7 Key Aspects of Normal Age-Related Changes With Aging: Immune System

Changes	Effects
Reduced immunity	Increased risk for infections
Delayed immune response	Decrease in those signs of illness seen in younger adults (e.g., fever)

when in fact it is a hearing loss. Hearing loss of some kind affects more than 80% of those older than age 85; the major type is SNL (Wallings & Dickson, 2012).

Immune

The immune system functions to protect the host from the invasion of foreign substances and organisms. To do so, it must be able to differentiate the self from a foreign body (Kishiyama, 2009). The immune system includes elements of many of the systems already discussed, as well as white blood cells, bone marrow, thymus, lymph nodes, and spleen.

A number of age-related changes have been implicated in the increased risk for infection in the older adult (Table 3.7). For example, the skin is thinner and therefore less resistant to bacterial invasion. The reduced number of cilia in the lungs leads to the increased risk for pneumonia. The friability of the urethra increases the risk for urinary tract infections, especially in women. But perhaps the most important of all is the reduced immunity at the cellular level, which is now understood to have a significant genetic underpinning.

Late life brings a reduction in T-cell function that results from a decrease in both innate immunity and adaptive immunity. Being alert for signs and symptoms of autoimmune changes is especially important to gerontological nursing, as part of the responsibility to promote disease prevention and protect older adults from infection. Goals for healthy aging related to the reduction of potentially preventable infections are provided in the document *Healthy People 2020* (Box 3.5). An immunization for the prevention of the life-threatening streptococcal pneumonia became available December 2014 (Prevnar). It is covered by Medicare with no co-pay, as are the annual influenza and the original pneumonia (Pneumovax) vaccinations (see Chapter 7).

The changes in immune function affect the older person's response to illness consistent with the immunological theory of aging. Early studies by Stengel (1983) found oral temperature norms in well elders significantly lower than those in younger adults. Older men

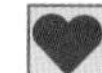 BOX 3.5 ***Healthy People 2020***

Goals to Reduce Potentially Preventable Infections

Objective IID-4: Reduce New Invasive Pneumococcal Infections—Persons 65 Years of Age and Older

Baseline: 40.4 confirmed new cases per 10,000 persons 65 years of age and older (2008)

Target: 31 new cases per 10,000 persons 65 years of age and older

Objective IID-4.4: Reduce New Cases of Penicillin-Resistant Invasive Pneumococcal Infections

Baseline: 2.6 confirmed new cases per 10,000 persons 65 years of age and older (2008)

Target: 2 new cases per 10,000 persons 65 years of age and older

Data from USDHHS: *Healthy People 2020: Immunizations and infectious disease: objectives.* Available at http://healthypeople.gov/2020/topicsobjectives2020/objectiveslist.aspx?topicId=23.

consistently had an even lower temperature than women of comparable age. This means that a febrile response suggestive of infection is no longer restricted to a temperature greater than 98.6° or 99° F. Instead, an older adult may have a core temperature elevation at much lower numbers. The very old may have an average normal temperature of 96° F, with an average range of 95° to 97° F. These findings emphasize the need to carefully evaluate the basal temperature of older adults and recognize that even low-grade fevers (99° F) in later life may signify serious illness. When this is combined with the age-related delay in the increases in the white blood cell count compared to younger adults, early detection of serious illness is difficult in many cases. A lack of fever (temperature greater than 98.6° F) or a normal white blood count cannot be used to rule out an infection. Instead, the nurse must consider the person as a whole—mood, level of consciousness, or other signs such as a recent fall or change in level of cognitive abilities.

Based on the current biological theories of aging, with support of clinical evidence, it can be concluded that complex functions of the body decline before simple body processes; that coordinated activity, which relies on interacting systems such as nerves, muscles, and glands, has a greater detrimental loss than single-system activity; and that a uniform and perhaps predictable loss of cell function occurs in all vital organs. Yet many older adults are able to function effectively within the physical dictates of their body and continue to live to a healthy old age, capable of wisdom, judgment, and satisfaction.

The physical changes that accompany aging affect every body system, and the theories of why they occur are many. Although there are numerous ways nurses can promote healthy aging in the presence of these changes, when nurses are able to begin to differentiate these normal changes from signs and symptoms of potential health problems, the positive effect of the nurse's interventions is multiplied.

KEY CONCEPTS

- The rapid advancement in understanding the biological basis of aging is in large part due to advances in genomic science.
- Although there continue to be a number of theories of aging, a commonality is in the recognition that over time the cell loses the ability to reproduce.
- There are many physical changes that accompany aging; however, a number of these are relatively insignificant in the absence of disease or unusual stress.
- There are enormous individual variations in the rate of aging of body systems and functions.
- Many of the normal changes with aging may be misinterpreted as being pathological, and some pathological conditions may be mistaken for normal changes of aging.
- Careful assessment of individual aging changes, lifestyle, and desires is fundamental to caring and quality nursing care of persons in later life.
- The nurse cannot rely on the "typical" signs of infection in the older adult but must use a more holistic approach.

ACTIVITIES AND DISCUSSION QUESTIONS

1. Identify at least two normal changes that accompany aging for each body system.
2. Discuss the changes of aging you find, or would find, most difficult to accept.

REFERENCES

Abdollahi M, Ranjbar A, Shadnia S, et al: Pesticides and oxidative stress: A review, *Med Sci Monit* 10(6):RA141–RA147, 2004.

Akintola AA, van Heemst D: Insulin, aging, and the brain: Mechanisms and implications, *Front Endocrinol (Lausanne)* 6:13, 2015. Epub available at http://www.ncbi.nlm.nih.gov/pmc/articles/PMC4319489. Accessed October 2015.

Borghini A, Cervelli T, Galli A, et al: DNA modifications in atherosclerosis: From the past to the future, *Atherosclerosis* 230(2):202–209, 2013.

Brashers VL, Jones RE, Huether SE: Alterations in hormonal regulation. In McCance KL, Huether SE, Brashers VL, et al, editors: *Pathophysiology: The biologic basis for disease in adults and children*, ed 7, St Louis, 2014, Mosby.

Brooks-Wilson AR: Genetics of healthy aging and longevity, *Hum Genet* 132(12):1323–1338, 2013.

Brown WJ, McCarthy MS: Sarcopenia: What every NP should know, *J Nurs Practioners* 11(8):753–759, 2015.

Burke M, Laramie JA: *Primary care of the older adult: A multidisciplinary approach*, ed 2, St Louis, 2003, Mosby.

Campisi J: Aging, cellular senescence, and cancer, *Annu Rev Physiol* 75:685–705, 2013.

Carnes BA, Staats DO, Sonntag WE: Does senescence give rise to disease?, *Mech Ageing Dev* 129:693–699, 2008.

Castelo-Branco C, Soveral I: The immune system and aging: A review, *Gynecol Endocrinol* 30(10):16–22, 2014.

Cefalu CA: Theories and mechanisms of aging, *Clin Geriatr Med* 27:491–506, 2011.

Chen Z, Miao L, Gao X, et al: Effect of obesity and hyperglycemia on benign prostatic hyperplasia in elderly patients with newly diagnosed type 2 diabetes, *Int J Clin Exp Med* 8(7):11289–11294, 2015.

Choudhury D, Levi M: Kidney aging—inevitable or preventable?, *Nat Rev Nephrol* 7(12):706–717, 2011.

Crowther-Radulewicz CL: Structure and function of the musculoskeletal system. In McCance KL, Huether SE, Brashers VL, et al, editors: *Pathophysiology: The biologic basis for disease in adults and children*, ed 7, St Louis, 2014, Mosby.

Cunningham GR, Kadmon D: *Epidemiology and pathogenesis of benign prostatic hyperplasia*, UpToDate September 2015. Available at http://www.uptodate.com/contents/epidemiology-and-pathogenesis-of-benign-prostatic-hyperplasia. Accessed October 2015.

Cunningham SG, Brashers VL, McCance KL: Structure and function of the cardiovascular system. In McCance KL, Huether SE, Brashers VL, et al, editors: *Pathophysiology: The biologic basis for disease in adults and children*, ed 7, St Louis, 2014, Mosby.

Dato S, Crocco P, D'Aquila P, et al: Exploring the role of genetic variability and lifestyle in oxidative stress response for healthy aging and longevity, *Int J Mol Sci* 14:16443–16472, 2013.

Dehbi AZ, Radstake TR, Broen JC: Accelerated telomere shortening in rheumatic disease: Cause or consequence? *Expert Rev Clin Immunol* 9(12):1193–1204, 2013.

Delves PJ: *Overview of the immune system*. In *The Merck manual of geriatrics*, on-line version, 2016. Available at http://www.merckmanuals.com/professional/resourcespages/about-the-merck-manuals. Accessed August 13, 2016.

Doig AK, Huether SE: Structure and function of the digestive system. In McCance KL, Huether SE, Brashers VL, et al, editors: *Pathophysiology: The biologic basis for disease in adults and children*, ed 7, St Louis, 2014, Mosby.

Einstein A: *Relativity: The special and the general theory*, New York, 1920, Henry Holt.

Friedman S: Integumentary function. In Meiner SE, editor: *Gerontologic nursing*, ed 4, St Louis, 2011, Mosby.

Fulop T, Wiltkowski JM, Pawelec G, et al: On the immunological theory of aging, *Interdiscip Top Gerontol* 39:163–176, 2014.

Goldsmith TC: Arguments against non-programmed theories of aging, *Biochemistry (Mosc)* 78(9):971–978, 2013.

Gosain A, DiPietro LA: Aging and wound healing, *World J Surg* 28(3):321–326, 2004.

Grune T, Shringarpure R, Sitte N, et al: Age-related changes in protein oxidation and proteolysis in mammalian cells, *J Gerontol Ser A Biol Sci Med Sci* 56:B459, 2001.

Hall KE: Effect of aging on gastrointestinal function. In Halter B, Ouslander J, Tinetti M, et al, editors: *Hazzard's principles of geriatric medicine and gerontology*, ed 6, New York, 2009, McGraw-Hill.

Harman D: Aging: A theory based on free radical and radiation chemistry, *J Gerontol* 11:298, 1956.

Hayflick L, Moorehead PS: The serial cultivation of human diploid cell strains, *Exp Cell Res* 25:585, 1981.

Hornsby PJ: Senescence and life span, *Pflügers Arch* 459:291, 2010.

Huether SE, Rodway G, DeFriez C: Pain, temperature regulation, sleep, and sensory function. In McCance KL, Huether SE, Brashers VL, et al, editors: *Pathophysiology: The biologic basis for disease in adults and children*, ed 7, St Louis, 2014, Mosby.

Jang Y, Van Remmen H: The mitochondrial theory of aging: Insight from transgenic and knockout mouse models, *Exp Gerontol* 44:256–260, 2009.

Kamel H, Dornbrand L: Health issues of the aging male. In Landefeld CS, Palmer R, Johnson MA, et al, editors: *Current geriatric diagnosis and treatment*, New York, 2004, McGraw-Hill.

Kee JL, Paulanka BJ: Fluids and their influence on the body. In Kee JL, Paulanka BJ, editors: *Handbook of fluids, electrolytes and acid-base imbalances*, Albany, NY, 2000, Delmar.

Kishiyama JL: Disorders of the immune system. In McPhee SJ, Hammer GD, editors: *Pathophysiology of disease: An introduction to clinical medicine*, ed 6, New York, 2009, McGraw-Hill Lange.

Lagouge M, Larsson N-G: The role of mitochondrial DNA mutations and free radicals in disease and aging, *J Intern Med* 273:529–543, 2013.

Lodovici M, Bigagli E: Oxidative stress and air pollution exposure, *J Toxicol* 2011. E journal article available at http://www.hindawi.com/journals/jt/2011/487074/. Accessed October 2015.

Luggen AS: Rapunzel no more: Hair loss in older women, *Adv Nurse Pract* 13(10):28–33, 2005.

Macias-Nunez JF, Cameron JS: The ageing kidney. In Davison AM, et al, editors: *Oxford textbook of clinical nephrology*, ed 3, New York, 2005, Oxford University Press.

Marin-Garcia J: *Aging and the heart: A post genomic view*, New York, 2008, Springer.

Meisami E, Brown CM, Emerle HF: Sensory systems: Normal aging, disorders, and treatments of vision and hearing in humans. In Timiras PS, editor: *Physiological basis of aging and geriatrics*, ed 3, New York, 2007, CRC Press.

Murphy MP: How mitochondria produce reactive oxygen species, *Biochem J* 417:1–13, 2009.

National Center for Complementary and Alternative Medicine (NCCAM): *Antioxidants and health: an introduction*, 2013, Available at http://nccam.nih.gov/health/antioxidants/introduction.htm. Accessed October 2015.

National Institute of Dental and Craniofacial Research (NIDCR): *Periodontal (gum) disease: Causes, symptoms, and treatments*, 2013. Available at http://www.nidcr.nih.gov/oralhealth/Topics/GumDiseases/PeriodontalGumDisease.htm#canPeriodontal. Accessed September 2015.

Nomellini V, Gomez CR, Kovacs EJ: Aging and impairment of innate immunity, *Contrib Microbiol* 15:188, 2008.

Pashkow FJ: Oxidative stress and inflammation in heart disease: Do antioxidants have a role in treatment and/or prevention? *Int J Inflam* 2011. E Pub available at http://www.hindawi.com/journals/iji/2011/514623/. Accessed October 2015.

Price S, Wilson L: *Pathophysiology: Clinical concepts of disease processes*, ed 6, St Louis, 2002, Mosby.

Shammas MA: Telomeres, lifestyle, cancer, and aging, *Curr Opin Clin Nutr Metab Care* 14(1):28–34, 2011.

Sheahan SL, Musialowski R: Clinical implications of respiratory system changes in aging, *J Gerontol Nurs* 27(5):26, 2001.

Shi Y, Buffenstein R, Pulliam DA, et al: Comparative studies of oxidative stress and mitochondrial function in aging, *Integr Comp Biol* 50(5):869–879, 2010.

Short KR, Bigelow ML, Kahl J, et al: Decline in skeletal muscle mitochondrial function with aging in humans, *Proc Natl Acad Sci USA* 102(15):5618, 2005.

Skin Cancer Foundation: *Skin cancer facts*. Available at http://www.skincancer.org/skin-cancer-information/skin-cancer-facts. Accessed September 2015.

Spector RE: *Cultural diversity in health and illness*, ed 8, Upper Saddle River, NJ, 2012, Prentice Hall.

Stengel GB: Oral temperature in the elderly, *Gerontologist* 23(special issue):306, 1983.

Strait JB, Lakatta EG: Aging-associated cardiovascular changes and their relationship to heart failure, *Heart Fail Clin* 8(1):143–164, 2012.

Sugarman RA: Structure and function of the neurologic system. In McCance KL, Huether SE, Brashers VL, et al, editors: *Pathophysiology: The biologic basis for disease in adults and children*, ed 7, St Louis, 2014, Mosby.

Swain SL, Nikolich-Zugich J: Key research opportunities in immune system aging, *J Gerontol Ser A Biol Sci Med Sci* 64:183, 2009.

Tufts G, Rodway G, Huether SE, et al: Structure and function of the reproductive systems. In McCance KL, Huether SE, Brashers VL, et al, editors: *Pathophysiology: The biologic basis for disease in adults and children*, ed 7, St Louis, 2014, Mosby.

Wallings AD, Dickson GM: Hearing loss in older adults, *Am Fam Physician* 85(12):1150–1156, 2012.

Walston J: Aging. In Durson SC, Price JD, Smith SC, editors: *Oxford American handbook of geriatric medicine*, New York, 2010, Oxford University Press.

World Health Organization (WHO): *The 10 leading causes of death in the world, 2000 and 2012*. Available at http://www.who.int/mediacentre/factsheets/fs310/en. Accessed October 2015.

Wiggins J, Patel S: Changes in renal function. In Halter B, Ouslander J, Tinetti M, et al, editors: *Hazzard's principles of geriatric medicine and gerontology*, ed 6, New York, 2009, McGraw-Hill.

Valko M, Morris H, Cronin M, et al: Metals, toxicity and oxidative stress, *Curr Med Chem* 12(10):1161–1208, 2005.

Vine J, Bores C, Abdul-Aziz KM, et al: The free radical theory of aging revisited, *Antiox Redox Sign* 19(8):779–787, 2013.

Yu S, Umapathysivan K, Visvanathan R: Sarcopenia in older people, *Int J Evid Based Healthc* 12(4):227–243, 2014.

4

Psychosocial, Spiritual, and Cognitive Aspects of Aging

Theris A. Touhy

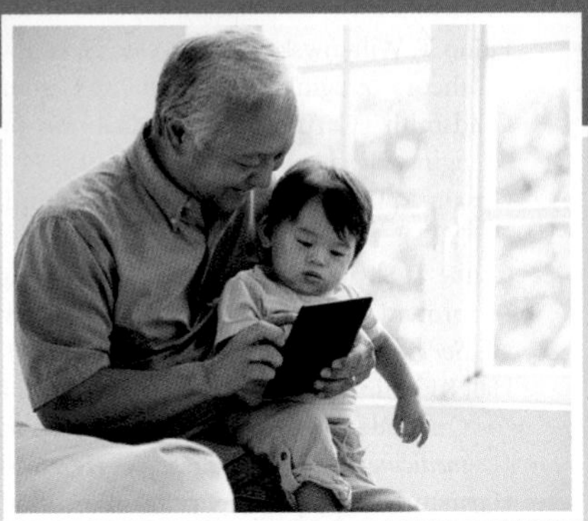

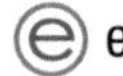 evolve.elsevier.com/Touhy/gerontological

LEARNING OBJECTIVES

Upon completion of this chapter, the reader will be able to:

- Explain the major psychosocial theories of aging.
- Discuss the importance of spirituality to healthy aging.
- Explain cognitive changes with age and strategies to enhance cognitive health.
- Discuss factors influencing learning in late life and appropriate teaching and learning strategies.

THE LIVED EXPERIENCE

If I Had My Life to Live Over

I'd dare to make more mistakes next time, I'd relax, I would limber up. I would be sillier than I've been this trip. I would take fewer things seriously. I would take more chances. I would climb more mountains and swim more rivers. I would eat more ice cream and less beans. I would perhaps have more actual troubles, but I'd have fewer imaginary ones.

You see, I'm one of those people who live sensibly and sanely hour after hour, day after day. Oh, I've had my moments, and if I had to do it over again, I'd have more of them. In fact, I'd try to have nothing else. Just moments, one after another, instead of living so many years ahead of each day. I've been one of those persons who never goes anywhere without a thermostat, a hot water bottle, a raincoat, and a parachute. If I had it to do again, I would travel lighter than I have.

If I had my life to live over, I would start barefoot earlier in the spring and stay that way later in the fall. I would go to more dances. I would ride more merry-go-rounds. I would pick more daisies.

Nadine Stair (1992)

Each individual has unique life experiences and because of this must be seen holistically, through the lens of his or her time, place, culture, gender, and personal history. The close relationship among biological, social, and psychological development that exists through childhood and adolescence varies more in adulthood because of the greater variations in life experiences and demands as one matures. This chapter provides the reader with information on the psychosocial, spiritual, and cognitive aspects of aging. The importance of the life story, reminiscence, and life review in coming to know elders is included. Factors influencing learning in later life and appropriate teaching and learning strategies are also discussed.

PSYCHOSOCIAL THEORIES OF AGING

A person is not just a biological being but a multidimensional whole. Only when life is considered in its totality can we begin to truly understand aging. Here we discuss the psychosocial theories of aging and acknowledge that most are more accurately conceptual models or approaches to understanding. Because they are most often referred to as theories in the gerontological literature, we will do so here for the ease of discussion. They can be classified as first-, second-, and third-generation theories (Hooyman & Kiyak, 2011).

First Generation

Early psychosocial theories of aging were an attempt to explain and predict the changes in middle and late life with an emphasis on adjustment. Adjustment was seen as an indication of success, at least by the academic theoreticians who developed them. The majority of these theories began appearing in the gerontological literature in the 1940s and 1950s. They were not based on extensive research; instead, they primarily developed as a consequence of "face validity," that is, emerging from the personal and professional experience of both scientists and clinicians and appearing to be reasonable explanations of aging. This set of theories has varied very little since they were first proposed. The major theories in the first generation were those of *role* and *activity*.

Role Theory

Role theory was one of the earliest explanations of how one adjusts to aging (Cottrell, 1942). Self-identity is believed to be defined by one's role in society (e.g., nurse, teacher, banker). As individuals evolve through the various stages in life, so do their roles. Successful aging means that as one role is completed it is replaced by another one of comparative value to the individual and society. For example, the wage-earning work role is replaced by that of a volunteer, or a parent becomes a grandparent. The ability of an individual to adapt to changing roles is a predictor of adjustment to aging.

Role theory is operationalized in the phenomenon of *age norms.* They are culturally constructed expectations of what is deemed acceptable behavior in society and are internalized by the individual. Age norms are based on the assumption that chronological age and gender, in and of themselves, imply roles; for example, one may hear, "If only they would act their age," or "You are too old to do/say/behave like that," or "That is unbecoming to a woman of your age." In each of these examples, the behavior challenged long-established age norms for white middle-aged and older individuals. With the aging of the "baby boomers," popular culture is challenging age norms; for example, from advertisements for genital lubricants featuring actors with graying hair to news of the availability of medications to treat erectile dysfunction, "older persons" are now depicted as still sexually active. These images replace the historical view that persons become asexual as they age (or so their grandchildren hope!) (see Chapter 26). Both men and women are assuming roles and engaging in behaviors today that were unimaginable when role theory was first proposed.

Activity Theory

In 1953 Havighurst and Albrecht proposed that successful aging was based on the individual's ability to maintain an *active lifestyle.* It is expected that the productivity and activities of middle life are replaced with equally engaging pursuits in later life (Maddox, 1963). The theory was based on the assumption that it is better to be active (and young) than inactive (Havighurst, 1972). *Activity theory* is consistent with Western society's emphasis on work, wealth, and productivity and therefore continues to influence the perception of unsuccessful aging (Wadensten, 2006).

The first-generation theories of aging have been criticized because of their limited applicability. Problems of intersubjectivity of meaning, testability, and empirical adequacy have persisted. Consistent with the historical period of their development, they failed to consider social class, education, health, and economic and cultural diversity as influencing factors (Hooyman & Kiyak, 2011).

Second Generation

Second-generation theories expanded or questioned those of the first generation. These include the *disengagement, continuity, age-stratification, social exchange, modernization, developmental,* and *gerotranscendence theories.*

Disengagement Theory

Disengagement theory is in contrast to both role and activity theories. In 1961, Cumming and Henry proposed that in the natural course of aging the individual does, and should, slowly withdraw from society to allow the transfer of power to the younger generations. The transfer is viewed as necessary for the maintenance of social equilibrium (Wadensten, 2006). A belief in the appropriateness of disengagement provided the basis of age discrimination for many years when an older employee was replaced by a younger one. Although this practice was overtly accepted in the past, it is still present more covertly but is now being challenged socially and legally. An elder's withdrawal is no longer an indicator of successful aging, is not *necessarily* a good thing for society, and does not take into account the needs of the individual or culture in which one lives.

Continuity Theory

Also in contrast with role theory but similar to activity theory is *continuity theory.* Havighurst and colleagues (1968) proposed that individuals develop and maintain a consistent pattern of behavior over a lifetime. Aging, as an extension of earlier life, reflects a *continuation of the patterns* of roles, responsibilities, and activities. Personality influences the roles and activities chosen and the level of satisfaction drawn from these. Successful aging is associated with one's ability to maintain and continue previous behaviors and roles or to find suitable replacements (Wadensten, 2006).

Age-Stratification Theory

Age-stratification theory is based on the belief that aging can be best understood by considering the experiences of individuals as members of cohorts with similarities to others in the same group (Riley, 1971). The importance of the similarities exceeds that of the differences. An example of age stratification is the traditional conceptualization of "young-old," "middle-old," and "old-old" (Neugarten, 1968). The cohort of baby boomers born between approximately 1947 and 1964 is presenting a significant challenge to this theory in the developed world. The range of experiences and the variability in age when some of these experiences occurred to individuals within this cohort have resulted in substratifications within baby boomers themselves. The wide range of socioeconomic and educational levels furthers this diversity (see Chapter 2).

Social Exchange Theory

Social exchange theory is conceptualized from an economic perspective. The presumption is that as one ages, one has fewer and fewer economic resources to contribute to society. This paucity results in loss of social status, self-esteem, and political power (Hooyman & Kiyak, 2011). Only those who are able to maintain control of their financial resources have the potential to remain fully participating members of society and anticipate successful aging. Although this may have some applicability in the communities in the world that have been able to develop a stable economy for its citizens, this theory marginalizes those in communities and underdeveloped countries who struggle for the barest necessities now and into the foreseeable future (World Health Organization [WHO], 2014).

Modernization Theory

Although not usually associated with social exchange theory, *modernization theory* can be used to consider nonmaterial aspects of exchange. This theory is an attempt to explain the social changes that have resulted in devaluing the contributions of elders. In the United States before about 1900, material and political resources were controlled by the older members of a society (Achenbaum, 1978). The resources included their knowledge, skills, experience, and wisdom (Fung, 2013). In agricultural cultures and communities, the oldest members held power through property ownership and the right to make decisions related to food distribution. Older men and women often held valuable religious and cultural roles of instructing youth and controlling ceremonies.

According to modernization theory, the status and value of elders are lost when their labors are no longer considered useful, their kinship networks are dispersed, their knowledge is no longer pertinent to the society in which they live, and they are no longer revered simply because of their age (Hendricks & Hendricks, 1986). Modernization has had a notable effect on cultures such as those in China and Japan where filial duty predominated as an underlying construct of eldercare (Fung, 2013). As more and more adult children enter the marketplace or emigrate for social or economic reasons, conflicts between traditional values mount (see *The Bonesetter's Daughter* by Amy Tan, 2001). It is proposed that these changes are the result of advancing technology, urbanization, and mass education (Cowgill, 1974). In some cultures or family structures and in underdeveloped areas of the world, "modernization" as described may not yet be applicable.

Developmental Theories

Psychologist Erik Erikson's theory of psychosocial development is one of the best known theories of personality in psychology. He theorized a predetermined order of developmental and specific tasks that were associated with specific periods in one's life course. The task of the last stage of life is ego integrity versus self-despair. Erikson saw the last stage of life as a vantage point from which one could look back with ego integrity or despair on one's life. Successfully completing this phase means looking back with few regrets and a general feeling of satisfaction. These individuals will attain wisdom, even when confronting death.

In later years, Erikson modified the "either-or" stance of each of the tasks. Thus ego integrity is tinged with some regrets, wisdom is balanced with frivolity, and letting go is balanced with hanging on (Erikson et al., 1986).

Gerotranscendence Theory

This theory is similar to that of disengagement yet the reason for the withdrawal is not for societal needs but to give the person time for self-reflection, exploration of the inner self, contemplation of the meaning of life, and movement away from the material world (Tornstam, 1989, 2000, 2005). Aging is viewed as movement from birth to death and maturation toward wisdom, an ever-evolving process that alters one's view of reality, sense of spirituality, and meaning beyond the self. Inasmuch, gerotranscendence implies achieving wisdom through personal transformation. With aging, time becomes less important, as do superficial relationships. Transcendence is viewed as a universal goal, the highest goal any person can achieve and a marker of successful aging. This theory is based on a highly egocentric approach to aging. It is less likely to be applicable in cultures based on the quality of interpersonal relationships (see Chapter 2). It also does not account for differences in economic resources, which may or may not provide the individual the "luxury" of time for introspection.

Third Generation

The third generation of theoretical development related to aging is also referred to as the "second transformation" occurring since the 1980s. The goal is "understanding the human meanings of social life in the context of everyday life rather than the explanation of facts" (Hooyman & Kiyak, 2011, p. 326). This may or may not rise to the level of a theory.

A phenomenological approach is used to achieve a qualitative understanding of the individual as an aging person. Aging is personally interpreted rather than socially or culturally constructed. In other words, to understand how an individual views aging, one has to come to know the individual by listening to his/her unique story rather than relying on stereotypical views of aging. This level is particularly useful in the application of nursing care and the incorporation of recognition of the aging person as unique and valuable in any circumstance and within the context of any culture. It can be used to promote healthy aging as the person is supported on the wellness continuum.

The Life Story

The life story as constructed through reminiscing, journaling, life review, or guided autobiography has held great fascination for gerontologists in the last 30 years. The universal appeal of the life story as a vehicle of culture, a demonstration of caring and generational continuity, and an easily stimulated activity has held allure for many professionals. "One of the few universals is that humans in all known cultures use language to tell stories" (Ramírez-Esparza & Pennebaker, 2006, p. 216).

The most exciting aspect of working with older adults is being a part of the emergence of the life story: the shifting and blending patterns. When we are young, it is important for our emotional health and growth to look forward and plan for the future. As one ages, it becomes more important to look back, talk about experiences, review and make sense of it all, and end with a feeling of satisfaction with the life lived.

Storytelling is a complementary and alternative therapy nurses can use with older adults to enhance communication (Moss, 2014). The nurse can learn much about an older adult's history, communication style, relationships, coping mechanisms, strengths, fears, affect, and adaptive capacity by listening thoughtfully as the life story is constructed.

Reminiscing

Reminiscing is an umbrella term that can include any recall of the past. Reminiscing occurs from childhood onward, particularly at life's junctures and transitions. Reminiscing cultivates a sense of security through recounting of comforting memories, belonging through sharing, and promotion of self-esteem through confirmation of uniqueness. Robert Butler (2003) emphasized that in the past, reminiscing was thought to be a sign of senility or what we now call Alzheimer's disease. Older people who talked about the past and told the same stories again and again were said to be boring and living in the past. From Butler's landmark research (1963), we now know that reminiscence is the most important psychological task of older people.

For the nurse, reminiscing is a therapeutic intervention important in assessment and understanding. The work of several gerontological nursing leaders, including Irene Burnside, Priscilla Ebersole, and Barbara Haight, has contributed to the body of knowledge about reminiscence and its importance in nursing. The International Institute for Reminiscence and Life Review (University of Wisconsin, Superior, WI), an interdisciplinary organization uniting participants to study reminiscence and life review, is another valuable resource for nurses and members of other disciplines involved in research or practice. This group also publishes a journal, the *International Journal of Reminiscence and Life Review.*

Reminiscence can have many goals. It not only provides a pleasurable experience that improves quality of life but also increases socialization and connectedness with others, provides cognitive stimulation, improves communication, facilitates personal growth, and can decrease depression scores (see Chapter 24) (Bohlmeijer et al., 2003; Grabowski et al., 2010; Haight & Burnside, 1993; Pinquart & Forstmeier, 2012; Stinson, 2009). The process of reminiscence can occur in individual conversations with older people, can be structured as in a nursing history, or can occur in a group where each person shares his or her memories and listens to others sharing their memories. Intergenerational reminiscence activities could have benefits for both older and younger individuals. Reminiscence can also be used by caregivers to enhance communication with family members experiencing cognitive impairment (Latha et al., 2014). Box 4.1 provides some suggestions for encouraging reminiscence, and group work is discussed later in this chapter.

Stinson (2009) offers a protocol for structured reminiscence based on research from earlier studies and the Nursing Interventions Classification (NIC) recommendations. Mudiwa (2010) reports on an innovative use of "YouTube" reminiscence therapy in Ireland and proposes that this medium can be easily used in reminiscence interventions. "In-the-Moment" recording of reminiscence episodes via new mobile devices also holds promise, and results of life review therapy for depression in older adults in a face-to-face setting with additional computer use are promising (Cappeliez, 2013; Preschl et al., 2012). Although further research on the effectiveness of reminiscence and the development of evidence-based protocols is needed, nurses can have confidence in using this technique in work with older people (Latha et al., 2014; Stinson, 2009).

Cognitive impairment does not necessarily preclude older adults from participating in reminiscence or storytelling groups. Opportunities for telling the life story, enjoying memories, and achieving ego integrity should not be denied to individuals on the basis of their cognitive status. Modifications must be made according to the cognitive abilities of the person, and although individual life review from a psychotherapeutic approach is not an appropriate modality, individuals with mild to moderate memory impairment can enjoy and benefit from group work focused on reminiscence and storytelling.

When the nurse is working with a group of persons who are cognitively impaired, the emphasis in reminiscence groups is on sharing memories in any way they can be expressed, rather than relying on specific recall of events. There should be no pressure to answer

BOX 4.1 Suggestions for Encouraging Reminiscence

- Listen without correction or criticism. Older adults are presenting their version of their reality; our version belongs to another generation.
- Encourage older adults to discuss various ages and stages of their lives. Use questions such as, "What was it like growing up on that farm?", "What did teenagers do for fun when you were young?", or "What was WWII like for you?"
- Be patient with repetition. Sometimes people need to tell the same story often to come to terms with the experience, especially if it was meaningful to them. If they have a memory loss, it may be the only story they can remember, and it is important for them to be able to share it with others.
- Be attuned to signs of depression in conversation (dwelling on sad topics) or changes in physical status or behavior, and provide appropriate assessment and intervention.
- If a topic arises that the person does not want to discuss, change to another topic.
- If individuals are reluctant to share because they do not feel their life was interesting, reassure them that everyone's life is valuable and interesting and tell them how important their memories are to you and others.
- Keep in mind that reminiscing is not an orderly process. One memory triggers another in a way that may not seem related; it is not important to keep things in order or verify accuracy.
- Keep the conversation focused on the person reminiscing, but do not hesitate to share some of your own memories that relate to the situation being discussed. Participate as equals, and enjoy each other's contributions.
- Listen actively, maintain eye contact, and do not interrupt.
- Respond positively and give feedback by making caring, appropriate comments that encourage the person to continue.
- Use props and triggers such as photographs, memorabilia (e.g., a childhood toy or antique, short stories or poems about the past, favorite foods, YouTube videos, old songs).
- Use open-ended questions to encourage reminiscing. If working with a group, you can prepare questions ahead of time, or you can ask the group members to pick a topic that interests them. One question or topic may be enough for an entire group session.
- Consider using questions such as the following:
  - How did your parents meet?
  - What do you remember most about your mother? Father? Grandmother? Grandfather?
  - What are some of your favorite memories from childhood?
  - What was the first house you remember?
  - What were your favorite foods as a child?
  - Did you have a pet as a child?
  - What do you remember about your first job?
  - How did you celebrate birthdays or other holidays?
  - If you were married, what are your memories of your wedding day?
  - What was your greatest accomplishment or joy in your life?

questions such as "Where were you born?" or "What was your first job?" Rather, discussions may center on jobs people had and places they have lived. Displaying additional props, such as music, pictures, familiar objects (e.g., an American flag, an old coffee grinder), and doing familiar activities that trigger past memories (e.g., having a tea party, folding linens) can prompt many recollections and sharing. The leader of a group with participants who have memory problems must assume a more active approach.

The TimeSlips program (Bastings, 2003, 2006; Fritsch et al., 2009) is an evidence-based innovation, cited by the Agency for Healthcare Research and Quality (AHRQ, 2014), that uses storytelling to enhance the lives of people with cognitive impairment. Positive outcomes associated with the program include enhanced verbal skills and provider reports of positive behavioral changes, increased communication, increased sociability, and less confusion. TimeSlips is a beneficial and cost-effective therapeutic intervention that can be used in many settings.

Using the TimeSlips format, group members looking at a picture are encouraged to create a story about the picture. The pictures can be fantastical and funny, such as from greeting cards, or more nostalgic, such as Norman Rockwell paintings. All contributions are encouraged and welcomed, there are no right or wrong answers, and everything that the individuals say is included in the story and written down by the scribe. Stories are read back to the participants during the session, using their names to identify their contributions. At the beginning of each session, the story from the last session is read to the participants. Care is taken to compliment each member for his or her contribution to the wonderful story. The stories that emerge are full of humor and creativity and often include discussions of memories and reminiscing.

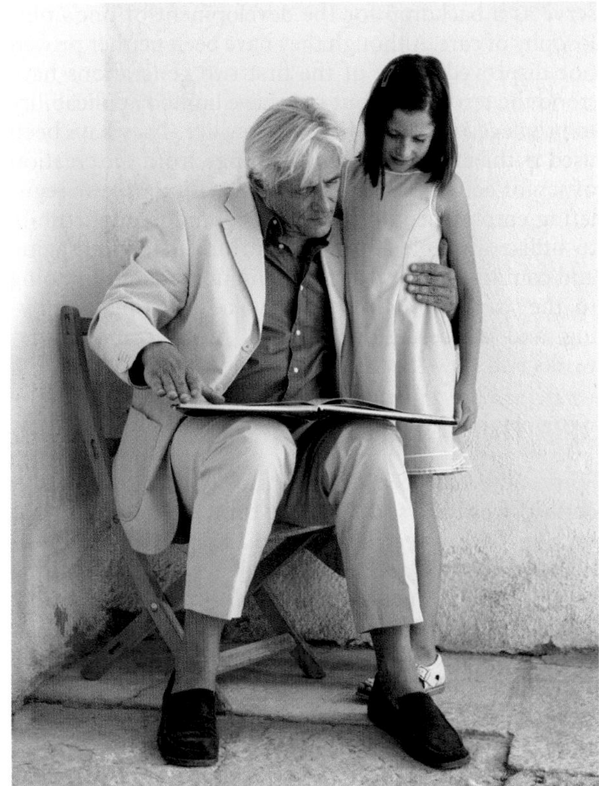

Grandfather sharing stories with his granddaughter. (© iStock.com/IS_ImageSource.)

Life Review

Robert Butler (1963) first noted and brought to public attention the review process that normally occurs in the older person as the realization of his or her approaching death creates a resurgence of unresolved conflicts. Butler called this process *life review*. Life review occurs quite naturally for many persons during periods of crisis and transition. However, Butler (2003) noted that in old age, the process of putting one's life in order increases in intensity and emphasis. Life review occurs most frequently as an internal review of memories, an intensely private, soul-searching activity.

Life review is considered more of a formal therapy technique than reminiscence and takes a person through his or her life in a structured and chronological order. Life review therapy (Butler & Lewis, 1983), guided autobiography (Birren & Deutchman, 1991), and structured life review (Haight & Webster, 2002) are psychotherapeutic techniques based on the concept of life review. Life review may be especially important for older people experiencing depressive symptoms and those facing death (Chan et al., 2014; Pot et al., 2010).

Life review should occur not only when we are old or facing death but also frequently throughout our lives. This process can assist us to examine where we are in life and change our course or set new goals. Butler (2003) commented that ongoing life review by an individual may help avoid the overwhelming feelings of despair that may surface for some individuals at the end of life when there may not be time to make changes.

❖ IMPLICATIONS FOR GERONTOLOGICAL NURSING AND HEALTHY AGING

Psychosocial theories and perspectives of aging provide the gerontological nurse with useful information to serve as a backdrop for the development of one's philosophy of care. Although they have been neither proved nor disproved, some of the first two generations have stood the test of time but may have limited applicability to privileged persons wherever they live. They have been used as the rationale for many things, from the creation of senior activity centers to the formation of laws regulating employment. Nurses have a unique opportunity to utilize multiple approaches to understanding aging and coming to know the person in uniqueness. In doing so, they can have an important voice in testing, modifying, and discussing psychosocial theories and frameworks and how they apply to worldwide diversity.

SPIRITUALITY AND AGING

Spirituality has been defined as a "quality of a person derived from the social and cultural environment that involves faith, a search for meaning, a sense of connection with others, and a transcendence of self, resulting in a sense of inner peace and well-being" (Delgado, 2007, p. 230). The spiritual aspect of people's lives transcends the physical and psychosocial to reach the deepest individual capacity for love, hope, and meaning. Erickson's concept of ego integrity seems closely related to development of a spiritual self.

Aging as a biological process has been studied extensively. Less attention has been paid to the study of aging as a spiritual process. As people age and move closer to death, spirituality may become more important. Declining physical health, loss of loved ones, and a realization that life's end may be near often challenge older people to reflect on the meaning of their lives. Spiritual belief and practices often play a central role in helping older adults cope with life challenges and are a source of strength in the lives of older adults (Hodge et al., 2010).

Distinguishing between religion and spirituality is a concern for many health professionals. Religious beliefs and participation in religious obligations and rites are often the avenues of spiritual expression, but they are not necessarily interchangeable. "Religion can be described as a social institution that unites people in a faith in God, a higher power, and in common rituals and worshipful acts. A god, divinity, and/or soul is always included in the concept" (Strang & Strang, 2002, p. 858). Each religion involves a particular set of beliefs.

Spirituality is a broader concept than religion and encompasses a person's values, beliefs, or search for meaning as well as their relationships with a higher power, with nature, and with other people. The concept of spirituality is found in all cultures and societies. For some people, particularly older people, formalized religion helps them feel fulfilled. The majority of older adults describe themselves as both spiritual and religious (Hodge et al., 2010).

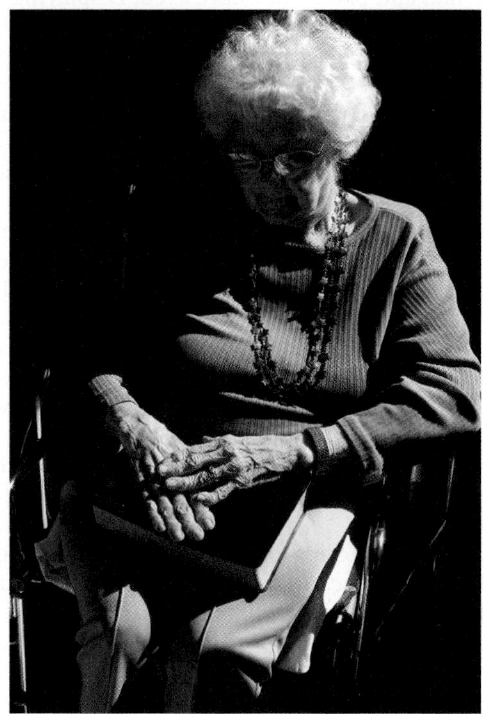

Prayer. (© iStock.com/Lisa Thornberg)

Spirituality is also a significant factor in understanding healthy aging. Rowe and Kahn's (1998) model of successful aging includes active engagement in life, minimal risk and disability, and high cognitive and physical function. Crowther and colleagues (2002) maintain that spirituality must be the fourth element of the model and is interrelated with all of the other elements (Edlund, 2014). The ultimate goal for promoting spirituality is to support and enhance quality of life.

Spiritual well-being may be considered the ability to experience and integrate meaning and purpose in life through connectedness with self, others, art, music, literature, nature, or a power greater than oneself (Gaskamp et al., 2006). Spirituality may be particularly important to healthy aging in "historically disadvantaged populations who display remarkable strengths despite adversities in their lives" (Hooyman & Kiyak, 2005, p. 213).

A nursing evidence-based guideline for promoting spirituality in the older adult (Gaskamp et al., 2006) provides a framework for spiritual assessment and interventions. The guideline identifies older adults who may be at risk for spiritual distress and who might be most likely to benefit from use of the guideline

BOX 4.2 Identifying Elders at Risk for Spiritual Distress

- Individuals experiencing events or conditions that affect the ability to participate in spiritual rituals
- Diagnosis and treatment of a life-threatening, chronic, or terminal illness
- Expressions of interpersonal or emotional suffering, loss of hope, lack of meaning, need to find meaning in suffering
- Evidence of depression
- Cognitive impairment
- Verbalized questioning or loss of faith
- Loss of interpersonal support

Data from Gaskamp C, Sutter R, Meraviglia M, et al: Evidence-based guideline: Promoting spirituality in the older adult, *J Gerontol Nurs* 32(11):8–11, 2006.

(Box 4.2). Spiritual distress or spiritual pain is "an individual's perception of hurt or suffering associated with that part of his or her person that seeks to transcend the realm of the material. Spiritual distress is manifested by a deep sense of hurt stemming from feelings of loss or separation from one's God or deity, a sense of personal inadequacy or sinfulness before God and man, or a pervasive condition of loneliness" (Gaskamp et al., 2006, p. 9). Spiritual distress may be manifested by anger, guilt, blame, hatred, expressions of alienation (such as turning away from family and friends), inability to derive pleasure, and inability to participate in religious activities that have previously provided comfort.

❖ IMPLICATIONS FOR GERONTOLOGICAL NURSING AND HEALTHY AGING

◆ Assessment

Assessment of spirituality is as important as assessment of physical, emotional, and social dimensions (Edlund, 2014). A spiritual history opens the door to a conversation about the role of spirituality and religion in a person's life. People often need permission to talk about these issues. Without a signal from the nurse, patients may feel that such topics are not welcome. Patients welcome a discussion of spiritual matters and want health professionals to consider their spiritual needs.

Nurses may neglect to explore this issue with elders because religion and spirituality may not seem high priority. The client should be assured that religious longings and rituals are important and that opportunities will be made available as desired. Nurses need to be knowledgeable and respectful about the rites and rituals of varying religions, cultural beliefs, and values

BOX 4.3 Brief Assessment of Spiritual Resources and Concerns

Instructions: Use the following questions as an interview guide with the older adult (or caregiver if the older adult is unable to communicate).

- Does your religion/spirituality provide comfort or serve as a cause of stress? (Ask to explain in what ways spirituality is a comfort or stressor.)
- Do you have any religious or spiritual beliefs that might conflict with health care or affect health care decisions? (Ask to identify any conflicts.)
- Do you belong to a supportive church, congregation, or faith community? (Ask how the faith community is supportive.)
- Do you have any practices or rituals that help you express your spiritual or religious beliefs? (Ask to identify or describe practices.)
- Do you have any spiritual needs you would like someone to address? (Ask what those needs are and if referral to a spiritual professional is desired.)
- How can we (health care providers) help you with your spiritual needs or concerns?

From Gaskamp C, Sutter R, Meraviglia M, et al: Evidence-based guideline: Promoting spirituality in the older adult, *J Gerontol Nurs* 32(11):10, 2006. Adapted from Meyer CL: How effectively are nurse educators preparing students to provide spiritual care? *Nurse Educ* 28(4):185–190, 2003; Koenig HG, Brooks RG: Religion, health and aging: Implications for practice and public policy, *Public Policy Aging Rep* 12:13–19, 2002.

(see Chapter 2). Religious and spiritual resources, such as pastoral visits, should be available in all settings where older people reside. It is important to avoid imposing one's own beliefs and to respect the person's privacy on matters of spirituality and religion (Touhy & Zerwekh, 2006).

Simply listening to patients as they express their fears, hopes, and beliefs is important. Spiritual assessments are intended to elicit information about the individual's core spiritual needs and about ways the nurse and other members of the health care team can respond to them. These include the Faith or Beliefs, Importance and Influence, Community, and Address (FICA) Spiritual History (Puchalski & Romer, 2000) and the Brief Assessment of Spiritual Resources and Concerns (Koenig & Brooks, 2002; Meyer, 2003) (Box 4.3). The Joint Commission requires spiritual assessments in hospitals, nursing homes, home care organizations, and many other health care settings providing services to older adults. The process of spiritual assessment is more complex than completing a standardized form and must be done within the context of the nurse-patient relationship. Simply listening to patients as they express their fears, hopes, and beliefs is important.

For older people with cognitive impairment, information about the importance of spirituality and religious beliefs can be obtained from family members. Nurses often see cognitive impairments as obstacles or excuses to providing spiritual care to people with dementia. Nurturing mind, body, and spirit is part of holistic nursing, and nurses must provide opportunities to all elders, no matter how impaired, to live life with meaning, purpose, and hope (Touhy, 2001).

◆ Interventions

The caring relationship between nurses and persons nursed is the heart of nursing that touches and supports the spirit. Knowing persons in their complexity, responding to that which matters most to them, identifying and nurturing connections, listening with one's being, using presence and silence, and fostering connections to that which is held sacred by the person are spiritual nursing responses that arise from within the caring, connected relationship (Touhy et al., 2005). Suggestions for spiritual care interventions are presented in Box 4.4.

BOX 4.4 Spiritual Nursing Interventions

- Relieving physical discomfort, which permits focus on the spiritual
- Creating a peaceful environment
- Using comforting touch, which fosters nurse-patient connection
- Providing an authentic presence
- Using attentive listening
- Knowing the patient as a person
- Listening to life stories
- Sharing fears and listening to self-doubts or guilt
- Fostering forgiveness and reconciliation
- Validating the person's life and assuring the person that he/she will be remembered
- Sharing caring words and love
- Encouraging family support and presence
- Fostering connections to that which is held sacred by the person
- Praying with and for the patient
- Respecting religious traditions and providing access to religious objects and rituals
- Referring the person to a spiritual counselor

From Gaskamp C, Sutter R, Meraviglia M, et al: Evidence-based practice guideline: Promoting spirituality in the older adult, *J Gerontol Nurs* 32(11):8–11, 2006; Touhy T, Brown C, Smith C: Spiritual caring: End of life in a nursing home, *J Gerontol Nurs* 31(9):27–35, 2004; Touhy T, Zerwekh H: Spiritual caring. In Zerwekh J, editor: *Nursing care at the end of life: palliative care for patients and families,* Philadelphia, 2006, FA Davis.

Nurturing the Spirit of the Nurse

"Because spiritual care occurs over time and within the context of relationship, probably the most effective tool at the nurse's disposal is the use of self" (Soeken & Carson, 1987, p. 607). Thinking about what gives your own life meaning and value helps in developing your spiritual self and assists you in being able to offer spiritual support to patients. Examples of activities include finding quiet time for meditation and reflection; keeping your own faith traditions; being with nature; appreciating the arts; spending time with those you love; and journaling (Touhy & Zerwekh, 2006). Find ways to nourish your own spirit. Nurses often do not take the time to do so and become dispirited. This is especially true for nurses who work with dying patients and experience grief and loss repeatedly. Having someone to talk to about feelings is important. Practicing compassion for oneself is essential to authentic practice of compassion for others (Touhy & Zerwekh, 2006).

ADULT COGNITION

Cognition is the process of acquiring, storing, sharing, and using information. Components of cognitive function include language, thought, memory, executive function (planning, organizing, remembering, paying attention, solving problems), judgment, attention, and perception (Desai et al., 2010). The determination of intellectual capacity and performance has been the focus of a major portion of gerontological research. Emerging research suggests that cognitive function and intellectual capacity is a complex interplay of age-related changes in the brain and nervous system and many other factors such as education, environment, nutrition, life experiences, physical function, emotions, biomedical and physiological factors, and genetics (Glahn et al., 2013; National Institutes of Health, 2004).

Before the development of sophisticated neuroimaging techniques, conclusions about brain function as we age were based on autopsy results (often on diseased brains) or results of cross-sectional studies conducted with older adults who were institutionalized or had coexisting illnesses. Changes seen were considered unavoidable and the result of the biological aging process rather than disease. As a result, the bulk of research has focused on the inevitable cognitive declines rather than on cognitive capacities. There are many old myths about aging and the brain that may be believed by both health professionals and older adults. It is important to understand cognition and memory in late life and dispel the myths that can have a negative effect on wellness and may, in fact, contribute to unnecessary cognitive decline (Box 4.5).

BOX 4.5 Myths About Aging and the Brain

MYTH: People lose brain cells every day and eventually just run out.

FACT: Most areas of the brain do not lose brain cells. Although you may lose some nerve connections, it can be part of the reshaping of the brain that comes with experience.

MYTH: You can't change your brain.

FACT: The brain is constantly changing in response to experiences and learning, and it retains this "plasticity" well into aging. Changing our way of thinking causes corresponding changes in the brain systems involved; that is, your brain believes what you tell it.

MYTH: The brain doesn't make new brain cells.

FACT: Certain areas of the brain, including the hippocampus (where new memories are created) and the olfactory bulb (scent-processing center), regularly generate new brain cells.

MYTH: Memory decline is inevitable as we age.

FACT: Many people reach old age and have no memory problems. Participation in physical exercise, stimulating mental activity, socialization, healthy diet, and stress management help maintain brain health. The incidence of dementia does increase with age, but when there are changes in memory, older people need to be evaluated for possible causes and receive treatment.

MYTH: There is no point in trying to teach older adults anything because "you can't teach an old dog new tricks."

FACT: Basic intelligence remains unchanged with age, and older adults should be provided with opportunities for continued learning. Minimizing barriers to learning such as hearing and vision loss and applying principles of geragogy enhance learning ability.

Modified from American Association of Retired Persons: *Myths about aging and the brain* (2007). Available at http://www.aarp.org/health/brain/aging/myths_about_aging_and_the_brain.html.

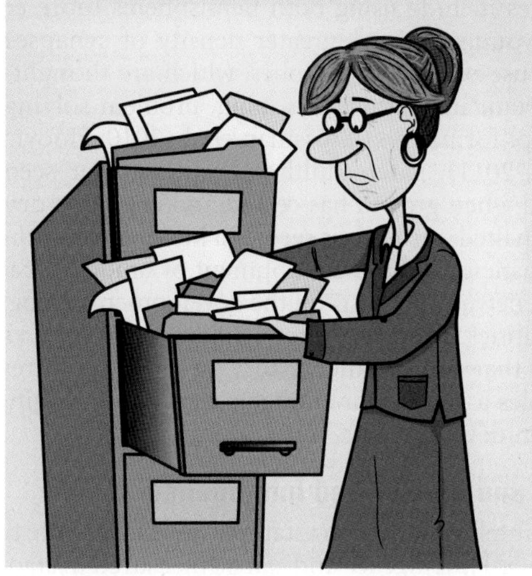

Alex Comfort, an early gerontologist, described the slower response time of an older adult: By the time you are 80, you have a lot of files in the file cabinet. Your secretary is 80 so it also takes her a lot longer to locate the files, go through them, find the one you want, and bring it to you.

Changes in the aging nervous system (see Chapter 3) cause a general slowing of many neural processes, but they are not consistent with deteriorating mental function, nor do they interfere with daily routines. Age-related changes in brain structure, function, and cognition are also not uniform across the whole brain or across individuals. Recent research suggests that the reason older brains respond more slowly is because they take longer to process constantly increasing amounts of information (Ramscar et al., 2014).

Cognitive functions may remain stable or decline with increasing age. The cognitive functions that remain stable include attention span, language skills, communication skills, comprehension and discourse, and visual perception. The cognitive skills that decline are verbal fluency, logical analysis, selective attention, object naming, and complex visuospatial skills. Overall cognitive abilities remain intact, and it is important to remember that if brain function becomes impaired in old age, it is the result of disease, not aging (Crowley, 1996).

Neuroplasticity

It is very important to know that the aging brain maintains resiliency or the ability to compensate for age-related changes. Developing knowledge refutes the myth that the adult brain is less plastic than the child's brain and less able to strengthen and increase neuronal connections (Petrus et al., 2014). The old adage "use it or lose it" applies to cognitive and physical health. Stimulating the brain increases brain tissue formation, enhances synaptic regulation of messages, and improves the development of cognitive reserve (CR).

CR is based on the concept of neuroplasticity and refers to the strength and complexity of neuronal/dendrite connections from which information is transmitted and cognition/mentation emerges. The greater the strength and complexity of these connections, the more the brain can absorb damage before cognitive functioning is compromised. To maximize brain plasticity and CR, it is important to engage in challenging cognitive, sensory, and motor activities, as well as meaningful social interactions, on a regular basis throughout life.

Changes in the brain with aging, once seen only as compensation for declining skills, are now thought to indicate the development of new capacities. These changes include using both hemispheres more equally than younger adults, greater density of synapses, and more use of the frontal lobes, which are thought to be important in abstract reasoning, problem solving, and concept formation (Grossman et al., 2010; Hooyman & Kiyak, 2011). Later adulthood is no longer seen as a period when growth has ceased and cognitive development halted; rather, it is seen as a life stage programmed for plasticity and the development of unique capacities. The renewed emphasis on the development of cognitive capabilities that can develop with age provides a view of aging that reflects the history of many cultures and provides a much more hopeful view of both aging and human development.

Fluid and Crystallized Intelligence

Fluid intelligence and crystallized intelligence are factors of general intelligence and can be measured in standardized IQ tests. Fluid intelligence (often called *native intelligence*) consists of skills that are biologically determined, independent of experience or learning. It involves the capacity to think logically and solve problems in novel situations, independent of acquired knowledge. Fluid intelligence has been likened to "street smarts." Crystallized intelligence is composed of knowledge and abilities that the person acquires through education and life ("book smarts") and is demonstrated largely through one's vocabulary and general knowledge. Crystallized intelligence is long-lasting and improves with experience.

Older people perform more poorly on performance scales (fluid intelligence), but scores on verbal scales (crystallized intelligence) remain stable. This is known as the classic aging pattern. The tendency to do poorly on performance tasks may be related to age-related changes in sensory and perceptual abilities, as well as psychomotor skills. Speed of cognitive processing, slower reaction time, and testing methods also affect performance.

Memory

Memory is defined as the ability to retain or store information and retrieve it when needed. Memory is a complex set of processes and storage systems. Three components characterize memory: immediate recall; short-term memory (which may range from minutes to days); and remote or long-term memory. Biological, functional, environmental, and psychosocial influences affect memory development throughout adulthood. Recall of newly encountered information seems to decrease with age, and memory declines are noted in connection with complex tasks and strategies. Even though some older adults show decrements in the ability to process information, reaction time, perception, and capacity for attentional tasks, the majority of functioning remains intact and sufficient. Familiarity, previous learning, and life experience compensate for the minor loss of efficiency in the basic neurological processes.

In unfamiliar, stressful, or demanding situations (e.g., hospitalization), however, these changes may be more marked. Healthy older adults may complain of memory problems, but their symptoms do not meet the criteria for mild or major neurocognitive impairment (see Chapter 23). The term *age-associated memory impairment (AAMI)* has been used to describe memory loss that is considered normal in light of a person's age and educational level. This may include a general slowness in processing, storing, and recalling new information, as well as difficulty remembering names and words. However, these concerns can cause great anxiety in older adults who may fear dementia. Many medical or psychiatric difficulties (delirium, depression) also influence memory abilities, and it is important for older adults with memory complaints to have a comprehensive evaluation (see Chapters 8 and 23).

❖ IMPLICATIONS FOR GERONTOLOGICAL NURSING AND HEALTHY AGING

Healthy cognitive aging (healthy brain aging) is comprehensive and proactive; it implies that cognitive health is much more than simply a lack of decline with aging (Desai et al., 2010). A healthy brain is "one that can perform all mental processes that are collectively known as cognition, including the ability to learn new things, intuition, judgment, language, and remembering" (Centers for Disease Control and Prevention [CDC], 2014). Attention to cognitive health, beginning at conception and continuing throughout life, is just as important as attention to physical and emotional health.

Nurses need to educate people of all ages about effective strategies to enhance cognitive health and vitality and to promote cognitive reserve and brain plasticity (Box 4.6). A healthy diet, physical activity, social engagement, and brain exercises may improve or maintain cognitive functioning in older people at risk for dementia (Ngandu et al., 2015). Playing games (e.g., Scrabble, Trivial Pursuit, cards), solving puzzles, learning a new language, developing a new hobby, reading books, and engaging in interesting conversations are other forms of cognitive-stimulating activities. Among the various types of cognitive-stimulating activities, games such as cards or puzzles seem to be particularly useful (Rebok et al., 2014; School of Medicine and Public Health, University of Wisconsin-Madison, 2014). There is no evidence that computerized cognitive training programs (brain games)

BOX 4.6 Tips for Best Practice

Cognitive Health

- Dispel myths about brain aging and teach about cognition and aging.
- Educate people of all ages about factors that influence cognitive health.
- Be aware of cultural differences in perceptions of cognitive health and adapt education accordingly.
- Advise older adults to have comprehensive assessment if they are experiencing cognitive decline.
- Encourage socialization and participation in intellectually stimulating activities, exercise, healthy diets (e.g., Mediterranean diet, DASH diet).
- Teach chronic illness prevention strategies and ensure good management of chronic illnesses.
- Share resources for cognitive training (memory enhancing techniques, puzzles, card games).

prevent dementia, and experts suggest that these games be considered entertainment and not a disease-prevention activity (Ratner and Atkinson, 2015). The Centers for Disease Control and Prevention and the National Institute on Aging have large-scale programs focused on healthy brain aging and provide resources nurses can use in health-promotion education.

LEARNING IN LATER LIFE

Basic intelligence remains unchanged with increasing years, and older adults should be provided with opportunities for continued learning. Adapting communication and teaching to enhance understanding requires knowledge of learning in late life and effective teaching-learning strategies with older adults. *Geragogy* is the application of the principles of adult learning theory to teaching interventions for older adults.

The older adult demands that teaching situations be relevant; new learning must relate to what the person already knows and should emphasize concrete and practical information. Aging may present barriers to learning, such as hearing and vision losses and cognitive impairment. Pain and discomfort can also interfere with learning. Moreover, the process of aging may accentuate other challenges that had already been factors in a person's life, such as cultural and cohort variations and education. Many older adults may have special learning needs based on educational deprivation in their early years and consequent anxiety about formalized learning.

Attention to literacy level and cultural variations is important to enhance learning and the usefulness of

BOX 4.7 Tips for Best Practice

Guiding Older Adult Learners

- Ensure individual is ready to learn. Watch for signs of fatigue, anxiety, or inability to pay attention.
- Ensure comfort (appropriate seating, room temperature). Provide pain medication if needed.
- Pay attention to vision and hearing deficits (face individual, speak slowly, keep pitch of voice low, eliminate background noise).
- Adapt materials for culture, language, and health literacy.
- Allow adequate time, provide regular feedback, and avoid distractions.
- Emphasize concrete material rather than abstract; connect new learning to past experiences.
- Use plain language and readable font (e.g., Arial, 16 to 18 points), with both uppercase and lowercase letters.
- Use high contrast on printed materials (dark colors for text and lighter for background; black print on white, dark blue on pale yellow).
- Use gestures, demonstrations, and pictures in addition to printed materials.
- Use "teach-back" methods to enhance understanding.

what is learned (see Chapter 2). Mood is extremely important in terms of what individuals (both young and old) will recall. In other words, when we attempt to measure recall of events that may have occurred in a crisis situation or an anxiety state, recall will be impaired. This is significant for health care professionals who give information to older adults who are ill or upset, particularly at times of crisis such as hospital discharge. Box 4.7 presents Tips for Best Practice in guiding older learners.

Learning Opportunities

Opportunities for older adults to learn are available in many formal and informal modes: self-teaching, college attendance, participation in seminars and conferences, public television programs, CDs, Internet courses, and countless others. In most colleges and universities, older people are taking classes of all types. Fees are usually lower for individuals older than 60 years of age, and elders may choose to work toward a degree or audit classes for enrichment and enjoyment. Senior centers and local school districts often provide a wide array of adult education courses as well. The Road Scholar (formerly Elderhostel) program is an example of a program designed for older people that combines continued learning with travel. The program offers trips to 90 countries and presents learning programs in the United States and Canada. Road Scholar offers intergenerational programs for grandparents and grandchildren ages 4 and older.

Information Technology and Older Adults

Older adults comprise the fastest growing population using computers and the Internet. According to data from the Pew Research Center, 58% of American adults ages 65 and older use the Internet. One-quarter of older adults use social networks, and older women comprise the fastest growing group using social networking sites such as Facebook, Twitter, and Myspace (Pew Research Center, 2015). More than any other age group, older adults perceive the Internet as a valuable resource to help them more easily obtain information and connect to loved ones. This could range from using a cell phone to set medication reminders to using Skype and FaceTime to interact with long-distance grandchildren. Many individuals are also using email to communicate with their health care providers. Organizations such as Cyber-Seniors and AARP provide basic computer and Internet training for older people.

With the aging of the baby boomers and the young tech-savvy adults, the future of technology in care and services for older adults can only be imagined. Technology has the potential to improve the quality of life for older adults across settings by enhancing access to health information and resources, making communication with family and friends easier, providing cognitive stimulation and enjoyable activities, and alleviating isolation among community-dwelling older adults and those in nursing homes (Culley et al., 2013; Tak et al., 2007) (see Chapter 16).

❖ IMPLICATIONS FOR GERONTOLOGICAL NURSING AND HEALTHY AGING

Traditional ways of providing health information and services are changing, and both public and private institutions are increasingly using the Internet and other technologies. This presents challenges for people with limited experience using computers and for those with limited literacy. Nurses can share resources available for older adults who want to learn computer skills and adaptations that can be made to make computers as user-friendly as possible (e.g., touch screens, voice systems) for those who may have limitations (Choi & Dinitto, 2013).

Nurses and other health professionals need to develop skills in the understanding and use of consumer health information and teach clients how to evaluate the reliability and validity of health information on the Internet. Using social media as a platform for health promotion and health education presents exciting possibilities (Kolanowski et al., 2013). Continued attention to access to technology, especially among disadvantaged groups, and also efforts to enhance culturally and language-appropriate materials are important (Culley et al., 2013). *Healthy People 2020* has set goals for information technology that include improving health literacy and access to the Internet, increasing the proportion of reliable health-related websites, and encouraging use of the Internet to organize health data and communicate with health care providers.

KEY CONCEPTS

- The impact of gender, culture, and cohort must always be considered when discussing the validity of psychosocial theories of aging.
- Spirituality must be considered a significant factor in understanding healthy aging.
- Late adulthood is no longer seen as a period when growth ceases and cognitive development halts; rather, it is seen as a life stage programmed for plasticity and the development of unique capacities.
- Cognitive stimulation and attention to brain health is just as important as attention to physical health.
- Learning in late life can be enhanced by utilizing principles of geragogy and adapting teaching strategies to minimize barriers such as hearing and vision impairment.

ACTIVITIES AND DISCUSSION QUESTIONS

1. How well do the psychological and sociological theories of aging "fit" within your own cultural perspective?
2. Review the myths about aging and the brain (Box 4.5). Were any of the facts surprising to you?
3. What types of health teaching would you provide to a young adult to enhance brain health in aging? How would the teaching differ for an older adult with mild neurocognitive disorder?
4. How would you respond to the following myth of aging: "You can't teach an old dog new tricks"?
5. Discuss some ways that nurses can respond to the spiritual needs and concerns of older adults.

REFERENCES

Achenbaum WA: *Old age in a new land*, Baltimore, 1978, Johns Hopkins University Press.

Agency for Healthcare Research and Quality: *Weekly group storytelling enhances verbal skills, encourages positive behavior change, and reduces confusion in patients with Alzheimer's and related dementias*, AHRQ Innovations Exchange, 2014. Available at https://innovations.ahrq.gov/profiles/weekly-group-storytelling-enhances-verbal-skills-encourages-positive-behavior-change and https://innovations.ahrq.gov/. Accessed October 2014.

Bastings A: Reading the story behind the story: Context and content in stories by people with dementia, *Generations* 27:25–29, 2003.

Bastings A: Arts in dementia care: "This is not the end… it's the end of this chapter," *Generations* 30:16–20, 2006.

Birren JE, Deutchman DE: *Guiding autobiography groups for older adults: Exploring the fabric of life*, Baltimore, 1991, Johns Hopkins University Press.

Bohlmeijer E, Smit F, Cuijpers P: Effects of reminiscence and life review on late-life depression: A meta-analysis, *Int J Geriatr Psychiatry* 18:1088–1094, 2003.

Butler R: The life review: An interpretation of reminiscence in the aged, *Psychiatry* 26:65–76, 1963.

Butler R: Age, death and life review. In Doka K, editor: *Living with grief: Loss in later life*, Washington, DC, 2003, Hospice Foundation.

Butler R, Lewis M: *Aging and mental health: Positive psychosocial approache*, ed 3, St Louis, MO, 1983, Mosby.

Cappeliez P: Neglected issue and new orientations for research and practice in reminiscence and life review, *Int J Reminiscence Life Rev* 1(1):19–25, 2013.

Centers for Disease Control and Prevention (CDC): *Healthy brain initiative,* 2014. Available at http://www.cdc.gov/aging/healthybrain/index.htm. Accessed October 2015.

Chan M, Leong K, Heng B, et al: Reducing depression among community-dwelling older adults using life-story review: A pilot study, *Geriatr Nurs* 35:105–110, 2014.

Choi N, Dinitto DM: The digital divide among low-income homebound older adults: Internet use patterns, eHealth literacy, and attitudes toward computer/Internet use, *J Med Internet Res* 15(5):e93, 2013.

Cottrell L: The adjustment of the individual to his age and sex roles, *Am Sociol Rev* 7:617–620, 1942.

Cowgill D: Aging and modernization: A revision of the theory. In Gubrium J, editor: *Late life communities and environmental policy*, Springfield, IL, 1974, Charles C Thomas.

Crowley SL: Aging brain's staying power, *AARP Bulletin* 37:1, 1996.

Crowther M, Parker M, Achenbaum W, et al: Rowe and Kahn's model of successful aging revisited: Positive spirituality—the forgotten factor, *Gerontologist* 42(5):613, 2002.

Culley J, Herman J, Smith D, et al: Effects of technology and connectedness on community-dwelling older adults, *Online J Nurs Inform* 17(3):2013.

Cumming E, Henry W: *Growing old*, New York, 1961, Basic Books.

Delgado C: Sense of coherence, spirituality, stress and quality of life in chronic illness, *J Nurs Scholarsh* 39(3):229–234, 2007.

Desai A, Grossberg G, Chibnall J: Healthy brain aging: A road map, *Clin Geriatr Med* 26:1, 2010.

Edlund B: Revisiting spirituality in aging, *J Gerontol Nurs* 40(7):4–5, 2014.

Erikson EH, Erikson JM, Kivnick HQ: *Vital involvement in old age: The experience of old age in our time*, New York, 1986, WW Norton.

Fritsch T, Kwak J, Grant S, et al: Impact of TimeSlips, a creative expression intervention program, on nursing home staff and residents with dementia and their caregivers, *Gerontologist* 49:117–127, 2009.

Fung HH: Aging in culture, *Gerontologist* 53(3):369–377, 2013.

Gaskamp C, Sutter R, Meraviglia M, et al: Evidence-based guideline: Promoting spirituality in the older adult, *J Gerontol Nurs* 32(11):8–11, 2006.

Glahn D, Kent J Jr, Sprooten E, et al: Genetic basis of neurocognitive decline and reduced white-matter integrity in normal human brain aging, *Proc Natl Acad Sci USA* 110(47):19006–19011, 2013. Available at http://www.pnas.org/content/early/2013/10/30/1313735110.abstract. Accessed October 2015.

Grabowski D, Aschbrenner K, Tome V, et al: Quality of mental health care for nursing home residents: A literature review, *Med Care Res Rev* 67:627–656, 2010.

Grossman I, Na J, Varnum M, et al: Reasoning about social conflicts improves into old age, *Proc Natl Acad Sci USA* 107(16):7246–7250, 2010.

Haight B, Burnside IM: Reminiscence and life review: Explaining the differences, *Arch Psychiatr Nurs* 7:91–98, 1993.

Haight B, Webster J: *Critical advances in reminiscence work: From theory to application*, New York, 2002, Springer.

Havighurst RJ: *Developmental tasks and education*, ed 3, New York, 1972, Longman.

Havighurst RJ, Albrecht R: *Older people*, New York, 1953, Longmans, Green.

Havighurst RJ, Neugarten BL, Tobin SS: Disengagement and patterns of aging. In Neugarten BL, editor: *Middle age and aging*, Chicago, 1968, University of Chicago Press.

Hendricks J, Hendricks CD: *Aging in mass society: Myths and realities*, Boston, 1986, Little, Brown.

Hodge D, Bonifas R, Chou R: Spirituality and older adults: Ethical guidelines to enhance service provision, *Adv Soc Work* 11:1, 2010.

Hooyman N, Kiyak H: *Social gerontology*, ed 7, Boston, 2005, Pearson.

Hooyman N, Kiyak H: *Social gerontology*, ed 9, Boston, 2011, Pearson.

Koenig HG, Brooks RG: Religion, health and aging: Implications for practice and public policy, *Public Policy Aging Rep* 12:13–19, 2002.

Kolanowski A, Resnick B, Beck C, et al: Advances in nonpharmacological interventions 2011-2012, *Res Gerontol Nurs* 6(1):5–8, 2013.

Latha K, Bhandury P, Tejaswini S, et al: Reminiscence therapy: An overview, *Middle East J Age Ageing* 11(1):18–22, 2014.

Maddox G: Activity and morale: A longitudinal study of selected elderly subjects, *Soc Forces* 42:195–204, 1963.

Meyer CL: How effectively are nurse educators preparing students to provide spiritual care?, *Nurse Educ* 28(4):185–190, 2003.

Moss M: Storytelling. In Lindquist R, Snyder M, Tracy M, editors: *Complementary and alternative therapies in nursing*, ed 7, New York, 2014, Springer, pp 215–228.

Mudiwa L: The online future of reminiscence therapy, *Irish Medical Times* November 24, 2010. Available at http://www.imt.ie/features-opinion/2010/11/the-online-future-of-reminiscence-therapy.html.

National Institutes of Health: *Cognitive and emotional health project: The healthy brain,* 2004. Available at http://trans.nih.gov/CEHP. Accessed October 19, 2015.

Neugarten BL: *Middle age and aging*, Chicago, 1968, University of Chicago Press.

Ngandu T, Lehtisaio J, Solomon A, et al: A 2 year multidomain intervention of diet, exercise, cognitive training, and vascular risk monitoring versus control to prevent cognitive decline in at-risk elderly people (FINGER): A randomised controlled trial, *Lancet* 35(9984):2255–2263, 2015.

Petrus E, Isaiah A, Jones A, et al: Crossmodal induction of thalamocortical potentiation leads to enhanced information processing in the auditory cortex, *Neuron* 51(3):664–673, 2014.

Pew Research Center: *Social media usage 2000-2015*. Available at http://www.pewinternet.org/2015/10/08/social-networking-usage-2005-2015/. Accessed July 30, 2016.

Pinquart M, Forstmeier S: Effects of reminiscence on psychosocial outcomes: A meta-analysis, *Aging Ment Health* 16:1–18, 2012.

Pot A, Bohlmeijer E, Onrust S, et al: The impact of life review on depression in older adults: A randomized controlled trial, *Int Psychogeriatrics* 1–10, 2010. doi: 10.1017/S104161020999175X.

Preschl B, Maercker A, Wagner B, et al: Life-review therapy with computer supplements for depression in the elderly: A randomized control trial, *Aging Ment Health* 16:964–974, 2012.

Puchalski C, Romer A: Taking a spiritual history allows clinicians to understand patients more fully, *J Palliat Med* 3:129–137, 2000.

Ramírez-Esparza N, Pennebaker J: Do good stories produce good health? Exploring words, language and culture, *Narrat Inq* 16(11):211–219, 2006.

Ramscar M, Hendrix P, Shaoul C, et al: The myth of cognitive decline: Non-linear dynamics of lifelong learning, *Top Cogn Sci* 6(1):5–42, 2014.

Ratner E, Atkinson D: Why cognitive training and brain games will not prevent or forestall dementia, *JAGS* 63(12):2612–2614, 2015.

Rebok G, Ball K, Guey I, et al: Ten-year effects of the advanced cognitive training for independent and vital elderly cognitive training trial on cognition and everyday functioning in older adults, *J Am Geriatr Soc* 62:16–24, 2014.

Riley MW: Social gerontology and the age of stratification of society, *Gerontologist* 11:79–87, 1971.

Rowe JW, Kahn RL: *Successful aging*, New York, 1998, Pantheon-Random House.

School of Medicine and Public Health, University Wisconsin-Madison: *Cognitive activities may help protect brain from Alzheimer's,* 2014. Available at http://www.med.wisc.edu/news-events/cognitive-activities-may-help-protect-the-brain-from-alzheimers/43886. Accessed October, 2015.

Soeken K, Carson V: Responding to the spiritual needs of the chronically ill, *Nurs Clin North Am* 22:603–611, 1987.

Stair N: If I had my life to live over. In Martz S, editor: *If I had my life to live over I would pick more daisies*, Watsonville, CA, 1992, Papier Mache Press.

Stinson C: Structured group reminiscence: An intervention for older adults, *J Contin Educ Nurs* 40(11):521–528, 2009.

Strang S, Strang P: Questions posed to hospital chaplains by palliative care patients, *J Palliat Med* 5:887, 2002.

Tak S, Beck C, McMahon E: Computer and Internet access for long-term care residents, *J Gerontol Nurs* 33:32, 2007.

Tan A: *The bonesetter's daughter*, ed 1, New York, 2001, Putnam Adult.

Tornstam L: Gerotranscendence: A meta-theoretical reformulation of the disengagement theory, *Aging Clin Exper Res* 1:55–64, 1989.

Tornstam L: Transcendence in later life, *Generations* 23:1014, 2000.

Tornstam L: *Gerotranscendence: A developmental theory of positive aging*, New York, 2005, Springer.

Touhy T: Touching the spirit of elders in nursing homes: Ordinary yet extraordinary care, *Int J Human Caring* 6(1):12–17, 2001.

Touhy T, Brown C, Smith C: Spiritual caring: End of life in a nursing home, *J Gerontol Nurs* 31:27–35, 2005.

Touhy T, Zerwekh J: Spiritual caring. In Zerwekh J, editor: *Nursing care at the end of life: Palliative care for patients and families*, Philadelphia, 2006, FA Davis.

Wadensten B: An analysis of the psychosocial theories of ageing and their relevance to practical gerontological nursing in Sweden, *Scand J Caring Sci* 20:347–354, 2006.

World Health Organization: *Global financial crisis and the health of older people,* 2014. Available at http://www.who.int/ageing/economic_issues/en/. Accessed October 2015.

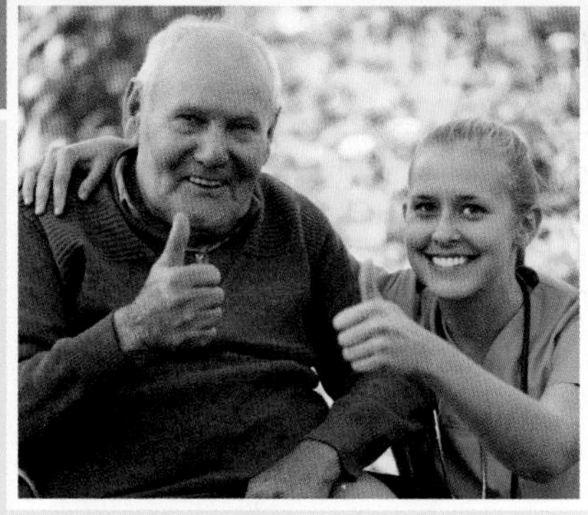

5

Gerontological Nursing and Promotion of Healthy Aging

Theris A. Touhy

evolve.elsevier.com/Touhy/gerontological

LEARNING OBJECTIVES

Upon completion of this chapter, the reader will be able to:

- Discuss the implications of a growing older adult population on nursing education, practice, and research.
- Identify several factors that have influenced the development of gerontological nursing as a specialty practice.
- Examine the American Nurses Association *Gerontological Nursing: Scope and Standards of Practice* and the recommended educational competencies for gerontological nursing practice.
- Discuss several formal gerontological organizations and describe their significance to the gerontological nurse.
- Compare various gerontological nursing roles and requirements across the health-wellness continuum.

THE LIVED EXPERIENCE

I don't think I will work in gerontological nursing; it seems depressing. I don't know many older people, but they are all sick without much hope to get better. I'll probably go into labor and delivery or the emergency room where I can really make a difference.

Student Nurse, age 24

Because geriatric nursing especially offers nurses the unique opportunity to dramatically impact people's lives for the better and for the worst, it demands the best that you have to offer. I am very optimistic about the future of geriatric nursing. Increasing numbers of older adults are interested in marching into old age as healthy and involved. Geriatric nursing offers a unique opportunity to help older adults meet these aspirations while at the same time maintaining a commitment to the oldest and frailest in our society.

Mathy Mezey, Professor Emeritus and Retired Founding Director, The Hartford Institute for Geriatric Nursing, New York University College of Nursing
(Ebersole & Touhy, 2006, p. 142)

CARE OF OLDER ADULTS: A NURSING IMPERATIVE

Older people today are healthier, are better educated, and expect a much higher quality of life as they age than did their elders. Healthy aging is now an achievable goal for many. It is essential that nurses have the knowledge and skills to help people of all ages, races, and cultures to achieve this goal. Enhancing health in aging requires attention to health throughout life, as well as expert care from nurses.

Most nurses care for older people during the course of their careers. Estimates are "that by 2020, up to 75% of nurses' time will be spent with older adults" (Holroyd et al.,

2009, p. 374). In addition, the public will look to nurses to have the knowledge and skills to assist people to age in health. Every older person should expect care provided by nurses with competence in gerontological nursing. Knowledge of aging and gerontological nursing is core knowledge for the profession of nursing (Young, 2003).

The terms *geriatric nursing* and *gerontological nursing* are both used in the literature and in practice to describe the specialty of caring for older adults. While both terms are used in the text, we prefer the term *gerontological nurse* because this reflects a more holistic approach encompassing both health and illness.

Who Will Care for an Aging Society?

By 2040 the number of older people in the world will be at least 1.3 billion (Tolson et al., 2011) (see Chapter 1). It is a critical health and societal concern that gerontological nurses, other health professionals, and direct care workers are prepared to deliver care in all settings across the globe. The aging workforce is in shortage in most of the developed world, and the increased aging population is posing challenges for many countries to meet the expanding need for care services for older people (European Economic and Social Committee, 2012). The developing countries are experiencing the most rapid growth in numbers of older people and at the same time they lack systems of care and services.

In the United States, eldercare is projected to be the fastest growing employment sector in health care. In spite of demand, the number of health care workers who are interested and prepared to care for older people remains low (Institute of Medicine [IOM], 2008). Less than 1% of registered nurses and less than 3% of advanced practice nurses (APNs) are certified in geriatrics (Cortes, 2012; IOM, 2008; Robert Wood Johnson Foundation, 2012). "We do not have anywhere close to the number of nurses we need who are prepared in geriatrics, whether in the field of primary care, acute care, nursing home care, or in-home care" (Christine Kovner, RN, PhD, FAAN, as cited in Robert Wood Johnson Foundation, 2012).

Geriatric medicine faces similar challenges with about 7000 prepared geriatricians, 1 for every 2546 older Americans; and this number is falling with the trend predicted to be less than 5000 by 2040 (Cortes, 2012; IOM, 2008). Other professions such as social work, physical therapy, and psychiatry have similar shortages. It is estimated that by 2030 nearly 3 million additional health care professionals and direct care workers will be needed to meet the care needs of a growing older adult population (Eldercare Workforce Alliance, 2014). Improving the competency and adequacy of the eldercare workforce is essential to meet the needs and demands of a burgeoning aging population (Bardach & Rowles, 2012). *Healthy People 2020* includes goals related to geriatric education (Box 5.1).

BOX 5.1 *Healthy People 2020*

Older Adults

- Increase the proportion of the health care workforce with geriatric certification (physicians, geriatric psychiatrists, registered nurses, dentists, physical therapists, dietitians)

From U.S. Department of Health and Human Services, Office of Disease Prevention and Health Promotion: *Healthy People 2020,* 2012. Available at http://www.healthypeople.gov/2020.

HISTORY OF GERONTOLOGICAL NURSING

Historically, nurses have always been in the frontlines of caring for older people. They have provided hands-on care, supervision, administration, program development, teaching, and research and are, to a great extent, responsible for the rapid advancement of gerontology as a profession. Gerontological nurses have made substantial contributions to the body of knowledge guiding best practice in care of older people. Nurses have been, and continue to be, the mainstay of care of older adults (Mezey & Fulmer, 2002).

Gerontological nursing has emerged as a circumscribed area of practice only within the past 6 decades. Before 1950, gerontological nursing was seen as the application of general principles of nursing to the older adult with little recognition of this area of nursing as a specialty similar to obstetric, pediatric, or surgical nursing. Whereas most specialties in nursing developed from those identified in medicine, this was not the case with gerontological nursing because health care of the older adult was traditionally considered within the domain of nursing.

The foundation of gerontological nursing as we know it today was built largely by a small cadre of nurse pioneers, many of whom are now deceased. The specialty was defined and shaped by those innovative nurses who saw, early on, that older individuals had special needs and required the most subtle, holistic, and complex nursing care. This history is similar to the development of pediatric nursing and the recognition that pediatric nursing is "not med-surg nursing on little people" (Taylor, 2006, p. E128) and nurses needed special skills to care for children. In examining the history of gerontological nursing, one must marvel at the advocacy and perseverance of nurses who have remain committed to improving the care of older adults despite struggling against great odds over the years.

Box 5.2 presents the views of some of the geriatric nursing pioneers, as well as those of current leaders, on the practice of gerontological nursing and the reasons they are attracted to this specialty. For a comprehensive

BOX 5.2 Reflections on Gerontological Nursing From Gerontological Nursing Pioneers and Current Leaders in the Field

Mary Opal Wolanin, Gerontological Nursing Pioneer

"I believe that one of the most valuable lessons I have learned from those who are older is that I must start with looking inside at my own thinking. I was very guilty of ageism. I believed every myth in the book, was sure that I would never live past my seventieth birthday, and made no plan for my seventies. Probably the most productive years of my career have been since that dreaded birthday and I now realize that it is very difficult, if not impossible, to think of our own aging." (From interview data collected by Priscilla Ebersole between 1990 and 2001.)

Terry Fulmer, Dean, College of Nursing, New York University, and Co-Director, John A. Hartford Institute for Geriatric Nursing

"I soon realized that in the arena of caring for the aged, I could have an autonomous nursing practice that would make a real difference in medical outcomes. I could practice the full scope of nursing. It gave me a sense of freedom and accomplishment. With older patients, the most important component of care, by far, is nursing care. It's very motivating." (From Ebersole P, Touhy T: *Geriatric nursing: Growth of a specialty*, New York, 2006, Springer, p. 129.)

Jennifer Lingler, PhD, FNP

"When I was in high school, a nurse I knew helped me find a nursing assistant position at the residential care facility where she worked. That experience sparked my interest in older adults that continues today. I realized that caring for frail elders could be incredibly gratifying, and I felt privileged to play a role, however small, in people's lives. At the same time, I became increasingly curious about what it means to age successfully. I questioned why some people seemed to age so gracefully, while others succumbed to physical illness, mental decline, or both. As a Building Academic Geriatric Nursing Capacity (BAGNC) alumnus, I now divide my time serving as a nurse practitioner at a memory disorders clinic, teaching an ethics course in a gerontology program, and conducting research on family caregiving. I am encouraged by the realization that as current students contemplate the array of opportunities before them, seek counsel from trusted mentors, and gain exposure to various clinical populations, the next generation of geriatric nurses will emerge. And, I am confident that in doing so, they will set their own course for affecting change in the lives of society's most vulnerable members." (Jennifer Lingler as cited in Fagin C, Franklin P: Why choose geriatric nursing? Six nursing scholars tell their stories, *Imprint*, September/October, 2005, p. 74.)

review of the history of the specialty, including Dr. Ebersole's interviews with geriatric nursing pioneers, the reader is referred to *Geriatric Nursing: Growth of a Specialty* (Ebersole & Touhy, 2006).

Nursing was the first of the professions to develop standards of gerontological care and the first to provide a certification mechanism to ensure specific professional expertise through credentialing (Ebersole & Touhy, 2006). The most recent edition of *Gerontological Nursing: Scope and Standards of Practice* (American Nurses Association [ANA], 2010) provides a comprehensive overview of the scope of gerontological nursing, the skills and knowledge required to address the full range of needs related to the process of aging, and the specialized care of older adults as a group and as individuals. The document also identifies levels of gerontological nursing practice (basic and advanced) and standards of clinical gerontological nursing care and gerontological nursing performance.

Current Initiatives

The most significant influence in enhancing the specialty of gerontological nursing has been the work of The Hartford Institute for Geriatric Nursing, established in 1996 and funded by the John A. Hartford Foundation. It is the only nurse-led organization in the country seeking to shape the quality of the nation's health care for older Americans by promoting geriatric nursing excellence to both the nursing profession and the larger health care community. Initiatives in nursing education, nursing practice, nursing research, and nursing policy include enhancement of geriatrics in nursing education programs through curricular reform and faculty development and development of the National Hartford Centers of Gerontological Nursing Excellence, predoctoral and postdoctoral scholarships for study and research in geriatric nursing, and clinical practice improvement projects to enhance care for older adults (http://www.hartfordign.org).

Another significant influence on improving care for older adults was the Nurse Competence in Aging (NCA) project. This initiative provided grant and technical assistance to more than 50 specialty nursing organizations, developed a free web-based comprehensive gerontological nursing resource center (ConsultGeriRN.org) where nurses can access evidence-based information on topics related to the care of older adults, and conducted a national gerontological nursing certification outreach program (Stierle et al., 2006). There are also two iPad/iPhone apps that give access to information and tools to treat common problems encountered in the care of older adults, including one specific to dementia (https://consultgeri.org/).

Sigma Theta Tau's Center for Nursing Excellence in Long-Term Care was launched in 2009. The Center sponsors the Geriatric Nursing Leadership Academy

(GNLA) and offers a range of products and services to support the professional development and leadership growth of nurses who provide care to older adults in long-term care. In 2013, The Hartford Institute for Geriatric Nursing, in collaboration with several other organizations, began several initiatives focusing on interprofessional education, leadership, and team building skills, as well as improving the knowledge and skill sets of primary care providers caring for older adults.

GERONTOLOGICAL NURSING EDUCATION

According to the ANA's *Gerontological Nursing: Scope and Standards of Practice* (2010), "Nurses require the knowledge and skills to assist older adults in a broad range of nursing care issues, from maintaining health and preventing illnesses, to managing complex, overlapping chronic conditions and progressive/protracted frailty in physical and mental functions, to palliative care" (pp. 12, 13).

Essential educational competencies and academic standards for care of older adults have been developed by national organizations such as the American Association of Colleges of Nursing (AACN) for both basic and advanced nursing education (ANA, 2010). *The Essentials of Baccalaureate Education for Professional Nursing Practice* (AACN, 2008) specifically address the importance in the education of students of geriatric content and structured clinical experiences with older adults across the continuum.

In 2010 AACN and The Hartford Institute for Geriatric Nursing, New York University, published the *Recommended Baccalaureate Competencies and Curricular Guidelines for the Nursing Care of Older Adults,* a supplement to the *Essentials* document. In addition, gerontological nursing competencies for advanced practice graduate programs have also been developed. All of these documents can be accessed from the AACN website. "Despite these lists of competencies, however, there remains a lack of consistency among nursing schools in helping students gain needed gerontological nursing information and skills" (ANA, 2010, p. 12).

There has been some improvement in the amount of geriatrics-related content in nursing school curricula, but it is still uneven across schools and hampered by lack of faculty expertise in the subject (IOM, 2011; Robert Wood Johnson Foundation, 2012). Faculty with expertise in gerontological nursing are scarce and there is a critical need for nurses with master's and doctoral preparation and expertise in the care of older adults to assume faculty roles. Most schools still do not have freestanding courses in the specialty similar to courses in maternal/child or psychiatric nursing. This means that a substantial number of graduating nurses have not had the education needed to competently meet the needs of the burgeoning number of older adults for whom they will care. "In the past, nursing education has been dogged about assuring that every student has the opportunity to attend a birth, but has never insisted that every student have the opportunity to manage a death, even though the vast majority of nurses are more likely to practice with clients who are at the end of life" (AACN, 2007, p. 7). Best practice recommendations for nursing education include provision of a standalone course, as well as integration of content throughout the curriculum "so that gerontology is valued and viewed as an integral part of nursing care" (Miller et al., 2009, p. 198).

It is important to provide students with nursing practice experiences caring for elders across the health-wellness continuum. For clinical practice sites, one is not limited to the acute care setting or the nursing home. Experiences with well elders in the community and opportunities to focus on health promotion should be the first experience for students. This will assist them to develop more positive attitudes, understand the full scope of nursing practice with older adults, and learn nursing responses to enhance health and wellness. Rehabilitation centers, post–acute care and skilled nursing facilities, and hospice settings provide opportunities for leadership experience, nursing management of complex problems, interprofessional teamwork, and research application for more advanced students (Fox, 2013; Neville et al., 2014).

ORGANIZATIONS DEVOTED TO GERONTOLOGY RESEARCH AND PRACTICE

The Gerontological Society of America (GSA) demonstrates the need for interdisciplinary collaboration in research and practice. The divisions of Biological Sciences, Health Sciences, Behavioral and Social Sciences, Social Research, Policy and Practice, and Emerging Scholar and Professional Organization include individuals from myriad backgrounds and disciplines who affiliate with a section based on their particular function rather than their educational or professional credentials. Nurses can be found in all sections and occupy important positions as officers and committee chairs in the GSA.

This mingling of the disciplines based on practice interests is also characteristic of the American Society on Aging (ASA). Other interdisciplinary organizations have joined forces to strengthen the field. The Association for Gerontology in Higher Education (AGHE) has partnered with the GSA, and the National Council on Aging (NCOA) is affiliated with the ASA. These organizations and others have encouraged the blending of ideas and functions, furthering the understanding of aging and the interprofessional collaboration necessary for optimal care. International gerontology associations, such as the International Federation on Aging and the International Association of Gerontology and Geriatrics, also have interdisciplinary membership and offer the opportunity to study aging internationally.

Organizations specific to gerontological nursing include the National Gerontological Nursing Association (NGNA), the Gerontological Advanced Practice Nurses Association (GAPNA), the National Association Directors of Nursing Administration/Long Term Care (NADONA/LTC) (also includes assisted-living RNs and LPNs/LVNs as associate members), the American Association of Directors of Nursing Services (AADNS), the International Consortium on Professional Nursing Practice in Long Term Care Homes, and the Canadian Gerontological Nursing Association (CGNA). In 2001 the Coalition of Geriatric Nursing Organizations (CGNO) was established to improve the health care of older adults across care settings. The CGNO represents more than 28,500 geriatric nurses from 8 national organizations and is supported by The Hartford Institute for Geriatric Nursing and located at New York University College of Nursing (New York, NY).

RESEARCH ON AGING

Inquiry into and curiosity about aging is as old as curiosity about life and death itself. Gerontology began as an inquiry into the characteristics of long-lived people, and we are still intrigued by them. Anecdotal evidence was used in the past to illustrate issues assumed to be universal. Only in the past 60 years have serious and carefully controlled research studies on aging flourished.

The impact of disease morbidity and impending death on the quality of life and the experience of aging have provided the impetus for much of the study by gerontologists. Much that has been thought about aging has been found to be erroneous, and early research was conducted with older people who were ill. As a result, aging has been inevitably seen through the distorted lens of disease. However, we are finally recognizing that aging and disease are separate entities although frequent companions.

Aging has been seen as a biomedical problem that must be reversed, eradicated, or controlled for as long as possible. The trend toward the medicalization of aging has influenced the general public as well. The biomedical view of the "problem" of aging is reinforced on all sides. A shift in the view of aging to one that centers on the potential for health, wholeness, and quality of life, and the significant contributions of older people to society, is increasingly the focus in the research, popular literature, the public portrayal of older people, and the theme of this text.

The National Institute on Aging (NIA), the National Institute of Nursing Research (NINR), the National Institute of Mental Health (NIMH), and the Agency for Healthcare Research and Quality (AHRQ) continue to make significant research contributions to our understanding of older people. Ongoing and projected budget cuts are of concern in the adequate funding of aging research and services in the United States.

Nursing Research

Nursing research draws from its own body of knowledge, as well as from other disciplines, to describe, monitor, protect, and evaluate the quality of life while aging and the services more commonly provided to the aging population, such as hospice care. Nurses have generated significant research on the care of older adults and have established a solid foundation for the practice of gerontological nursing. Research with older adults receives considerable funding from the National Institute of Nursing Research (NINR), and their website (http://www.ninr.nih.gov) provides information about results of studies and funding opportunities.

Gerontological nurse researchers publish in many nursing journals and journals devoted to gerontology such as *The Gerontologist* and *Journal of Gerontology* (GSA), and there are several gerontological nursing journals including *Journal of Gerontological Nursing, Research in Gerontological Nursing, Geriatric Nursing,* and the *International Journal of Older People Nursing.*

Nursing research has significantly affected the quality of life of older people and gains more prominence each decade. Federal funding for gerontological nursing research is increasing, and more nurse scholars are studying nursing issues related to older people. Some of the most important nursing studies have investigated methods of caring for individuals with dementia, reducing falls and the use of restraints, pain management, delirium, care transitions, and end-of-life care.

Knowledge about aging and the lived experience of aging has changed considerably and will continue to change in the future. Past ideas and current practices will not be acceptable to present and current cohorts of older individuals. Nursing research will continue to examine the best practices for care of older people who are ill and living in institutions, but increasing emphasis will be placed on strategies to maintain and improve health while aging, especially in light of the increasing numbers of older individuals across the globe.

Current research priorities include a focus on community and home-care resources for older adults, an emphasis on family caregiving issues, and a shift from the attention on illness and disease to the expectation of wellness, even in the presence of chronic illness and functional impairment. Improving quality of life for individuals with chronic illness an End-of-Life and Palliative Care: The Science of Compassion are two areas of scientific focus in the NINR Strategic Plan (2016). Translational research and continued attention to interprofessional studies are increasingly important.

GERONTOLOGICAL NURSING ROLES

Gerontological nursing roles encompass every imaginable venue and circumstance. The opportunities are limitless because we are a rapidly aging society. "Nurses have the potential to improve elder care across settings through effective screening and comprehensive assessment, facilitating access to programs and services, educating and empowering older adults and their families to improve their health and manage chronic conditions, leading and coordinating the efforts of members of the health care team, conducting and applying research, and influencing policy" (Young, 2003, p. 9).

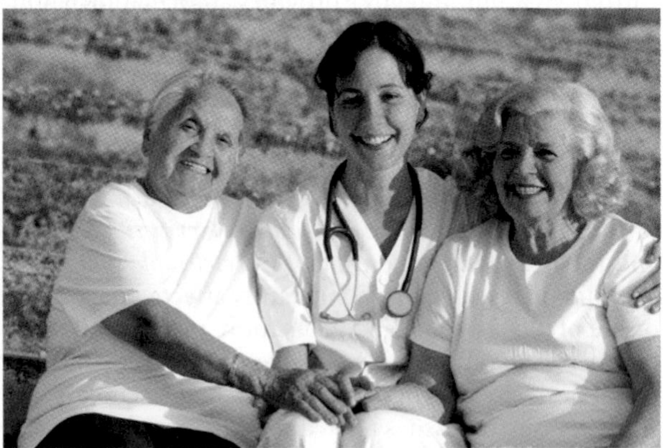

Gerontological nursing is important in this rapidly aging society. (© iStock.com/DianaHirsch.)

A gerontological nurse may be a generalist or a specialist. The generalist functions in a variety of settings (primary care, acute care, home care, post–acute and long-term care, and the community), providing nursing care to individuals and their families. National certification as a gerontological nurse is a way to demonstrate one's special knowledge in care for older adults and should be encouraged (http://www.nursecredentialing.org/GerontologicalNursing).

The gerontological nursing specialist has advanced preparation at the master's level and performs all of the functions of a generalist but has developed advanced clinical expertise, as well as an understanding of health and social policy and proficiency in planning, implementing, and evaluating health programs.

Specialist Roles

Under the *Consensus Model for APRN Regulation: Licensure, Accreditation, Certification & Education* (2008), advanced practice registered nurses (APRNs) must be educated, certified, and licensed to practice in a role and a population. APRNs are educated in one of four roles, one of which is adult–gerontology. This population focus encompasses the young adult to the older adult, including the frail elder. Titles of APRNs educated and certified across both areas of practice will include the following: Adult–Gerontology Acute Care Nurse Practitioner, Adult–Gerontology Primary Care Nurse Practitioner, and Adult–Gerontology Clinical Nurse Specialist. Certification is available for all of these levels of advanced practice; in most states this is a requirement for licensure.

Advanced practice nurses with certification in adult–gerontology will find a full range of opportunities for collaborative and independent practice both now and in the future. Direct care sites include geriatric and family practice clinics, long-term care, acute care and post–acute care facilities, home health care agencies, hospice agencies, continuing care retirement communities, assisted living facilities, managed care organizations, and specialty care clinics (e.g., Alzheimer's disease, heart failure, diabetes). Gerontological nursing specialists are also involved with community agencies such as local Area Agencies on Aging, public health departments, and national and worldwide organizations such as the Centers for Disease Control and the World Health Organization. They function as care managers, eldercare consultants, educators, and clinicians.

One of the most important advanced practice nursing roles that emerged over the last 40 years is that of the gerontological nurse practitioner (GNP) and the gerontological clinical nurse specialist (GCNS) in skilled nursing facilities. The education and training programs arose from evident need, particularly in the long-term care (LTC) setting (Ploeg et al., 2013). Nurse practitioners have been providing care in nursing homes in the United States since the 1970s, in Canada since 2000, and only recently in the United Kingdom. Numbers remain small and there is a need for continued attention at the policy and funding level for increased use of nurse practitioners in LTC. Recommendations from expert groups in the United States and Canada have called for

BOX 5.3 Outcomes of APNs Working in LTC Settings

- Improvement in or reduced rate of decline in incontinence, pressure ulcers, aggressive behavior, and loss of affect in cognitively impaired residents
- Lower use of restraints with no increase in staffing, psychoactive drug use, or serious fall-related injuries
- Improved or slower decline in some health status indicators including depression
- Improvements in meeting personal goals
- Lower hospitalization rates and costs
- Fewer ED visits and costs
- Improved satisfaction with care

Data from Ploeg J, Kaasalainen S, McAiney C, et al: Resident and family perceptions of the nurse practitioner role in long term care settings, *BMC Nurs* 12(1):24, 2013.

a nurse practitioner in every nursing home (Harrington et al., 2000; Ploeg et al., 2013). This role is well established and there is strong research to support the impact of advanced practice nurses working in LTC settings (Bakerjian, 2008; Oliver et al., 2014; Ploeg et al., 2013) (Box 5.3).

Generalist Roles

Acute Care

Older adults often enter the health care system with admissions to acute care settings. Older adults comprise 60% of the medical-surgical patients and 46% of the critical care patients. Acutely ill older adults frequently have multiple chronic conditions and comorbidities and present many challenges. Even though most nurses working in acute care are caring for older patients, many have not had gerontological nursing content in their basic nursing education programs and few are certified in the specialty. "Only a small number of the country's 6000 hospitals have institutional practice guidelines, educational resources, and administrative practices that support best practice care of older adults" (Boltz et al., 2008, p. 176).

Kagan (2008) reminds us that "older adults are the work of hospitals but most nurses practicing in hospitals do not say they specialize in geriatrics ... We, as a profession and a force in an aging society, must make the transformation to understanding care of older adults is acute care nursing ... Care of older adults would be the rule instead of the exception" (2008, p. 103). Kagan goes on to suggest that such a transformation would mean that acute care nurses would proudly describe themselves as geriatric nurses with subspecialties (geriatric vascular nurses, geriatric emergency nurses) and, along with geriatric nurse generalists, would populate hospital nursing services across the country.

Nurses caring for older adults in hospitals may function in the direct care provider role; or as care managers, discharge planners, care coordinators, or transitional care nurses; or in leadership and management positions. Many acute care hospitals are adopting new models of geriatric and chronic care to meet the needs of older adults. These include geriatric emergency departments and specialized units such as acute care for the elderly (ACE), geriatric evaluation and management units (GEMs), and transitional care programs. This will increase the need for well-prepared geriatric professionals working in interprofessional teams to deliver needed services.

NICHE. The Nurses Improving Care for Healthsystem Elders (NICHE), a program developed by the Hartford Geriatric Nursing Institute in 1992, was designed to improve outcomes for hospitalized older adults. The vision of NICHE is for all patients 65 and older to be given sensitive and exemplary care. NICHE, based at New York University College of Nursing, has more than 620 hospitals and health care facilities in 46 states, Canada, Bermuda, and Singapore (http://www.nicheprogram.org).

The mission of NICHE is to provide principles and tools to stimulate a change in the culture of health care facilities to achieve patient-centered care for older adults. NICHE offers many opportunities for new roles for acute care nurses such as the geriatric resource nurse (GRN). The GRN role emphasizes the pivotal role of the bedside nurse in influencing outcomes of care and coordination of interprofessional activities.

NICHE especially targets the prevention of iatrogenic complications, which occur in as many as 29% to 38% of hospitalized older adults, a rate three to five times higher than that seen in younger patients (Inouye et al., 2000). Common iatrogenic complications include functional decline, pneumonia, delirium, new-onset incontinence, malnutrition, pressure ulcers, medication reactions, and falls. Recognizing the impact of iatrogenesis, both on patient outcomes and on the cost of care, the Centers for Medicare and Medicaid Services (CMS) has instituted changes that will reduce payment to hospitals relative to these often preventable outcomes (https://www.cms.gov/medicare/medicare-fee-for-service-payment/hospitalacqcond/hospital-acquired_conditions.html). The changes target hospital-acquired conditions (HACs) that are high cost or high volume, result in a higher payment when present as a secondary diagnosis, are not present on admission, and could have reasonably been prevented through the use of evidence-based guidelines. Targeted conditions include several of the common geriatric syndromes such as catheter-associated urinary tract infections (CAUTIs), pressure ulcers, and falls (see Chapters 12, 14, and 15). Expertise in gerontological nursing is essential in prevention of these conditions.

NICHE has been the most successful acute care geriatric model in recruiting hospital membership and contributing to the depth of geriatric hospital programming.

Community- and Home-Based Care

Nurses will care for older adults in hospitals and long-term care facilities, but the majority of older adults live in the community. Community-based care occurs through home and hospice care, provided in persons' homes, independent senior housing complexes, retirement communities, residential care facilities such as assisted living facilities, and adult day health centers. It also takes place in primary care clinics and public health departments. Care will continue to move out of hospitals and long-term care institutions into the community because of rapidly escalating health care costs and the person's preference to "age in place" (see Chapters 6 and 16). Gerontological nurses will find opportunities to create practices in community-based settings with a focus not only on care for those who are ill but also on health promotion and community wellness.

Nurses in the home setting provide comprehensive assessments including physical, functional, psychosocial, family, home, environmental, and community. Care management and working with interprofessional teams are integral components of the home health nursing role. Nurses may provide and supervise care for elders with a variety of care needs (including chronic wounds, intravenous therapy, tube feedings, unstable medical conditions, and complex medication regimens) and for those receiving rehabilitation and palliative and hospice services.

Schools of nursing must increase education and practice experiences for nursing students in home- and community-based care. Advances in technology for remote monitoring of health status and safety and the development of point-of-care testing devices show promise in improving outcomes for elders who want to age in place. These technologies present exciting opportunities for registered nurses in the management and evaluation of care (see Chapter 16).

Case and Care Management Roles

Nurses are especially well suited for roles as case managers and care managers. There are increasing opportunities for these roles both in care of individuals with chronic illnesses and in transitional care (see Chapter 6). Although the terms case manager and care manager have slightly different connotations, in real practice the roles are seldom that clear and there is much overlap. Both of these roles include that of advocate, broker, leader, manager, counselor, negotiator, administrator, and communicator. Ideally the care manager follows the person through the entire continuum of care. Care managers must be experts regarding community resources and understand how these can best be used to meet the person's needs. They are expected to make appropriate referrals within the person's expectations and abilities and to monitor the quality of arranged services. The care or case manager is a resource person whom the elder or caregiver can seek for advice and counsel and for brokering (negotiating, arranging) the flow of services. As a gatekeeper, the care or case manager controls the entrances and exits to services to make sure that the elder gets what is needed without wasting resources.

Care managers are usually paid privately. Those who cannot afford the out-of-pocket expenses of purchased care management services must rely on services available through Medicaid–managed care plans or nonprofit community agencies, such as Catholic Senior Services, if available. Access to publicly funded programs varies by state and areas within the state and is dependent on state, county, and agency budget and priorities. Hospitals, skilled nursing facilities, and insurance agencies also utilize care/case managers. Care that is well managed is believed to be a solution to both the spiraling costs and the fragmentation of care experienced by elders with multiple needs. The care manager works to optimize the resources and outcome for the client and the agency or community in which the person resides. There are Standards of Practice and certifications available for care/case manager roles (Box 5.4) and Chapter 6 provides more information on transitional care.

Certified Nursing Facilities (Nursing Homes)

Certified nursing facilities, commonly called nursing homes, have evolved into a significant location where health care is provided across the continuum. Estimates are that 37% of all acute hospitalizations require

BOX 5.4 Resources for Best Practice

Care/Case Management

American Association of Managed Care Nurses: Certification, educational resources

Case Management Society of America: Standards of Practice, certification, educational resources

RNCaseManager.com: Resources, education, job assistance for job seekers and employers post–acute care services and older adults now enter nursing homes with increasingly acute health conditions. The old image of nursing homes caring for older adults in a custodial manner is no longer valid. Today, most facilities have post–acute care units that more closely resemble the general medical-surgical hospital units of the past. Most people enter nursing homes for short stays that last no more than 1 week to 3 months (Toles et al., 2014). "Nursing homes are no longer just a destination but rather a stage in the recovery process" (Thaler, 2014). Post–acute care in nursing facilities will continue to grow with health care reform, and there are many new roles and opportunities for professional nursing in this setting. The American Health Care Association (2010) predicts a 41% increase in the need for RNs in long-term care between 2000 and 2020.

Roles for professional nursing include nursing administrator, manager, supervisor, charge nurse, educator, infection control nurse, Minimum Data Set (MDS) coordinator, case manager, transitional care nurse, quality improvement coordinator, and direct care provider. Professional nurses in nursing facilities must be highly skilled in the complex care concerns of older people, ranging from post–acute care to end-of-life care. Excellent assessment skills; ability to work with interprofessional teams in partnership with residents and families; skills in acute, rehabilitative, and palliative care; and leadership, management, supervision, and delegation skills are essential.

Practice in this setting requires independent decision-making and is guided by a nursing model of care because there are fewer physicians and other professionals on-site at all times. In addition, stringent federal regulations governing care practices and greater use of licensed practical nurses and nursing assistants influence the role of professional nursing in this setting. Many new graduates will be entering this setting upon graduation so it is essential to provide education and practice experiences to prepare them to function competently in this setting, particularly leadership and management skills. See Chapter 6 for more information on long-term care.

❖ IMPLICATIONS FOR GERONTOLOGICAL NURSING AND HEALTHY AGING

With the promise of a healthier old age, health care professionals, particularly nurses, will play a significant role in creating systems of care and services that enhance the possibility of healthy aging for an increasingly diverse population. In times of health, illness, rehabilitation, and end-of-life care, outcomes for older adults most often depend on the nursing care received. Nurses have the skills needed to create a more person-centered, coordinated health care system and improve outcomes in health and illness. Continued attention must be paid to the recruitment and education of health professionals and direct care staff prepared to care for older people to meet the critical shortages that threaten health and safety can be attained.

Exciting roles for nurses with preparation in gerontological nursing are increasing across the continuum of care and eldercare is projected to be the fastest growing employment sector in health care. Nursing education is called upon to prepare graduates to assume positions across the continuum of care, with increasing emphasis on community-based and post–acute care settings. Dare we say that gerontological nursing will be the most needed specialty in nursing as the number of older people continues to increase and the need for our specialized knowledge becomes even more critical in every specialty and every health care setting?

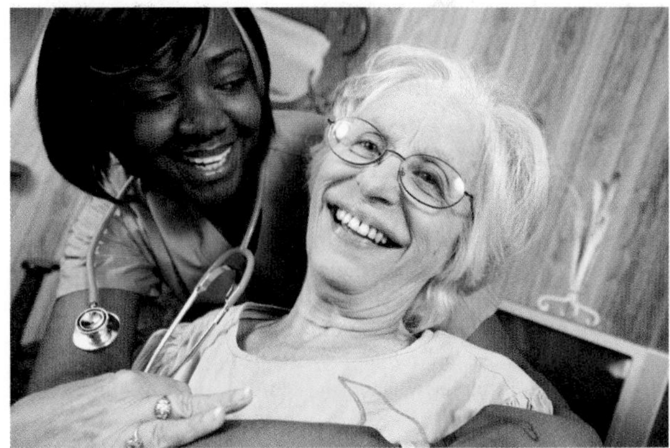

Gerontological nurses have a significant role in the healthy aging of older adults. (© iStock.com/Pamela Moore.)

KEY CONCEPTS

- The major changes in health care delivery and the increasing numbers of older adults have resulted in numerous revised, refined, and emergent roles for nurses in the field of gerontological nursing. There is a critical shortage of nurses prepared in the care of older adults.
- Nursing has led the field in gerontology, and nurses were the first professionals in the nation to be certified as geriatric specialists.
- Certification assures the public of nurses' commitment to specialized education and qualification for the care of older people.
- Advanced practice role opportunities for nurses are numerous and are seen as potentially cost-effective

in health care delivery while facilitating more holistic health care.

- All students graduating from nursing programs and all practicing nurses working with older adults should have competency in gerontological nursing.

ACTIVITIES AND DISCUSSION QUESTIONS

1. Consider and discuss with classmates the various gerontological nursing roles that you find most interesting and stimulating.
2. Discuss the gerontological organizations of today and their significance to the practicing nurse.
3. Why do you think more students do not choose gerontological nursing as a specialty? What would increase interest in this area of nursing?
4. What do you think are the most important issues in gerontological nursing education at this time?
5. Discuss your clinical education experiences and reflect on how they have influenced your views about care of older people and gerontological nursing.

REFERENCES

American Association of Colleges of Nursing (AACN): *White paper on the education and role of the clinical nurse leader*, Feb 2007. Available at http://www.nursing.vanderbilt.edu/msn/pdf/cm_AACN_CNL.pdf. Accessed September 16, 2014.

American Association of Colleges of Nursing (AACN): *The essentials of baccalaureate education for professional nursing practice*, 2008. Available at http://www.aacn.nche.edu/education-resources/baccessentials08.pdf.

American Health Care Association: *U.S. long term care workforce at a glance*, 2010. Available at http://www.ahcancal.org/research_data/staffing/Documents/WorkforceAtAGlance.pdf.

American Nurses Association: *Gerontological nursing: Scope and standards of practice*, Silver Springs, MD, 2010, Nursesbooks.org.

APRN Consensus Work Group & National Council of State Boards of Nursing APRN Advisory Committee: *Consensus model for APRN regulation: Licensure, accreditation, certification & education*, March 2008. Available at http://www.nursingworld.org/EspeciallyForYou/AdvancedPracticeNurses/Consensus-Model-Toolkit. Accessed October 1, 2015.

Bakerjian D: Care of nursing home residents by advanced practice nurses: A review of the literature, *Res Gerontol Nurs* 1:177, 2008.

Bardach S, Rowles G: Geriatric education in the health professions: Are we making progress?, *Gerontologist* 52(5):607–618, 2012.

Boltz M, Capezuti E, Bower-Ferres S, et al: Changes in the geriatric care environment associated with NICHE (Nurses Improving Care for Health System Elders), *Geriatr Nurs* 29(3):176–185, 2008.

Cortes T: *Out of the ashes, Hot Issues in Geriatrics Now: HIGN blog*, May 30, 2012. Available at http://hartfordinstitute.wordpress.com/?s=Out+of+the+Ashes. Accessed October 1, 2015.

Ebersole P, Touhy T: *Geriatric nursing: Growth of a specialty*, New York, 2006, Springer.

Eldercare Workforce Alliance: *Geriatrics workforce shortage: A looming crisis for our families* (Issue brief), 2014. Available at http://www.eldercareworkforce.org/files/Issue_Brief_PDFs/EWA_Issue.Supplydemand.final-3.pdf. Accessed October 1, 2015.

European Economic and Social Committee: *Active ageing and solidarity between generations*, 2012. Available at http://www.eesc.europa.eu/resources/docs/eesc-12-16-en.pdf. Accessed October 1, 2015.

Fox J: Educational strategies to promote professional nursing in long-term care: An integrative review, *J Gerontol Nurs* 39(1):52–60, 2013.

Harrington C, Kovner C, Mezey M, et al: Experts recommend minimum nurse staffing for nursing facilities in the United States, *Gerontologist* 40(1):5–16, 2000.

Holroyd A, Dahlke S, Fehr C, et al: Attitudes towards aging: Implications for a caring profession, *J Nurs Educ* 48(7):374–380, 2009.

Inouye S, Bogardus S, Baker D, et al: The Hospital Elder Life Program: A model of care to prevent cognitive and functional decline in older hospitalized patients, *J Am Geriatr Soc* 48:1657–1706, 2000.

Institute of Medicine (IOM): *Retooling for an aging America: Building the health care workforce*, 2008. Available at http://nationalacademies.org/hmd/reports/2008/retooling-for-an-aging-america-building-the-health-care-workforce.aspx. Accessed August 18, 2016.

Institute of Medicine (IOM): *The future of nursing: leading change, advancing health*, 2011. Available at http://nationalacademies.org/HMD/Reports/2010/The-Future-of-Nursing-Leading-Change-Advancing-Health.aspx. Accessed August 18, 2016.

Kagan S: Moving from achievement to transformation, *Geriatr Nurs* 203:102–104, 2008.

Mezey M, Fulmer T: The future history of gerontological nursing, *J Gerontol A Biol Sci Med Sci* 57:M438–M441, 2002.

Miller J, Coke L, Moss A, et al: Reluctant gerontologists: Integrating gerontological nursing content into a prelicensure program, *Nurse Educ* 34(5):198–203, 2009.

National Institute of Nursing Research: *The NINR strategic plan: Advancing science: improving lives.* NIH publication #16-NR-7783. Printed September 2016. Available at https://www.ninr.nih.gov/newsandinformation/newsandnotes/strategicplan2016#.V9x7JvkrJrS. Accessed September 2016.

Neville C, Dickie R, Goetz S: What's stopping a career in gerontological nursing? Literature review, *J Gerontol Nurs* 40(1):18–27, 2014.

Oliver G, Pennington L, Revelle S, et al: Impact of nurse practitioners on health outcomes of Medicare and Medicaid patients, *Nurs Outlook* 2014. doi: 10.1016/j.outlook.201407.004. [Epub ahead of print].

Ploeg J, Kaasalainen S, McAiney C, et al: Resident and family perceptions of the nurse practitioner role in long term care settings: A qualitative descriptive study, *BMC Nurs* 12(1):24, 2013. Available at http://www.biomedcentral.com/content/pdf/1472-6955-12-24.pdf. Accessed October 1, 2015.

Robert Wood Johnson Foundation: *United States in search of nurses with geriatrics training*, 2012. Available at http://www.rwjf.org/en/about-rwjf/newsroom/newsroom-content/2012/02/

united-states-in-search-of-nurses-with-geriatrics-training.html. Accessed February 5, 2014.

Stierle L, Mezez M, Schumann M, et al: Professional development: The nurse competence in aging initiative: Encouraging expertise in the care of older adults, *Am J Nurs* 106(9):93–96, 2006.

Taylor M: Mapping the literature of pediatric nursing, *J Med Libr Assoc* 92(2 Suppl):E128–E136, 2006.

Thaler M: *The need for SNFs for baby boomers. McKnight's long-term care news and assisted living*, 2014. Available at http://www.mcknights.com/the-need-for-snfs-for-baby-boomers/article/327724/. Accessed October 1, 2015.

Toles M, Anderson R, Massing M, et al: Restarting the cycle: Incidence and predictors of first acute care use after nursing home discharge, *J Am Geriatr Soc* 62(1):79–85, 2014.

Tolson D, Rolland Y, Andrieu S, et al: International Association of Gerontology and Geriatrics: A global agenda for clinical research and quality of care in nursing homes, *J Am Med Dir Assoc* 12:184–189, 2011.

U.S. Department of Health and Human Services, Office of Disease Prevention and Health Promotion: *Healthy People 2020*, 2012. Available at http://www.healthypeople.gov/2020.

Young H: Challenges and solutions for care of frail older adults, *Online J Issues Nurs* 8(2):1–13, 2003.

6

Gerontological Nursing Across the Continuum of Care

Theris A. Touhy

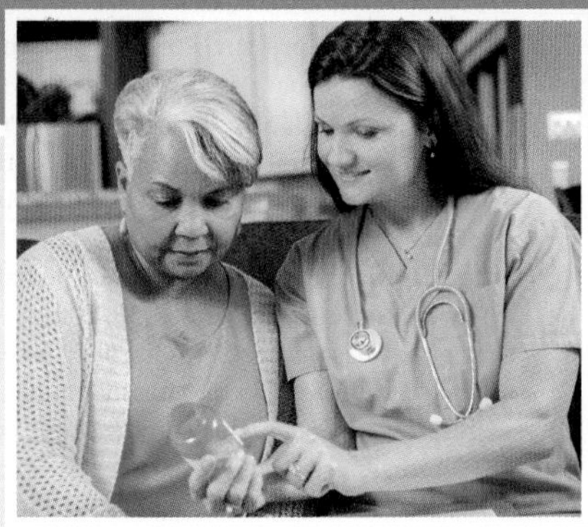

evolve.elsevier.com/Touhy/gerontological

LEARNING OBJECTIVES

Upon completion of this chapter, the reader will be able to:

- Compare the major features, advantages, and disadvantages of several residential options available to the older adult.
- Discuss long-term care as a component of health care systems.
- Discuss interventions to improve care for older adults in skilled nursing facilities, including quality improvement and culture change.
- Identify interventions to improve outcomes for older adults during transitions between health care settings.

THE LIVED EXPERIENCE

We are dealing with some really tough decisions for my parents. They insist on staying in their own home but I don't think it's safe anymore. They need quite a bit of help and I cannot do it all. We talked about assisted living and nursing home but they don't want that and would have to use all of their savings to pay for care. Coming to my home is not an option with 3 active teenagers and only 3 small bedrooms. I worry constantly about what to do.

Marianne, age 55

This chapter discusses residential and long-term care options across the continuum and transitions between health care settings with related implications for nursing practice. Long-term care (LTC) as a component of the health care system and the role of skilled nursing facilities (SNFs) in the provision of post–acute care are also discussed.

Most people would prefer to stay in their own home (age in place) but there are many factors that can affect decision-making about where to live as one ages (see Chapter 20). Some older people, by choice or by need, move from one type of residence to another. A number of options exist, especially for those with the financial resources that allow them to have a choice. Residential options range along a continuum from remaining in one's private house or apartment; to senior retirement communities; to shared housing with family members, friends, or others; to residential care communities such as assisted living settings; to nursing facilities for those with the most needs. It is important for nurses in all practice settings to be knowledgeable about the range of options so that they can assist older adults and their families who may need to make decisions about relocation.

COMMUNITY CARE

Program for All-Inclusive Care for the Elderly

An innovative long-standing community-based service program is the Program of All-Inclusive Care for the Elderly (PACE). PACE provides community services to people age 55 or older who meet the criteria for nursing home admission, prefer to remain in the community, and are eligible for Medicare and Medicaid. PACE provides a comprehensive continuum of primary care, acute care, home care, adult day health care, nursing facility care, and specialty care by an interdisciplinary team. Outcomes of the PACE program include "increased use of ambulatory care services, lower rate of nursing home use, lower rates of functional decline, and better reported health status and quality of life than among comparison populations" (Cortes & Sullivan-Marx, 2016, p. 11).

PACE is a capitated system in which the team is provided with a monthly sum to provide all care to the enrollees, including medications, eyeglasses, and transportation to care, as well as urgent and preventive care. PACE is now recognized as a permanent provider under Medicare and a state option under Medicaid. In 2016 there were 120 PACE programs operational in 31 states. Nursing has been central to the PACE care model since its beginning 40 years ago. The PACE Innovation Act 2015 provided authority to expand the program to individuals younger than 55 years with disabilities and at risk of needing a nursing home (Cortes & Sullivan-Marx, 2016). Models such as PACE are innovative care delivery models, and continued development of such models is important as the population ages (Casiano, 2015; National PACE Association, 2016).

Adult Day Services

Adult day services (ADSs) are community-based group programs designed to provide social and some health services to adults who need supervised care in a safe setting during the day. They also offer caregivers respite from the responsibilities of caregiving, and most provide educational programs, support groups, and individual counseling for caregivers. ADSs are increasingly being utilized to provide community-based care for conditions like Alzheimer's disease and for transitional care and short-term rehabilitation following hospitalization. Staff ratios in ADSs are one direct care worker to six clients. Almost 80% of centers have professional nursing staff, 50% have a social worker, and 60% offer case management services. Most also offer transportation services (National Adult Day Services Association, n.d.).

Some ADSs are private pay, and others are funded through Medicaid home and community-based waiver programs, state and local funding, and the Veterans Administration. Pilot programs have been implemented through Medicare and are being evaluated. Adult day services are an important part of the long-term care continuum and a cost-effective alternative or supplement to home care or institutional care (Table 6.1). Continued expansion and funding are expected. Although further research is needed on patient and caregiver outcomes, findings suggest that ADSs improve health-related quality of life for participants and improve caregiver well-being (National Adult Day Services Association, n.d.).

TABLE 6.1 Costs of U.S. Long-Term Care Services and Support Programs

Service	Cost
Homemaker services	National median hourly rate: $20
Home health aide	National median hourly rate: $20
Adult day health	National median daily rate: $68
Assisted living facility	National median monthly rate: $3628
Skilled nursing facility	National median daily rate: $225 (semiprivate room); $250 (private)

From Genworth: *Cost of care survey, 2015*. Available at https://www.genworth.com/dam/Americas/US/PDFs/Consumer/corporate/131168_050516.pdf. Accessed June 8, 2016.

Continuing Care Retirement Communities

Life care communities, also known as continuing care retirement communities (CCRCs), provide the full range of residential options, from single-family homes to skilled nursing facilities all in one location. Most of these communities provide access to these levels of care for a community member's entire remaining lifetime, and for the right price, the range of services may be guaranteed. Having all levels of care in one location allows community members to make the transition between levels without life-disrupting moves. For married couples in which one spouse needs more care than the other, life care communities allow them to live nearby in a different part of the same community. Most CCRCs are managed by not-for-profit organizations.

Choosing to live in a CCRC is a costly endeavor, and individuals with low or even middle incomes and assets usually cannot afford this senior housing option. Payment plans differ at each CCRC, but a large entrance fee is usually required. This fee can be as little as $10,000 and as much as $500,000. With most continuing care retirement communities, the residence purchased usually belongs to the community after the death of the owner. Residents must also pay a monthly maintenance fee, which can range from roughly $200 to more than $2000 (A Place for Mom, 2015).

Residential Care/Assisted Living

Residential care/assisted living (RC/AL) is a long-term care option that provides housing and services for close to 1 million older adults in the United States and is the fastest growing housing option for older adults (Beeber et al., 2014). RC/AL is known by more than 30 different names across the country, including adult congregate facilities, foster care homes, personal care homes, homes for the elderly, domiciliary care homes, board and care homes, rest homes, family care homes, retirement homes, and assisted living facilities.

RC/AL is viewed as more cost-effective than nursing homes while providing more privacy and a homelike environment. Medicare does not cover the cost of care in these types of facilities. Eighty-six percent of individuals in RC/AL pay for their care from their personal resources, but there is some assistance for low-income individuals through Medicaid and state programs of waivers. Private and long-term care insurance may also cover some costs (Assisted Living Federation of America, 2015). The rates charged and the services those rates include vary considerably, as do regulations and licensing (Table 6.1).

Assisted Living

Assisted living facilities (ALFs), also called *board and care homes* or *adult congregate living facilities,* are a popular type of RC/AL. Assisted living is a residential long-term care choice for older adults who need more than an independent living environment but do not need the 24 hours/day skilled nursing care and the constant monitoring of a nursing home. Box 6.1 presents information about the typical assisted living resident. Assisted living settings may be a shared room or a single-occupancy unit with a private bath, kitchenette, and communal meals. They all provide some support services.

BOX 6.1 Profile of a Resident in an Assisted Living Facility

- 86.9 years old
- Female (74%)
- Needs help with two to three activities of daily living
- 87% need help with meal preparation
- 81% need help managing medications
- 45% to 67% have Alzheimer's disease or other dementia types of diagnoses
- Average length of stay: 22 months
- 59% move to a nursing facility
- 33% die while a resident of an assisted living facility

Assisted living is more expensive than independent living and less costly than skilled nursing home care, but it is not inexpensive. Costs vary by geographical region, size of the unit, and relative luxury. Most ALFs offer two or three meals per day, light weekly housekeeping, and laundry services, as well as optional social activities. Each added service increases the cost of the setting but also allows for individuals with resources to remain in the setting longer, as functional abilities decline. Consumers are advised to inquire as to exactly what services will be provided and by whom if an ALF resident becomes more frail and needs more intensive care.

Many seniors and their families prefer ALFs to nursing homes because they cost less, are more homelike, and offer more opportunities for control, independence, and privacy. However, many residents of ALFs have chronic care needs and over time may require more care than the facility is able to provide. Services (e.g., home health, hospice, homemakers) can be brought into the facility, but some persons question whether this adequately substitutes for 24-hour supervision by registered nurses (RNs). Not all states require a nurse in assisted living facilities, but between 47% and 70% of these settings employ an RN or licensed practical nurse (LPN)/licensed vocational nurse (LVN). In the ALF, there is no organized team of providers such as that found in nursing homes (i.e., nurses, social workers, rehabilitation therapists, pharmacists).

With the growing numbers of older adults with dementia residing in ALFs, many are establishing dementia-specific units. It is important to investigate services available as well as staff training when making decisions about the most appropriate placement for older adults with dementia. The Alzheimer's Association has issued a set of dementia care practices for ALFs and nursing homes (Alzheimer's Association, 2009) (Box 6.2).

The Joint Commission and the Commission for Accreditation of Rehabilitation Facilities have published standards for accreditation of ALFs, but many people are advocating for more comprehensive federal and state standards and regulations. The nonmedical nature of ALFs is a primary factor in keeping costs more reasonable than those in nursing facilities, but costs are still high for those without adequate funds. Appropriate standards of care must be developed, and care outcomes monitored to ensure that residents are receiving quality care in this setting, which is almost devoid of professional nursing. Further research is needed on care outcomes of residents in ALFs and the role of unlicensed

BOX 6.2 Resources for Best Practice

Advancing Excellence in America's Nursing Home Campaign: https://www.nhqualitycampaign.org/
Alzheimer's Association: Dementia Care Practice Recommendations for ALFs and Nursing Homes
American Assisted Living Nurses Association: Certification, Scope and Standards of Practice
Argentum (formerly Assisted Living Federation of America): Information, educational resources, guide to choosing an assisted living facility
Centers for Medicare and Medicaid Services: Guide to choosing a nursing home; Nursing Home Compare; Nursing Home Quality Care Collaborative (NHQCC) Learning; Partnership to Improve Dementia Care in Nursing Homes
National Adult Day Services Association
National Center for Assisted Living: Information, educational resources, guide to choosing an assisted living facility
National PACE Association
Pioneer Network: Culture change information and toolkit

assistive personnel, as well as RNs, in these facilities (Kaskie et al., 2015).

Advanced practice gerontological nurses are well suited to the role of primary care provider in ALFs, and many have assumed this role. The American Assisted Living Nurses Association has established a certification mechanism for nurses working in these facilities and Argentum (formerly Assisted Living Federation of America) and the National Center for Assisted Living provide a consumer guide for choosing an assisted living residence (Box 6.2).

SKILLED NURSING FACILITIES (NURSING HOMES)

Nursing homes are complex health care settings that are a mixture of hospital, rehabilitation facility, hospice, and dementia-specific units. Nursing facilities most often include up to two levels of care: a *skilled nursing care* (also called *sub–acute or post–acute care*) facility is required to have licensed professionals with a focus on the management of complex medical needs; and a *chronic care* (also called *long-term* or *custodial*) facility is required to have 24-hour personal assistance that is supervised and augmented by professional and licensed nurses. Often, both kinds of services are provided in one facility. There are significant differences in focus of care, staffing, level of reimbursement, and regulatory guidelines between these two kinds of services. There are approximately 15,655 skilled nursing care centers in the United States and most are for-profit organizations (American Health Care Association, 2015).

BOX 6.3 Interprofessional Teams in Nursing Homes

Patient
Family/significant others
Nurse
Primary care provider: physician, nurse practitioner
Physical, occupational, speech therapists
Social worker
Dietitian
Discharge planner/case manager
Psychologist
Prosthetist and orthotist
Audiologist
Chaplain

Sub–Acute Care (Short-Term)

The old concept of nursing home has dramatically changed with the increase in the number of patients with complex medical needs being cared for in this setting. Skilled nursing facilities are the most frequent site of post–acute care in the United States. Post–acute care is more intensive than traditional nursing home care and several times more costly, but far less costly than care in a hospital. With continued health care reform and cost-saving measures, this trend will continue.

The expectation in post–acute care settings is that the patient will be discharged home or to a less intensive setting. Length of stay is usually no more than 1 to 3 months and is largely reimbursed by Medicare. In addition to skilled nursing care, rehabilitation services are an essential component of post–acute care units. Patients are usually younger and less likely to be cognitively impaired than those in chronic (custodial) care. Generally, professional nurse staffing levels are higher than those in the traditional nursing home setting because of the acuity of the patient's condition. Roles for professional nursing in this setting are increasing, and nurses with expert skills in rehabilitation nursing and acute and long-term care will be needed (Camicia et al., 2014) (see Chapter 5).

Skilled nursing facilities (both post–acute and long-term chronic) utilize interprofessional teams, working with the resident and family, to assess, plan, and implement care (Box 6.3). Rehabilitation and restorative care is increasingly important in light of shortened hospital stays that may occur before conditions are stabilized and the older adult is unable to function independently. The opportunity to work collaboratively with an interprofessional team is one of the most exciting aspects of nursing practice in long-term care facilities (see Box 6.3).

Chronic Care (Long-Term)

Nursing homes also care for patients who may not need the intense care provided in post–acute care units but still need ongoing 24-hour care. Long-term care residents represent the frailest of all older adults. Their need for 24-hour care could not be met in the home or residential care setting, or may have exceeded what the family was able to provide. This may include individuals with severe strokes, dementia, or Parkinson's disease as well as persons receiving hospice care. Residents of long-term facilities are predominantly women, 80 years or older, widowed, and dependent in activities of daily living (ADLs) and instrumental activities of daily living (IADLs).

About 50% of residents in nursing homes are cognitively impaired, and nursing homes are increasingly caring for people at the end of life. Twenty-three percent of Americans die in nursing homes, and this figure is expected to increase to 40% by 2040 (Agency for Healthcare Research and Quality, 2011; Teno et al., 2013). While the percentage of older people living in nursing homes at any given time is low (4% to 5%), those who live to age 85 will have a 50% chance of spending some time in a nursing home. This could be for post–acute care, ongoing long-term care, or end-of-life care.

Cost of care for individuals in nursing homes with chronic long-term health conditions is expensive. Many people think that Medicare covers long-term nursing home care but Medicare is not designed to provide coverage for long-term chronic care either in institutions or in the community. If the older person was admitted because of a dementia diagnosis and the need for assistance with ADLs and maintenance of safety, Medicare would not cover the cost of care unless there was some skilled need. Of long-term nursing home care, 57% is paid by Medicaid, 14% by Medicare, and 29% by private insurance plans, other payers, and the patients and families themselves (see Chapter 7) (American Health Care Association, 2015).

LONG-TERM CARE AND THE U.S. HEALTH CARE SYSTEM

The term long-term care (LTC) is often only associated with nursing homes and with care of older people. However, long-term care describes a variety of services, including medical and nonmedical care, provided on an ongoing basis to people of all ages who have a chronic illness or physical, cognitive, or developmental disabilities. Long-term and post–acute care services (LTPAC) can be provided informally or formally in a range of environments, from an individual's home to the home of a friend or relative, an adult day health center, independent and assisted living facilities, continuing care retirement communities, skilled nursing facilities, and hospice (Applebaum et al., 2013). Most people with LTC needs live in their own home with family, friends, and volunteers (as well as hired personnel) providing most of the care. However, the bulk of long-term care throughout the developed world is informal unpaid care provided by family members. More than 80% of individuals needing long-term care support and services receive help informally from friends and relatives (Frank, 2012). Without family caregivers, the present level of LTC could not be sustained (see Chapter 27).

The U.S. health care system has been focused on delivering acute care and addressing time-limited and specific illnesses and injuries as they occur in episodes. Such a system does not address the increasingly complex and long-term needs of people with chronic conditions. There has been little recognition of LTC as an integral part of the continuum of care. Today, the spectrum of care has been expanded to include long-term and post–acute care services (LTPAC), which includes nursing facilities, assisted living facilities, home care, and hospice (Golden & Shier, 2012–2013) (Fig. 6.1). The LTC system is complex and fragmented, isolated from other service providers, and poorly funded; it is confusing for the individual and the caregiver to access and negotiate. There is no comprehensive approach to care coordination, which results in unmet needs, risk for injuries, and

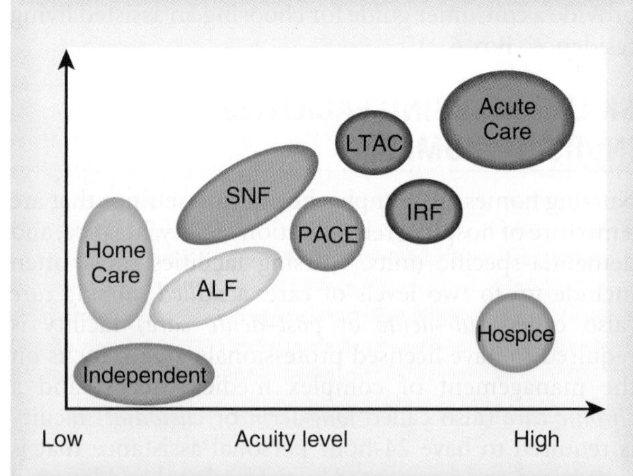

FIGURE 6.1 LTPAC spectrum of care. *ALF,* Assisted living facility; *IRF,* inpatient rehabilitation facility; *LTAC,* long-term acute care; *PACE,* Program of All-Inclusive Care for the Elderly; *SNF,* skilled nursing facility. (From John F. Derr, RPh; JD and Associates Enterprises, Inc.)

BOX 6.4 Focus of Acute and Long-Term Care

Acute Care Orientation

- Illness
- High technology
- Short term
- Episodic
- One-dimensional
- Professional
- Medical model
- Cure

Long-Term Care Orientation

- Function
- High touch
- Extended
- Interdisciplinary model
- Ongoing
- Multidimensional
- Paraprofessional and family
- Care

Adapted from Ouslander J, Osterweil D, Morley J: *Medical care in the nursing home,* New York, 1997, McGraw-Hill.

BOX 6.5 Goals of Long-Term Care

1. Provide a safe and supportive environment for chronically ill and functionally dependent people.
2. Restore and maintain highest practicable level of functional independence.
3. Preserve individual autonomy.
4. Maximize quality of life, well-being, and satisfaction with care.
5. Provide comfort and dignity at the end of life for residents and their families.
6. Provide coordinated interdisciplinary care to sub–acutely ill residents who plan to return to home or to a less restrictive level of care.
7. Stabilize and delay progression, when possible, of chronic medical conditions.
8. Prevent acute medical and iatrogenic illnesses, and identify and treat them rapidly when they do occur.
9. Create a homelike environment that respects the dignity of each resident.

Adapted from Ouslander J, Osterweil D, Morley J: *Medical care in the nursing home,* New York, 1997, McGraw-Hill.

adverse outcomes (Nazir et al., 2014; United States Senate, 2013).

Health care professionals who have not had experience in the long-term care system are often unaware of the many differences between acute and long-term care. Unless they have experienced the problems in their own families, they may be unaware of the challenges associated with obtaining quality care for individuals with long-term needs. It is important for health care professionals, especially nurses, to understand the total spectrum of care and the differences between acute and long-term care (Boxes 6.4 and 6.5).

Costs of LTC

Long-term care is expensive and becoming more expensive; costs have outpaced inflation since 2003. The number of older people needing long-term care services and support is dramatically increasing year after year. Worldwide, the number of people older than age 80, those most likely to need long-term care services, will increase by 233% between 2008 and 2040 (Applebaum et al., 2013). A fivefold increase in spending on LTC is projected by 2045 in the United States (Frank, 2012). Long-term care coverage in the United States is overly reliant on institutional care (the most expensive) and primarily financed by Medicaid and individuals themselves (Markkanen et al., 2012). The United States and the United Kingdom (excluding Scotland) are the only two countries in the developed world that do not have some system for universal long-term care.

LTC is the largest expenditure for older adults in the United States (Markkanen et al., 2012). Finding a way to pay for long-term care is a growing concern for people of all ages. Most people have not planned for their LTC needs and are not knowledgeable about resources (Harris-Kojetin et al., 2013). State and federal governments cannot continue to support the costs of the Medicaid program. The reimbursement levels of both Medicare and Medicaid do not cover actual costs, and there is fear that if further cuts are made, quality of care will be more drastically compromised. Health care reform measures will continue to address rising health care costs across the continuum and develop programs to decrease costs while enhancing quality. Medical (health) homes and accountable care organizations (ACOs) are examples of these types of programs (see Chapter 7).

QUALITY OF CARE IN SKILLED NURSING FACILITIES

Nursing homes are one of the most highly regulated industries in the United States. The Omnibus Budget Reconciliation Act (OBRA) of 1987 and its frequent revisions and updates are designed to improve the quality of resident care and have had a positive impact.

Some of the requirements of OBRA and subsequent legislation include the following: comprehensive resident assessments (Minimum Data Set [MDS]) (see Chapter 8), increased training requirements for nursing assistants, elimination of the use of medications and restraints for the purpose of discipline or convenience, higher staffing requirements for nursing and social work staff, standards for nursing home administrators, and quality assurance activities.

The Affordable Care Act (ACA) provided additional legislation to support quality and performance improvement in nursing homes. The Quality Assurance and Performance Improvement (QAPI) approach requires all nursing homes participating in Medicare or Medicaid programs to implement a QAPI program to assess quality of care provided to residents and to improve outcomes (Box 6.2). The Centers for Medicare and Medicaid Services (CMS) has activities underway with regard to pay-for-performance based on quality indicators for both the nursing home and the home health settings. Box 6.6 presents quality measures.

Nursing homes were the first to publish on-line quality information, which is now available for hospitals and other health care organizations. In 2007 CMS instituted the skilled nursing facility scorecard, known as Nursing Home Compare, which provides a 5-star rating system for ranking all licensed facilities. Nursing Home Compare helps professionals, consumers and their families, and caregivers compare nursing homes (http://www.medicare.gov/NHCompare). This rating system is based on the nursing home's most recent health inspection (highest weight), staffing, and quality measures.

Although the national rating system for nursing homes is helpful for evaluating quality, CMS advises consumers to use additional sources of information before choosing a facility. The rating report is only a "snapshot" of the care in individual nursing homes based on the annual survey (Nazir et al., 2014). The most appropriate method of choosing a nursing home is to personally visit the facility, meet with the director of nursing, observe care routines, and discuss the potential resident's needs. CMS provides a nursing home checklist on its website, and the National Citizens Coalition for Nursing Home Reform also provides resources for choosing a nursing home and understanding quality measures (Box 6.2).

Quality of care in skilled nursing facilities is improving. From 2011 to 2014, 11 out of 13 long-stay and all 5 short-stay quality measures improved (American Health Care Association, 2014). Advanced practice nurses, either on-site or in consultation, are linked to improved quality of care in nursing homes (Dyck et al., 2014) (see Chapter 5).

BOX 6.6 Quality Measures for LTC Facilities

Short Stay Quality Measures

- Percentage of residents who self-report moderate to severe pain
- Percentage of residents with pressure ulcers that are new or worsened
- Percentage of residents who were assessed and appropriately given the seasonal influenza vaccine
- Percentage of residents assessed and appropriately given the pneumococcal vaccine
- Percentage of residents who newly received an antipsychotic medication
- Percentage of residents who were successfully discharged to the community (claims-based)
- Percentage of residents who have had an outpatient emergency department visit (claims-based)
- Percentage of residents who were re-hospitalized after a nursing home admission (claims-based)
- Percentage of residents who made improvements in function (MDS-based)

Long Stay Quality Measures

- Percentage of residents experiencing one or more falls with major injury
- Percentage of residents who self-report moderate to severe pain
- Percentage of high-risk residents with high risk and develop pressure ulcers
- Percentage of residents assessed and appropriately given the seasonal influenza vaccine
- Percentage of residents assessed and appropriately given the pneumococcal vaccine
- Percentage of residents with a urinary tract infection
- Percentage of low-risk residents who lose control of their bowels or bladder
- Percentage of residents who have/had a catheter inserted and left in their bladder
- Percentage of residents who were physically restrained
- Percentage of residents whose need for help with activities of daily living has increased
- Percentage of residents who lose too much weight
- Percentage of residents who have depressive symptoms
- Percentage of residents who received an antianxiety or hypnotic medication (MDS-based)
- Percentage of residents whose ability to move independently worsened (MDS-based)

MDS, Minimum data set.

From *Medicare.gov: Why quality measure are important to you.* Available at https://www.medicare.gov/NursingHomeCompare/About/Short-Stay-Residents.html. Accessed September 2016.

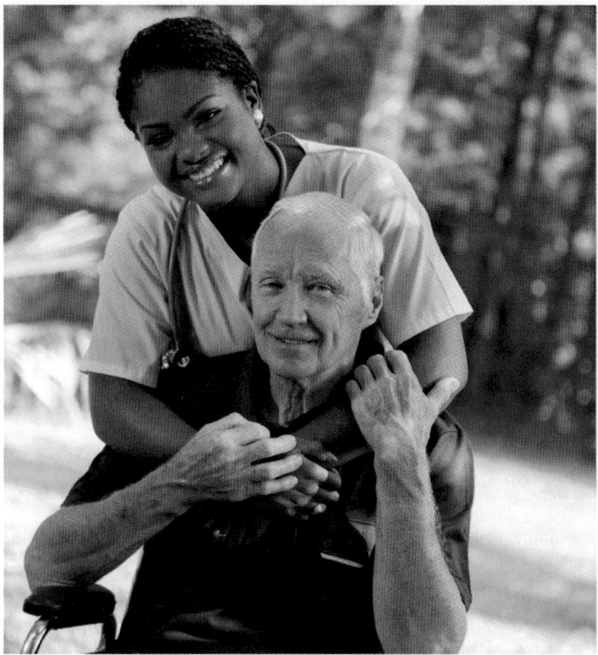

Caring relationships between staff and residents in long-term care enhance quality of care. (© iStock.com/Pamela Moore.)

❖ IMPLICATIONS FOR GERONTOLOGICAL NURSING AND HEALTHY AGING

Nurses play an important role in helping individuals and their family/significant others understand the discharge process and their posthospital needs, particularly if discharge to a skilled nursing facility is planned. CMS recommends that an evaluation of discharge needs be performed at least 48 hours before discharge, but ideally, discharge planning should begin on admission (Nazir et al., 2014). Patient and family education should include the role of skilled nursing facilities in rehabilitation, role of members of the interprofessional team, interpretation of five-star ratings, and other information on how to choose a facility.

Resident Bill of Rights

Quality is also promoted through regulations to protect the rights of the residents of nursing homes. Residents in long-term care facilities have rights under both federal and state laws. The staff of the facility must inform residents of these rights and protect and promote their rights. The rights to which the residents are entitled should be conspicuously posted in the facility (Box 6.7). Also, the Long-Term Care Ombudsman Program is a nationwide effort to support the rights of both the residents and the facilities. In most states, the program provides trained volunteers to investigate resident rights and examine quality complaints or conflicts. All reporting is anonymous. Each facility is required to post the name and contact information of the ombudsman assigned to the facility.

BOX 6.7 Bill of Rights for Long-Term Care Residents

- The right to voice grievances and have them remedied
- The right to information about health conditions and treatments and to participate in one's own care to the greatest extent possible
- The right to choose one's own health care providers and to speak privately with one's health care providers
- The right to consent to or refuse all aspects of care and treatments
- The right to manage one's own finances, if capable, or to choose one's own financial advisor
- The right to be transferred or discharged only for appropriate reasons
- The right to be free from all forms of abuse
- The right to be free from all forms of restraint to the extent compatible with safety
- The right to privacy and confidentiality concerning one's person, personal information, and medical information
- The right to be treated with dignity, consideration, and respect in keeping with one's individuality
- The right to immediate visitation and access at any time for family, health care providers, and legal advisors; the right to reasonable visitation and access for others

NOTE: This list of rights is a sampling of federal and several states' lists of rights of residents or participants in long-term care. Nurses should check the rules of their own state for specific legal rights.

Advancing Excellence in America's Nursing Homes

Another quality improvement initiative is the Advancing Excellence in America's Nursing Homes. This is an ongoing, voluntary campaign to help nursing homes achieve measurable improvement in the quality of care and quality of life for residents and staff. The campaign works with CMS to identify national goals for improvement and publish free downloadable quality improvement (QI) resources. The National Partnership to Improve Dementia Care in Nursing Homes is an important initiative as well (see Chapter 25). The quality indicators of restraint use have shown the greatest improvement, but the presence of pain and pressure ulcers and use of antipsychotic medications have also shown improvement (Bakerjian & Zisberg, 2013) (see Chapter 25).

The Culture Change Movement

Across the United States, as well as internationally, the movement to transform nursing homes from the typical medical model into "homes" that nurture quality of life for older people and support and empower frontline caregivers is changing the face of long-term care. Begun by the Pioneer Network, a national not-for-profit organization that serves the culture change movement, many facilities are changing from a rigid institutional approach to one that is person centered. CMS has endorsed culture change and has also released a self-study tool for nursing homes to assess their own progress toward culture change. The Affordable Care Act includes a national demonstration project on culture change to develop best practices and the development of resources and funding to undertake culture change.

Culture change is the "process of moving from a traditional nursing home model—characterized as a system unintentionally designed to foster dependence by keeping residents, as one observer put it, 'well cared for, safe, and powerless'—to a regenerative model that increases residents' autonomy and sense of control" (Brawley, 2007, p. 9). The ultimate vision of culture change is to improve the lives of residents and staff by centering the facility's philosophies, organizational structures, environmental designs, and care around practices that support residents' needs and preferences (Hartmann et al., 2013).

Older people in need of long-term care want to live in a homelike setting that does not look and function like a hospital. They want a setting that allows them to make decisions they are used to making for themselves, such as when to get up, take a bath, eat, or go to bed. They want caregivers who know them and understand and respect their individuality and their preferences. Box 6.8 presents some of the differences between an institution-centered culture and a person-centered culture.

Although further research is needed, some results suggest that person-centered care is associated with improved organizational performance, including higher resident and staff satisfaction, better workforce performance, and higher occupancy rates (Hartmann et al., 2013). Examples of philosophies and programs of culture change are the Eden Alternative (companion animals, indoor plants, frequent visits by children, involvement with the community), the Green House Project (small homes designed for 10 to 12 residents), and the Wellspring Model. The Eden Alternative is best known for the addition of animals, plants, and children to nursing homes. However, cats and dogs are not the heart of culture change. Truly transforming a nursing home starts at the top and requires involvement from all levels of staff and changes in values, attitudes, structures, and management practices. The principles central to culture change are presented in Box 6.9.

BOX 6.8 Institution-Centered Versus Person-Centered Culture

Institution-Centered Culture

- Schedules and routines are designed by the institution and staff, and residents must comply.
- Focus is on tasks that need to be accomplished.
- Rotation of staff among units occurs.
- Decision-making is centralized with little involvement of staff or residents and families.
- There is a hospital environment.
- Structured activities are provided to all residents.
- There is little opportunity for socialization.
- Organization exists for employees rather than residents.
- There is little respect for privacy or individual routines.

Person-Centered Culture

- Emphasis is on relationships between staff and residents.
- Individualized plans of care are based on residents' needs, usual patterns, and desires.
- Staff members have consistent assignments and know the residents' preferences and uniqueness.
- Decision-making is as close to that of the resident as possible.
- Staff members are involved in decisions and plans of care.
- Environment is homelike.
- Meaningful activities and opportunities for socialization are available around the clock.
- There is a sense of community and belonging—"like family."
- There is involvement of the community—children, pets, plants, outings.

Adapted from the Pioneer Network. Available at http://www.pioneernetwork.net. Accessed August 8, 2008.

TRANSITIONS ACROSS THE CONTINUUM

Care transition refers to the movement of patients from one health care practitioner or setting to another as their condition and care needs change. Older people have complex health care needs and often require care in multiple settings across the health-wellness continuum. This makes them and their families and/or caregivers vulnerable to poor outcomes during transitions (Naylor, 2012). An older person may be treated by a family practitioner or internist in the community and by a hospitalist and specialists in the hospital; discharged to a post–acute care setting and followed by another practitioner; and then discharged home or to a less care-intensive setting (e.g., assisted living facilities/residential care settings) where the person's original providers may

BOX 6.9 Principles of Culture Change

- Care and activities are directed by the residents.
- The environment and care practices support a homelike atmosphere.
- Relationships among staff and residents are supported and fostered.
- Increased attention to respect of staff and the value of caring are promoted.
- Staff is empowered to respond to the residents' needs and desires.
- The organizational hierarchy is flattened to support collaborative decision-making for staff.
- Comprehensive and continuous quality improvement underscores all activities and decisions to sustain a person-directed organizational culture.

Adapted from Mueller C, Burger S, Rader J, et al: Nurse competencies for person-directed care in nursing homes, *Geriatr Nurs* 34:101–104, 2013.

BOX 6.10 Patient Story

John is a 68-year-old retired farm laborer who was readmitted for heart failure 10 days after hospital discharge. He lives alone in a rural community and has no friends or family to assist in his care and was not given a referral for home health care follow-up. His medical records document teaching about medication usage and his ability to repeat back the instructions correctly. He brought all of his pill bottles in a bag; all of the bottles were full, not one was opened. When questioned why he had not taken his medication, he looked away and began to cry, explaining he had never learned to read and could not read the instructions on the bottles.

Adapted from The Joint Commission: *Hot topics in health care: Transitions of care: The need for a more effective approach in continuing patient care*, 2012. Available at http://www.jointcommission.org/assets/1/18/Hot_Topics_Transitions_of_Care.pdf. Accessed February 10, 2014.

or may not resume care. Most health care providers practice in only one setting and are not familiar with the specific requirements of other settings. Each setting is seen as a distinct provider of services and little collaboration exists. The purpose of health care reform initiatives (ACOs, medical homes, bundled care) is to improve coordination and communication among providers so that the individual receives the most appropriate care in the most appropriate setting (see Chapter 7).

Readmissions: The Revolving Door

One in five older patients is readmitted to the hospital within 30 days of discharge. Some readmissions may be predictable but many can and should be prevented. Ninety percent of these readmissions for Medicare patients are unplanned, resulting in annual costs of more than $17 billion, paying for return trips that need not happen if patients received the appropriate care. CMS has identified avoidable readmissions as one of the leading problems facing the U.S. health care system and penalizes hospitals (with fines) that have high readmission rates for patients with heart failure, heart attack, and pneumonia (Robert Wood Johnson Foundation, 2013).

Additionally, one in four Medicare patients admitted for post–acute care in skilled nursing facilities is rehospitalized within 30 days and up to 67% of these readmissions may have been preventable, futile, or directly related to diagnoses that could have been treated in the SNF. The cost of these avoidable admissions has been estimated as high as $4 billion annually. Penalties for skilled nursing facilities with high rates of hospital readmissions are expected to go into effect in 2018 (Camahan et al., 2016; Mor et al., 2010). There are several CMS demonstration projects, funded by the Patient Protection and Affordable Care Act (2010), designed to address avoidable readmissions and care transitions. Many hospitals and nursing homes have also begun programs to address the issue with transitional care programs and there has been some improvement. The average hospital was fined less for high readmission rates in the second year of the penalty program but ongoing efforts are needed (Ness, 2013).

Factors Contributing to Poor Transitional Care Outcomes

Multiple factors contribute to poor outcomes during transitions: patient, provider, and system. Many are the result of a fragmented system of care that too often leaves discharged patients to their own devices, unable to follow instructions they did not understand, and not taking medications or getting the necessary follow-up care (Box 6.10). Patient characteristics such as age, diagnoses, language, literacy, and cultural and socioeconomic factors are contributing factors to hospital readmissions. Place of residence and the health care system providing care also influence readmission rates. Many patients are readmitted because they live in an area where the hospital is used more frequently as a site for illness care or there are limited resources for community-based care (Robert Wood Johnson Foundation, 2013).

Improving Transitional Care

Transitional care "refers to a broad range of time limited services to ensure health care continuity, avoid preventable poor outcomes among at-risk populations, and

SAFETY ALERT

Medication discrepancies are the most prevalent adverse event following hospital discharge and the most challenging component of a successful hospital-to-home transition (Foust et al., 2012; Hain et al., 2012; Pincus, 2013). Nurses' attention to an accurate prehospital medication list; medication reconciliation during hospitalization, at discharge, and after discharge; and patient and family education about medications are required to enhance safety.

promote the safe and timely transfer of these patient groups from one level of care (e.g., acute to post-acute) or setting (e.g., hospital to home) to another" (Naylor, 2012, p. 116). National attention to improving patient safety during transfers is increasing, and a growing body of evidence-based research provides data for design of care to improve transition outcomes.

Nurses play a very important role in ensuring the adequacy of transitional care, and many of the successful models involve the use of advanced practice nurses and registered nurses in roles such as transition coaches, care coordinators, and care managers (Chalmers & Coleman, 2008; Naylor, 2012). Nurse researchers Dorothy Brooten and Mary Naylor, along with their colleagues, have significantly contributed to knowledge in the area of transitional care and the critical role of nurses in transitional care improvement. One of the most rigorously studied acute care approaches, the Transitional Care Model (TCM), has demonstrated reductions in preventable hospital readmissions, improvements in health outcomes, enhancement in patient satisfaction, and reductions in total health care costs (Naylor, 2012) (see Box 6.2).

In the post–acute and long-term care setting, QAPI program improvement requirements include attention to improving transitional care processes and effectively managing acute changes in an individual's condition. Interventions to Reduce Acute Care Transfers (INTERACT) is an exemplar program for reducing the frequency of transfers to the acute hospital from nursing homes. INTERACT is a quality improvement program with communication tools, care paths or clinical tools, and advance care planning tools to assist nursing homes in identifying and managing acute changes in condition without hospital transfer when safe and feasible (interact2.net). Other successful interventions include the use of nurse practitioners working in collaborative teams with physicians, standardized admission assessments, palliative care consultations for residents with recurrent hospitalizations, and interprofessional case conferences (Toles et al., 2014).

Nursing interventions such as medication management, patient and family caregiver education, comprehensive discharge planning, and adequate and timely communication between providers and sites of service are also important. "Pilot studies have demonstrated that when a nurse with an understanding of care transitions is integrated into the process, unplanned 30-day hospital readmission rates decline and other quality outcomes are improved" (Camicia et al., 2014, p. 6).

Box 6.11 presents Resources for Best Practice and Box 6.12 gives Tips for Best Practice for transitional care nursing. Further research is needed to evaluate which Transitional Care Models are most effective in various settings and for which group of patients, particularly those who are most frail or cognitively impaired and for medically underserved populations (Golden & Shier, 2012–2013).

❖ IMPLICATIONS FOR GERONTOLOGICAL NURSING AND HEALTHY AGING

Nurses in all practice settings play a key role in improving care for older people across the continuum. New roles for nursing are emerging in the era of health care reform and heightened attention to improved patient outcomes. Nurses in all settings need to increase awareness of the roles and responsibilities of nursing practice across the continuum and work collaboratively to improve care outcomes, particularly during times of transition. We can no longer work in our individual "silos" and not be concerned with what happens after the patient is out of our particular unit or institution. Nurses are well positioned "to create services and

BOX 6.11 Resources for Best Practice

Transitional Care

Hospital Admission Risk Profile (HARP): Hartford Institute for Geriatric Nursing (Try This, General Assessment Series)

INTERACT: A quality improvement program designed to improve the early identification, assessment, documentation, and communication about changes in the status of residents in skilled nursing facilities (https://interact2.net/)

The Joint Commission: Transitions of Care Portal: http://www.jointcommission.org/toc.aspx

Transitional Care Model (TCM): http://www.nursing.upenn.edu/media/transitionalcare/Documents/Information%20on%20the%20Model.pdf

Transitional Care Model (TCM): Hospital Discharge Screening Criteria for High Risk Older Adults: Hartford Institute for Geriatric Nursing (Want to Know More: Transitional Care)

BOX 6.12 Tips for Best Practice

Transitional Care

- Identify patients at high risk for poor outcomes (e.g., low literacy, living alone, frequent hospitalizations, complex chronic illness, cognitive impairment, socioeconomic deprivation).
- Coach patient in self-care skills and encourage active involvement in care.
- Educate and support family caregivers and informal and formal caregivers.
- Adapt patient teaching for health literacy, language, culture, cognitive function, and sensory deficits.
- Prepare patient and family for what to expect at next site of care.
- Provide a complete and updated medication record; explain purpose of all medications, side effects, correct dosing, and how to obtain more medication.
- Assist in establishing regimen for proper administration of medication.
- Discuss symptoms that should be reported after discharge and how to contact provider; provide follow-up plan for how outstanding tests and follow-up appointments will be completed.
- Be aware of community resources in your area to assist with needs following discharge and how to link patient to resources.

environments that embrace values that are at the core of this profession—patient/caregiver centered care, communication and collaboration, and continuity" (Naylor, 2012, p. 140).

KEY CONCEPTS

- Nurses must be knowledgeable about the range of residential options for older people so they can assist the elder and the family to make appropriate decisions.
- The old concept of nursing home has dramatically changed with the increase in the number of patients with complex medical needs being cared for in this setting. Skilled nursing facilities are the most frequent site of post–acute care in the United States.
- Quality of care in skilled nursing facilities is improving. Nationwide, the average performance has improved in 12 of the 15 reported clinical outcome quality measures over the past 5 years.
- Culture change in nursing homes is a growing movement to develop models of person-centered care and improve care outcomes and quality of life.
- LTC can be provided informally or formally in a range of environments, from an individual's home to the home of a friend or relative, an adult day health center, independent and assisted living facilities, continuing care retirement communities, skilled nursing facilities, and hospices.
- LTC coverage in the United States is expensive and fragmented, overly reliant on institutional care, and primarily financed by individuals or their families or by Medicaid.
- Professional nursing involvement is an essential component in models to improve transitions across the continuum.

ACTIVITIES AND DISCUSSION QUESTIONS

1. Identify three objects in your living space that are important to you, and explain why these are significant. Would you take these with you whenever you relocate?
2. Ask an older relative about the items or conditions in his or her home that make him or her feel secure and comfortable.
3. Discuss with the elder from Question 2 the various moves he or she has made and how he or she felt about them.
4. How might the care needs of an older adult in assisted living, sub–acute care, and a nursing home differ? What is the role of the professional nurse in each of these settings?
5. Select three places listed in your phone book as assisted living facilities, and make inquiries regarding possible placement of an older adult parent. What questions did you ask? Suggestions include: What is the cost? What are the provisions for health care? What types of activities and assistance are available? After your review, which would you select for your grandmother and why?
6. In your experience in the acute care setting, what improvements would you suggest to improve transitions to other care settings? Discuss any experience you or your friends or family may have had with transitions after hospital discharge.
7. If you were the director of nursing, what would your nursing home be like (design, staffing, quality of care, training)?

REFERENCES

Agency for Healthcare Research and Quality: *Comparison of characteristics of nursing homes and other residential long-term care settings for people with dementia,* 2011. Available at http://effectivehealthcare.ahrq.gov/index.cfm/search-for-guides-reviews-and-reports/?pageaction=display product&productid=832. Accessed October 2015.

Alzheimer's Association: *Dementia care practice: Recommendations for assisted living residences and nursing homes,* 2009. Available at http://www.alz.org/national/documents/brochure_DCPRphases1n2.pdf.

American Health Care Association: *2014 Quality report,* Washington, DC, 2014, Author. Available at http://www.ahcancal.org/qualityreport/Pages/default.aspx. Accessed October 2015.

American Health Care Association: *Fast facts,* 2015. Available at http://www.ahcancal.org/research_data/trends_statistics/Pages/Fast-Facts.aspx. Accessed October 6, 2015.

A Place for Mom: *Continuing care retirement communities (CCRC),* April 22, 2015. Available at http://www.aplaceformom.com/senior-care-resources/articles/continuing-care-retirement-communities. Accessed October 5, 2014.

Applebaum R, Bardo A, Robbins E: International approaches to long-term services and supports, *Generations* 37(1):59–65, 2013.

Assisted Living Federation of America: *Assisted living,* 2015. Available at http://www.alfa.org/alfa/Assisted_Living_Information.asp. Accessed October 2015.

Bakerjian D, Zisberg A: Applying the advancing excellence in America's nursing homes circle of success to improving and sustaining quality, *Geriatr Nurs* 34:402–411, 2013.

Beeber A, Cohen L, Zimmerman S, et al: Differences in assisted living staff perceptions, experience, and attitudes, *J Gerontol Nurs* 40(1):41–49, 2014.

Brawley E: What culture change is and why an aging nation cares, *Aging Today* 28:9–10, 2007.

Camahan J, Unroe K, Torke A: Hospital readmission penalties: Coming soon to a nursing home near you!, *JAGS* 64(3):614–618, 2016.

Camicia M, Black T, Farrell J, et al: The essential role of the rehabilitation nurse in facilitating care transitions: A white paper by the Association of Rehabilitation Nurses, 2013, *Rehabil Nurs* 39(1):3–15, 2014.

Casiano A: PACE: A model of care for individuals with multiple chronic conditions, *Ann Longterm Care* 23(7):41–45, 2015.

Chalmers S, Coleman E: Transitional care. In Capezuti E, Swicker D, Mezey M, et al, editors: *The encyclopedia of elder care,* ed 2, New York, 2008, Springer.

Cortes T, Sullivan-Marx E: A case exemplar for national policy leadership, *J Gerontol Nurs* 42(3):9–14, 2016.

Dyck M, Schwinderhammer T, Butcher H: Quality improvement in nursing homes, *J Gerontol Nurs* 40(7):21–31, 2014.

Foust JB, Naylor MD, Bixby MB, et al: Medication problems occurring at hospital discharge among older adults with heart failure, *Res Gerontol Nurs* 5(1):26–33, 2012.

Frank R: Long-term care financing in the United States: Sources and institutions, *Appl Econ Perspect Policy* 34(2):333–345, 2012.

Genworth: *Cost of care survey,* 2015. Available at https://www.genworth.com/dam/Americas/US/PDFs/Consumer/corporate/131168_050516.pdf. Accessed June 8, 2016.

Golden R, Shier G: What does "care transitions" really mean?, *Generations* 36(4):6–12, 2012–2013.

Hain D, Tappen R, Diaz S, et al: Characteristics of older adults rehospitalized within 7 and 30 days of discharge: Implications for nursing practice, *J Gerontol Nurs* 38(8):32–44, 2012.

Harris-Kojetin L, Sengupta M, Park-Lee E, et al: *Long-term care services in the United States: 2013 overview,* Hyattsville, MD, 2013, National Center for Health Statistics.

Hartmann C, Snow A, Allen R, et al: A conceptual model for culture change evaluation in nursing homes, *Geriatr Nurs* 34:388–394, 2013.

Kaskie B, Nattinger M, Potter A: Policies to protect persons with dementia in assisted living: Déjà vu all over again?, *Gerontologist* 55(2):199–209, 2015.

Markkanen P, Abdallah L, Lee J, et al: Long-term care in the United States and Finland: Policy and lessons to be learned, *J Gerontol Nurs* 38(12):16–21, 2012.

Mor V, Intrator I, Feng Z, et al: The revolving door of hospitalization from skilled nursing facilities, *Health Aff* 29(1):57–64, 2010.

National Adult Day Services Association: *About adult day services.* Available at http://nadsa.org/learn-more/about-adult-day-services. Accessed August 2016.

National PACE Association: *What is PACE?* 2016. Available at http://www.npaonline.org/website/article.asp?id=12&title=Who,_What_and_Where_Is_PACE. Accessed August 2016.

Naylor M: Advancing high value transitional care: The central role of nursing and its leadership, *Nurs Admin Q* 36(2):115–126, 2012.

Nazir A, Little M, Arling G: More than just location: Helping patients and families select an appropriate skilled nursing facility, *Ann Longterm Care* 22(11):30–34, 2014.

Ness D, Kramer W: Reducing hospital readmissions: It's about improving patient care, *Health Affairs Blog* 2013. Available at http://healthaffairs.org/blog/2013/08/16/reducing-hospital-readmissions-its-about-improving-patient-care/. Accessed August 2016.

Pincus K: Transitional care management services, *J Gerontol Nurs* 39(10):10–15, 2013.

Robert Wood Johnson Foundation: *The revolving door: A report on U.S. hospital readmission,* 2013. Available at http://www.rwjf.org/content/dam/farm/reports/reports/2013/rwjf404178. Accessed October 2015.

Teno J, Gozato P, Bynum J, et al: Change in end-of-life care Medicare beneficiaries, *JAMA* 309(5):470–477, 2013.

Toles M, Anderson R, Massing M, et al: Restarting the cycle: Incidence and predictors of first acute care use after nursing home discharge, *J Am Geriatr Soc* 62(1):79–85, 2014.

United States Senate, Commission on Long-Term Care: *Report to the Congress,* September 13, 2013. Available at http://www.gpo.gov/fdsys/pkg/GPO-LTCCOMMISSION/content-detail.html. Accessed September 2014.

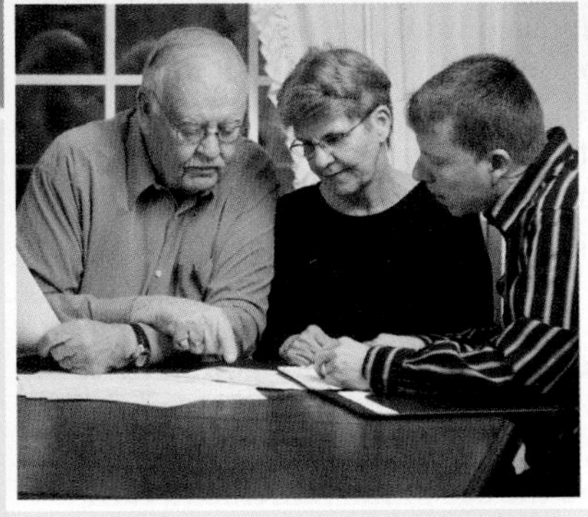

7

Economic and Legal Issues

Kathleen Jett

evolve.elsevier.com/Touhy/gerontological

LEARNING OBJECTIVES

Upon completion of this chapter, the reader will be able to:

- Describe the major methods of financing health care for older adults in the United States.
- Explain the fundamentals of Medicare, Medicaid, and TRICARE sufficiently to assist elders in accessing the services needed.
- Discuss the potential impact of health care financing in long-term and home health care.
- Compare the major forms of legal protection for elders with limited capacity.

THE LIVED EXPERIENCE

When I was growing up life was hard. We were so poor we couldn't do much but to hold on tight. When I was lucky I could get work plowing a field and make $1.00 an acre. You work hard, and you make do. When I turned 65 I got a little check from the government and a red, white, and blue insurance [Medicare] card. The check isn't much, only about $564 a month, but you know I just consider myself blessed. And now I don't worry about my health, I will be taken care of.

Aida, age 74, 1993

People living in the United States represent all levels of education, experience, and income. It is rare to meet an older adult who does not have experience with the health care system in his or her country of origin. Health care in the United States is in a state of flux in the face of skyrocketing costs, financial constraints, and the increasing number of older adults.

This chapter will review the major mechanisms by which eligible elders (beneficiaries) in the United States receive a basic income and health insurance in place at the time of this writing. It is recognized that the Affordable Care Act of the Obama administration has affected the health of older adults in at least two major ways already. The first is expanded access to preventive care and the second is reduced medication costs discussed later in this chapter. These benefits may no longer be available by the time this edition is published.

The chapter concludes with a discussion of common key legal issues related to a person's capacity to make informed health care decisions.

LATE LIFE INCOME

Until the early 1900s most families lived in agricultural areas. An elder usually worked in some way until death. If care was needed, an extended network of family, friends, and community members could provide whatever support was necessary (Achenbaum, 1978).

The social and financial basis of the family changed when people moved from rural areas to cities, seeking work in factories. Whole families worked to survive, including very young children. The work was onerous and fraught with demands that became increasingly difficult to meet as one aged. The family was no longer available to provide care or support for older and disabled family members.

In 1935 the Social Security Act was passed and has been considered by many to be one of the most successful federal programs. Its primary function was to provide monetary (but not medical) benefits to lift the burden on families (SSA, n.d.a).

Social Security

Social Security was designed as a pay-as-you-go system. Payroll taxes collected from employees and employers are immediately distributed to beneficiaries (retirees, the disabled, eligible spouses, or children). Although individually deposited, the revenues are not reserved for any one individual; that is, no one has an account reserved in his or her name. All funds that are not immediately paid to beneficiaries are "borrowed" by the federal government for regular operating expenses.

At the time of its inception the system was constructed to transfer funds from those believed to be relatively prosperous (workers) to those believed to be relatively poor (e.g., the elderly). Social Security and a number of programs that followed were established as "age-entitlement" programs. This meant that they are available to persons at a certain age regardless of other sources of personal income or assets. They were and are, however, limited to U.S. citizens and legal residents older than a designated age who have previously earned the required amount of "credits" or to a dependent of someone who has met these criteria. Credits are based on income from sources in which Social Security taxes were withheld. One credit was equivalent to $1260 in 2016 with a maximum of four credits in a year for an income of $5040. Special rules apply for earnings of less than $400. Persons born in 1929 or later must have 40 credits (in 10 years) to be eligible for Social Security retirement benefits (referred to as "Social Security"); the number of required credits decreases for those born before 1929. Eligibility further takes into account a number of circumstances, including disability, spousal income, dependent parents, and survivors of different ages (SSA, 2015a).

The amount of Social Security received is calculated in part on the person's average salary during 10 of his or her working years. If one did not earn the requisite credits, the "nonworking years" count as zero in the calculation. This has been most beneficial to older white men, who are more likely to have worked the most consistently at higher salaries than any other group. It has been most disadvantageous for persons of color and for many women who took time off for child or parent care or were paid in cash (Hooyman & Kiyak, 2008). The average Social Security monthly stipend in 2016 was $2212 for a couple when both are receiving benefits.

Except under special circumstances, 62 is the earliest age when one may begin receiving Social Security. However, the amount received is less than it would be at "full retirement age" (i.e., 65 years of age for those born later than 1938). The age of eligibility for full benefits is increasing (Table 7.1). For those who choose or need to work beyond the age of full retirement, earnings continue to increase one's record of earnings and there will be higher benefits at retirement. This increase will continue until the age of 70.

Overall, a person's highest median income occurs between ages 45 and 55 years, after which it declines each decade to age 65, from $70,832 to $36,895, respectively. However, there is great variation by race and ethnic group, with those of Asian descent having the highest income and African Americans having the lowest. Compared with wages paid to male employees for a specific occupation, female workers have consistently earned 79% of that value, which is translated into lower Social Security upon retirement (DeNavas-Walt & Proctor, 2015).

The amount of benefit a person receives potentially increases each year on January 1 in the form of a

TABLE 7.1 Full Retirement Age

Year of Birth*	Full (Normal) Retirement Age
1937 or earlier	65
1938	65 and 2 months
1939	65 and 4 months
1940	65 and 6 months
1941	65 and 8 months
1942	65 and 10 months
1943–1954	66
1955	66 and 2 months
1956	66 and 4 months
1957	66 and 6 months
1958	66 and 8 months
1959	66 and 10 months
1960 and later	67

*Persons whose birthday is January 1 should refer to the previous year.
Data from Social Security Administration: *Retirement planner: Benefits by year of birth.* Available at http://www.socialsecurity.gov/retire2/agereduction.htm. Accessed June 2016.

cost-of-living adjustment (COLA) based on the consumer price index (CPI) for the previous year. Since the CPI was lower in 2015 than that in 2014, a COLA for 2016 was not allocated (SSA, n.d.b).

Supplemental Security Income (SSI)

Not all older persons living in the United States have Social Security benefits adequate to provide even the most basic necessities of life. This has been especially true for many of today's older adults. If they spent their lives employed in the agricultural industry, as domestic workers, or in the service industry and were paid very low wages, Social Security taxes were not withheld by their employers, or they were paid on a cash basis. SSI was established in 1965 to provide a minimum level of economic support to older adults and select others. Of the 9.1 million people who received SSI for at least 1 month in 2015 older adults comprised only 2.1 million of these (SSA, 2015b; SSA, 2015c).

Among the eligibility requirements are a very low income and few resources ($2000 per individual and $3000 per couple) excluding one's home and prepaid burial expenses. The maximum SSI benefit to persons at least 65 years of age was $733 for an individual and $1100 for an eligible couple, with an average of $526 per person in 2016. There is potential supplementation to the maximum benefit allowed by the state of residence. Unlike Social Security, the amount is reduced by any countable income such as cash or in-kind contributions, including housing or food (SSA, 2015b).

Other Late Life Income

Finally, late life income may come from private retirement investments or employer pensions. Monies are held for the beneficiary until such a time when he or she must begin to "withdraw" all or a portion of the money at the age determined by the fund. Often the beneficiary can elect to take his or her pension in one lump sum or in a monthly amount based on his or her own anticipated life expectancy, or based on the life expectancy of a spouse or partner. In other words, a person may establish a plan so that he or she receives all or most of the benefit during his or her expected lifetime rather than providing for any survivor benefit. Notification of the potential survivor of such a choice is now required, but was not always so in the past. This may still affect some older survivors (Box 7.1).

The median income of married couples 65 years and older was $52,772 in 2013 but only $18,643 for individuals. Since women continue to earn significantly less than their male counterparts (about $29,327 for males and $16,301 for females, generalized from all racial and ethnic groups), this can have significant implications for poverty rates among women (10.4%) (DeNavas-Walt & Proctor, 2015; SSA, 2015b).

BOX 7.1 A Surprising Change of Income

Mrs. Jones lived in a small rural community. Her husband had worked for the same company from the time he was 18 until he died. His pension and Social Security benefits were small due to a lifetime of low wages. When Mr. Jones died suddenly, Mrs. Jones was informed that she would no longer receive support from his pension. When he enrolled, he had opted for the "no survivor benefit," meaning that all benefits would cease upon his death.* Because she had never worked outside of the home, Mrs. Jones was dependent solely on her husband's Social Security as his widow. She was in danger of losing her home because she could not afford her taxes.

*NOTE: This is no longer legal without the express permission of the potentially surviving spouse.

The major sources of income as reported by older persons in 2014 were Social Security benefits (84% of older persons), income from assets (51%), private pensions (27%), government employee pensions (14%), and earnings (28%). Social Security constituted 90% or more of the income received by 36% of beneficiaries, of which 22% were married couples and 47% were nonmarried beneficiaries, especially women (SSA, 2015b).

HEALTH CARE INSURANCE PLANS IN LATER LIFE

Until 1965 there were only a few successful insurance plans for wealthier working people. In most cases health care was on a fee-for-service, out-of-pocket basis. This meant that each health care service could only be obtained if delivered by the provider, bartered, or purchased for cash (or "out-of-pocket"). When costs were reasonable, many older adults could continue to pay for their care. However, as people began to live longer with more chronic health problems, advances in technology escalated, and costs for health care increased, paying for health care out-of-pocket became harder and even impossible for many older adults who were entirely dependent on limited incomes.

In today's economy there is an increasingly large disparity in income levels; there is a rising number of people with very high incomes and a rising number of people with low and very low incomes. Greater wealth enables persons to obtain any type of health care they desire, primarily through purchased insurance policies. For those older than 65 years of age, the primary plans in the United States are Medicare and Medicaid.

Medicare

With few exceptions health care has always been a purchased service in the United States. It is not considered a universal right. However, the federal government is the major purchaser of health care through its insurance plans (Medicare, Railroad Medicare, Medicaid, and TRICARE) or through direct care provided by Veterans Services. The major plan available to and used by eligible older adults (≥65 years of age) living in the United States is Medicare. Those with very low incomes may also be eligible for Medicaid, an insurance plan that is jointly funded by state and federal resources (referred to as "joint eligibility"). Although the cost is still beyond the reach of some, many younger adults have been able to purchase insurance in an exchange system within the U.S. health care "Market Place" through the Affordable Care legislation of 2010. These health insurance benefits are not available to persons eligible for Medicare.

In 1934 President Franklin D. Roosevelt tried to create a plan to provide universal health insurance for U.S. citizens. This was met with unbeatable opposition from groups such as the American Medical Association and, by poll, the majority of the American public (Cantril, 1951).

In 1965, through the efforts of President Lyndon B. Johnson, legislation (Social Security Act) was passed creating an insurance plan for all persons eligible for Social Security, SSI, or railroad retirement benefits. The U.S. Department of Health and Human Services created the Centers for Medicare and Medicaid Services (CMS) to administer these benefits. In 2013, 43.5 million people at least 65 years of age were enrolled in Medicare. The average benefit per enrollee was $11,910 a year (National Committee to Preserve Social Security and Medicare, 2016).

To be eligible for Medicare today, one must be eligible for Social Security. Otherwise, coverage must be purchased. Medicare only covers select services and requires that such services are medically necessary. This means that the prescribed treatments and services are needed for the prevention, diagnosis, or treatment of a medical condition; meet the standards of good medical practice; and are not performed for the convenience of the health care provider. The costs related to Medicare are covered by a total employer and employee tax of 2.9% and by the beneficiary in the form of premiums, deductibles, and co-pays (National Committee, 2016).

Medicare Part B is a subsidized insurance plan to cover the costs of seeing health care providers and several other services. Medicare Part C was created as an alternative to Medicare Part B. The costs of outpatient medications were not covered by Medicare until 2006, when an elective drug plan (Medicare Part D) was created under President G. W. Bush's administration. The Affordable Care Act added the Annual Wellness Visit (Box 7.2) to the "Welcome to Medicare Visit" established under President G. W. Bush (Box 7.3).

Further services, several of which are relevant to older adults, were added through the Affordable Care Act under the Obama administration (Table 7.2).

Between October 15 and December 7 (open enrollment) of each year, persons with Medicare may make changes to any of the component Parts B, C, or D (see below). Medicare Part A does not change. If new coverage is elected, it will begin on January 1 of the next year (e.g., a change made on December 6, 2017, becomes effective January 1, 2018).

BOX 7.2 Annual "Wellness" Visit*

Completion of a "Health Risk Assessment"

- A review of medical and family history
- Developing or updating a list of current providers and prescriptions
- Height, weight, blood pressure, and other routine measurements
- Detection of any cognitive impairment and depression
- A list of person-specific health advice risk factors and treatment options
- A screening schedule for appropriate preventive services

*The first Annual Wellness Visit must be at least 12 months after the "Welcome to Medicare" visit. This is a component of the Affordable Care Act and therefore subject to change.

Data from https://www.medicare.gov/coverage/preventive-visit-and-yearly-wellness-exams.html.

BOX 7.3 The "Welcome to Medicare" Exam

Must be obtained within 12 months of enrolling in Medicare Part B and includes:

- Review of medical record
- Review of social history related to your health
- Education and counseling about preventive services
- Health screenings, immunizations, or referrals for other care as needed
- Height, weight, and blood pressure measurements
- Calculation of body mass index
- Simple vision test
- Review of risk for depression and level of safety
- An offer to discuss advance directives
- Written preventive health plan

Data from https://www.medicare.gov/people-like-me/new-to-medicare/welcome-to-medicare-visit.html.

TABLE 7.2 Major Components of the Affordable Care Act That Affect Older Adults

Component	Description
Primary care	Incentives to providers based on quality and not just quantity of care ("evaluation of quality based indicators")
Bundled payments	Payment to hospital for entire "bundle of care," which will include both the hospital stay and the medical needs for a period of time after discharge
Demonstration projects	Welcoming of creative proposals to improve quality and control cost
Five-star programs	Yearly evaluation and ranking of Medicare Parts C and D plans, nursing homes and acute care hospitals, home health agencies, and a growing number of other sources for health care
Decreasing out-of-pocket costs for prescription medications	Reduce current size of donut-hole and decrease the co-pay in the donut-hole from 100% to 25%; donut-hole planned to be eliminated by 2020
No co-pays for preventive services with most evidence of usefulness*	Increased access to preventive services

*See http://www.medicare.gov/coverage/preventive-visit-and-yearly-wellness-exams.html for "Is my test, item, or service covered?"
Adapted from Byman JPW: Financing and organization of health care. In Ham RJ, Sloane PD, Warshaw GA, et al, editors: *Primary care geriatrics: A case-based approach,* ed 6, pp 92–101, Philadelphia, 2014, Elsevier.

BOX 7.4 Health Services Provided Through Medicare Part A (2016 Figures)

1. Acute care
   a. There is a $1288 deductible (each stay) for days 1 to 60 but no co-pay (each stay)
   b. Days 60 to 90 co-pay $322/day
   c. One lifetime reserve of 60 additional days at $644/day
   d. No coverage after 150 days
   e. Deductibles and co-pays increase every year
   f. The deductibles and co-pays are either paid out-of-pocket or reimbursed by Medicaid or Medigap policies
2. Skilled rehabilitative nursing care in a health care facility (only when care by a licensed nurse or physical or occupational therapist is needed):
   a. Only after a minimum 72-hour acute care hospital admission
   b. The first 20 days are covered at 100%
   c. Days 21 to 100 with a daily co-pay of more than $161
   d. No coverage after 100 days
   e. Coverage ceases the day skilled care is no longer needed
3. Home health services requiring skilled care (only when care by a licensed nurse or physical or occupational therapist is needed):
   a. Intermittent skilled care for the purpose of rehabilitation provided in the home
   b. The person must be ill enough to be considered homebound
   c. Medicare pays 80% of allowable costs
4. Hospice care (provided for terminally ill persons expected to live less than 6 months who elect to forgo traditional medical treatment for the terminal illness):
   a. No co-pay
   b. Co-pay of 5% for limited respite or pain management stays
   c. Replaces Medicare Parts A and B for all costs associated with the terminal condition
5. Inpatient psychiatric care:
   a. $1288 deductible for each stay
   b. Day 1-60: no co-pay
   c. Day 61-90: $322/day co-pay
   d. After day 90 start using lifetime reserves of 60 days with co-pay of $644/ day
   e. 20% of physician services while inpatient

Data from Centers for Medicare and Medicaid Services: *Your Medicare coverage,* n.d. Available at https://www.medicare.gov/coverage/is-your-test-item-or-service-covered.html. Accessed August 14, 2016.

Medicare Part A

Medicare Part A is free to those who receive Social Security. As an "age entitlement" program, it provides insurance to eligible beneficiaries regardless of their personal financial status. Medicare Part A is a plan covering acute hospital care, short-term acute rehabilitative care, and costs associated with hospice and home health care under certain circumstances. Unless already a Medicare recipient for some other reason (e.g., end-stage renal disease), a person is automatically enrolled in Medicare Part A on the first day of the month of his or her 65th birthday. The deductible and co-payments under Part A vary by setting and can be quite high (Box 7.4).

For any Part A coverage in skilled nursing homes or acute rehabilitation hospitals, the transfer must be directly from an acute care facility after at least a 72-hour *admission.* Extended hours spent in an emergency department or even on a hospital unit for the purpose of *observation* do not apply (CMS, 2015a). As a result of the significant financial ramifications, this important distinction should be made very clear so that the individual and/or caregivers can plan accordingly. When the assistance needed is limited to personal care or medication supervision, it is not covered by Medicare at all.

There are no prehospitalization requirements for the receipt of skilled home health care. To be considered a covered service, however, nursing care or physical, occupational, or speech therapy must be required on an intermittent basis with the goal of restoring the person to a prior level of functioning and preventing the necessity of 24-hour skilled care. The care must be provided at the written direction of a physician and by a Medicare-certified agency.

Medicare Part B

A person who is eligible for Part A must apply for Part B through the local Social Security Administration office in the 6 months surrounding his or her 65th birthday (from 3 months before to 3 months after the birth month) (Box 7.5). At the time of enrollment the person will be asked to choose either the *"Original"* Medicare Part B plan (Box 7.6) *or* one of the alternative plans available in the person's geographical area. If beneficiaries do not apply during their initial eligibility period, they must wait for the next "open enrollment period" and significant penalties may be levied.

The *Original Medicare Part B plan* is based on a traditional fee-for-service arrangement. The patient buys the insurance policy and receives services from a provider, a bill for the costs of care is sent to Medicare, and the patient is billed for the associated co-pays and deductible. Medicare reimburses physicians at a rate of 80% of what it considers an "allowable charge" for necessary medical services (CMS, n.d.). The patient is responsible for the remaining 20% of the charge. A provider who "accepts assignment" cannot charge a patient any more than the 20% of the "allowable charge." The number of physicians and nurse practitioners who accept assignment is decreasing rapidly. Providers who do not accept assignment may charge the patient up to 15% more than the allowable charge and are not required to bill Medicare directly. As the "allowable" for mental health services is very low, those who accept assignment are rare.

With the Original Medicare Part B plan, the patient is responsible for a monthly premium (usually deducted directly from the monthly Social Security check), an annual deductible, and co-pays. The premium is now based on income and marital status and was $104.90 in 2016 for individuals with incomes less than $85,000, increasing slowly until one's individual income is $335,000 (premium of $214 per month).

The advantages of the Original Medicare plan include choice and access. The person can seek the services of any provider of choice and without a referral from one's primary care provider. Some providers are members of Accountable Care Organizations (ACOs). The only difference when a person uses an ACO in conjunction with the Original Medicare Part B plan is that a group of providers have elected to work together and are able to share information about the patient to help provide the most coordinated care possible while maintaining

BOX 7.5 An Exception to the Late Enrollment Penalties

On April 3, 2014, the U.S. Department of Health and Human Services announced that the Social Security Administration was now able to process requests for Medicare Parts A and B and that the late enrollment penalties, under certain circumstances, would be waived for same-sex partners. This was based on the June 26, 2013, Supreme Court ruling that Medicare is no longer prevented from recognizing same-sex marriages for entitlement to, and eligibility for, benefits.

From U.S. Department of Health and Human Services: *HHS announces important Medicare information for people in same-sex marriages* (Press release), April 3, 2014. Available at https://www.medicare.gov/sign-up-change-plans/same-sex-marriage.html. Accessed November 2015.

BOX 7.6 Health Services Provided Through Medicare Part B

Designed to cover some of the costs associated with outpatient or ambulatory services. Deductibles and co-pays are required in most cases.

1. Physician, nurse practitioner, or physician assistant medically necessary services
2. Limited prescribed supplies
3. Medically necessary diagnostic tests
4. Physical, occupational, and speech therapy for the purpose of rehabilitation
5. Limited durable medical equipment if prescribed by a physician and indicated as documented medical necessity
6. Outpatient hospital treatment, bloodwork, and ambulatory surgical services
7. Some preventive services (many with no co-pay or deductible)
8. Diabetic supplies (excluding insulin and other medications) (see Chapter 20)

From Centers for Medicare and Medicaid Services: *Medicare: How much does Medicare cost?* n.d. Available at https://www.medicare.gov/your-medicare-costs/part-a-costs/part-a-costs.html. Accessed November 2015.

patient choice. There is no penalty for seeking care outside of the ACO (CMS, 2015b). Many people with the Original plan purchase Medigap (supplemental) policies to cover the deductibles and co-pays (see Supplemental Insurance/Medigap Policies).

Medicare Part C

Medicare Part C (also referred to as *Medicare Advantage Plans* or *MAP*) replaces both Medicare Part A and Medicare Part B; Part C plans are privately managed care plans similar to what we know as health maintenance organizations (HMOs) and preferred provider organizations (PPOs). The type and availability of such plans depend on location. All Part C plans are required to provide at least all of those benefits provided by the original Medicare Part B and may include extra benefits as well. Co-pays and deductibles, if any, vary considerably and extra premiums may be required for added services. All Medicare Part C plans have special rules that must be followed or services are only covered partially (PPOs) or not covered at all (HMOs).

The PPO plans work like the Original Medicare except that only specific providers can be used (those in the network) and the allowable charges are preset. Any additional services and fees or co-pays vary by plan. If a patient chooses to be seen by a provider outside the PPO, the services received may not be covered by the plan.

In HMOs the consumer "enrolls" to receive services at specific locations and from assigned primary health care providers. There are fewer out-of-pocket costs, but care received from providers outside of the network is not covered. Specialists cannot be seen without a referral from one's primary care provider. Medicare contracts with the private HMO to provide comprehensive services, financed by Medicare premiums paid directly to the company. The best of these are complete health care systems with highly trained physicians, nurse practitioners, and other health care professionals working out of single or regional completely equipped medical centers. Medical services are expected to emphasize preventive medicine, comprehensive care, periodic physical examinations, and immunizations. Aetna and Humana, the largest of these plans, have recently merged.

Capitation is imposed on HMOs by Medicare; this means that the plan is paid a fixed amount each day for each enrollee regardless of the amount of care needed and provided. Although the intention of this design was to increase preventive care, in some cases it has created abuse and there are horror stories in which elders were denied necessary treatments, presumably motivated by the plan's desire to lower its costs. Patient protection laws now allow consumers to lodge complaints and initiate legal action against the HMO. The Center for Patient Advocacy supported a much needed bill that became law in October 1999; this bill allows appeals when a managed care plan (MCP) denies care, guarantees access to specialists when needed, ensures that health-related decisions are made by health care providers rather than bureaucrats, and holds MCPs legally accountable for medical decisions that cause harm.

The supplemental services offered may save the participant a considerable amount in the costs of medications, assistive devices, and professional consultation charges. Some HMOs provide extensive health education services, support groups, and telephone support services to homebound persons. The potential negative aspects of HMOs and PPOs include limited choice of, and acess to, providers.

Alternatives to Medicare Part C. Health care finance is changing in the United States and several new programs have emerged. One of these is the Private Fee-For-Service Medical Savings Account. In this plan, the federal government makes monthly payments directly into the person's own private savings account and when health services are obtained the individual pays for them directly. This program has high deductibles and the fees charged by the providers are predetermined on a contractual basis between the provider and Medicare. Although no contracted provider can deny services at the agreed rate, noncontracted providers are under no obligation to accept the rate. For information about the range of existing and pending plans, see http://www.medicare.gov.

Medicare Part D

Medicare Part D was created as part of the Medicare Modernization Act of 2003 and is an optional prescription coverage plan. For those interested in purchasing this plan, they must enroll within the same 6 months of initial Medicare eligibility to prevent paying possible penalties and waiting until the next open enrollment period. Medicare Part D is not one plan but is a designation for dozens of private plans that have met certain criteria and are approved by the CMS (Box 7.7). The premiums vary by company and reflect the range of medications covered and the person's income. At this time Medicare Part D has a "donut-hole." In other words, it is possible that after spending a certain amount in prescription co-pays the person may be faced with very limited coverage, and then higher ("catastrophic") coverage resumes. Changes to Medicare Part D as a result of the Affordable Care Act have included capping the maximum amount that pharmaceutical companies can charge. There is also a reduction in the size of the donut-hole, with it expected to no longer exist by 2020 (CMS, 2015c).

BOX 7.7 Medicare Prescription Drug Plans (PDPs)

Most PDPs are organized in a similar way with deductibles and co-pays; however, to be a provider in Medicare Part D, the insurance plan must meet the following specific guidelines (2016 figures):

1. Premiums based on the plan
2. Annual deductible as low as zero but no greater than $360
3. Co-pay of medications dependent on plan until $3310 has been spent
4. Uncovered period ("donut-hole"): out-of-pocket cost is 45% for brand name drugs and 58% for generic medications
5. After $4850 in any single year, "catastrophic coverage" begins with about 5% copays of all remaining medications for year

From *Drug coverage (Part D)*. Available at https://www.medicare.gov/part-d/index.html. Accessed August 14, 2016.

As with Medicare Part B and C plans there is an open enrollment period every year. Recipients should be encouraged to annually examine their current plan to ensure they are enrolled in the plan that provides the best coverage for their medications. Most plans change to some extent every year. There is a straightforward calculator comparing the medications needed, the plans available, and the associated costs at http://www.medicare.gov/part-d.

Supplemental Insurance/Medigap Policies

Because of potentially high deductibles and co-payments, people who have the financial resources to do so often purchase supplemental insurance plans, referred to as Medigap. Some are part of a person's retirement benefit or are available to members of organizations such as the American Association of Retired Persons (AARP). A monthly premium is paid and in exchange all or part of the co-pays and deductibles not covered by the "primary insurance" (e.g., Medicare) are paid. The gerontological nurse can refer persons searching for an appropriate plan to the Medicare website or can request a printed copy of the standard plans (available at http://www.cms.gov).

Medicaid

Another amendment to the Social Security Act of 1965 created a second form of insurance for the elderly, the disabled, and children with very low incomes, known as *Medicaid*. Medicaid was designed to help states defray expenses of the very poor; this included elders who did not qualify for or could not afford to purchase Medicare Parts B/C and Medicare Part D or to pay the required deductibles or co-payments. Nearly all of these elders are "dually eligible" or qualify for both Medicare and Medicaid.

For a person who requires the financial support of Medicaid for a nursing home stay and has a spouse who is able to remain in the community, Congress enacted provisions in 1988 to protect him or her from "spousal impoverishment." Burial funds and only half of the combined value of the household goods, including the automobile (up to a limit), are counted as belonging to the patient, are used to determine eligibility, and are not expected to be used to pay for care. After the death of *both* spouses, it is expected that the amount Medicaid has spent on the care (and only up to that point) be reimbursed with any remaining funds in the couple's estate.

Within the broad guidelines established by the federal government, each state establishes its own eligibility criteria, determines the types and extent of services to be covered, sets the payment rates to providers, and administers its own programs. States pay about 40% of the costs with the federal government paying the remainder. This means that the Medicaid services available to the poorest of the elderly are dependent on the affluence and the policy of a given state. Alabama, with one of the highest percentages of poor residents, also has one of the lowest state incomes and therefore one of the lowest levels of Medicaid services. In most cases, Medicaid covers more services than Medicare, including custodial care in nursing homes.

More states are turning to Medicaid MCPs and HMOs and requiring persons who are dually eligible to enroll in these plans in an attempt to control costs. Waiver programs (that is, alternative and sometime innovative models) are used in some states to further control costs by providing extra support to help keep Medicaid-eligible elders in their own homes and out of nursing homes. Medicaid does not help the near-poor: those who cannot qualify for aid but cannot afford basic health care.

In some states there have been "Medically Needy" and Medicare saving plan programs, with month-to-month Medicaid coverage provided only during the months the elders' medical expenses exceed a preset threshold. With the financial crisis that states have been experiencing, many of these programs have been abandoned and services under Medicaid have been reduced. The Affordable Care Act (referred to as "Obamacare") has created some alternatives for these lost services but the programs are in great dispute at the time of this writing.

The premise of Medicare and Medicaid managed care is that better outcomes will result from systems of care that integrate professionals in responsive teams, maximize the use of sub–acute care, and provide incentives to reduce the reliance on institutional acute care.

Managed care systems are most effective for individuals enrolled over a long period who use ongoing primary care and preventive strategies to maintain health and avoid high-cost emergency services and intensive treatment.

Other Means to Finance Health Care

In some parts of the country (and for some persons), alternative plans have been developed to both finance and provide for health needs while aging.

Indian Health Services

The Indian Health Service (IHS) is a federal health program for and with American Indians and Alaskan Natives (http://www.ihs.gov). Services are provided both at the Tribal level and through Urban Indian Health Programs. Traditional IHS is available to documented members of one of the Indian Nations who have no other source of care (e.g., Medicare, Medicaid, TRICARE). There are a number of programs in development and implementation intended to promote health promotion at all ages, ranging from those who are aging healthfully to those caring for aging and debilitated elders (see http://www.ihs.gov/ElderCare).

Care for Veterans

The Veterans Health Administration (VA) system has long held a leadership role in gerontological research, medical care, and extended care. A great deal of the research that has guided gerontologists was generated through the VA system. It has been a model for continuity of care with a variety of care provider systems in place. Since its inception, these included VA-run nursing homes, home care and community-based primary care programs, respite care, blindness rehabilitation, mental health, and numerous other services in addition to acute medical-surgical hospitals. As a result of a combination of budget cuts and an increasing number of veterans in need of care, services have become more restricted, but the needs of veterans, especially those who were active in a war zone, have remained a priority.

At one time, veterans' hospitals and services were available on an as-needed basis for anyone who had served at any time. It was not necessary for individuals to use their Medicare benefits. However, this system has undergone significant change. One of the first changes was the placement of restrictions on the use of veterans' hospitals and services. Instead of coverage for any health problem, priorities were set for those problems that were in some way deemed "service-connected"; in other words, the problem had to be linked to the time the person was on active duty. In addition, those receiving Medicare benefits are expected to apply for and use that payment mechanism first before the VA will cover medical expenses, usually through TRICARE.

TRICARE for life. TRICARE for Life (TFL) is the health care insurance program provided by the Department of Defense; it is available for active duty and retired military/uniformed service personnel and their dependents. This plan requires the person to enroll in both Medicare Part A and Medicare Part B and pay the premiums for Part B. As a Medigap policy, TFL covers those expenses not covered by Medicare, such as co-pays and prescription medicines. Dependent parents or parents-in-law may be eligible for pharmacy benefits if they turned 65 years of age on or after April 1, 2001, and are already enrolled in Medicare Part B. For more information, see http://www.tricare.mil.

Veteran aid and dependence. For those veterans who served in a war zone and receive a military pension, there is additional monetary support available to them if they need assistance with daily personal needs. The application process to the program, which is called "Aid and Attendance Pension," is quite cumbersome but may be especially helpful for those who need custodial care at home or in an assisted living facility. The veteran may qualify for monetary help for his or her own care or for care of a spouse, depending on circumstances. Other benefits change over time, such as the recent availability of funds to reimburse a veteran for travel to and from a physician's office. For those living in rural areas or dependent on companion transport services, this can be quite helpful. The nurse is encouraged to learn more about these services to promote care for the most indigent veterans (VeteranAid, 2015).

Long-Term Care Insurance

Some persons are electing to purchase additional insurance (long-term care insurance [LTCI]) for their potential long-term care needs. Ideally these policies cover the expenses related to co-pays both for nursing home and home care and for what is called custodial care, which is help with activities of daily living (ADLs). Traditionally these policies were limited to care in long-term care facilities and provided a flat-rate reimbursement to residents to help cover their costs. However, these policies are becoming more creative and innovative and may cover home care costs instead, or both LTC costs and home care costs under some circumstances. Because they do not receive any governmental subsidies, the premiums can be prohibitive.

Many plans are being marketed at present, although many do not reach the ideal benefits. The purchaser must be cautioned to read the policy carefully and understand all the details, limitations, and exclusions. There are particular concerns related to Alzheimer's disease because many policies exclude these individuals from home benefits and include very limited institutional benefits. The best LTCI packages have been negotiated by a large employer or state organization or association (see http://www.ANA.org). A useful resource for persons considering the purchase of long-term care insurance can be found at http://longtermcare.gov/costs-how-to-pay/what-is-long-term-care-insurance/.

LEGAL ISSUES IN GERONTOLOGICAL NURSING

In the day-to-day practice of caring for older adults, gerontological nurses face questions and situations that have legal components. While nurses (unless also attorneys) cannot provide any legal advice, it is imperative that they are aware of several key legal issues frequently encountered in their work. This basic knowledge is as important as the financial issues just discussed. Legal concerns are most often related to an individual's ability to make health care decisions and consent to treatment or research. Although this section is not intended to provide legal advice or encourage nurses to do so, it is intended to provide background into common protective issues the gerontological nurse will be exposed to in caring for older persons, especially those who are vulnerable.

Decision-Making

In the Western model of health care, decisions are expected to be based on the ethical concepts of autonomy and informed consent. The provider has a responsibility to inform the individual of the decision needed and the individual has the right and responsibility to make his or her decisions. In many cultures, decision-making responsibilities, including decisions related to health care, are shared or delegated (see Chapter 2). Regardless of the culture, the responsibility to obtain informed consent often falls on the nurse. This task can be particularly difficult and complex because of a multitude of factors but can be made easier through advance planning if this acceptable in the person's culture (Box 7.8).

BOX 7.8 Factors Affecting the Responsibility of Nurses in Obtaining Informed Consent

1. Impaired sensory functioning
2. Low educational level
3. Low or limited health literacy
4. Low literacy of any kind
5. Questionable cognitive status
6. Complexity of procedure (e.g., surgery of any kind)
7. Participation in research

Capacity

Informed consent in health care is only possible with the assumption that adults have decision-making capacity. Decisional capacity means that a person is able to understand a problem, the risks and benefits of a decision, the alternative options, and the consequences of the decision. *Capacity is presumed when the legal age of "adult" is reached, unless the person has been adjudicated (decided by a court) to lack such capacity.* However, even in the absence of such adjudication, it is sometimes necessary to make professional judgments that influence accepting consent from a particular person, especially those with limited cognitive capacity or advanced frailty for any other reason.

Capacity is multifaceted. It ranges from the ability to accomplish instrumental activities of daily living (e.g., handle finances and daily business), to the capacity to complete one's most basic personal needs, to the capacity to make medical and specific health-related decisions. Capacity includes the ability to accept or decline complex health care treatments and procedures (e.g., consent to a surgical procedure). Giving consent to participate in research is more complex because it may or may not directly benefit the individual.

When the capacity of an individual to make informed decisions is believed to be impaired, only the courts can declare the person "incapacitated." He or she may be determined to have no or limited capacity in one area of his or her life but to have ability in another. For example, a person may be unable to adequately take care of day-to-day personal business such as bill paying but may still be able to make personal health care decisions. For those who are unable to speak for themselves or are unable (for any reason) to understand the consequences of their decisions, legal protection may be needed. Guiding principles are that protection is provided to those with questionable capacity in a manner that ensures that the person's needs are met, personal rights are protected to the extent possible, and the least restrictive type of protection necessary is used.

These types of protection include power of attorney, appointment of a health care proxy, conservatorship, and guardianship. It is important that nurses understand the differences and meaning of each.

Advance Care Planning

Gerontological nurses have the responsibility to encourage their patients, neighbors, and family members to discuss their wishes regarding potential incapacity, otherwise referred to as advance care planning. It is always advisable to appoint a legal surrogate or proxy (see following sections) and formally document one's wishes. The use of living wills is addressed in Chapter 28.

Power of Attorney

A *power of attorney* (POA) is a legal document in which one person designates another person (e.g., family member, friend) to act on his or her behalf. The two types are a general POA and a durable POA. The appointed person becomes known as the *attorney-in-fact*. The attorney-in-fact named in a general POA usually has rights such as to make financial decisions and pay bills in defined circumstances, but not necessarily to make decisions related to health care. The attorney-in-fact appointed in a durable POA usually has additional rights and responsibilities to make health-related decisions for persons when they are unable to do so themselves. This person is known as the *health care surrogate* or *proxy*.

POAs are in effect only at the specific request of the elder or, in the case of the durable POA, in the event that the person is unable to act on his or her own behalf. As soon as the person regains abilities, the POA is no longer in force unless the individual requests it to continue. The elder retains all of the rights and responsibilities afforded by usual law. This is the least restrictive form of protection and assistance, providing decision-making for persons with impaired capacity. An important aspect of the POA is that persons who are given decision-making rights are those who have been chosen by the elder rather than by a court. Because gerontological nurses work with people who are making decisions about the selection of a surrogate, they can encourage persons to carefully consider someone who is willing to uphold their wishes or holds similar values.

Health Care Proxy

Most state statutes and cultures provide a "hierarchy" of those who have the authority to act on a person's behalf when capacity has been either temporarily or permanently lost and preferences have not been documented or expressed in advance. For example, in the state of Florida this is written into Statute 765.401 and all health care facilities have the legal responsibility to follow this "order of decision-maker" (Box 7.9). The decision-making responsibilities proceed down the list until a willing proxy is obtained.

Both surrogates and proxies are expected to use "substituted judgment"; that is, decisions are made on the basis of what they believe the person would decide if able to do so and not the surrogate's choice in a similar situation (Zorowitz, 2014). The gerontological nurse can support the surrogate in following the person's wishes (Box 7.10).

BOX 7.9 Hierarchy of Appointments of Health Care Proxy by Florida State Statute, From First to Last

Guardian
Spouse
Majority of adult children
Parents
Majority of adult siblings reasonably available for consultation
Adult relative who has exhibited special care and has regular contact
Close friend
Licensed clinical social worker appointed by a bioethics committee

BOX 7.10 "I Know That Is What She Would Want but That Is Not What I Want"

Mr. and Mrs. Jones had been married for 60 years. She had developed Alzheimer's disease a number of years earlier and reached a point where she did not always know what to do with food in her mouth. She no longer recognized her husband and did not respond in any verbal way. In almost daily distress, her husband intermittently pleaded that a "feeding tube" be placed into her so she could "eat." However, Mrs. Jones had made it very clear to her husband and to all who knew her that she "never wanted artificial nutrition" or to do anything to stop a natural death when she worsened. When Mr. Jones asked for a feeding tube, the only thing we could say was that we were very sorry but her wishes had been made very clearly and that is what we were bound to follow. He agreed that those indeed were her wishes and started to cry.

Guardians and Conservators

Guardians and conservators are individuals, agencies, or corporations that have been appointed by the court to have care, custody, and control of a disabled person (ward) and manage his or her personal or financial affairs (or both) when the person has been found (adjudicated) to lack capacity.

Whereas a *conservator* is appointed specifically to control the finances of the ward, the person appointed to be responsible for the ward is usually called the *guardian*, although these terms are sometimes used interchangeably. The conservator or guardian continues in that role until the court rescinds the order. The appointment is made at a court hearing in which a person demonstrates the incapacity of the elder (who may not be present) and he or she is declared *incapacitated* (formerly called *incompetent*). How this is handled differs by state. In many states the ward is unable to petition the courts to have his or her rights restored.

In some states, limits are set according to the degree of protection needed. Total dependency means the person cannot meet basic needs for survival and is unable to manage the environment in any self-sustaining way. Some dependency means the person may be able to manage certain challenges of life; health or judgment may interfere with management of other needs. In the latter situation, a limited guardian may be appointed to protect the person in very specific ways.

There are considerable pros and cons in the use of conservatorships and guardianships, including risk for exploitation. The use of these mechanisms of care is the most restrictive and in most cases the person loses all rights to self-determination; therefore, appointment of conservators and guardians should only be considered in cases of severe impairment, such as advanced dementia. Nurses working with older adults and their families can encourage the use of advance planning to find alternatives that are less restrictive, noting that the definitions and rules vary among states.

❖ IMPLICATIONS FOR GERONTOLOGICAL NURSING AND HEALTHY AGING

Gerontological nurses have long been helping their older patients deal with financial issues, such as the following: Are adequate funds available for needed food and medication or for the co-payments for needed health care? Does the Medicare plan in which they are currently enrolled (Part B, C, or D) best meet their needs, or can the nurse refer them to a community organization to help them find a plan that will be better for next year (Box 7.11)? These questions may be part of the comprehensive assessment as described in Chapter 8 or be a specific issue under special circumstances. Nurses are able to use their well-known expert advocacy and negotiation skills in these situations.

Although nursing has long recognized the need for gerontological specialization, the law and lawyers have done so as well. The National Elder Law Foundation (NELF) is one of the few specialty organizations that certify lawyers who have demonstrated knowledge pertinent to the legal needs of older adults (http://www.naela.org).

Nurses and nurses' aides may be the first persons to notice the subtle changes signifying a potential change in capacity, indicating the need for an evaluation for reversible causes and then consideration of the extent of impairment. These concerns are first discussed with the individual; only when this is not possible are those legally designated as decision-makers involved. It is vital for the nurse to work within the applicable statutes of his or her state, province, or country. Nurses who are consulted by elders about legal issues should not attempt to provide legal advice, but instead should refer their clients to a NELF-certified attorney. The state or local bar association is a resource both for nurses and for elders and their advocates.

BOX 7.11 Tips for Best Practice

Helping Your Patients Enroll in Medicare Plans That Best Suit Their Needs

When it is time for the person to enroll in Medicare he or she can be referred to the Medicare website (http://www.cms.gov). At this website, the person will find not only information about plans available in his or her area but also information about the procedures for changing from one plan to another according to personal choice or change in needs. If the person has limited literacy or health literacy, he or she should be referred to the nearest Area Agency on Aging for guidance (for locations, see http://www.n4a.org).

KEY CONCEPTS

- Health care and its systems are undergoing profound changes, including an increase in the number of managed care organizations and changes in the roles of health care providers. All of these changes affect the care of the older adult.
- A combination of Social Security and Supplementary Security Income payments provides eligible persons with a regular income after the age of 65, or earlier if the person is disabled. The total amount varies greatly and is dependent on qualified income earned during the working years.
- There may be substantial out-of-pocket costs associated with the receipt of health care today.
- In order for Medicare to pay for the expenses related to long-term care or home health care, strict criteria of medical necessity must be met.
- The nurse can encourage and to some extent guide the person toward advance care planning.
- In the Western culture of health care, informed consent is based on the ethical principle of autonomy, which requires the capacity to understand a situation, the choices that are available, and the consequences of a decision.
- In the health care setting, an individual may be legally competent but have diminished or varying levels of capacity to make health-related decisions.

- Varying levels of protection are available to protect persons with diminished capacity to ensure their previously expressed wishes are followed.
- The nurse has a responsibility to ensure the safety and security of those persons to whom care is provided. This responsibility does not change with a change in the persons' legal status or capacity.

ACTIVITIES AND DISCUSSION QUESTIONS

1. Describe the role of the nurse advocate in relation to health and consumer protection.
2. Explain the fundamentals of Medicare and Medicaid sufficiently to assist elders in obtaining more specific information.
3. Interview an elder in a rehabilitation center or in an adult day health or senior center and ask about his or her experience in the setting and across settings.
4. Identify a person at least 70 years of age who has Medicare. Ask the person how Medicare does or does not meet his or her needs. Write a brief summary, and present it to the class.

REFERENCES

Achenbaum WA: *Old age in a new land*, Baltimore, 1978, Johns Hopkins University Press.

Cantril H: *Public opinion 1935–1946*, Princeton, NJ, 1951, Princeton University Press.

Centers for Medicare and Medicaid Services (CMS): *Medicare and you, 2016*, Baltimore, MD, 2015a, Author.

Centers for Medicare and Medicaid Services (CMS): *Accountable care organizations and you: Frequently asked questions (FAQs) for people with Medicare*, 2015b. Available at https://www.medicare.gov/Pubs/pdf/11588.pdf. Accessed November 2015.

Centers for Medicare and Medicaid Services (CMS): *Closing the coverage gap—Medicare Prescription drugs are becoming more affordable*, 2015c. Available at https://www.medicare.gov/Pubs/pdf/11493.pdf. Accessed November 2015.

Centers for Medicare and Medicaid Services (CMS): *Medicare: How much does Medicare cost?* n.d. Available at https://www.medicare.gov/your-medicare-costs/part-a-costs/part-a-costs.html. Accessed November 2015.

DeNavas-Walt C, Proctor BD: *Income and poverty in the United States: 2014*, Current Population Reports, Series P60-252, Washington, DC, 2015, U.S. Census Bureau.

Hooyman N, Kiyak H: *Social gerontology: A multidisciplinary approach*, New York, 2008, Pearson.

National Committee to Preserve Social Security and Medicare: *Fast facts about Medicare*, 2016. Available at http://www.ncpssm.org/Medicare/MedicareFastFacts. Accessed August 14, 2016.

Social Security Administration (SSA): *Social Security: How you earn credit*, 2015a. Available at https://www.ssa.gov/pubs/EN-05-10072.pdf. Accessed November 2015.

Social Security Administration (SSA): *Fast facts and figures about Social Security*, 2015b. Available at https://www.ssa.gov/policy/docs/chartbooks/fast_facts/2015/fast_facts15_text.html#page6. Accessed November 2015.

Social Security Administration (SSA): *Annual report of the supplemental security income program*, 2015c. Available at https://www.socialsecurity.gov/OACT/ssir/SSI15/ssi2015.pdf. Accessed November 2015.

Social Security Administration (SSA): *Social Security history*, n.d.a. Available at https://www.socialsecurity.gov/history/index.html. Accessed November 2015.

Social Security Administration (SSA): *Cost-of-living adjustment (COLA) information for 2016*, n.d.b. Available at https://www.socialsecurity.gov/news/cola/. Accessed 2015.

VeteranAid: *Find senior care options for veterans*, 2015. Available at http://www.veteranaid.org. Accessed November 2015.

Zorowitz RA: Ethics. In Ham RJ, Sloane D, Warshaw GA, et al, editors: *Primary care geriatrics: A case-based approach*, ed 6, Philadelphia, 2014, Elsevier, pp 77–91.

8

Assessment and Documentation for Optimal Care

Kathleen Jett

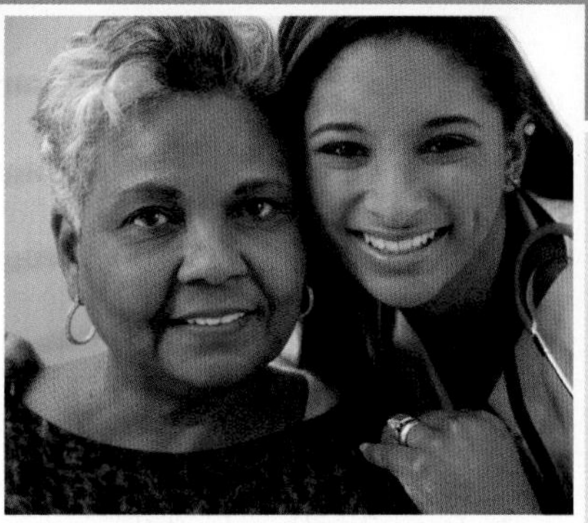

evolve.elsevier.com/Touhy/gerontological

LEARNING OBJECTIVES

Upon completion of this chapter, the reader will be able to:

- Identify key differences in assessing older adults and younger adults.
- Describe the range of tools that may be used in gerontological assessment.
- Discuss the advantages and disadvantages of the use of standardized assessment tools in gerontological nursing.
- Discuss the impact of common normal changes with aging on the assessment.
- Identify ways in which errors in documentation and communication are especially dangerous when caring for older adults.
- Compare the major documentation methods used in acute, long-term, and home care.

THE LIVED EXPERIENCE

I was so happy to be able to make a big difference in Mrs. Jones's life. She was 97 and had grown slowly confused over the years. She was also profoundly hard of hearing. She spent the majority of time calling for "Mary," her deceased sister. We really could not communicate effectively with her; we could only show her we cared and keep her safe. Eventually she became acutely ill, and a decision had to be made about CPR (cardiopulmonary resuscitation). When we tried to find out what her wishes were, we could not immediately find any record of them, and she had no living relatives or friends, just an attorney. I searched and searched and finally found documentation about her wishes. We were able to provide her the comfort she wanted because of a nurse's careful documentation years before.

Kathleen, GNP, at age 45

Gerontological nurses conduct skilled and detailed assessments of and with persons who entrust themselves to their care. Although many of the techniques used in the physical assessment of younger and older adults are the same, the overall process of working with the latter is strikingly different primarily because of the medical, psychological, and social complexity of late life. Older adults vary greatly in their health and function, from active and independent to medically fragile and dependent, making the assessment even more challenging.

Assessment of the older adult requires special abilities: to listen patiently, to allow for pauses, to ask questions that are not often asked and to obtain data from all available sources, and to understand that not all positive findings will require interventions. The nurse must be able to recognize normal changes of aging (see

Chapter 3) and atypical presentations to appropriately and effectively conduct assessments and interpret findings. The assessment must be paced according to the stamina of both the person and the nurse. If the elder is physically frail or cognitively impaired, is unable to speak, or does not speak the same language as the nurse, the health assessment becomes particularly difficult but even more important. The quality and speed of the assessment with complex older adults are a reflection of experience. Novice nurses should expect improvement in both of these assessment factors over time. According to Benner (1984), assessment is a task for the expert. However, an expert is not always available. By following some basic guidelines and learning how to use the wide range of assessment tools and resources now available, consistent quality is possible.

The assessment is not complete until it is documented. Nursing documentation is an age-old practice of making a permanent record of the conditions of our patients, our actions, and the patients' responses to our actions or those of others. Probably all of today's nurses know the mantra, "If you didn't document it—you didn't do it!" Further, if you did not document your findings then you cannot determine their efficacy.

In this chapter the basic concepts of the general assessment process as it applies to working with elders are reviewed as well as discussions of several of the most commonly used instruments that are used today. The chapter further provides the reader with basic information about documenting the assessment and other pertinent data in the health records of older adults in specific care settings. The instruments included are those most nurses may encounter in their day-to-day practice at some time. Those used in specialty situations can be found elsewhere in the text.

THE ASSESSMENT PROCESS

At a minimum, health assessment includes the collection of physical data and the integration of spiritual and psychosocial factors within an individual's cultural context. When working with older adults, additional assessment areas further include functional and cognitive status, caregiver stress or burden, patterns of health and health care, advance care planning, and the presence or absence of any of the *geriatric syndromes* (e.g., delirium, falls, dizziness, syncope, and urinary incontinence [see Chapter 17]). Areas or problems frequently not addressed by the care provider or mentioned by the elder that should be addressed are sexual function, depression, alcoholism, hearing loss, oral health, and environmental safety. Although not usually conducted by a nurse, a driving assessment may be recommended any time there is a question of ability. Questions regarding genetic background in this age group, especially for those in the younger range, have most relevance as they relate to Alzheimer's disease, stroke, diabetes, and several types of cancer.

BOX 8.1 Key Points to Consider in Observing Cultural Rules and Etiquette

- Be aware of past experiences in the health care setting.
- Ask if there are persons (e.g., males in the family) that need to be present or involved in some way with the exam.
- Respect the communication style used, especially in the health care setting.
- Do not intrude into personal space without permission.
- Be aware of general health orientation related to time (past, present, future).
- Inquire as to appropriate wording reference to the person; presume using last name unless otherwise welcomed.
- Inquiry as to acceptable level of touch and gender of provider.

Conducting an assessment begins with establishing rapport. It is never appropriate to address the patient by the first name unless invited to do so. The assumption of familiarity of any kind including the use of the first name in addressing an elder can easily be perceived as condescending, especially when the nurse is younger than the patient or of a different ethnic background (Box 8.1) (see Chapter 2).

There are three approaches used for collecting assessment data: self-report, report-by-proxy, and observation. In the self-report format, either questions are asked directly or the person is expected to respond to written questions about his or her health status. Patients tend to overestimate their own abilities, and older adults in particular have been found to under-report symptoms, often because of the erroneous belief that their symptoms are normal parts of aging. When assessment information is obtained indirectly (report-by-proxy) the nurse asks another person to report his or her observations. This approach is used extensively with persons who are cognitively impaired; the elder's abilities and health are often underestimated. In the observational approach the nurse collects and records objective and subjective data using parameters considered to be objective for performance-based functional assessments (e.g., the distance the person can walk).

The usual physical examination includes measurement of objective data such as blood pressure, pulse rate, and respirations, as well as subjective data such as the patient's appearance and level of awareness. Observation and the use of previously developed tools are probably the most accurate assessment methods but they are limited because they only represent a snapshot in time. It is especially dangerous to base conclusions regarding the health of older adults on these snapshots, because changes can and often do occur very rapidly.

Certain guidelines should be followed regardless of the approach used in the data collection:

- Whenever possible, conduct the assessment at a time when the patient is at his or her best.
- If a standard tool is being used, be sure it is used correctly; training may be required.
- To avoid biasing the response, do not direct the way the question will be answered.
- Attempt to obtain additional information only if it is needed to complete the assessment.
- Approach questions that are more personal (such as sexual functioning) in a matter-of-fact, but nonetheless sensitive, manner.
- Record the responses accurately, using the patient's own words whenever possible; do not analyze at the same time the data are being collected. For example, if the patient says "I have a runny nose," this is not recorded as "Patient has a cold."

The use of these guidelines is especially important when working with very frail elders who have particularly limited physical or cognitive stamina.

Ideally, the assessment should be used to gather baseline data before the older adult has a health crisis (e.g., the Welcome to Medicare Visit) (see Chapter 7). Persons free of chronic diseases or who are very stable can have an annual review of their health status and the preventive strategies they use at the time of their Annual Wellness Visit (see Chapter 7). For example, a person who has an altered mental status as a result of an illness or medication *(delirium)* should be reassessed when the underlying problem has been resolved.

The appropriate and accurate use of assessment and documentation instruments will increase the likelihood of obtaining reliable, useful data, especially data that can be used to monitor changes over time. This implies that data collection is always followed by analysis to determine the person's needs, which is followed by the development of nursing interventions. By accomplishing both, the nurse contributes to the nation's goal of increasing the quality of life for all Americans and the health of older adults (see Chapter 1).

Assessment instruments exist that can broadly categorize physical health, mood, motor capacity, manual ability, self-care ability, more complex instrumental abilities, and cognitive and social function. Assessments are completed in every setting. The assessments used depend both on the setting and on the purpose. Sometimes these tools are available directly from the gerontological literature or from payer sources like Medicare, and other times they are modified to meet a particular need.

Fortunately, we have a number of excellent instruments at our disposal. Several are discussed or referred to in this chapter. We ask the reader to note that those described herein serve only as examples of what is available. The *Try This: Series* available from the Hartford Institute for Geriatric Nursing is one of the sources for ever-evolving information, tools, and evidence-based protocols. There are videos and detailed instructions at the ConsultGeriRN website (https://consultgeri.org/education-training/e-learning-resources). Complete descriptions of the instruments, techniques for optimal use of the instruments with older adults, and access to the instruments themselves are usually available on-line for educational or clinical nonprofit use. Additional information about using any of the instruments as well as finding research related to any of the tools discussed throughout this text can be easily found through sources such as PubMed.

THE HEALTH HISTORY

The initiation of the health history marks the beginning of the assessment process. It begins with a review of what the *person* reports as a problem, known as the "chief complaint." This is considered subjective data that are documented in the patient's own words. In older populations, the "complaint" is often very vague because the interaction of the numbers of chronic diseases, medications used, and other factors obscures what may be a specific or even multifactorial problem. For example, it is not unusual for the person to say, "I just don't feel well."

The health history is best collected either verbally in a face-to-face interview or using the interview to review a written history completed by the patient or by the patient's trusted proxy beforehand. The written format should never be used if the person has limited vision, questionable reading level, or limited health fluency, or if it is written in a language or at a level in which the patient does not have reading fluency. Although it takes more time for patients to complete written formats, they are more advantageous for nurses because written formats permit the nurse to review patient data and then concentrate on specific information when meeting the patient. Whether collecting the history verbally or reviewing a previously written document, the nurse uses techniques that optimize communication. If the elder has limited language proficiency, a trained medical interpreter is needed and about twice the typical time must be scheduled for the visit. If the person has limited health fluency, special attention will need to be paid to wording of questions and answers to the patient's questions. If the person is cognitively impaired, he or she should be included to the extent possible with additional information obtained from a proxy who knows the person well (Box 8.2).

Any health history form or interview includes a patient profile, a medical history, a review of systems (Box 8.3), a medication history (see Chapter 9), and a nutritional history (see Chapter 10) as well as any other factors that influence the person's quality of life. The nurse should be aware that with an older adult the traditional review of systems may be quite lengthy because of the number of years the person has had the opportunity to be affected by illness or disease. It may be easier and more appropriate to begin with reviewing the symptoms (i.e., ROS = review of symptoms) the person is currently having and then guide the review

BOX 8.2 Speaking to the Wrong Person

Madame DuBois came to the clinic for a checkup related to her diabetes and hypertension, both of which were out of control. She spoke no English. At the first visit the nurse spent a long time explaining the plan of care through an interpreter, making the interaction especially time-consuming for the patient, the nurse, and the person accompanying Mdm DuBois. Few questions were asked. A different person accompanied Mdm DuBois at her next visit and asked the same questions that had been addressed in the first visit. The nurse then discovered that the woman at the second visit was actually the person who helped Mdm DuBois. The person at the first visit was a neighbor who happened to have time to accompany Mdm DuBois and thought it was impolite to question the nurse.

BOX 8.3 Tips for Best Practice

Areas of Emphasis When Conducting a Review of Systems With an Older Adult

Constitutional
- Change in the level of energy

Senses
- Changes in vision or hearing acuity and situations in which changes occur, or complaints of others related to these changes
- Increase in dental caries, changes in taste, presence of bleeding gums, level of current dental care
- Changes in smell

Respiratory
- Shortness of breath and, if present, circumstances in which this occurs
- Frequency of respiratory problems
- Need to sleep in chair or with head elevated on pillows

Cardiac
- Chest, shoulder, or jaw pain and circumstances in which pain occurs
- If already taking antianginal medication such as nitroglycerin, how often is it needed
- Sense of heart palpitations
- If using anticoagulants, any evidence of bruising or bleeding

Vascular
- Cramping of extremities, decreased sensation (see also Neurological), edema (including time of day and amount)
- Change of color to the skin, especially increased pigmentation of the lower extremities, cyanosis, or any other change in color

Urinary
- Changes in urine stream and length of time condition has been present; difficulty starting stream
- Incontinence and, if present, under what circumstances and degree; personal strategies used to address urinary incontinence (e.g., pads)

Sexual
- Desire and ability to continue physical sexual activity
- Ability to express other forms of intimacy
- Changes with aging that may affect sexual functioning (e.g., vaginal dryness, erectile dysfunction)

Musculoskeletal
- Pain in joints, back, or muscles
- Changes in gait and sense of safety in ambulation
- If stiffness is present, when it is the worst and when it is relieved by activity
- If limited, effect on day-to-day life

Neurological
- Changes in sensation, especially in extremities
- Changes in memory other than very minimal
- Ability to continue usual cognitive activities
- Changes in sense of balance or episodes of dizziness
- History of falls, trips, slips

Gastrointestinal
- Continence, constipation, bloating, anorexia

Integument
- Dryness, frequency of injury, and speed of healing
- Itching, history of skin cancer, sun exposure

accordingly. In the oldest older adult, family history in and of itself becomes less important as the person ages, and it is replaced with the increasing importance of the social history. The social history includes current living arrangements, economic resources to meet current health-related or food expenses, level of family and friend support, and community resources available if needed. Tools to adequately measure social networks have been in development for a number of years. However, the many nuances and configurations of social support networks make standardized measurements difficult.

Finally, to meet the needs of our increasingly diverse population of elders, the use of questions related to the LEARN Model is highly recommended to complement the health history (see Chapter 2). The responses will better enable the nurse to understand the perception of the problem and to plan culturally and individually appropriate and effective interventions.

PHYSICAL ASSESSMENT

Nurses learn to conduct a complete "head-to-toe" when conducting a physical assessment. Although this is usually done when assessing younger persons, it is rarely possible when working with an older adult, especially one who is medically complex or fragile. To do so would be excessively time-consuming and burdensome to all involved. Instead the assessment is first directed to that which is most likely associated with the presenting problem or major diagnoses and progresses from there. When performing a physical assessment the gerontological nurse must be able to quickly prioritize what is the most necessary to know (based on the chief complaint) and proceed to what would be "nice to know."

If the chief complaint is not known, such as in persons with moderate to advanced dementia, in persons who are unable to express themselves (such as those with expressive aphasia), or in the presence of any other type of language barrier, a more thorough assessment is always necessary. When the focus is on health promotion and disease prevention, the emphasis is on the major preventable health problems, especially obesity, cardiovascular disease, and illnesses associated with smoking.

The collection of data for the physical assessment begins the moment the nurse sees the person, noting skin color and texture and presence or absence of lesions. If the person "looks ill," this should be noted in the medical record with an explanation of this observation. Is the person able to ambulate alone or does he or she hold on to the walls along the way to the exam room, dining room, or bathroom? Are assistive devices used? Is the person able to follow directions when the nurse uses a normal voice volume or is an elevated one needed? If unable to follow directions at all or only with difficulty, it will be necessary to determine whether this is related to sensory losses or indicates cognitive impairment.

While considering the expected findings related to normal age changes discussed in Chapter 3, the manual techniques used in the physical exam are applicable to any age group and the reader is referred to any number of excellent textbooks solely dedicated to this. However, extra time is usually needed for dressing and undressing older patients, and some positions (e.g., lying flat for an abdominal exam) may not be possible. Several modifications may be necessary due to common changes seen in later life (Table 8.1).

Most often the physical exam is only one part of the evaluation of one or more other aspects of the person and his or her life. Because of the complexity of life and health in later life, this elevates the responsibility of the nurse. The nurse working in the geriatric setting must have a considerable repertoire of physical assessment skills and be able to draw upon these as the circumstance arises; in some cases this may need to be done quickly. In most circumstances the quality of care the elder receives is dependent on the quality of the assessment conducted.

Comprehensive Physical Assessment of the Frail and Medically Complex Elder

The mnemonic *FANCAPES* stands for Fluids, Aeration, Nutrition, Communication, Activity, Pain, Elimination, and Socialization. The guide was developed by Barbara Bent (2005) in her work as a geriatric resource nurse at Missouri Hospital in Asheville, North Carolina. It has broad applicability in any setting. It is a model for a comprehensive yet prioritized, primarily physical assessment that is especially useful for the frail elder (Resnick & Mitty, 2009). It emphasizes the determination of very basic needs and the individual's functional ability to meet these needs independently. It can be used in all settings, may be used in part or whole depending on the need, and is easily adaptable to functional pattern grouping if nursing diagnoses are used.

F—Fluids

What is the current state of hydration (see Chapter 11)? Does the person have the functional capacity to consume adequate fluids to maintain optimal health? This includes the abilities to sense thirst, mechanically obtain the needed fluids, swallow them, and excrete them. Medications are reviewed to identify those with the potential to affect intake. This is especially important when working with older adults who are not able to

TABLE 8.1 Considerations of Common Changes in Late Life During the Physical Assessment

Height and weight	Monitor for changes in weight. *Weight gain:* Especially important if the person has any heart disease; be alert for early signs of heart failure. *Weight loss:* Be alert for indications of malnutrition from dental problems, depression, or cancer. Check for mouth lesions from ill-fitting dentures.
Temperature	Even a low-grade fever could be an indication of a serious illness. Temperatures as low as 100° F may indicate pending sepsis.
Blood pressure	Positional blood pressure readings should be obtained because of the high occurrence of orthostatic hypotension. Both arms should be checked (at heart level) and the arm with the highest measurement should be recorded. Isolated systolic hypertension is common.
Skin	Check for indications of solar damage, especially among persons who worked outdoors or live in sunny climates. Because of thinning of skin, "tenting" cannot be used as a measure of hydration status.
Ears	Cerumen impactions are common. These must be removed before hearing can be adequately assessed or tympanic membrane visualized.
Hearing	High-frequency hearing loss (presbycusis) is common. The person often complains that he or she can hear but not understand because some, but not all, sounds are lost. The person with severe but unrecognized hearing loss may be incorrectly thought to have dementia.
Eyes	Lids sag and position of lids may change. Reduced pupillary responsiveness (miosis) occurs (normal if equal bilaterally). Gray ring around the iris (arcus senilis) may develop.
Vision	Person exhibits increased glare sensitivity, decreased contrast sensitivity, and need for more light to see and read. Ensure that waiting rooms, hallways, and exam rooms are adequately lit. Decreased color discrimination may affect ability to self-administer medications safely.
Mouth	Excessive dryness is common and exacerbated by many medications. Cannot use mouth moisture to estimate hydration status. Periodontal disease is common. Decreased sense of taste occurs. Tooth surface may be abraded.
Neck	Because of loss of subcutaneous fat it may appear that carotid arteries are enlarged when they are not.
Chest	Any kyphosis will alter the location of the lobes, making careful assessment more important. Risk for aspiration pneumonia is increased, increasing the importance of the lateral exam and the need for measurement of oxygen saturation. Evidence of pneumonia may not be evident if the person is dehydrated. Third heart sound indicative of pathology.
Heart	Listen carefully for third and fourth heart sounds. Faint fourth heart sounds may be heard. Determine if this was present in the past or is new. Up to 50% of persons have a heart murmur.
Extremities	Dorsalis pedis and posterior tibial pulses are very difficult or impossible to palpate. Must look for other indications of vascular integrity.
Abdomen	Because of deposition of fat in the abdomen, auscultation of bowel sounds may be difficult.
Musculoskeletal	Osteoarthritis is very common and pain is often undertreated. Ask about pain and function in joints. Conduct very gentle passive range of motion if active range of motion not possible. Do not push past comfort level. Observe for gait disorders. Observe the person get in and out of chair in order to assess independent function and fall risk.
Neurological	Although there is a gradual decrease in muscle strength, it still should remain equal bilaterally. Greatly diminished or absent ankle jerk (Achilles) tendon reflex is common and normal. Decreased or absent vibratory sense of the lower extremities is common, making testing unnecessary.
Genitourinary: male	Men have pendulous scrotum with less rugae. Have thin and graying pubic hair.
Genitourinary: female	Women have nonpalpable ovaries; short, dryer vagina; decreased size of labia and clitoris; sparse pubic hair. **NOTE**: Use utmost care with exam to avoid trauma to the tissues.

independently access fluids because of functional limitations, or for anyone with a reduced sense of thirst, a common change with aging (see Chapter 3).

A—Aeration

Because of the close relationship between pulmonary function (aeration) and cardiovascular function, they are assessed simultaneously. Is the person's oxygen exchange adequate for full respiratory functioning (see Chapter 22)? Measurement of the oxygen saturation rate is a part of this exam and easily done in any setting with a small, inexpensive fingertip device, familiar to most nurses. Persons with any amount of peripheral cyanosis will have artificially low readings. Is supplemental oxygen required and, if so, is the person able to obtain it? What is the respiratory rate and depth at rest and during activity, talking, walking, and exercising and while performing activities of daily living? What sounds are auscultated, what is learned from palpation and percussion, and what do they suggest? For the older person, it is particularly important to carefully assess lateral and apical lung fields.

N—Nutrition

What mechanical and psychological factors affect the person's ability to obtain and benefit from adequate nutrition (see Chapter 10)? What is the type and amount of food consumed? Does the person have the abilities to bite, chew, and swallow? What is the oral health status and what is the impact of periodontal disease if present? For edentulous persons, do their dentures fit properly and are they worn? If a special diet is recommended, has it been designed so that it is consistent with the person's eating and cultural patterns? Can the person afford the special foods needed? Is the person at risk for aspiration? Have preventive strategies been taught or provided, including meticulous oral hygiene?

C—Communication

Is the person able to communicate his or her needs adequately? Do the persons who provide care understand the patient's form of communication? What is the person's ability to hear in various environments? Are there any situations in which understanding of the spoken word is inadequate? If the person depends on lip-reading, is his or her vision adequate? Is the person able to clearly articulate words that are understandable to others? Does the person have either expressive or receptive aphasia (see Chapter 23), and if so has a speech therapist been made available to the person and significant others? What is the person's reading and comprehension levels? The impoverished childhoods of some individuals and the racist educational practices for others, even in developed countries, have resulted in very low or no literacy levels in these groups. It is best to assume that an elder's literacy is no greater than at a fifth-grade level in most settings. Inadequate assessment of communication by the nurse will lead to erroneous conclusions and significantly reduce the quality of care.

A—Activity

The ability to continue to participate in enjoyable activities is an important part of healthy aging. However, activity assessment is exceedingly complex because of the range of abilities among those referred to as "older adults." As more baby boomers join this group, the complexity of assessment increases. It ranges from the risk for falling and the need for, and correct use of, assistive devices to the degree to which one can participate in aerobic exercises. Assessment of activity abilities may be accomplished by the combined efforts of nurses, physical therapists, and personal trainers (see Chapters 13 and 15).

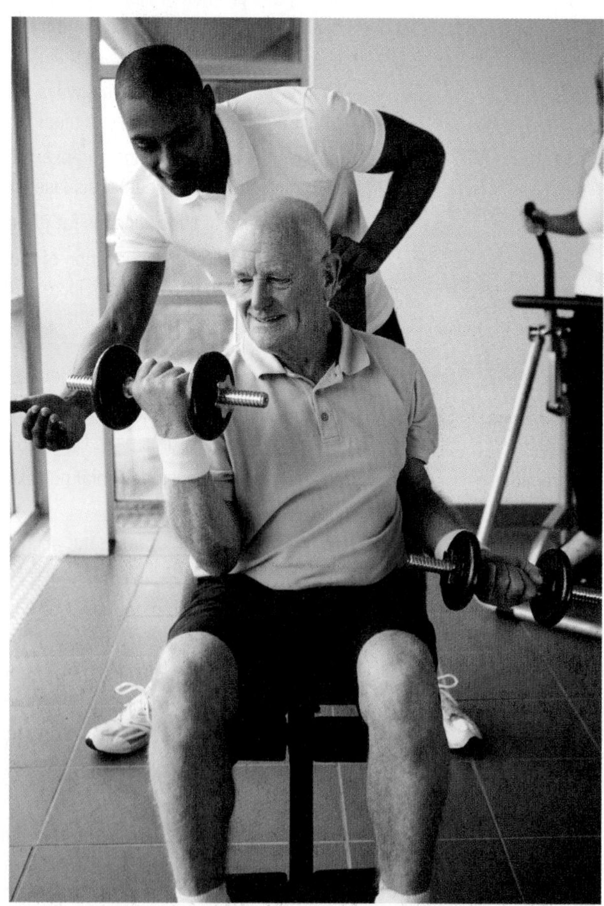

(©iStock.com/Dean Mitchell.)

P—Pain

Is the person experiencing physical, psychological, or spiritual pain? Rarely does one type of pain occur in isolation. Is the person able to express pain and relief of pain? Are there cultural barriers between the nurse and the patient that make the assessment or expression of pain difficult? Do cognitive limitations provide further barriers? How does the person customarily attain pain relief (see Chapter 18)? As a result of the increasing amount of pain common with each decade of life (e.g., progression of arthritis or number of losses), this deserves particular attention by gerontological nurses.

E—Elimination

While difficulties with bowel and bladder functioning are not normal parts of aging, they are more common than they are in younger adults and can be triggered by such things as immobility attributable to physical limitations (e.g., following a stroke) or medications (e.g., diuretics). Incontinence can result from cognitive changes that may cause reduction, or even absence, of the sensation indicating a need to void or defecate. There are many elimination problems for older adults living in institutional settings where they are dependent on others for assistance to maintain continence (e.g., getting to the toilet in time). Is the person having difficulty with bladder or bowel elimination (see Chapter 12)? Is there a lack of control? Does the environment interfere with elimination and related personal hygiene (e.g., are toileting facilities adequate and accessible)? Are any assistive devices used, such as a high-rise toilet seat or bedside commode, and if so, are they available and functioning? If there are problems, how are they affecting the person's social functioning and self-esteem?

S—Socialization and Social Skills

Socialization and social skills include the individual's ability to negotiate in society, to give and receive love and friendship, and to feel self-worth. The selection of persons included in one's social network is highly culturally influenced (Box 8.4). Assessment focuses on the individual's ability to deal with loss and to interact with other people in give-and-take situations. It is addressed in more detail in Chapters 16 and 28.

ASSESSMENT OF MENTAL STATUS

With increases in age there is an increased rate of neurocognitive illnesses, such as Alzheimer's disease and Lewy body dementia. Cognitive ability is also easily threatened by any disturbance in physical health, such as an electrolyte disturbance. Altered or impaired mental status may be the first sign of anything from a heart attack to a urinary tract infection. The gerontological nurse must be aware of the need to conduct an assessment of mental status, especially cognitive abilities and mood, whenever there is a change in an elder's condition or safety. Several of the most commonly used instruments are described here, with more details in Chapters 24 and 25. The nurse working in the geriatric setting is often expected to be proficient in their use. To ensure that the results are valid and reliable, they must be administered exactly as they have been created and tested.

> **BOX 8.4 Culturally Constructed Support**
>
> **Helen, Age 52**
>
> I grew up in a large extended Catholic family. As a growing child, all of our activities and even lives, revolved around the Church and the family. Now my cousins have grown and have families of their own. While we have been able to hold on to our affection, we live scattered across the country. Over the years I have also been apart from the Church. Now that I need support, I don't really have any experience reaching out for it—it was "just always there." I stay connected with my family through Facebook, but it is not the same.

Cognitive Measures

Mini-Mental State Examination

For many years the 30-item Mini-Mental State Examination (MMSE) has been the mainstay for the gross screening of cognitive status (Folstein et al., 1975; Mitchell, 2009). It is used to screen and monitor orientation, short-term memory and attention, calculation ability, language, and ability to correctly copy a figure (Wattmo et al., 2011). There is now a revised 16-item instrument, the *MMSE-2,* and a slightly longer *Expanded Version.* Both are reported to be equivalent to the original instrument and are available in multiple languages. To ensure reliability, the nurse must be able to administer them correctly each time they are used. The instruments, permission for use, and instructions for use can be purchased from Psychological Assessments Resources (PAR, http://www.parinc.com).

Clock Drawing Test

In use since 1992, the *Clock Drawing Test* is reported to be second in frequency of use to the MMSE across the world (Aprahamian et al., 2010; Ehreke et al., 2010). It is not appropriate for use with those who are blind or who have limiting conditions such as tremors, or a stroke that affects their dominant hand. Although reading fluency is not necessary, completion of the Clock Drawing Test requires number fluency, adequate

BOX 8.5 Clock Drawing Test

Instructions

Provide the person with a piece of paper with a predrawn large circle on it. Ask the person to:

1. Place the numbers 1–12 inside the circle as for a clock.
2. Place the hands so that the clock reads 10 minutes after 4.

Scoring

Draws closed circle	1 point
Places numbers in correct position	1 point
Includes all 12 correct numbers	1 point
Places hands in correct position	1 point

Interpretation

There are several viewpoints by psychologists about how the clocks are scored. All consider the following:

1. Executive functioning: The symmetry of the numbers, indicating ability to plan ahead: Are all numbers included? Are any numbers repeated or missed? Are the numbers inside or outside of the circle? Do they look like numbers?
2. Abstract thinking: Are there hands on the clock? Are they in the correct place relative to the numbers?

Data from Mendez MF, Ala T, Underwood KL: Development of scoring criteria for the clock drawing task in Alzheimer's disease, *J Am Geriatr Soc* 40(11):1095–1099, 1992; Tuokko H, Hadjistavropoulos T, Miller J, et al: The clock test: A sensitive measure to differentiate normal elderly from those with Alzheimer disease, *J Am Geriatr Soc* 40(6):579–584, 1992.

vision and hearing, manual dexterity sufficient to hold a pencil, and experience with analog clocks (Box 8.5). This tool cannot be used as the sole measure for dementia but it does test for constructional apraxia, an early indicator (Shulman, 2000) (Fig. 8.1). The Clock Drawing Test is an evidence-based instrument that has been found to be useful across cultures and languages and is a sensitive instrument to differentiate among those with and without some level of dementia (Borson et al., 1999; Tuokko et al., 1992).

The Mini-Cog

In some settings the use of the *Mini-Cog* has replaced the MMSE as a screening tool for cognitive impairment (Borson et al., 2000). It has been found to be as accurate and reliable as the MMSE but less biased, easier to administer, and possibly more sensitive to dementia (Mitchell & Malladi, 2010). The Mini-Cog combines the test of short-term memory in the original MMSE with the Clock Drawing Test (Box 8.6). It has been found to be equally reliable with English-speaking and non–English-speaking individuals (Borson et al., 2003).

BOX 8.6 The Mini-Cog

1. Tell the person that you are going to name three objects (e.g., apple, table, coin) and ask the person to repeat the objects after you and remember them (maximum of 3 tries).
2. Administer the Clock Drawing Test (see Box 8.5).
3. Ask the person to repeat the objects back to you.
4. Give 1 point for each recalled word, 2 points for a normal clock, and 0 points for an abnormal clock.

Score

0 recall	Indication of dementia
0–2 recall	Indication of dementia
3–5 recall	No indication of dementia

From Borson S: The mini-cog: A cognitive "vital signs" measure for dementia screening in multi-lingual elderly, *Int J Geriatr Psychiatry* 15(11):1021, 2000.

It serves as an indicator of the need for more detailed assessments leading to diagnosis. It requires the same basic skills as the Clock Drawing Test (Doerflinger, 2013).

The Global Deterioration Scale

The *Global Deterioration Scale* (Reisberg et al., 1982) is a classic measure of the levels of cognitive changes as one passes through the process of dementia (Table 8.2). It uses an ordinal scale from stage 1 (no cognitive decline; i.e., no dementia) to 7 (late-stage dementia; i.e., very severe cognitive decline) and is sensitive enough to show therapeutic changes (e.g., those related to medication adjustments) (Reisberg, 2007). It is commonly used in the United States, Canada, and many other countries (Alzheimer Society of Canada, 2016). It is useful to both the nurse and the family to develop appropriate interventions to help the person optimize his or her health and anticipate future needs and changes.

Mood Measures

Assessment of mood is especially important because of the high rate of depression in late life; it can occur as a side effect of a medication or develop in association with several health conditions, including stroke and Parkinson's disease (Bowker et al., 2012). Persons with untreated depression are more functionally impaired and will have prolonged hospitalizations and nursing home stays, lowered quality of life, and shortened length of life. They may appear as if they have dementia, and many persons with dementia are also depressed. The interconnection between depression and dementia necessitates skill and sensitivity in the nurse to ensure

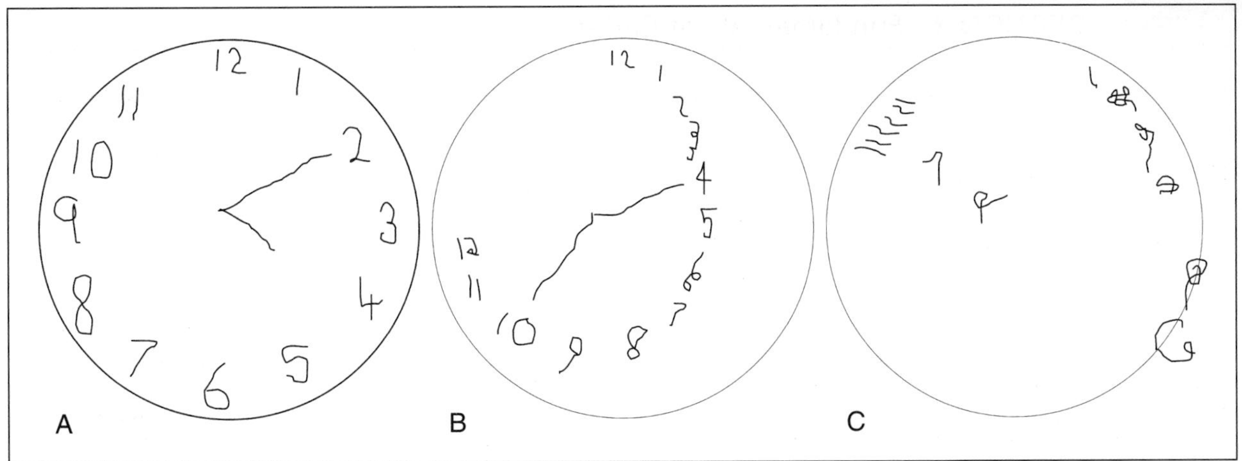

FIGURE 8.1 Examples of results of a clock drawing test. **A,** Unimpaired. **B** and **C,** Impaired. (From Stern TA, Rosenbaum JF, Fava M, et al: *Massachusetts General Hospital comprehensive clinical psychiatry,* St Louis, 2008, Mosby.)

TABLE 8.2 The Global Deterioration Scale

Diagnosis	Stage	Signs and Symptoms
No dementia	Stage 1: no cognitive decline	In this stage the person functions normally, has no memory loss, and is mentally healthy. People with no subjective or other thinking problems would be considered to be in Stage 1.
No dementia	Stage 2: very mild cognitive decline	This stage is used to describe normal forgetfulness associated with aging; for example, forgetfulness of names and where familiar objects were placed. Symptoms are not evident to loved ones or the physician.
No dementia	Stage 3: mild cognitive decline	This stage includes increased forgetfulness, slight difficulty concentrating, decreased work performance. People may get lost more often or have difficulty finding the right words. At this stage, a person's loved ones may begin to notice a cognitive decline. Average duration: 7 years before onset of dementia.
Early stage	Stage 4: moderate cognitive decline	This stage includes difficulty concentrating, decreased memory of recent events, and difficulties managing finances or traveling alone to new locations. People have trouble completing complex tasks efficiently or accurately and may be in denial about their symptoms. They may also start withdrawing from family or friends because socialization becomes difficult. At this stage a physician can detect clear cognitive problems during a patient interview and exam. Average duration: 2 years.
Midstage	Stage 5: moderately severe cognitive decline	People in this stage have major memory deficiencies and typically require some assistance to choose the proper clothing to wear. Memory loss is more prominent and may include major relevant aspects of current life; for example, people may not remember their address or phone number and may not know the date or the season. Average duration: 1.5 years.
Midstage	Stage 6: severe cognitive decline (middle dementia)	People in Stage 6 require assistance to carry out daily activities. They start to forget names of close family members and have little memory of recent events. Many people can remember only some details of earlier life. They also have difficulty counting down from 10 and finishing tasks. Incontinence (loss of bladder or bowel control) becomes a problem in the course of this stage. Personality changes—such as delusions (believing something to be true that is not), obsessions (repeating a simple behavior, such as cleaning), and/or anxiety and agitation—may occur. Average duration: 2.5 years.
Late stage	Stage 7: very severe cognitive decline (late dementia)	People in this stage have little or no ability to speak or communicate. They require assistance with most activities (e.g., using the toilet, eating). They eventually lose psychomotor skills, for example, the ability to walk. Average duration: 2 to 5 years.

From Reisberg B, Ferris SH, de Leon MJ, et al: The Global Deterioration Scale for assessment of primary degenerative dementia, *Am J Psychiatry* 139:1136–1139, 1982.

that elders receive the assessment and care they need (see Chapter 24).

Geriatric Depression Scale

The most commonly used mood measure in both middle-aged and older adults is the *Geriatric Depression Scale (GDS)*, developed by Yesavage and colleagues (1982). The GDS has been extremely successful in determining depression because it deemphasizes physical complaints, sex drive, and appetite—those things most affected by medications. It has been tested extensively with translations in multiple languages (Ortiz & Romero, 2008). A shortened 15-item version is now used (Table 8.3), with the free resources provided by Drs. Yesavage and Brink. The instrument can be completed on an iPhone or ANDROID with an automatic calculation of the results, which can be downloaded to a computer. It cannot be used in persons with dementia or cognitive impairment. Dr. Yesavage may be contacted directly at Stanford University for more information and a description of the products he has available. See also http://www.stanford.edu/~yesavage/GDS.html.

TABLE 8.3 Geriatric Depression Scale (Short Form)

Are you basically satisfied with your life?	Yes	No*
Have you dropped many of your activities and interests?	Yes*	No
Do you feel that your life is empty?	Yes*	No
Do you often get bored?	Yes*	No
Are you in good spirits most of the time?	Yes	No*
Are you afraid that something bad is going to happen to you?	Yes*	No
Do you feel happy most of the time?	Yes	No*
Do you often feel helpless?	Yes*	No
Do you prefer to stay at home, rather than going out and doing new things?	Yes*	No
Do you feel you have more problems with memory than most?	Yes*	No
Do you think it is wonderful to be alive?	Yes	No*
Do you feel pretty worthless about the way you are now?	Yes*	No
Do you feel full of energy?	Yes	No*
Do you feel that your situation is hopeless?	Yes*	No
Do you think that most people are better off than you?	Yes*	No

*Each answer indicated by an asterisk counts as 1 point. Scores greater than 5 indicate need for further evaluation. Contact Dr. Yesavage directly at Stanford University in Palo Alto, CA, or see http://www.stanford.edu/~yesavage/GDS.html.

From Yesavage J, Brink TL, Rose TL, et al: Development and validation of a Geriatric Depression Screening Scale: A preliminary report, *J Psychiatr Res* 17:37, 1982–1983.

FUNCTIONAL ASSESSMENT

A determination of functional status is part of the usual gerontological assessment. If the person is healthy and active, a simple statement may be all that is needed, such as "Patient is active and independent; denies functional difficulties." However, if any potential problems exist, such as for a person who has Parkinson's disease or for a person who recently fell, a more detailed assessment is conducted.

A thorough functional assessment includes the following:

- Identifying the specific areas in which help is needed
- Identifying changes in abilities from one period of time to another
- Assisting in the determination of the need for specific service(s)
- Providing information that may be useful in determining the safety of the current living situation

Functional abilities have been divided between those associated with the ability to perform the tasks needed for self-care (i.e., needed to maintain one's health), referred to as activities of daily living (ADLs), and those tasks needed for independent living, referred to as instrumental activities of daily living (IADLs). ADLs are most often identified as eating, toileting, ambulation, bathing, dressing, and grooming. Three of these tasks (grooming, dressing, and bathing) entail higher cognitive function than the others. The IADLs such as cleaning, yard work, shopping, and money management are considered to be more complex activities necessitating higher physical and cognitive functioning than the ADLs. For persons with dementia, the progressive loss of abilities begins with IADLs and progresses to the higher level ADLs. The nurse must keep in mind that both the willingness and the ability to perform skills are influenced by sociocultural factors unique to the person.

Numerous tools are available that describe, screen, assess, monitor, and predict functional ability. Like the health history, functional ability is measured by observation, self-report, or report-by-proxy. Most of the tools result in an arbitrary score of some kind—a rating of the person's ability to do the task alone, with assistance, or not at all. When such an assessment is conducted, the use of existing and established tools is recommended. However, most tools do not divide a task

BOX 8.7 Examples of Activities of Daily Living

- Bathing
- Dressing
- Using the toilet
- Transferring oneself
- Feeding oneself
- Controlling bowel and bladder function (continence)

From Katz S, Down TD, Cash HR, et al: Progress in the development of the index of ADL, *Gerontologist* 10(1):20–30, 1970.

into its component parts, such as picking up a spoon or cup and swallowing when assessment of eating is done; instead, eating is seen as a total task. The tools are useful in that they serve the purposes noted earlier. However, the ratings are not usually sensitive enough to show small changes in function and are more global in nature.

Activities of Daily Living

Activities of daily living (ADLs) were first classified by Sidney Katz and colleagues in 1963 (Katz et al., 1963). The *Katz Index* has served as a basic framework for most of the subsequent measures (Box 8.7). On the *Katz Index,* the ADLs are considered only in dichotomous terms: the ability to complete the task independently (1 point) or the complete inability to do so (0 points). Over the years this instrument has been refined to afford more sensitivity to the nuances of, and changes in, functional status (Nikula et al., 2003). Despite these limitations, the tool is useful because it creates a common language about patient function for all caregivers involved in planning overall care.

Barthel Index

The *Barthel Index (BI)* (Mahoney & Barthel, 1965; Wade & Collin, 1988) is a quick and reliable instrument for the assessment of both mobility and the ability to perform ADLs. The items are rated in various ways, depending on the item. The BI has been found to be sensitive enough to identify when a person first needs help and to measure progress or decline, especially following a stroke (Quinn et al., 2011).

Functional Independence Measure

The *Functional Independence Measure (FIM)* was designed to assess a person's need for assistance with ADLs during inpatient stays and for discharge planning, especially following a stroke (Cournan, 2011). In some studies the BI and FIM were found to be comparable. In other studies, the FIM was deemed preferable (Kidd et al., 1995). The FIM is a highly sensitive functional assessment tool and includes measures of ADLs, mobility, cognition, and social functioning. The tasks are rated using a seven-point scale that ranges from totally independent to totally dependent. Although the FIM is commonly used in acute rehabilitation and Veteran's Administration hospitals in the United States and several other countries, it cannot yet be applied across all countries (Lundgren-Nilsson et al., 2005; Ottenbacher et al., 1996). For information about training, certification, and purchasing agreements in the use of the FIM, see http://www.udsmr.org.

BOX 8.8 Examples of Instrumental Activities of Daily Living

- Ability to use the telephone (look up numbers, dial, make calls)
- Ability to travel (alone [e.g., drive], with another, unable)
- Ability to shop for necessities (alone even if needs someone to provide transportation, cannot do without help, unable)
- Ability to prepare meals (plan and prepare full meals safely, can prepare light meals but cannot cook full meals, unable)
- Ability to do housework (heavy housework, limited to light housework, unable)
- Ability to self-administer medication (independently take medications in the right dose at the right time, able to take medications but needs reminding or someone to prepare them, unable)
- Ability to manage money (independently manage money [e.g., write checks, pay bills], needs some help, unable)

From Lawton MP, Brody EM: Assessment of older people: Self-maintaining and instrumental activities of daily living, *Gerontologist* 9(3):179–186, 1969.

Instrumental Activities of Daily Living

The original tool for the assessment of IADLs was developed by Lawton and Brody (1969) (Box 8.8). Both the original tool and the subsequent variations use the self-report, report-by-proxy, and observed formats with three levels of functioning (independent, assisted, and unable to perform). A copy of this instrument for individual use is available through the *Try This: Series* (http://www.nursingign.org). The advantages and disadvantages of using these tools are the same as those for the measures of ADLs.

COMPREHENSIVE GERIATRIC ASSESSMENTS

In some cases an integrated approach is used rather than a collection of separate tools and assessments. The original integrated assessment tool was probably the *Older American's Resources and Services (OARS)* and later the *Older American's Resources and Services*

Multidimensional Functional Assessment Questionnaire (OMFAQ) created by Eric Pfeiffer and his colleagues at Duke in 1979. It can be found at the site for the U.S. Library of Congress (http://id.loc.gov/authorities/sh88002554).The OMFAQ has served as the basis of many subsequent measures. All are quite comprehensive and therefore quite lengthy. Completion of these assessments requires a collaborative and interdisciplinary approach and training. When completed, they serve as a resource for a detailed plan of care. Related instruments discussed herein are the Fulmer SPICES (Fulmer & Wallace, 2012), the Minimum Data Set used in skilled nursing facilities, and the OASIS used in certified home care agencies.

The OARS Multidimensional Functional Assessment Questionnaire (OMFAQ)

The classic instrument, the *Older Americans Resources and Services (OARS),* was developed at the Center for the Study of Aging and Human Development at Duke University. It was later updated as the *OMFAQ* (Duke University Center for the Study of Aging and Human Development, 2014). The areas evaluated in the OMFAQ include social and economic resources, mental and physical health, and ADLs. The person's functional capacity in each area is rated on a scale of 1 (excellent functioning) to 6 (totally impaired functioning). At the conclusion of the assessment, a cumulative impairment score (CIS) is calculated ranging from the most capable (6) to total disability (30). An analysis of the data results in (1) an evaluation of the ability, disability, and capacity level at which the person is able to function, and (2) the determination of the extent and intensity of utilization of resources.

The OMFAQ and training materials can be purchased for a nominal fee from the Center for the Study of Aging and Human Development at Duke University (http://centerforaging.duke.edu/services/141).

Fulmer SPICES

The *Fulmer SPICES* is a simple and overall assessment tool of older adults focusing on geriatric syndromes (Fulmer & Wallace, 2012) (see Chapter 17). It has proved reliable and valid when used with older persons either in health or with illness, regardless of the setting. The acronym *SPICES* refers to the sometimes vague but nonetheless very important problems that require nursing interventions: Sleep disorders, Problems with eating or feeding, Incontinence, Confusion, Evidence of falls, and Skin breakdown. Nurses are encouraged to use this acronym as a reference when caring for older adults (see http://www.hartfordign.org). It is a system that alerts the nurse to the most common problems that occur in the health and well-being of older adults, particularly those who have one or more medical conditions.

Resident Assessment Instrument (RAI)/Minimum Data Set (MDS 3.0)

In 1986 the Institute of Medicine (IOM; now called the Health and Medicine Division of the National Academy of Medicine) completed a study indicating that although considerable variation existed, residents in skilled nursing facilities in the United States were receiving an unacceptably low quality of care (IOM, 1986). As a result, nursing home reform was legislated as part of the Omnibus Budget Reconciliation Act (OBRA) of 1987. The creators of OBRA recognized the challenging work of caring for increasingly ill persons discharged from acute care settings to nursing homes and, along with this, the need for comprehensive assessments, complex decision-making, and documentation regarding the care that was needed, planned, implemented, and evaluated.

In 1990 a Resident Assessment Instrument (RAI) was created and mandated for use in all skilled nursing facilities that receive compensation from either Medicare or Medicaid (see Chapter 7) (CMS, 2014a; Dellefield, 2007). In March 2014, Quality Measures were updated to provide a standardized measure of the quality of care provided. This includes consideration of 992 different measures, ranging from postoperative infection to fall prevention strategies (Box 8.9) (CMS, 2015).

The Quality Indicators, along with the RAI, are used in several countries outside of the United States, including provinces in Canada, and have been found to provide a foundation for quality care (Touhy et al., 2012). Now in its third version, the 450-item *Minimum Data Set* (MDS 3.0) is the basis for the assessment within the RAI (CMS, 2014a). As the MDS is analyzed, specific areas of need are identified that guide development and revisions in the plan of care. The most recent revision has been found to be more reliable, efficient, and clinically relevant than previous versions; evidence-based assessment tools are included whenever possible (Saliba & Buchanan, 2008). In a significant change, care recipient interviews have been added.

The RAI/MDS provides a comprehensive health, social, and functional profile of persons as they enter skilled nursing facilities and at designated times thereafter. The initial assessment serves as the framework for the initial goals and outcomes for the individual. As reassessments are done, the nurse and other members of the care team have the opportunity to track the progress toward the resolution of identified problems and make changes to the plan of care as appropriate. As goals are met and resources are made available, the assessment leads to discharge to a lower level of care, such as

BOX 8.9 Examples of Quality Measures Highly Relevant to Persons Receiving Care in Skilled Nursing Facilities

Short Stay Residents	Long-Term Stay Residents
Self-report severe pain	All of the indicators for short stays **plus:**
Pressure ulcers: new or worsened	Developed a urinary tract infection
One or more falls with major injury	Developed incontinence
Assessed for/given seasonal influenza vaccination	Has/had catheter inserted into bladder
	Is physically restrained
Assessed for/given pneumococcal vaccine	Has increased need for assistance with ADLs
Newly received antipsychotic medication	Has/had excessive weight loss
	Shows depressive symptoms
	Received an antipsychotic medication

From CMS: *Quality measures,* 2014, Available at http://www.cms.gov/Medicare/Quality-Initiatives-Patient-Assessment-Instruments/NursingHomeQualityInits/NHQIQualityMeasures.html. Accessed August 2016.

BOX 8.10 Risk for Hospitalization From the OASIS Assessment

- ☐ 1. History of falls (2 or more falls—or any fall with an injury—in the past 12 months)
- ☐ 2. Unintentional weight loss of a total of 10 pounds or more in the past 12 months
- ☐ 3. Multiple hospitalizations (2 or more) in the past 6 months
- ☐ 4. Multiple emergency department visits (2 or more) in the past 6 months
- ☐ 5. Decline in mental, emotional, or behavioral status in the past 3 months
- ☐ 6. Reported or observed history of difficulty complying with any medical instructions (e.g., medications, diet, exercise) in the past 3 months
- ☐ 7. Currently taking 5 or more medications
- ☐ 8. Currently reports exhaustion
- ☐ 9. Other risk(s) not listed in 1–8
- ☐ 10. None of the above

returning home or to an assisted living facility. For a person whose condition is one of progressive decline, the RAI leads to a plan of care focused on comfort. The RAI process is dynamic and solution-oriented. It is used to gather definitive information and promote healthy aging in a specific care setting and in a holistic manner. The RAI is coordinated by a nurse and requires his or her signature attesting to its accuracy.

Outcome and Assessment Information Set (OASIS-C1)

The skilled care provided in the home is based on, and documented in, the Outcome and Assessment Information Set (OASIS) (CMS, 2012). Now in its third revision (OASIS-C), further modifications were effective October 1, 2014 (OASIS-C1). The assessment is very comprehensive and focuses on the development of interventions to prevent rehospitalization and ensure safety in the home setting. Among the items on the instrument are those that identify the person's risk for hospitalization (Box 8.10). The majority of the documentation takes place in the patient's home and is entered into a laptop or tablet for transmission to the agency database, and ultimately to the Centers for Medicare and Medicaid Services. Completion is required for all care that is compensated by Medicare or Medicaid, and forms the basis for the level of reimbursement. As with other instruments, the assessment is completed at the time the care is begun and at intervals thereafter. Nurses supplement the OASIS data with information necessary to personalize the care provided. It is exceedingly complex and training is required. For more information, see http://www.cms.gov or search OASIS-C.

DOCUMENTATION FOR QUALITY CARE

Clinical documentation chronicles, supports, and communicates the results of the assessment. The recorded assessment provides the data needed for the careful development of the individualized plan of care and the evaluation of patient outcomes. Good documentation will help the nurse identify, monitor, and evaluate interventions. It also provides the communication needed to ensure continuity of care—from one shift to another, from one caregiver to another, and across various settings. The nurse who provides care to a patient for whom the previous nurse did not document is very familiar with the potential errors that can be made and the added risk to the patient and legal liability for the nurse. At the same time, documentation is the major means for the nurse to demonstrate the quality of care he or she provides. In any setting, documentation is a means to more quickly identify iatrogenic problems and hospital-acquired conditions (HACs) that frequently complicate recovery.

Since the Patient Self-Determination Act was passed in 1991, all persons entering a health care facility or who begin to receive skilled home care are asked if they have an advance directive and, if not, are provided information about them (see Chapters 7 and 28). The nursing records supplement this documentation with more details regarding persons' wishes and include who persons want involved in their care, who persons want to have access to their records, and persons' wishes related to everything from organ donation to the use of cardiopulmonary resuscitation (CPR) to the handling of their bodies after death. Patients often discuss these issues with nurses during quiet moments. By noting these conversations in the clinical record, nurses are able to both officially document this important information and share it with other members of the health care team to ensure that the patient's wishes are respected.

Documentation in Acute Care and Acute Rehabilitation Care Settings

Documentation in the acute care setting has undergone a significant change in recent years, especially with the mandates for upgrading to the electronic medical record (EMR). Computers can be found at the bedside, in nurses' pockets, and in strategic locations around the unit. Nurses are given passwords that may be more important than their name tags or the bar codes on their name tags. In some settings, fingerprints are scanned for anything from access to records and supplies, to administration of treatments and medications, to identification of patients. The use of checklists, flow sheets, and standardized tools has become the norm, all documented electronically. A care map of some kind is used to predict and document the care provided within a preestablished trajectory and to anticipate the day of discharge.

Documentation in Long-Term Care Facilities

The term long-term care facility is applied to a number of settings, including family care homes, assisted living facilities (board and care homes), nursing facilities, skilled nursing facilities (SNFs), and "swing beds" in rural hospitals (beds that serve for either acute or long-term care, depending on the patient's needs) (see Chapter 6). The level of documentation required varies by setting and is prescribed by state or jurisdiction statutes. In family care homes and assisted living facilities, documentation (usually written) generally occurs only if a nurse has been hired or is under contract with the facility. This service is always limited to administration of medications or the delegation of this act to nursing aides.

Both nursing facilities and skilled nursing facilities are making the transition to the electronic medical record but still lag considerably behind acute care facilities. In addition to nursing observations, documentation in these facilities encompasses the recording of daily care (such as eating status and presence or absence of bowel movements) as well as vital signs, periodic assessment, medication and treatment administration, assessment of any unusual event or change in condition, and periodic mandated comprehensive assessments. Documentation in SNFs includes narrative progress notes, flow sheets, checklists, and the RAI as already discussed. The RAI data are transmitted to Medicare electronically and subsequently into a national database. When a resident's care is not considered "skilled" and therefore no longer covered by Medicare, narrative notes are reduced to "problem-oriented only" and are completed on an "as-needed" and weekly or monthly basis depending on the facility and licensing body. Good documentation is an expectation of all care staff. The nurse is ultimately responsible for both the quality of the care provided and the completeness and accuracy of the documentation of the care and serves as a means of monitoring functional and medical conditions and promoting healthy aging.

Documentation in Home Care

The majority of the nonskilled care provided in the home is by informal caregivers such as family members and hired "private duty attendants." They will often develop documentation systems of their own to track appointments, medication administration, and health care provider instructions. If used, this system increases the continuity of care. Nurses may need to assist the family in developing and using effective systems.

Documentation and Reimbursement

When care is covered by Medicare, Medicaid, or another insurer (see Chapter 7) the reimbursement in all settings is based on the assessment and the documentation of care. In skilled nursing facilities this is through the analysis of the MDS and the subsequent calculation of resources needed for care (RUG or resource utilization group) when Medicare is the payer (CMS, 2013). Reimbursement is similarly calculated in skilled home care through the OASIS assessment.

Although initial reimbursement in acute care settings (hospitals and acute rehabilitation) is preset by diagnosis codes (diagnosis-related groups [DRGs]), documentation of the assessment at admission, with any change in condition, at the time of specific preventable events (hospital-acquired condition [HAC]) (Box 8.11) in the hospital, and at re-admission for the same problem (within 30 days of discharge) have negative financial consequences for the facility. No payment is made for the HAC when the diagnosis was not present at the time of diagnosis, *documentation is necessary to determine if it was present,* or it cannot be determined clinically if it was present (CMS, 2014b).

BOX 8.11 Hospital-Acquired Conditions (HACs)

- Foreign object retained after surgery
- Air embolism
- Blood incompatibility
- Pressure ulcer stages III and IV
- Falls and trauma (e.g., fractures, burns, etc.)
- Catheter-associated urinary tract infections
- Vascular catheter-associated infections
- Manifestations of poor glycemic control
- Surgical site infection following
  - coronary artery bypass surgery
  - bariatric surgery for obesity
  - cardiac implantable device insertion
- Deep vein thrombosis and pulmonary embolism following certain orthopedic procedures
- Iatrogenic pneumothorax with venous catheterization

❖ IMPLICATIONS FOR GERONTOLOGICAL NURSING AND HEALTHY AGING

Communication of both assessment data and information needed in day-to-day care activities through documentation has become critical to ensure patients' rights, adequate patient care, and the economic survival of providers. It is the responsibility of the nurse to make sure that communication and documentation are of the highest quality so as to provide error-free and appropriate care and continuity and to maximize both patient outcomes and accurate reimbursement.

Whether the nurse is working with a standardized instrument or creating a new one, the goal of the gerontological nursing assessment is to promote healthy aging. To accomplish this it is necessary to collect the most accurate data in the most efficient, yet caring manner possible. The use of tools serves as a way to organize the collected data necessary for assessment and makes it possible to compare the data from time to time. As noted earlier, each tool has strengths and weaknesses. A number of factors complicate assessment of the older adult. These include the difficulty of differentiating the effects of aging from those originating from disease, the coexistence of multiple diseases, the underreporting of symptoms by older adults, the atypical presentation or nonspecific presentation of illnesses, and the increase in iatrogenic illnesses.

Overdiagnosis or underdiagnosis occurs when the normal age changes are not considered; these include both physical changes and psychosocial changes. Underdiagnosis is far more common in gerontological nursing. Many symptoms or complaints are ascribed to normal aging rather than to the possible development of a health problem. Assessing the older adult with multiple chronic conditions is a challenge. Symptoms of one condition can exacerbate or mask symptoms of another. The gerontological nurse is challenged to provide the highest level of excellence in the care of elders. If a particular tool will facilitate the achievement of this goal, it should be used. If the tool serves little purpose or is burdensome to either the nurse or the patient, it should be avoided or replaced. Without appropriate documentation neither the tool nor the assessment can contribute to the well-being of those who entrust themselves to our care.

KEY CONCEPTS

- Assessment of the physical, cognitive, psychosocial, and environmental status is essential to meeting the specific needs of the older adult and implementing appropriate interventions.
- The quality and quantity of data obtained for an assessment tool are affected by the manner used to gather the data, whether by self-report, report-by-proxy, or nurse observation.
- Knowledge of how to use a particular gerontological assessment tool is needed to accurately administer it.
- Anticipate that compensation may be necessary for the many older adults with hearing or visual impairments.
- Expect findings that are different from those for a younger adult and anticipate the need to begin to differentiate normal age-related changes from potential pathological conditions.
- For those with cognitive impairments, obtaining some assessment data from a proxy may be necessary but can only be done with the permission of the patient or legal representative.
- Excellence in documentation sets the stage for excellence in patient care.
- Standardized instruments for patient evaluation are integral to consistent determination of the needs and health status of patients and appropriate reimbursement for care provided.
- Documenting patient status and needs accurately is a key responsibility of the licensed and registered nurse.

ACTIVITIES AND DISCUSSION QUESTIONS

1. What is the importance of the measurement of ADLs and IADLs in older adults?

2. What makes an assessment tool effective?
3. Discuss problems you have experienced with incomplete data or poor documentation in a health facility.
4. Discuss the potential uses of the MDS 3.0 and OASIS-C.
5. Explain the reasons why documentation is critical to patient care.

REFERENCES

Alzheimer Society of Canada: *The stages of Alzheimer's disease*, 2016. Available at http://www.alzheimer.ca/en/About-dementia/Alzheimer-s-disease/Stages-of-Alzheimer-s-disease. Accessed November 2015.

Aprahamian I, Martinelli JE, Neri AL, et al: The accuracy of the Clock Drawing Test compared to that of standard screening tests for Alzheimer's disease: Results from a study of Brazilian elderly with heterogeneous educational backgrounds, *Int Psychogeriatr* 22:64, 2010.

Benner P: *From novice to expert*, Menlo Park, CA, 1984, Addison-Wesley.

Bent B: FANCAPES assessment: Increases in longevity lead to need for expertise in geriatric care, *Adv Healthcare Network Nurses* 7(14):10, 2005.

Borson S, Brush M, Gil E, et al: The Clock Drawing Test: Utility for dementia detection in multiethnic elders, *J Gerontol A Biol Sci Med Sci* 54(11):M534–M540, 1999.

Borson S, Scanlan J, Brush M, et al: The Mini-Cog: A cognitive "vital signs" measure for dementia screening in multi-lingual elderly, *Int J Geriatr Psychiatry* 15(11):1021–1027, 2000.

Borson S, Scanlan JM, Chen P, et al: The Mini-Cog as a screen for dementia: Validation in a population-based sample, *J Am Geriatr Soc* 51(10):141–144, 2003.

Bowker LK, Price JD, Smith SC, editors: *Oxford handbook of geriatric medicine*, ed 2, Oxford, UK, 2012, Oxford University Press.

Centers for Medicare and Medicaid Services (CMS): *Outcome and assessment information set (OASIS)*, 2012. Available at http://www.cms.gov/Medicare/Quality-Initiatives-Patient-Assessment-Instruments/OASIS/index.html?redirect=/OASIS. Accessed November 2015.

Centers for Medicare and Medicaid Services (CMS): *RUG refinement*, 2013. Available at https://www.cms.gov/Medicare/Medicare-Fee-for-Service-Payment/SNFPPS/RUGRefinement.html. Accessed November 2015.

Centers for Medicare and Medicaid Services (CMS): *MDS 3.0 for nursing homes and swing bed providers*, 2014a. Available at http://www.cms.gov/Medicare/Quality-Initiatives-Patient-Assessment-Instruments/NursingHomeQualityInits/NHQIMDS30.html. Accessed November 2015.

Centers for Medicare and Medicaid Services (CMS): *Hospital-acquired conditions and present on admission indicator reporting provision*, 2014b. Available at https://www.cms.gov/Outreach-and-Education/Medicare-Learning-Network-MLN/MLNProducts/Downloads/wPOAFactSheet.pdf. Accessed November 2015.

Centers for Medicare and Medicaid Services (CMS): *Quality measures*, 2015. Available at https://www.cms.gov/Medicare/Quality-Initiatives-Patient-Assessment-Instruments/QualityMeasures/index.html?redirect=/QUALITYMEASURES/. Accessed November 2015.

Cournan M: Use of the functional independence measure for outcomes measurement in acute inpatient rehabilitation, *Rehabil Nurs* 36(3):111–117, 2011.

Dellefield ME: Implementation of the resident assessment instrument/minimum data set in the nursing home as organization: Implications for quality improvement in RN clinical assessment, *Geriatr Nurs* 28(6):377–386, 2007.

Doerflinger DMC: *Mental status assessment of older adults: The mini-cog*, 2013. Available at http://consultgerirn.org/try-this/general-assessment/issue-3.1.pdf. Accessed September 2016.

Duke University Center for the Study of Aging and Human Development: *Older Americans resources and services*, 2013. Available at http://centerforaging.duke.edu/services/141. Accessed May 2014.

Ehreke L, Luppa M, König HH, et al: The Clock Drawing Test: A screening tool for the diagnosis of mild cognitive impairment? A systematic review, *Int Psychogeriatr* 22:56, 2010.

Folstein MF, Folstein SE, McHugh PR: Mini-mental state: A practical method for grading the cognitive state of patients for the clinician, *J Psychiatr Res* 12(3):189–198, 1975.

Fulmer T, Wallace M: *Fulmer SPICES: An overall assessment tool for older adults*, 2012. Available at https://consultgeri.org/education-training/e-learning-resources. Accessed November 2016.

Institute of Medicine (IOM): *Improving the quality of care in nursing homes: Consensus report*, 1986. Available at http://nationalacademies.org/hmd/reports/1986/improving-the-quality-of-care-in-nursing-homes.aspx. Accessed August 2016.

Katz S, Ford AB, Moskowitz RN, et al: Studies of illness in the aged: The index of ADL: A standardized measure of biological and psychosocial function, *JAMA* 185:914–919, 1963.

Kidd D, Stewart G, Baldry J, et al: The Functional Independence Measure: A comparative validity and reliability study, *Disabil Rehabil* 17:10, 1995.

Lawton MP, Brody EM: Assessment of older people: Self-maintaining and instrumental activities of daily living, *Gerontologist* 9(3):179–186, 1969.

Lundgren-Nilsson A, Grimby G, Ring H, et al: Cross-cultural validity of Functional Independence Measure items in stroke: A study using Rasch analysis, *J Rehabil Med* 37:23–31, 2005.

Mahoney FI, Barthel DW: Functional evaluation: The Barthel index, *Md State Med J* 14:61–65, 1965.

Mitchell AJ: A meta-analysis of the accuracy of the Mini-Mental Status Examination in the detection of dementia and mild cognitive impairment, *J Psychiatr Res* 43:411, 2009.

Mitchell AJ, Malladi S: Screening and case finding tools for the detection of dementia. 1. Evidence-based meta-analysis of multidomain tests, *Am J Geriatr Psychiatry* 18:759, 2010.

Nikula S, Jylha M, Bardage C, et al: Are ADLs comparable across countries? Sociodemographic associates of harmonized IADL measures, *Aging Clin Exp Res* 15(6):451–459, 2003.

Ortiz I, Romero L: Cultural implications for assessment and treatment of depression in Hispanic elderly individuals, *Ann Longterm Care* 16:45, 2008.

Ottenbacher KJ, Hsu Y, Granger CV, et al: The reliability of the functional independence measure: A quantitative review, *Arch Phys Med Rehabil* 77(12):1226–1232, 1996.

Quinn TJ, Langhorne P, Stott DJ: Barthel Index for stroke trials: Development, properties and application, *Stroke* 42:1146–1151, 2011.

Reisberg B: Global measures: Utility in defining and measuring treatment response in dementia, *Int Psychogeriatr* 19:421, 2007.

Reisberg B, Ferris S, de Leon MJ, et al: The global deterioration scale for assessment of primary progressive dementia, *Am J Psychiatry* 139(9):1136–1139, 1982.

Resnick B, Mitty E, editors: *Assisted living nursing: A manual for management and practice*, New York, 2009, Springer.

Saliba D, Buchanan J: *Development and validation of a revised nursing home assessment tool: MDS 3.0*, April 2008, The RAND Corp.

Shulman KI: Clock drawing: Is it the ideal cognitive screening test? *Int J Geriatr Psychiatry* 15:545, 2000.

Touhy TA, Jett KF, Boscart V, et al: *Ebersole and Hess' gerontological nursing and healthy aging*, ed 1, Canada, Toronto, 2012, Elsevier Canada.

Tuokko H, Hadjistavropoulos T, Miller J, et al: The clock test: A sensitive measure to differentiate normal elderly from those with Alzheimer disease, *J Am Geriatr Soc* 40(6):579–584, 1992.

Wade C, Collin C: The Barthel ADL Index: A standard measure of physical disability, *Int Disabil Stud* 10(2):64–67, 1988.

Wattmo C, Wallin AK, Londos E, et al: Long-term outcome and predictive models of activity of daily living in Alzheimer disease with cholinesterase inhibitor treatment, *Alzheimer Dis Assoc Disord* 25(1):63–72, 2011.

Yesavage JA, Brink TL, Rose T, et al: Development and validation of a geriatric depression screening scale: A preliminary report, *J Psychiatr Res* 17(1):37–49, 1982.

9

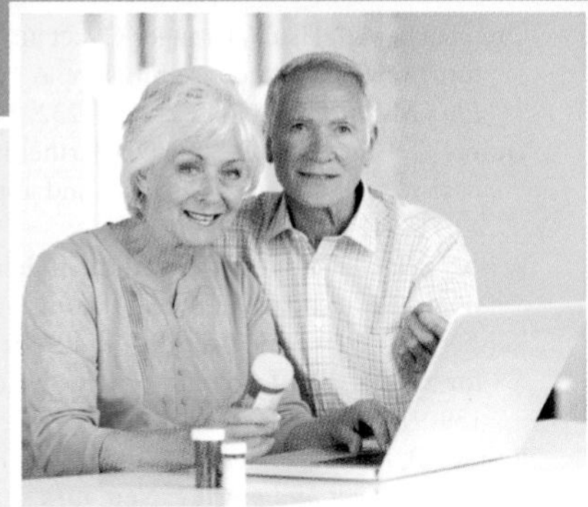

Safe Medication Use

Kathleen Jett

 evolve.elsevier.com/Touhy/gerontological

LEARNING OBJECTIVES

Upon completion of this chapter, the reader will be able to:

- Explain age-related pharmacokinetic and pharmacodynamics changes.
- Discuss potential use of chronotherapy.
- Describe drug use patterns and their implications for the older adult.
- Explain the roles of elder, caregiver, and social network in reducing medication misuse and polypharmacy.
- List interventions that can reduce medication misuse by older adults and their health care providers.
- Identify diagnoses or symptoms for which psychotropic drugs are prescribed.
- Discuss issues concerning psychotropic medication management in the older population.

THE LIVED EXPERIENCE

It is so hard to keep track of my medications. I try arranging them in little cups to take with each meal, but then there are the ones that I take at odd times. Those are the easiest to forget. I get really confused and think sometimes I have taken them twice and then think I must be going crazy. I really wish I didn't have to take so many pills, but I'm not sure what would happen if I stopped all of them. I don't even know why I'm taking most of them.

Geraldo, with hypertension, diabetes, and cardiac disease

In the United States, persons 65 years of age and older are prescribed more medications than any other age group. Although the exact statistics vary among studies, all findings indicate that as one ages, the number of prescribed medications, dietary supplements, and herbal products taken increases. When used appropriately, prescription medications can afford survival or even enhance quality of life for those with chronic conditions and disabilities. When they are used inappropriately, they threaten even the most basic level of physiological stability. Yet, at times, even when drugs are used appropriately, they may adversely affect health and well-being. Many factors influence how prescribed medicines and other bioactive products are used.

Gerontological nurses have a responsibility to help minimize the risks and maximize the safety of medication use in the persons who receive their care. A review of the effects of aging on drug pharmacokinetics and pharmacodynamics and the occurrence of medication-related problems in older adults is presented in this chapter. The final section addresses the use of psychotropic agents. These are frequently prescribed to frail elders and have the potential for both great benefit and significant risk, thereby requiring special attention.

PHARMACOKINETICS

The term *pharmacokinetics* refers to the movement of a drug in the body from the point of administration to excretion. During this process medications are absorbed, distributed, and metabolized. There is no conclusive evidence of an appreciable change in overall pharmacokinetics with aging; however, several normal age-related physiological changes have implications for safe drug use in later life (Fig. 9.1). In particular, these changes significantly increase the risk for adverse reactions or unpredictable effects.

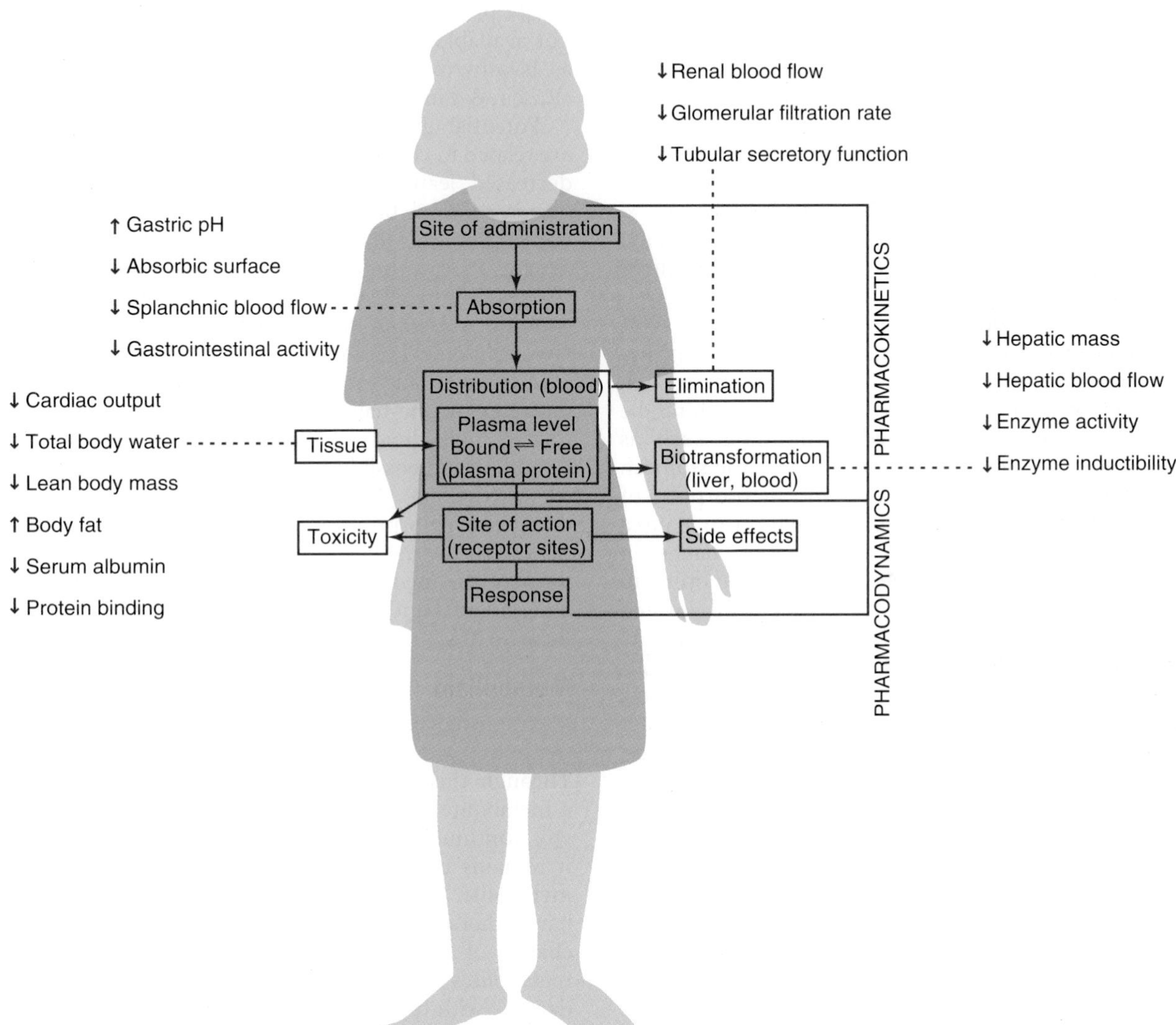

FIGURE 9.1 Physiological changes of aging and the pharmacokinetics and pharmacodynamics of drug use. (Data from Kane RL, Ouslander JG, Abrass IB: *Essentials of clinical geriatrics,* New York, 1984, McGraw-Hill; Lamy PP: Hazards of drug use in the elderly: Commonsense measures to reduce them, *Postgrad Med* 76[1]:50–53, 1984; Vestal RE, Dawson GW: Pharmacology and aging. In Finch CE, Schneider EL, editors: *Handbook of biology and aging,* New York, 1985, Van Nostrand Reinhold; Roberts J, Tumer N: Pharmacodynamic basis for altered drug action in the elderly, *Clin Geriatr Med* 4[1]:127–149, 1988; Montamat SC, Cusack BJ, Vestal RE: Management of drug therapy in the elderly, *N Engl J Med* 321[5]:303–309, 1989.)

This chapter is not intended to replace a pharmacology text, but to supplement it for the key associations between safe medication use and the aging process.

Absorption

For a drug to be effective it must be absorbed into the bloodstream. The amount of time between the administration of the drug and its absorption depends on a number of factors, including the route of introduction (i.e., intravenous, oral, parenteral, transdermal, or rectal) and the bioavailability and dose of the medication. The drug is delivered immediately to the bloodstream when administered by the intravenous route and is quickly delivered when using parenteral and transdermal routes or when mucous membranes, such as the rectum and the oral mucosa, are utilized. Compared to other routes of administration, orally administered drugs are absorbed the most slowly, especially those with enteric coatings.

Increased gastric pH retards the action of acid-dependent drugs. Delayed stomach emptying diminishes or negates the effectiveness of short-lived drugs such that they could become inactivated before reaching the small intestine. Enteric-coated medications such as aspirin are specifically designed to bypass the stomach and be absorbed by the small intestine. If absorption of these products is delayed, gastric irritation or nausea may result. Absorption is also influenced by changes in gastrointestinal motility. If there is increased motility in the small intestine, the effect of the drug is diminished because of shortened contact time, resulting in decreased absorption and effectiveness. Conversely, slowed intestinal motility increases the contact time, amount absorbed, and effect. Many medications commonly taken by older adults can also affect the absorption of other drugs. Antispasmodic drugs slow gastric and intestinal motility. In some instances the ingested drug's action may be useful, but when there are other medications involved, it is necessary to consider the problem of drug absorption alterations attributable to drug-drug interaction. Antacids or iron preparations affect the availability of some drugs for absorption by binding the drug with elements and forming chemical compounds.

Distribution

When a drug is absorbed it must be transported to the receptor site on a target organ to have the desired effect. Distribution depends on the availability of plasma protein in the form of lipoproteins, globulins, and especially albumin. As drugs are absorbed, they bind with the protein and are distributed throughout the body. Normally, a predictable percentage of the absorbed drug is inactivated as it binds to a protein. The remaining free drug is available in the blood and has a therapeutic effect when an adequate concentration is reached in the plasma. Many older adults have an insignificant reduction in the serum albumin level. However, serum albumin may become dramatically diminished in those who are frail, such as many adults needing long-term care. When this occurs, toxic levels of available free drug may accumulate unpredictably, especially highly protein-bound medications (because protein is not available) with narrow therapeutic windows, such as levothyroxine, phenytoin (Dilantin), and warfarin (Ruscin & Linnebur, 2014).

Potential alterations of drug distribution in late life are related to changes in body composition, particularly decreased lean body mass, increased body fat, and decreased total body water (see Fig. 9.1). Decreased body water leads to higher serum levels of water-soluble drugs, such as lithium, digoxin, ethanol, and aminoglycosides. With extended diarrhea, vomiting, or other conditions leading to dehydration, increased serum levels can quickly lead to toxicity.

Adipose tissue nearly doubles in older men and increases by one-half in older women; therefore drugs that are highly lipid-soluble are stored in the fatty tissue, extending and possibly elevating the drug effect (Masoro & Austed, 2003). This affects drugs such as lorazepam, diazepam, chlorpromazine, phenobarbital, and haloperidol. If the medication accumulates in excess it may increase the medication's effect and can even result in an accidental and potentially fatal overdose (Hughes & Beizer, 2014).

Metabolism

Metabolism (biotransformation) is the process by which the body modifies the chemical structure of the drug. Through this process the compound is converted to a metabolite that is later more easily excreted. A drug will continue to exert a therapeutic effect as long as it remains either in its original state or as an active metabolite. Active metabolites retain the ability to have a therapeutic effect, as well as the same or a greater chance of causing adverse effects. For example, the metabolites of acetaminophen (Tylenol) can cause liver damage with higher dosages (>4 g/24 hr, or more than eight extra-strength products). The duration of drug action is determined by the metabolic rate and is measured in terms of half-life, or the length of time one half of the drug remains active in the body. Because of the unpredictable nature of drug metabolism in the older body, it is probably safer to consider 3 g of acetaminophen in 24 hours (from all sources) as the maximum dosage. This is reached rapidly with the popular formulations of "extra strength" 500-mg tablets.

A number of enzymes play an active part in drug metabolism. Among these are a group known as the cytochrome P450 (CYP450) monooxygenase system. Although age does not appear to affect the functioning of the CYP450 system, we now know that genetics have a great effect (Box 9.1).

The liver is the primary site of drug metabolism. With aging, the liver's activity, mass, volume, and blood flow are reduced and hepatic clearance may decrease by up to 30% to 40% (Ruscin and Linnebur, 2014). These changes result in a potential decrease in the liver's ability to metabolize drugs such as benzodiazepines (e.g., the tranquilizer lorazepam [Ativan]) (Table 9.1). This reduction in liver function results in a significant increase in the half-life of these drugs. For example, the half-life of diazepam (Valium) in a younger adult is about 37 hours, but in an older adult it extends to as long as 82 hours. If the dose and timing are not adjusted, drugs can accumulate and the administration of a single dose can have significantly more effects (and longer) than those found in a younger person. As a result of this change, it is never appropriate to prescribe Valium to anyone older than 65 (American Geriatrics Society [AGS], 2015).

Excretion

Drugs and their metabolites are excreted in sweat, saliva, and other secretions, but their primary site of excretion is through the kidneys. However, because kidney function declines significantly with aging (up to a 50% decrease by the time one is 80 years old), so does the ability to excrete or eliminate drugs in a timely manner. The considerably decreased glomerular filtration rate (GFR) further prolongs the half-life of drugs, or the amount of time required to eliminate the drug, adding to the risk for accumulation and increasing the potential

BOX 9.1 Focus on Genomics

Pharmacogenomics (sometimes called pharmacogenetics) is a field of research focused on understanding how variations in the genes for proteins influence individual responses to medications. The proteins (in the form of enzymes) of special interest are those in the liver that convert medications into their active or inactive forms. One liver enzyme known as CYP2D6 has been found to act on 25% of all prescription drugs, including the painkiller codeine, which it converts into the drug's active form, morphine. The *CYP2D6* gene exists in more than 160 different versions, many of which vary by slight differences, although some have larger changes. The majority of these variants do not affect drug responses. Some people have hundreds or even thousands of copies of the *CYP2D6* gene instead of the typical two copies. These produce an overabundance of the CYP2D6 enzyme and drugs are metabolized very rapidly. As a result, codeine may be converted to morphine so quickly and completely that a standard dose of the drug can be an overdose. On the other end of the spectrum, some variants of the *CYP2D6* gene result in a nonfunctional enzyme. People with these variants metabolize codeine slowly, if at all, so they might not experience much pain relief. For these people, a different type of pain reliever is necessary.

The long-term goal of pharmacogenomics is to provide information ensuring that both the medication and the dosage best suit the individual.

From National Institute of General Medical Sciences: *Pharmacogenomics fact sheet*, 2015. Available at https://www.nigms.nih.gov/education/Pages/factsheet-pharmacogenomics.aspx. Accessed December 2015.

TABLE 9.1 Drugs to Watch: Examples of Commonly Used Medications Affected by Normal Changes With Aging

Class or Category	Affected by Decreased Hepatic Metabolism	Affected by Decreased Renal Excretion
Analgesic/ anti-inflammatory	Ibuprofen (Advil)* Nonsteroidal anti-inflammatories such as naproxen and Advil* Morphine	
Antibiotics		Cipro Macrobid
Cardiovascular	Amlodipine (Norvasc) Diltiazem (Cardizem) Verapamil (Calan)	Captopril (Capoten) Digoxin (Lanoxin) Enalapril (Vasotec) Lisinopril (Zestril)
Diuretics		Furosemide (Lasix) Hydrochlorothiazide (HCTZ)
Others	Levodopa	Glyburide Ranitidine (Axid)
Psychoactive drugs	Alprazolam (Xanax) Diazepam (Valium) Trazodone	Risperidone

*See Box 9.9 for new FDA warning related to the use of NSAIDs.
Adapted from *The Merck Manual of Diagnosis and Therapy*, edited by Robert Porter. Copyright 2016 by Merck Sharp & Dohme Corp., a subsidiary of Merck & Co., Inc., Whitehouse Station, NJ. Available at http://www.merckmanuals.com/professional/index.html. Accessed July 2016.

for toxicity or other adverse events. Although renal function is highly individualized and cannot be estimated by the serum creatinine level, we approximate it by calculating the creatinine clearance rate (see equation). Reductions in dosages for drugs excreted by the kidneys (e.g., allopurinol, vancomycin) are needed when the creatinine clearance rate is reduced. Reductions in dosages may also be necessary when the patient is very ill or dehydrated. Although there are several nomograms and algorithms available to estimate GFR, the most reliable tool to use for those at the extremes of age or with active diseases may be the Cockcroft-Gault equation (Hughes & Beizer, 2014).

Estimated creatinine clearance rate (the Cockcroft-Gault equation):

$$\frac{(140 - \text{age}) \times \text{wt(kg)} (\times 0.85 \text{ only if female})}{(\text{serum creatinine} \times 72)}$$

For automatic calculators, see http://www.nephron.com/cgi-bin/CGSI.cgi or http://www.niddk.nih.gov.

PHARMACODYNAMICS

Pharmacodynamics refers to the interaction between a drug and the body (see Fig. 9.1). The older the person becomes, the more likely there will be an altered or unreliable response of the body to the drug. Although it is not always possible to explain the change in response, several mechanisms are known. For example, the aging process causes a decreased response to beta-adrenergic receptor stimulators and blockers; decreased baroreceptor sensitivity; and increased sensitivity to a number of medications, especially anticholinergics, benzodiazepines, narcotic analgesics, warfarin, and the cardiac drugs diltiazem and verapamil (Briggs, 2005).

CHRONOPHARMACOLOGY

The relationship between the biological rhythms of the body and variations in pharmacokinetics and pharmacodynamics is referred to as chronopharmacology. For example, if a cortisone tablet (e.g., from a Medrol dose pack) is taken in the morning, it may have little or no effect on the adrenocortical system. If the same dose is taken in divided amounts over the day, unwanted effects of the drug may suppress the hormonal activities stemming from the hypothalamus-pituitary-adrenal axis.

As noted earlier, absorption is influenced by the pH of gastric acid, the level of motility of the gastrointestinal tract, and the degree of blood flow. All have been shown to have biorhythmical variations. Distribution of protein-bound drugs depends on levels of albumin and glycoproteins produced by the liver. During the day, albumin levels are high, but they are low in the early morning. Drug metabolism is also biorhythmical because of changes in the liver over the course of the day. Renal elimination depends on kidney perfusion, glomerular filtration, and urine acidity and has shown rhythmical variation. The brain, the heart, and blood cells have also been found to have varied rhythmicity, resulting in a cyclical response for beta blockers, calcium channel blockers, angiotensin-converting enzyme (ACE) inhibitors, nitrates, and other similar drugs (Table 9.2).

TABLE 9.2 Rhythmical Influences on Disease and Physiological Processes

Disease or Process	Rhythmical Influence
Allergic rhinitis	Symptoms worse in the morning
Arterial blood pressure	Circadian surge—morning hours
Asthma	Greatest respiratory distress overnight (during sleeping) Symptoms peak in early morning (4–5 AM)
Blood plasma volume	Plasma volume falls at night; thus hematocrit increases
Cancer	Tumor cells proliferate when normal cell miosis is low
Cardiac disease	Angina, myocardial infarction, thrombolytic stroke occur in the first 4 hours after waking (peak 9–10 AM) (Prinzmetal's angina—during sleep)
Catecholamines	Increase in early morning
Fibrinolytic activity	Increases in early morning
Gastric system	Gastric acid secretion peaks every morning (2–4 AM); circannual variability—incidence of gastric ulcers greater in winter
Osteoarthritis	Pain more severe in morning
Platelet activation	May result from abnormality in circadian rhythm, which affects cortisol levels, body temperature, sleep-wake cycle
Potassium excretion	Lowest in morning; highest in late afternoon
Rheumatoid arthritis	Pain more severe in late afternoon
Systemic insulin level	Highest in afternoon

As more is learned about chronotherapeutics, the potential for decreasing individual doses of medications and/or the frequency of administration is present. When we are able to do so we will be able to significantly decrease the potential for adverse drug events while maximizing therapeutic effects. Research has begun to produce promising results of understanding potential changes in circadian rhythm in aging (Ortiz-Tudela et al., 2014).

MEDICATION-RELATED PROBLEMS AND OLDER ADULTS

Polypharmacy

Polypharmacy has been defined in many ways: the use of approximately five or more medications or the use of multiple medications for the same problem (Fig. 9.2). Either way, it is extremely common among older adults and a source of potential morbidity and mortality. Gnjidic and colleagues (Gnjidic et al., 2012) concluded that when five or more medications were taken, for each additional medication there was a significantly increased risk for the development of frailty, disability, death, and falls. If the patient has multiple chronic conditions, simple polypharmacy may be necessary, even if the prescribing provider is following evidence-based guidelines. It may occur unintentionally, especially if an existing medication regimen is not considered when new prescriptions are given or if any number of the hundreds of over-the-counter (OTC) preparations, supplements, and herbs are added to those prescribed. Polypharmacy may occur "accidentally" if an existing drug regimen is not considered when new medications are prescribed.

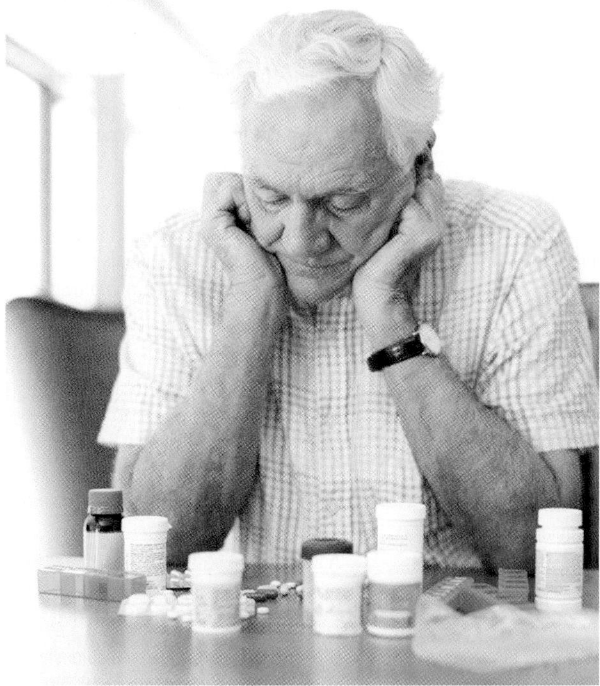

FIGURE 9.2 Polypharmacy. (From © iStock.com/Squaredpixels.)

Polypharmacy is exacerbated by the combination of a high use of health care specialists and a reluctance of prescribers to discontinue potentially unnecessary medications that have been prescribed by someone else. This can lead to the continued use of medications that may no longer be necessary (Rochon, 2014). When communication between patients, nurses, other health care providers, and caregivers becomes fragmented, the risk for duplicative medications, inappropriate medications, potentially unsafe dosages, and potentially preventable interactions is heightened. The two major concerns with polypharmacy are the increased risk for drug interactions and the increased risk for adverse events.

Drug Interactions

The more medications a person takes, the greater the possibility that one or more of them will interact with each other, with an herbal product, with a nutritional supplement, with food, or with alcohol. When two or more medications or foods are taken together or close together, the drugs may potentiate one another; that is, one may increase the effectiveness of the other.

An interaction may result in altered pharmacokinetic activity, that is, alterations in the absorption, distribution, metabolism, or excretion of one or any of the medications. Absorption can be delayed by drugs exerting an anticholinergic effect, a particular danger for frail elders. More than one drug may compete to simultaneously occupy the necessary binding receptors, preventing one of the drugs from reliably reaching the target organs and creating a varied bioavailability of one or both drugs.

Outside the body, interactions can develop whenever two medications or foods or herbs/supplements are mixed together before administration. For example, when delivering medications through a feeding tube, giving each one separately takes more time than is usually feasible. In haste the nurse may crush and deliver all of the medications simultaneously. The appropriate administration requires that the nurse knows those medications that are "crushable" and those that can be administered together.

Medication–Herb/Supplement Interactions

As the popularity of medicinal herbs and other dietary supplements rises, so does the risk for interactions with prescribed medications. Although much remains unknown, new knowledge is added almost daily upon which the gerontological nurse bases her or his practice. For example, a number of herbs have a direct effect on coagulability. When these herbs are taken with warfarin, the risk of bleeding increases significantly. The interactions presented in Table 9.3 represent only a small fraction of the many real and potential problems in prescribing medications and caring for persons who take an herb or a dietary supplement in addition to prescribed medications.

Medication-Food Interactions

Many foods interact with medications, producing increased, decreased, or variable effects such as inhibiting absorption (Table 9.4). For example, the calcium in dairy products will bind to levothyroxine, tetracycline,

TABLE 9.3 Selected* Herb-Medication and Herb-Disease Interactions

Herb	Medication	Complication	Nursing Action
Echinacea	**Any anticoagulant drug** such as warfarin sodium; digoxin	Risk of bleeding may increase; therapeutic digoxin level may be altered	Advise person not to take without provider approval
Garlic	**Any anticoagulant or antiplatelet drug** such as warfarin sodium, streptokinase, aspirin, other NSAIDs	Risk of bleeding may increase	Advise person not to take without provider approval
	Antihypertensives	Increased hypotensive effect	Advise provider approval with use
	Antivirals, such as ritonavir	Altered drug effect	Advise against use
	Antimetabolites such as cyclosporine	Risk of less effective response	Advise against use
	Insulin or oral hypoglycemic agent such as pioglitazone or tolbutamide	Serum glucose level control may improve; less antidiabetic drug needed	Monitor blood glucose levels
Ginkgo	Aspirin, other NSAIDs, heparin sodium, warfarin sodium, **any anticoagulant**	Risk of bleeding may occur	Teach person not to take without approval of provider
	Antiplatelet drugs such as ticlopidine		
	Antidiabetic drugs: insulin, oral DMT2 drugs such as metformin	May alter blood glucose levels	Monitor blood glucose level closely
	Antidepressants, MAOIs, SSRIs	May cause abnormal response or decrease effectiveness	Advise not to take with these drugs
	Antihypertensives	May cause increased effect	Monitor blood pressure
	Antiseizure drugs	Risk for seizure if history of seizure	Advise against use
Ginseng	Insulin and oral antidiabetic drugs	Blood glucose levels may be altered	Monitor blood glucose levels closely
	Anticoagulant and antiplatelet drugs	May increase bleeding	Advise use with caution and provider oversight
	Aspirin and other NSAIDs		
	MAOIs such as isocarboxazid	Headaches, tremors, mania	Advise against use
	Antihypertensives, cardiac drugs such as calcium channel blockers	May alter effects of drug	Advise against use unless provider monitors closely
	Immunosuppressants	May interfere with action	Advise against use
	Stimulants	May cause additive effect	Advise against use
	Fenugreek	Decreased blood glucose levels	Monitor closely
Green tea	**Warfarin sodium**	May alter anticoagulant effects	Advise against use
	Stimulants	May cause additive effect	Advise to use with care
Hawthorn	Digoxin	May cause a loss of potassium, leading to drug toxicity	Monitor blood levels
	Beta blockers and other drugs lowering blood pressure and improving blood flow	May be additive in effects	Monitor blood pressure meticulously; advise that this concern holds true for erectile dysfunction drugs also

TABLE 9.3 **Selected* Herb-Medication and Herb-Disease Interactions—cont'd**

Herb	Medication	Complication	Nursing Action
Red yeast rice	Fibrate drugs; other cholesterol drugs	May cause additive effects	Avoid concomitant use
	Drugs for diabetes management	May alter blood glucose levels	Monitor blood glucose levels carefully
	Anticoagulants, antiplatelet drugs, NSAIDs	May increase risk of bleeding	Warn patient and monitor carefully
St. John's wort	Triptans such as sumatriptan, zolmitriptan	May increase risks of serotonergic adverse effects, serotonin syndrome, cerebral vasoconstriction	Advise against use
	HMG-CoA reductase inhibitors	May decrease plasma concentrations of these drugs	Monitor levels of lipids
	MAOIs	May cause abnormal response or decrease effectiveness	Advise against use
	Digoxin	Decreases effects of the drug	Advise against use
	Alprazolam	May decrease effect of drug	Advise against use
	Ketoprofen	Photosensitivity	Advise sun block use
	Tramadol and some SSRIs	May increase risk of serotonin syndrome	Advise against use
	Olanzapine	May cause serotonin syndrome	Advise against use
	Paroxetine	Sedative-hypnotic intoxication	Advise against use
	Theophylline Albuterol	Increases metabolism; decreases drug blood level	Monitor drug effects
	Warfarin	May decrease anticoagulant effect	Advise against use
	Amlodipine	Lowers efficacy of calcium channel	Advise against use
	Estrogen or progesterone	May decrease effect of hormones	Advise that this effect may occur
	Protease inhibitors or nonnucleoside reverse transcriptase inhibitors in HIV/AIDS treatment; antivirals	May alter drug effects	FDA advises avoidance of this herb for patients taking these drugs

*The interactions listed represent only a few of the possible herb-drug interactions. Use of herbs that interfere with metabolism of drugs by the liver's cytochrome P450 enzyme system should be avoided or monitored closely by the provider.

AIDS, Acquired immunodeficiency syndrome; *DMT2,* diabetes mellitus type 2; *FDA,* U.S. Food and Drug Administration; *HIV,* human immunodeficiency virus; *HMG-CoA,* 3-hydroxy-3-methylglutaryl coenzyme-A; *MAOIs,* monoamine oxidase inhibitors; *NSAIDs,* nonsteroidal anti-inflammatory drugs; *SSRIs,* selective serotonin reuptake inhibitors.

Data from Natural Standard: *The authority on integrative medicine,* available at http://www.naturalstandard.com, accessed May 2014; Wilson BA, Shannon MT, Stang CL: *Nurse's drug guide,* Upper Saddle River, NJ, 2004, Pearson Prentice Hall; Yoon SL, Schaffer SD: Herbal, prescribed, and over-the-counter drug use in older women: Prevalence of drug interactions, *Geriatr Nurs* 27:118–129, 2006.

TABLE 9.4 **Common Drug-Food Interactions**

Food	Drug	Potential Effect
Fiber	Digoxin	Absorption of drug into fiber, reducing drug action
Foods with vitamin K	Warfarin	Decreased effect of drug
Any food	Many antibiotics	Reduced absorption rate of drug
Vitamin B_6 supplements	Levodopa-carbidopa	Reversed antiparkinsonian effect
Grapefruit juice	Multiple medications	Altered metabolism and elimination can increase concentration of drug
Citrus juice	Calcium channel blockers	Gastric reflux exacerbated

BOX 9.2 Top 10 Foods to Avoid When Taking Warfarin

Kale	Turnip greens
Spinach	Parsley
Collards	Broccoli
Swiss chard	Brussels sprouts
Mustard greens	Green tea

For expanded list and patient information, see http://www.cc.nih.gov/ccc/patient_education/drug_nutrient/coumadin1.pdf. Accessed December 2015.

BOX 9.3 Tips for Best Practice

Examples of Potential Medication-Medication Adverse Interactions

ACE* inhibitors and potassium-sparing diuretics
ACE inhibitors or ARBs and Septra (Bactrim)
Macrolide antibiotics (e.g., Cipro) and either calcium channel blockers or digoxin
Warfarin and any of the antibiotics or NSAIDs

**ACE*, Angiotensin-converting enzyme; *ARB*, alpha-receptor blocker; *NSAIDs*, nonsteroidal anti-inflammatory drugs.
From Hines LE, Murphy JE: Potentially harmful drug-drug interactions in the elderly: a review, *Am J Geriatr Pharmacother* 9(6):364–377, 2011.

and ciprofloxacin, greatly decreasing their absorption; lovastatin absorption is increased by a high-fat, low-fiber meal. All of these are medications frequently prescribed to older adults. Grapefruit juice contains substances that inhibit CYP3A4-mediated metabolism in the gut and bind with the statins used for cholesterol-lowering medications, clopidogrel, and many other medications. When a bisphosphonate (e.g., Fosamax) is taken with food of any kind, the absorption is reduced to only a few milligrams, and therefore the drug has no effect on the target organ, the bones.

The vitamin K in leafy green vegetables antagonizes (decreases) the anticoagulant effects of warfarin and may have a significant effect on the coagulability of the blood (Burchum, 2011). It is recommended that patients taking warfarin pay close attention to the regularity of their diet and especially green vegetables to avoid variations in their warfarin levels (Box 9.2).

Spironolactone, prescribed for end-stage heart failure, increases potassium (K^+) reabsorption. If a patient's diet is high in potassium (e.g., KCl salt substitute, molasses, oranges, bananas) or other potassium-sparing agents (e.g., Lisinopril) are taken at the same time, K^+ levels can rise significantly and quickly reach toxic levels.

Drug-Drug Interactions

The polypharmacy that may be a necessary part of health care in later life significantly increases both the risk for and the frequency of medication-medication interactions (Box 9.3). These may occur at any time from preparation to excretion. This can be especially dangerous for older adults when two or more drugs with the same effect are additive; that is, together they are more potent than when taken separately. Unless attention is paid to the components of the overall drug list, the time when each drug is administered, and the other products that are taken (such as over-the-counter medications, herbs, vitamins, and other supplements), an adverse drug event can occur.

For example, persons who cannot swallow after a stroke may receive all feedings and medications via the enteral route. Medications intended for oral administration must be converted to a soluble form for unobstructed passage through the tube and yet also remain in their original form. When several medications are crushed, mixed together, and then dissolved in water for administration, a new product is created and medication-medication interactions may have already begun. The nurse decreases the likelihood of this happening by monitoring the medications he or she administers and encouraging persons to do the same.

Adverse Drug Reactions

Polypharmacy, reduced organ function and physiological reserve, and varying levels of skills of health care providers put older adults at greater risk for adverse drug reactions (ADRs) and adverse drug events (ADEs) (Ajemigbitse et al., 2013). An ADR is an unwanted pharmacological effect such as a minor rash or nausea. When a reaction reaches the level of harm, it is referred to as an *adverse drug event* and includes adverse drug withdrawal and therapeutic failures. Many of these must be reported to the U.S. Food and Drug Administration or other regulatory bodies.

ADRs are most common in those over 65 years of age. The signs and symptoms are both typical and atypical. They can sometimes be predicted from the pharmacological action of the drug (e.g., bleeding from warfarin) and can also occur when a patient is started on a drug at a dosage that is inappropriately high. In addition, ADRs can occur when a patient takes a medication that necessitates laboratory monitoring (e.g., lithium, Coumadin) and adjustment of dosage but this is not done for whatever reason. The prevalence of associated hospitalizations is as high as 31% in some studies (Salvi et al., 2012).

In a study of almost 100,000 emergency hospitalizations among persons at least 65 years of age, almost 50% were older than 80. Nearly two-thirds of the hospitalizations were related to accidental overdoses (alone or in combination) of warfarin, insulins, antiplatelet medications, oral hypoglycemic agents, and psychotropics, all frequently prescribed to older adults (Budnitz et al., 2011–2012; Salvi et al., 2012).

One of the most troublesome ADRs for the older adult is drug-induced delirium and confusion. Polypharmacy with several psychoactive drugs exerting anticholinergic actions is perhaps the greatest precipitator of delirium. Too often delirium is unrecognized as an ADR and instead is viewed as a worsening of preexisting dementia or even new-onset dementia (see Chapter 25). Any time there is a change in the person's cognitive abilities or mental status, the possibility of a drug effect must be thoroughly evaluated (Box 9.4).

Another common adverse effect seen in older adults is lethargy, especially with the use of a number of the cardiovascular agents and antidepressants. Like confusion, lethargy can also be misinterpreted as a symptom of decline in cardiac, respiratory, or neurological conditions rather than as an ADR.

Although ADRs and ADEs continue to occur, there has been considerable progress in the development of strategies to reduce their likelihood, especially in the recognition of age-related pharmacokinetic and pharmacodynamic changes in later life. We now know that an older adult should be prescribed lower dosages of several medications, especially when they are first prescribed. To minimize the likelihood of an ADR, the dose can be slowly increased until it safely reaches a therapeutic level. A common adage related to medication dosing in older adults is, "Start low, go slow, but go." There has also been a recognition that the risk of ADEs is so high with some medications that the drugs are simply not recommended for use in persons as they age.

Misuse of Drugs

The more drugs taken, the more likely misuse will occur. Forms of drug misuse include overuse, underuse, erratic use, and contraindicated use. Misuse can occur for any number of reasons, from inadequate skills of the nurse or the prescriber to inadequate funds to purchase prescribed medications. What if a caregiver who administers the medications is not included in planning and education? Although this is often referred to as noncompliance or nonadherence, "misuse" is a term that is more descriptive of what is happening. For older adults without medication insurance coverage, such as older recent immigrants, the cost of necessary medication may be prohibitive.

Misuse by patients may be accidental, which often occurs through misunderstanding or inability to read labels or understand instructions (Box 9.5). It may be deliberate, such as in an attempt to make a prescription last longer for financial reasons or because of beliefs that the dose is either too low or too high or that the medication prescribed is the wrong/inappropriate treatment (see Chapter 2).

When a patient is labeled as noncompliant, the nurse and other health care personnel may become exasperated and angry at the individual for his or her failure to follow the established plan of care. In an attempt to help and do what they think is best for the patient, the nurse and other care providers tend to forget or ignore that one cannot and will not comply with a prescription or treatment plan under certain circumstances, such as when it is incompatible with the person's daily life. For example, the individual cannot follow the instruction "take medication three times per day with meals" if he or she eats only two meals each day.

Memory failures affect drug misuse in two major ways: forgetting the way to take medications correctly and forgetting the correct time(s) to take medications, which is called "prospective" recall failure (Miller, 2008). The more frequently a medication must be taken, the less anyone will comply. With more and more medications available in once-daily dosing rather than three or four times each day, we can expect more people to take their medications as instructed.

Problems with health literacy also limit the ability to correctly take medications. Many older adults, especially

BOX 9.4 Examples of Medications That Can Easily Impair Cognitive Function in Older Adults

Analgesics	Antiparkinsonian medications
Anticholinergics	Beta blockers
Antihistamines	Lanoxin
Benzodiazepines	

BOX 9.5 A Potentially Lethal Misunderstanding

I was making a visit to Mrs. Helena to enroll her in a research study. As we were reviewing her health and current medications she shared that she had not been feeling well and thought it was her heart, and that she had been told to "take the little white pills" until she felt better. When I looked at her pill bottle she had already taken five or more digoxin in the space of about 2 hours. I called an ambulance.

those from minority groups or new immigrants, are more likely to have low levels of literacy or no English literacy; written instructions should be at the third-grade level or below (see http://www.pfizerhealthliteracy.com). Limitations in vision will interfere with the reading of instructions, especially of bottle labels. One can ask the pharmacist to use large type or symbols. The tendency of nurses and physicians to give rapid-fire directions is not effective when addressing most persons, especially those with hearing impairments or with the normal age-related need for slightly slower verbalizations. In addition, the use of ambiguous terms such as "slowly increase" or "only in moderation" leads to further opportunities for misuse.

Unfortunately, it is also common for the nurse to explain the treatment and give directions concerning medications when the patient is physically uncomfortable or is about to be discharged from a care facility; to explain in English even when the person has limited English proficiency; or to explain in a noisy or busy place. Background noise or an unfamiliar accent of the nurse can significantly reduce comprehension for those with normal age-related hearing loss (see Chapter 19).

Potentially Inappropriate Medications: The "Beers Criteria"

The appropriate use of medications in the older adult means that such products are used only as needed, at the minimum dose necessary to achieve the desired effects, and in a manner in which the risks relative to benefits have been considered within the greater context of the person's life expectancy, health, lifestyle, and values. Beers first published a list of "potentially inappropriate medications (PIMs)" for nursing home settings in 1997 (Beers, 1997). It is now regularly evaluated and revised based on the latest knowledge (Box 9.6). The newest version includes lists of medications that have been demonstrated to cause harm, specific drug-drug interactions that are known to cause harm, medications that should only be used with caution, and medications that require dosage adjustments in the presence of altered kidney function (AGS, 2015).

The Beers Criteria have been incorporated into regulatory policy for long-term care facilities via their inclusion in regulations from the Centers for Medicare and Medicaid Services. They are a part of the quality measures for the National Committee for Quality Assurance (NCQA) and the Healthcare Effectiveness Data and Information Set (HEDIS) (AGS, 2012). When one of those medications on the "do not use" portion of the Beers list is prescribed in the long-term care (LTC) setting without documentation of an overwhelming benefit of its use, it can be considered a form of medication misuse by the prescribing practitioner. The American Geriatrics Society provides the entire list, a downloadable app, teaching slides, and a number of other tools at their website (http://www.americangeriatrics.org).

BOX 9.6 Examples of Potentially Inappropriate Medications (PIMs)

Sliding scale insulin
Proton pump inhibitors for longer than 8 weeks
Digoxin
Benzodiazepines
Tricyclic antidepressants
Medications with anticholinergic properties
Antispasmodics
Sulfonylureas

From American Geriatrics Society (AGS): American Geriatrics Society 2015 updated Beers Criteria for potentially inappropriate medication use in older adults, *J Am Geriatr Soc* 63(11): 2227–2246, 2015.

PSYCHOACTIVE MEDICATIONS

Psychoactive medications are those that affect mental function, which in turn affects behavior and how the world is experienced. The gerontological nurse, especially one working in a long-term care setting, is likely to be responsible for older adults who are receiving psychoactive medications, especially those for the treatment of depression, anxiety, bipolar disorders, and psychosis (see Chapter 24). Medications with psychoactive properties have a higher than usual risk for adverse events and must be prescribed and administered, with an acute awareness of how age-related changes in absorption, distribution, excretion, and hepatic function affect their overall concentration in the serum, especially in the older population. Some studies indicate that 35% to 53% of persons living in assisted living facilities were taking at least one psychoactive medication and more than half of older adults admitted from the community into a skilled nursing facility were prescribed at least one such drug within 2 weeks of admission (Lindsey, 2009).

In 1987 the Health Care Financing Administration mandated that residents of long-term care settings may only be prescribed psychotropic drugs for specific diseases or symptoms and that the use be monitored, reduced, or eliminated when possible. Prescribing physicians and nurse practitioners may exceed the recommended doses only if documentation reasonably explains the rationale for the benefit of the higher dose in restoring function or preventing dangerous behavior (Omnibus Budget Reconciliation Act [OBRA], 1987).

Since that time the concern over the potential misuse of psychotropic medications or their effects continues to grow. For example, at one time an atypical antipsychotic such as risperidone was commonly prescribed for the patient with dementia who exhibited neuropsychiatric symptoms, especially agitation. Unless the agitation is specifically related to psychosis, this use is no longer acceptable.

A patient should be prescribed a psychotropic medication only after thorough medical, psychological, and social assessments. Nursing assessment before medication intervention contributes knowledge and baseline information that can optimize the patient's medical and psychological improvement. At the same time, assessments should be done quickly to enable the patient to receive the appropriate treatment as soon as possible. Pharmacological interventions should always be supplemented by nonpharmacological measures such as providing counseling, making changes in the environment, and instituting other actions that promote healthy aging. Issues to consider include the patient's medical status (and other medications that might interact with a psychotropic), mental status, ability to carry out activities of daily living, and ability to participate in social activities and maintain satisfying relationships with others, as well as the potential for patient or caregiver compliance with any pharmacological or nonpharmacological recommendations.

The gerontological nurse, especially one working in a long-term care setting, is likely to care for older adults with psychiatric and cognitive problems, especially dementia, depression, anxiety, and psychosis. The rate of depression in older persons living in the community is significant and even more so for those living in long-term care facilities (see Chapter 24). Anxiety is also common, and when anxiety is treated with benzodiazepines, it significantly increases the older person's risk for adverse effects and drug interactions. Unfortunately, the use of psychotherapy is very limited, first because of the rarity of persons with specialty training in gerontologic psychiatry or counseling and second because of the very low reimbursement rates established by Medicare and other insurance plans.

Finally a small group of elders, especially those with neurological conditions or any one of the dementias, may develop psychosis at some time in their illnesses. Psychosis is also seen in delirium from an infection or from an ADR and in the few elders with schizophrenia. Persons with psychoses are often treated with antipsychotics that require special attention and skills from the gerontological nurse in cooperation with a psychiatrist or a psychiatric nurse practitioner specializing in geriatrics (see Chapter 24).

Antidepressants

Antidepressants, as the name implies, are drugs used to treat depression. In the past, the major drugs used were monoamine oxidase inhibitors (MAOIs) and tricyclic antidepressants (TCAs) (e.g., amitriptyline, doxepin). These drugs required high doses to be effective and had significant anticholinergic side effects such as dry mouth, constipation, sedation, and urinary retention. Since the development of the selective serotonin reuptake inhibitors (SSRIs), serotonin-norepinephrine reuptake inhibitors (SNRIs), and several other medications, the MAOIs and TCAs are rarely prescribed for the treatment of depression in older adults.

The SSRIs (e.g., Zoloft, Prozac, Lexapro, Celexa) have been found to be highly effective, with minimal or manageable side effects, and are the drugs of choice for use in older adults. Most of these medications cause initial problems with nausea or dry mouth. Although effective, these must be used with caution, especially with regard to serum sodium levels. The SSRIs should also be used with caution in persons with a history of falls because of the potential to produce ataxia or dizziness (AGS, 2015). One side effect of the SSRIs that does not resolve with time, if experienced, is sexual dysfunction. For elders who are sexually active, alternatives to the SSRIs are more appropriate. When sleep is a problem, the patient may be prescribed a low dose of the tetracyclic antidepressant mirtazapine (Remeron), which is often well tolerated in older adults and may also increase appetite. Trazodone is also an effective antidepressant with few anticholinergic side effects, making it more useful in older populations. It also has sedating effects suitable for those with sleep difficulties but can cause orthostatic hypotension. Many older adults are sensitive to these medications and may find significant relief from depression at low doses. Although it sometimes takes time to find the optimal dose, the nurse can help the elder monitor target symptoms and advocate for continued dose adjustments or changes until relief is obtained rather than the depression is simply reduced.

Antianxiety Agents

Drugs used to treat anxiety are referred to as *anxiolytics* or *antianxiety agents.* These agents include benzodiazepines, buspirone (BuSpar), and beta blockers. Antihistamines, especially diphenhydramine (Benadryl), are often self-administered (e.g., Tylenol PM) but *not recommended* because of their significant and highly dangerous anticholinergic effects. The decision to treat anxiety pharmacologically is based on the degree to which the anxiety interferes with the person's ability to function and subjective feelings of discomfort.

Although also usually contraindicated, the most frequently used agents are benzodiazepines. Older adults metabolize these drugs slowly and renal excretion is compromised. Even in health they persist in the bloodstream for long periods and can easily reach toxic levels more quickly than anticipated. Side effects include drowsiness, dizziness, ataxia, mild cognitive deficits, and memory impairment. Signs of toxicity include excessive sedation, unsteady gait, confusion, disorientation, cognitive impairment, memory impairment, agitation, and wandering. Because these symptoms resemble dementia, people can easily be misdiagnosed when they start taking benzodiazepines.

Benzodiazepines are highly addicting yet very popular because of their quick sedating effects for the highly anxious or agitated person. However, because of the problems noted earlier they should be avoided except in extreme cases. If necessary, lorazepam (Ativan) appears to be the least problematic, when prescribed in very low doses and for short periods. It has the shortest half-life of the benzodiazepines and no active metabolites.

BuSpar (buspirone) is a safer alternative. Although a side effect is dizziness, this is often dose-related and resolves with time. It is not addictive and may have an additive effect to some of the SSRIs, so lower doses can be used. No therapeutic effect may be felt by the patient or observed by the nurse for 5 to 7 days and the drug may be mistakenly discontinued because of its apparent lack of effect. BuSpar is best used for chronic anxiety and is not indicated for acute needs.

Mood Stabilizers

Mood stabilizers are the group of agents used for the treatment of a bipolar disorder, which are uncontrollable fluctuations in mood. The most common mood stabilizers include lamotrigine (Lamictal), lithium, and valproic acid (Depakote). Along with these, the anticonvulsants carbamazepine (Tegretol) and gabapentin (Neurontin) are used as well as several of the atypical antipsychotics (e.g., Abilify, Zyprexa, and Seroquel) even when psychosis is not present. Each drug has a very individualized drug-drug interaction profile and several medications require blood level monitoring. The nurse who is caring for a patient with a bipolar disorder or for a patient who is taking a mood stabilizer should seek guidance from the person's psychiatrist regarding specific strategies to enhance the person's quality of life and information regarding the drug's need for laboratory testing and dosage monitoring. If the patient is taking lithium, this is especially important. Lithium interacts with other medications and certain foods and has a narrow therapeutic window. For example, a low-salt diet will elevate the lithium level, and a high-salt diet will decrease it; dehydration can occur quickly and result in life-threatening toxicity. Likewise, thiazide diuretics and nonsteroidal anti-inflammatory drugs (NSAIDs) will elevate the serum lithium level. Side effects include the following: confusion, disorientation, and memory loss; flattening of T waves on the electrocardiogram; polyuria and polydipsia; nausea, vomiting, and diarrhea; fine resting tremor; benign goiter; and ataxia.

Antipsychotics (Neuroleptics)

The term "psychosis" covers a range of cognitive and behavioral disorders that are based on responses of the ill person to a private reality—a reality that may be distressing and problematic for the patient and those around him or her. Characteristically, psychosis occurs in schizophrenia but can also occur in mania, depression, delirium, dementia, and paranoid states. When psychosis occurs in the person with dementia it is often seen in a cluster of neuropsychiatric symptoms, especially agitation, physical aggression, and wandering.

Antipsychotics, formerly known as major tranquilizers, are also referred to as neuroleptics and are used as treatment both for psychotic symptoms and for mood stabilizing effects. Second-generation antipsychotics are referred to as atypical antipsychotics (e.g., risperidone [Risperdal], quetiapine [Seroquel], olanzapine [Zyprexa]). Because of their danger, especially risk of cardiovascular events, stroke, and even death, they are used as drugs of last resort and can only be prescribed following a careful assessment and search for any potential underlying cause of the problem. Inappropriate use of antipsychotic medications is a significant problem in long-term care settings. In addition to the risk for ADEs, they may mask a reversible cause for the problem, such as a thyroid disturbance, infection, dehydration, fever, electrolyte imbalance, an ADR, or a sudden change in the environment (Bullock & Saharan, 2002).

However, when no other approaches have been successful they may be necessary and must be used very cautiously in true psychiatric disorders. Antipsychotics can provide a person with relief from what may be frightening and distressing symptoms. When they are used, drugs with the lowest side effects' profile, at the lowest dose possible, and for the shortest length of time should be prescribed. In most states the prescribing and use of antipsychotics in long-term care settings is carefully monitored.

There are different classes and potencies of antipsychotics. First-generation antipsychotics (chlorpromazine [Thorazine], fluphenazine [Prolixin], thioridazine [Mellaril], and haloperidol [Haldol]) are less sedating than some of the second-generation drugs but cause more extrapyramidal reactions, are considered inappropriate medications, and are rarely used, except in emergencies (AGS, 2015). Patients who take first-generation antipsychotic medications are more susceptible to developing extrapyramidal reactions, particularly neuroleptic-induced parkinsonian symptoms and orthostatic hypotension. In older adults this means an increased risk for falls and other anticholinergic effects. A permanent side effect for this class of antipsychotics is tardive dyskinesia (see Tardive Dyskinesia).

Neuroleptic Malignant Syndrome

A rare but potentially life-threatening ADE to antipsychotics is *neuroleptic malignant syndrome* (NMS). The most typical symptoms are temperature greater than 100.4°F, muscle rigidity, autonomic instability (e.g., labile blood pressure, tachycardia), and altered mental status. Onset is rapid and unless treated appropriately death can occur quickly. The drug most associated with NMS is haloperidol (Haldol) but it has also developed when a person is taking chlorpromazine (Compazine) and promethazine (Phenergan). It occurs most often in the first 2 weeks of the start of treatment but must also be considered whenever a dose is increased. NMS is also seen if anti-Parkinson's medications are stopped abruptly. In most instances the person is hospitalized in an intensive care unit while being treated. The immediate response is to recognize that an adverse event is occurring, help the person obtain emergency medical assistance, and gently begin cooling the person.

Appropriate preventive interventions include ensuring adequate hydration, performing activities in a cool area away from direct sunlight, and using a fan or sponge bath if overheating should occur. The patient may or may not communicate his or her discomfort from the heat, so assessment for signs and symptoms may be left to the nurse or other caregiver. Any circumstance resulting in dehydration greatly increases the risk of heatstroke, with the morbidity and mortality increasing with age. Diuretics, coffee, alcohol, lithium, and uncontrolled diabetes decrease vascular volume, thereby decreasing the body's ability to handle antipsychotics. *Concurrent use of medications with anticholinergic properties is especially contraindicated.*

Extrapyramidal Reactions

Although neuroleptic malignant syndrome is not commonly seen, the most significant potential side effects of antipsychotics (especially first generation) are movement disorders, also referred to as *extrapyramidal syndrome (EPS)* reactions. These include acute dystonia, akathisia, parkinsonian symptoms, and tardive dyskinesia.

Acute dystonia. An acute dystonic reaction is an abnormal involuntary movement consisting of a slow and continuous muscular contraction or spasm. Involuntary muscular contractions of the mouth, jaw, face, and neck are common. The jaw may lock (trismus), the tongue may roll back and block the throat, the neck may arch backward (opisthotonos), or the eyes may close. In an oculogyric crisis, the eyes are fixed in one position. Often this creates a feeling of needing to look up constantly without the ability to make the eyes shift downward. Dystonias can be painful and frightening. An acute dystonic reaction may occur hours or days following antipsychotic medication administration, or after dosage increases, and last minutes to hours. It is considered a medical emergency.

Caregivers or others unfamiliar with these EPS reactions often become alarmed. Although frightening, acute dystonia is usually not dangerous and is quickly relieved by anticholinergic medication, such as benztropine (Cogentin), trihexyphenidyl (Artane), or diphenhydramine (Benadryl), providing relief within minutes if given intravenously, within 10 to 15 minutes if given intramuscularly, and within 30 minutes if given orally. These medications should be readily available to treat an EPS reaction for all persons taking antipsychotics. Although they are not recommended for use in persons more than 65 years of age, anticholinergics and amantadine (Symmetrel), a dopamine agonist, are sometimes prescribed to prevent dystonic reactions, but because of slow onset of action, they are not used for acute treatment.

Akathisia. Akathisia refers to the compulsion to be in motion and may occur at any time during therapy. Patients describe feeling restless, being unable to be still, having an unrelenting desire to move, and feeling "like crawling out of my skin." Often this symptom is mistaken for worsening psychosis instead of the ADR that it is. Pacing, aimless walking, fidgeting, shifting weight from one leg to the other, and marked restlessness are characteristic behaviors for a person experiencing akathisia. Safety is the primary concern.

Parkinsonian symptoms. The use of neuroleptics may cause a collection of symptoms that mimic Parkinson's disease. A bilateral tremor (as opposed to a unilateral tremor in true Parkinson's), bradykinesia, and rigidity may be seen, which may progress to the inability to move. The patient may have an inflexible facial expression and appear bored and apathetic, and mistakenly be diagnosed as depressed. More common with the higher-potency antipsychotics (e.g., Haldol), parkinsonian symptoms may occur within weeks to months of the initiation of antipsychotic therapy.

Tardive dyskinesia. When neuroleptics have been used continuously for at least 3 to 6 months, patients are at risk for the development of the irreversible movement disorder of *tardive dyskinesia (TD)*. Symptoms of TD usually appear first as wormlike movements of the tongue; other facial movements include grimacing, blinking, and frowning. Slow, maintained, involuntary twisting movements of limbs, trunk, neck, face, and eyes (involuntary eye closure) have been reported. There is no treatment that reverses the effect of TD; therefore it is essential that the nurse is attentive for early detection so that the health care provider can make prompt changes to the psychotropic regimen.

Response to treatment is the most important consideration when psychotropic medications are given. Subjective patient comments about feelings and symptoms and objective observations about the patient's behavior are important data for evaluating the effectiveness of a drug. Several tools are available to help the nurse monitor the patient taking antipsychotics. The Abnormal Involuntary Movement Scale (AIMS) was designed to quantify changes in movement. Other tools include the Barnes Rating Scale for Drug-Induced Akathisia (Barnes, 1989) and the Simpson-Angus Rating Scale for EPS (Simpson & Angus, 1970). All of these can be found on the Internet.

IMPLICATIONS FOR GERONTOLOGICAL NURSING AND HEALTHY AGING

Nurses in all inpatient settings and those who provide skilled home care are responsible for assessing, monitoring, evaluating, and educating persons regarding safe medication use (Planton & Edlund, 2010). The nurse and patient also decide together when a PRN or "as needed" medication is indicated.

Assessment

The initial step in ensuring that elders are using drugs safely and effectively is to conduct a comprehensive drug assessment. Although a clinical pharmacist may collect the medication history, it is more often completed through the combined efforts of the licensed or registered nurse and the prescribing health care provider.

In the outpatient, ambulatory care setting, it is best to use a "brown bag approach," or to ask the person to bring in all medications and other products he or she is currently taking. As each container is removed from the bag, the person is asked how he or she actually takes the medicine rather than depending on how the prescription is written. This provides an opportunity not only to determine if there is a misunderstanding but also to begin reconciliation between the labeling and any adjustments that may have been made by other clinicians. This is an important change in approach from what is too often used when the person is asked, "Has anything changed since you were last seen?"

An alternative approach is based on the "review of systems" discussed in Chapter 8. These questions will be something like, "What do you take for your heart, circulation, and breathing?" Assessments always end with questioning if there are any other medications/supplements taken, such as a vitamin, regular use of an antihistamine, or St. John's wort. Without the bag of medications or a list of some kind, patients often answer some of the preceding questions with descriptions (e.g., "a little blue pill" or "a bad-tasting one"), which is of little use.

In other settings obtaining accurate information is considerably more difficult. A person may arrive at an emergency department with no medication information. In transfers from one care setting to another such as from a skilled nursing center to the hospital, medical/medication records may be provided, but still cannot always be initially considered. When the patient returns to the long-term care setting the nurse is responsible for medication "reconciliation," wherein the previously prescribed medications are compared to the newly prescribed ones. This is often a laborious process and fraught with opportunities for error, from records not arriving with patients to physicians and nurse practitioners being asked to "approve" orders for unfamiliar patients without having access to patients' hospital medical records. In a cross-sectional study of medication reconciliation following transfers to nursing homes discrepancies were found in almost 75% of patients (Marcum et al., 2010).

Similar problems occur in the transfer between long-term care settings and home when the patient may have difficulty deciphering changes to previous drug regimens and may take his or her former medications instead of the new ones, or both. When electronic medical records become universal a significant number of errors are expected to decrease and the ease and accuracy of the assessment will increase.

Through this assessment the nurse can determine discrepancies between the prescribed dosage and the actual dosage, potential drug-drug and food-drug interactions, and potential or actual ADRs. When potentially inappropriate products are identified, the prescriber can be notified. See Box 9.7 for examples of the information needed that is particularly important when conducting a medication assessment with older adults.

Education

Because of the complex needs of the older patient, education can be particularly challenging. The following tips may be helpful when the goal of the nurse is to promote healthy aging related to safe medication use:

Key persons: Find out who, if anyone, assists the person with decision-making and administration and make

BOX 9.7 **Tips for Best Practice**

Components of a Medication Assessment With Special Emphasis for Older Adults

Ability to pay for prescription medications
Ability to obtain medications and refills
Persons involved in decision-making regarding medication use
Medications obtained from others
Recently discontinued medications or "leftover" prescriptions
Strategies used to remember when to take medications and when it has already been taken
Recent medication blood levels as appropriate
Recent measurement of liver and kidney functioning
Ability to remove packaging, manipulate medication, and store supply

BOX 9.8 **Knowing Who You Are Talking To**

M. François came to the clinic as a new patient with uncontrolled hypertension. The nurse practitioner, through an interpreter, spent a lot of time with M. François explaining how to take his medications, the purpose of the medications, and so on. M. François and his caregiver sat quietly and appeared to understand. When M. François returned a month later his blood pressure was still out of control. There was a different person with M. François and the new person asked all of the questions that were addressed at the first appointment. On further inquiry it was determined that the person who accompanied M. François to his first appointment was just a neighbor helping out and not involved in his day-to-day life at all! M. François' niece, who "takes care of things," had been unavailable during the previous appointment and was now available to take him to his appointment.

sure that the helper is present when any teaching is done (Box 9.8).

Environment: Minimize distraction, and avoid competition with television, grandchildren, or others demanding the person's attention; make sure the person is comfortable and is not hungry, thirsty, tired, too warm or too cold, in pain, or in need of the toilet.

Timing: Provide the teaching during the best time of the day for the person, when he or she is most engaged and energetic. Keep the education sessions short and succinct.

Communication: Communicate the information in a way that compensates for language differences and physical-sensory and cognitive changes so that the person understands. Use simple and direct language, and avoid medical or nursing jargon (e.g., "intake"). Speak clearly, facing the person at eye level and with light on the speaker's face. Make sure the person is wearing reading glasses or hearing aids if they are used. If the person has limited health fluency, plan for extra time. If the person has limited language proficiency in the country in which care is delivered, a trained medical interpreter is needed and up to twice the amount of time should be planned for the encounter.

Reinforce teaching: Although there is a wide array of teaching tools and medication reminders available on the market today, many older adults continue to use the strategies they have developed over the years to remember to take their medications. These may be as simple as a commercially available storage box or turning a bottle upside down once the medication has been taken for the day, or as intense as having a family member or friend call the person at designated times. Encourage the person to use techniques that have worked in the past or to develop new strategies to ensure correct and timely medication use when needed. All education is supported by written or graphic material in the language that the person (if literate) can read or in the language of the person who helps.

◆ Administration

Most elders who live in the community self-administer their own medications; others receive help from family, friends, or health care professionals. In nursing homes the administration of medications occupies nearly all of the "medication" nurses' time. In assisted living facilities, medication administration is an optional service and available only if permitted by local laws. Regardless of the setting or the persons involved, several skills are needed for safe administration.

Because of the high rate of arthritis and other debilitating conditions, it may be difficult or impossible for the person to remove a cap or break a tablet. If no children will have access to the medications, alternative bottle caps that are easier to open can be requested. Either the person or the nurse can also ask the pharmacist to pre-break the pills or dispense a smaller dose. Pill cutters are commercially available but still call for fine motor dexterity to place the pill for cutting in the correct place. Only pills that are "scored" can be cut. Some persons, especially those of low fixed incomes, will attempt to break unscored pills in an attempt to have them last longer, resulting in inconsistent dosing.

Most medications are taken orally but many tablets and capsules are difficult to swallow because of their size or because they stick to the tongue, especially if the mouth is dry due to anticholinergic drugs or dehydration. The person can be advised to first moisten the mouth and then place the pill or capsules on the front of the tongue and swallow a fluid or semisolid food, such as applesauce, chocolate syrup, or peanut butter—as long as the substances do not interact.

Enteric-coated, extended-release, or sustained-release products are all used to allow absorption at different places in the gastrointestinal tract. They can *never* be crushed because this will interfere with their pharmacological effects (causing either underdose or toxicity) or create problems in administration, such as injuring the mouth or gastrointestinal tract. However, since the formulation of medications is rapidly changing, the reader is advised to contact a clinical pharmacist or consult a very current drug handbook or package insert (found in the *Physicians' Desk Reference* [PDR]) for the changing list of "do-not-crush" products.

Administration of a drug in liquid form is sometimes preferable and allows for flexible dosing; concentrations can be varied so that quantities of solution can be prepared and taken by the teaspoon, tablespoon, or ounce, with simple and commonly used household tools. Because household spoons vary greatly in actual volume, the nurse should ensure that an accurate measurement is used. Liquid self-administration will not likely be an option for the person with any type of tremor.

More and more medications are becoming available in a transdermal route of delivery. Transdermal "patches" are not recommended for persons who are noticeably underweight because absorption is unpredictable owing to the reduced body fat. The patches may not be cut or altered in any way; gloves must be worn when they are being applied and the expired patch must be removed at the same time.

When medications are being administered directly into the stomach or duodenum via a feeding tube special precautions are needed. Safe administration is a time-consuming task resulting in a high risk for medication errors. To administer enteral medications safely a detailed knowledge of their formulation is needed along with the skills required to prepare them appropriately. The outcomes of the errors include occluded tube, reduced drug effect, drug toxicity, patient harm, or patient death. The three most common errors are incompatible route, improper preparation, and improper administration (see Safety Alert).

SAFETY ALERT

Administration of Medications Through Enteral Feeding Tubes: The Three Most Common Errors

Incompatible route: Medications must be appropriate for the oral route for immediate action. Watch for extensions such as CD, CR, ER, LA, SA, SE, TD, TR, XL, and XR as warnings for not crushable formulation of drugs (this list is not inclusive). See the "do-not-crush" lists available from the pharmacy or on-line (http://www.ismp.org/Tools/DoNotCrush.pdf).

Improper preparation: Medications administered via an enteral feeding tube must be fully dissolved in a liquid or in semiliquid form in order to pass through the tube and not clog the tube by adhering to its lining. Drug remaining on tubing means a reduced dose has been administered. This is a special concern when administering oral suspensions and tinctures.

Improper administration: Be sure to know where the distal end of the tube is resting. A drug that requires partial absorption in the stomach cannot be used when it will be administered directly into the duodenum or jejunum. Do not combine with a feeding product unless directions are to "administer with food." When more than one tablet is crushed (or more than one capsule is opened) and the contents are mixed before administration, a new "product" has been prepared and may not have the same pharmacotherapeutic effect as the two products taken separately. Find "compatibility information" from pharmacists to determine which medications may be mixed in this way.

See Medication Safety Alert at http://www.ismp.org/Newsletters/acutecare/articles/20100506.asp for more information.

◆ Monitoring

A significant part of the nurse's responsibilities is to monitor and evaluate the effectiveness of prescribed treatments and observe for signs of problems (e.g., ADRs)—either from a change in condition or from iatrogenic complications (i.e., problems that are the result of something the health care provider has done), especially misuse, interactions, or early and unreported adverse events (Table 9.5).

Monitoring involves making astute observations and documenting those observations, noting changes in physical and functional status (e.g., vital signs, performance of activities of daily living, sleeping, eating, eliminating) and mental status (e.g., attention and level of alertness, memory, orientation, behavior, mood). This is particularly important in gerontological nursing because of the medical complexity of the patient and the polypharmacy that often exists. Monitoring for iatrogenic effects means ensuring that blood levels are measured when they are needed, such as scheduled thyroid-stimulating hormone (TSH) levels for all persons taking thyroid replacement therapy, international normalized ratios (INRs) for all persons taking warfarin, and periodic hemoglobin A_{1c} levels for all persons with diabetes. Care of a patient also means that

TABLE 9.5 Indications of Toxicity

Medication(s)	Signs and Symptoms
Benzodiazepines (e.g., Ativan)	Ataxia, restlessness, confusion, depression, anticholinergic effect
Cimetidine (Tagamet)	Confusion, depression
Digitalis (Digoxin)	Confusion, headache, anorexia, vomiting, dysrhythmias, blurred vision or visual changes (halos, frost on objects, color blindness), paresthesia
Furosemide (Lasix)	Electrolyte imbalance, hepatic changes, pancreatitis, leukopenia, thrombocytopenia
Levodopa (L-Dopa)	Muscle and eye twitching, disorientation, asterixis, hallucinations, dyskinetic movements, grimacing, depression, delirium, ataxia
Nonsteroidal anti-inflammatory medications (NSAIDs) such as Advil and Naprosyn	Photosensitivity, fluid retention, anemia, nephrotoxicity, visual changes, bleeding, blood pressure elevations
Ranitidine (Zantac)	Liver dysfunction, blood dyscrasias
Sulfonylureas—first generation (e.g., Diabinese)	Hypoglycemia, hepatic changes, heart failure, bone marrow depression, jaundice

From Lexicomp: *Long term-care nursing drug handbook,* ed 14, Hudson, OH, 2013, Lexicomp.

BOX 9.9 FDA Warning: NSAIDs and Stroke

In July of 2015, the U.S. Food and Drug Administration (FDA) published a new, stronger alert related to the use of over-the-counter nonsteroidal anti-inflammatory medications (NSAIDs), such as ibuprofen and naproxen sodium. In detailed studies the following information has been found:

- The risk of heart attack or stroke can occur as early as the first weeks of using an NSAID. The risk may increase with longer use of the NSAID.
- The risk appears greater at higher doses.
- NSAIDs can increase the risk of heart attack or stroke in patients with or without heart disease or risk factors for heart disease.
- Patients with heart disease or risk factors for heart disease have a greater likelihood of heart attack or stroke following NSAID use than patients without these risk factors because they have a higher risk at baseline.
- Patients treated with NSAIDs following their first heart attack were more likely to die in the first year after the heart attack compared to patients who were not treated with NSAIDs after their first heart attack.
- There is an increased risk of heart failure with NSAID use.
- Patients taking NSAIDs should seek medical attention immediately if they experience symptoms such as chest pain, shortness of breath or trouble breathing, weakness in one part or side of their body, or slurred speech.

For more information, see http://www.fda.gov/Safety/MedWatch/SafetyInformation/SafetyAlertsforHumanMedicalProducts/ucm454141.htm. Accessed December 2015.

nurses promptly communicate their findings of potential problems to the patient's primary care provider.

The gerontological nurse is a key person in ensuring that the medications used are appropriate, effective, and as safe as possible. The nurse determines whether side effects are minimal and tolerable or serious. The knowledgeable nurse is alert for potential drug interactions and for signs or symptoms of ADRs. The nurse promotes the actions necessary to prevent drugs from becoming toxic and treats toxicity promptly should it occur. Nurses in the long-term care setting are responsible for monitoring the overall health of the residents, including being alert for the need for laboratory tests and other measures to ensure correct dosage of several medications (e.g., warfarin, vancomycin, levothyroxine). The nurse must give prompt attention to changes in physiological function that either are the result of the medication regimen or are affected by the regimen, such as potassium level to minimize the likelihood of adverse and toxic reactions (Box 9.9). The nurse is often the person to initiate assessment of medication use, evaluate outcomes, and provide the teaching needed for safe drug use and self-administration.

In most settings the nurse is also in a position to influence the timing of prescribed doses; therefore, some patients might benefit by understanding some of the findings emerging from the science of chronopharmacology (Barry et al., 2007). In all settings, a vital nursing function is to educate patients and to ensure that they understand the purpose and the side effects of medications as well as the time to call the provider regarding their medications. The analysis by the licensed practical nurse (LPN), registered nurse (RN), or advanced practice nurse (APN) should be centered on identifying unnecessary or inappropriate medications, establishing safe usage, determining the patient's self-medication management ability, monitoring the effect of current medications and other products (e.g., herbals), and evaluating the effectiveness of any education provided. Ideally, the nurse should be aware of the resources available for teaching about medications, such as access to a clinical pharmacist. The nurse is well situated to coordinate care, identify the patient's goals, determine what the patient needs to learn in order to understand his or her medications, and arrange for follow-up care to determine the outcome of medication teaching.

Medications occupy a central place in the lives of many older persons; cost, acceptability, interactions, unacceptable side effects, and the need to schedule medications appropriately all combine to create many difficulties. Although nurses, with the exception of advanced practice nurses, do not prescribe medications, we believe that having a basic understanding of issues specific to the safe administration and consumption of medications by persons in later life will reduce the use of inappropriate medications and allow the nurse to observe more closely for adverse side effects and interactions. In the roles of educator and advocate the nurse might promote safe medication use through personally and culturally appropriate instructions.

KEY CONCEPTS

- As we age, the way our body responds to medications changes.
- Any medication has side effects. The therapeutic goal is to reduce the targeted symptoms without undesirable side effects.
- Drug-drug, drug–herb/supplement, and drug-food interactions are increasing problems that require nurse awareness.
- Polypharmacy is one of the most serious problems of elders today, and this is usually the first area to investigate when adverse physiological or psychiatric findings are assessed.
- Drug misuse may be triggered by prescriber practices, individual self-medication, individual physiology, altered biodegradability, nutritional and fluid states, and inadequate assessment before prescribing or administering.
- Nurses must consider the occurrence of a possible adverse medication effect immediately if a change in the person's condition is observed, including mental status changes in an individual who is normally alert and aware, or increasing confusion. Many drugs cause temporary cognitive impairment in older persons.
- The side effects of psychotropic medications vary significantly; thus these medications must be carefully selected and prescribed for the older adult. This increases the nurse's responsibility in the administration and monitoring of these medications.
- The response of the elder to treatment with psychotropic medications should show reduced distress, clearer thinking, and more appropriate behavior.
- It is always expected that pharmacological approaches augment rather than replace nonpharmacological approaches.
- Older adults are particularly vulnerable to developing movement disorders (extrapyramidal symptoms, parkinsonian symptoms, akathisia, and dystonia) with the use of antipsychotics.
- The Omnibus Budget Reconciliation Act (OBRA) restricts the use of psychotropic drugs in the long-term care setting unless they are truly needed for specific disorders and to maintain or improve function.
- Any time a behavior change is noted in a person, reversible causes must be sought and treated before medications are used.
- Dosages of medications must be carefully titrated for the individual, and the individual's responses must be accurately and consistently recorded.

ACTIVITIES AND DISCUSSION QUESTIONS

1. What are the age-related changes that occur in the pharmacokinetics of the older adult?
2. What are the drug use patterns of older adults, and what can be done to correct or improve them?
3. Explain the roles of the elder, the care provider, and the social network in reducing medication misuse.
4. List a variety of measures that the nurse can suggest to assist older adults with their medication use and adherence to a medication regimen.
5. What are the most troublesome side effects of antipsychotic medications?
6. Mrs. J. is repeatedly asking for a nurse; other patients are complaining, and you simply cannot be available to Mrs. J. for long periods. Considering the setting and the OBRA guidelines, what would you do to manage the situation?

REFERENCES

Ajemigbitse AA, Omole MK, Erhun WO: An assessment of the rate, types and severity of prescribing errors in a tertiary hospital in southwestern Nigeria, *Afr J Med Sci* 42(4):339–346, 2013.

American Geriatrics Society (AGS): American Geriatrics Society updated Beers Criteria for potentially inappropriate medication use in older adults, *J Am Geriatr Soc* 60(4):616–631, 2012.

American Geriatrics Society (AGS): American Geriatrics Society 2015 updated Beers Criteria for potentially inappropriate medication use in older adults, *J Am Geriatr Soc* 63(11):2227–2246, 2015.

Barnes TR: A rating scale for drug-induced akathisia, *Br J Psychiatry* 154:672–676, 1989.

Barry PJ, O'Keefe N, O'Connor K, et al: Inappropriate prescribing in the elderly: A comparison of the Beers criteria and the improved prescribing in the elderly tool (IPET) in acutely ill elderly hospitalized patients, *J Clin Pharm Ther* 31(6):617–626, 2007.

Beers M: Explicit criteria for determining potentially inappropriate medication use by the elderly. An update, *Arch Intern Med* 157:1531–1536, 1997.

Briggs GC: Geriatric issues. In Younkgin E, Sawin KJ, Kissinger J, et al, editors: *Pharmacotherapeutics: A primary care guide*, Upper Saddle River, NJ, 2005, Prentice-Hall.

Budnitz DS, Lovegrove MC, Shehab N, et al: Emergency hospitalizations for adverse drug events in older persons, *N Engl J Med* 365(21):2002–2012, 2011.

Bullock R, Saharan A: Atypical antipsychotics: Experience and use in the elderly, *Int J Clin Pract* 56(7):515–525, 2002.

Burchum JLR: Pharmacologic management. In Meiner S, editor: *Gerontologic nursing*, ed 4, St Louis, MO, 2011, Elsevier.

Gnjidic D, Hilmer SN, Blyth FM, et al: Polypharmacy cutoff and outcomes: Five or more medications were used to identify community-dwelling older men at risk of different adverse outcomes, *J Clin Epidemiol* 65(9):989–995, 2012.

Hughes GJ, Beizer JL: Appropriate prescribing. In Ham RJ, Sloane PD, Warshaw GA, et al, editors: *Primary care geriatrics: A case-based approach*, ed 6, Philadelphia, 2014, Elsevier, pp 67–76.

Lindsey PL: Psychotropic medication use among older adults: What all nurses need to know, *J Gerontol Nurs* 35(9):28–38, 2009.

Marcum ZA, Handler SM, Boyce R, et al: Medication misadventures in the elderly: A year in review, *Am J Geriatr Pharmacother* 8(1):77–83, 2010.

Masoro EJ, Austed SN, editors: *Handbook of biology and aging*, ed 5, San Diego, 2003, Academic Press.

Miller CA: *Nursing for wellness in older adults*, ed 5, Philadelphia, 2008, Wolters Kluwer Health.

Omnibus Budget Reconciliation Act (OBRA) of 1987, House of Representatives, 100th Congress, 1st Session, Report 100-391, Washington, DC, 1987, U.S. Government Printing Office.

Ortiz-Tudela E, Martinez-Nicolas A, Diaz-Mardomingo C, et al: The characterization of biological rhythms in mild cognitive impairment, *Biomed Res Int* 2014. doi: 10.1155/2014/524971. Published online.

Planton J, Edlund BJ: Strategies for reducing polypharmacy in older adults, *J Gerontol Nurs* 36:8–12, 2010.

Rochon PA: *Drug prescribing for older adults*, 2014. UpToDate. Available at http://www.uptodate.com/contents/drug-prescribing-for-older-adults. Accessed December 2015.

Ruscin JM, Linnebur SA: *Introduction to drug therapy in the elderly*, 2014. Available at http://www.merckmanuals.com/professional/geriatrics/drug-therapy-in-the-elderly/introduction-to-drug-therapy-in-the-elderly. Accessed December 2015.

Salvi F, Machetti A, D'Angelo F, et al: Adverse drug events as a cause of hospitalization in older adults, *Drug Saf* Jan(Suppl 1):29–45, 2012.

Simpson GM, Angus JWS: A rating scale for extrapyramidal side effects, *Acta Psychiatr Scand* 212:11–19, 1970.

10

Nutrition

Theris A. Touhy

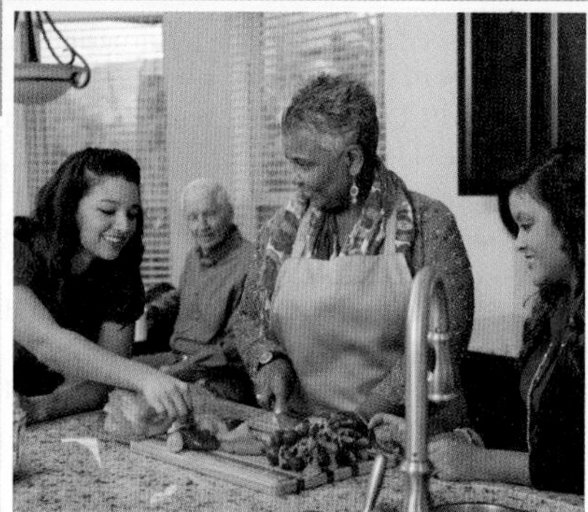

evolve.elsevier.com/Touhy/gerontological

LEARNING OBJECTIVES

Upon completion of this chapter, the reader will be able to:

- Discuss nutritional requirements and factors affecting nutrition for older adults.
- Describe a nutritional screening and assessment.
- Identify evidence-based interventions to promote adequate nutrition for older adults.
- Discuss assessment and interventions for older adults with dysphagia.

THE LIVED EXPERIENCE

If I do reach the point when I can no longer feed myself, I hope that the hands holding my fork belong to someone who has a feeling for who I am. I hope my helper will remember what she learns about me and that her awareness of me will grow from one encounter to another. Why should this make a difference? Yet, I am certain that my experience of needing to be fed will be altered if it occurs in the context of my being known. I will want to know about the lives of the people I rely on, especially the one who holds my fork for me. If she would talk to me, if we could laugh together, I might even forget the chagrin of my useless hands. We could have a conversation rather than a feeding.

From Lustbader (1999)

NUTRITION

The quality and quantity of diet are important factors in preventing, delaying onset, and managing chronic illnesses associated with aging. Results of studies provide growing evidence that diet can affect longevity and, when combined with lifestyle changes, reduce disease risk. "Of the top 10 leading causes of death in the United States, a lifetime of good nutrition would positively improve nine causes: heart disease, cancer, stroke, chronic respiratory disease, Alzheimer's disease, diabetes, influenza/pneumonia, nephritic syndrome/nephritis, and septicemia" (Amella & Aselage, 2012, p. 452). Additionally, about 87% of elders have diabetes, hypertension, dyslipidemia, or a combination of these diseases that have dietary implications (American Dietetic Association [ADA], American Society for Nutrition [ASN], and Society for Nutrition Education [SNE], 2010).

Proper nutrition means that all of the essential nutrients (i.e., carbohydrates, fat, protein, vitamins, minerals, and water) are adequately supplied and used to maintain optimal health and wellness. Although some age-related changes in the gastrointestinal system do occur (see Chapter 3), these changes are rarely the primary factors in inadequate nutrition. Fulfillment of nutritional needs in aging is more often affected by numerous other factors, including chronic disease, lifelong eating habits, ethnicity, socialization, income, transportation, housing, mood, food knowledge, functional impairments, health, and dentition. Data from the National Health and Nutrition Examination Survey (NHANES) showed that U.S. adults continue to fall short in meeting recommended dietary guidelines, and sociodemographic conditions influence food choices and overall diet quality (Ervin, 2011).

This chapter discusses the dietary needs of older adults, the risk factors contributing to inadequate nutrition, and the effects of obesity, diseases, functional and cognitive impairments, and dysphagia on nutrition. Several conditions warrant further discussion because they are frequently encountered in older adults and are related to adequate diet and nutritional status. Dehydration and oral health are discussed in Chapter 11 and the effect of neurocognitive disorders on nutrition is discussed in Chapter 25. Readers are referred to a nutrition text for more comprehensive information on nutrition and aging and disease.

United States Dietary Guidelines

The *2010 Dietary Guidelines for Americans,* published by the federal government, are designed to promote health, reduce the risk of chronic diseases, and decrease the prevalence of overweight and obesity through improved nutrition and physical activity. The guidelines focus on balancing calories with physical activity; encourage Americans to consume more healthy foods such as vegetables, fruits, whole grains, fat-free and low-fat dairy products, and seafood; and urge Americans to consume less sodium, saturated and trans fats, added sugars, and refined grains. In addition to the key recommendations, there are recommendations for specific population groups including older adults (U.S. Department of Health and Human Services [USDHHS] & U.S. Department of Agriculture [USDA], 2015). *Healthy People 2020* also provides goals for nutrition (Box 10.1).

MyPlate for Older Adults

Choose MyPlate is a visual depiction of daily food intake (www.ChooseMyPlate.gov). The USDA Human Nutrition Research Center on Aging at Tufts University has introduced the *MyPlate for Older Adults,* which calls attention to the unique nutritional and physical activity needs associated with advancing years. The illustration features different forms of vegetables and fruits that are convenient, affordable, and readily available. Other unique components of the *MyPlate for Older Adults* include addition of icons for regular physical activity and emphasis on adequate fluid intake, areas of particular concern for older adults (Fig. 10.1).

BOX 10.1 *Healthy People 2020*

Nutrition and Weight Status

- Promote health and reduce chronic disease through the consumption of healthful diets and achievement and maintenance of body weight.
- Increase the proportion of primary care physicians who regularly measure the body mass index in their adult patients.
- Increase the proportion of physician office visits made by adult patients who are obese that include counseling or education related to weight reduction, nutrition, or physical activity.
- Increase the proportion of physician visits made by all child and adult patients that include counseling about nutrition or diet.
- Increase the proportion of adults who are at a healthy weight.
- Reduce household food insecurity and in so doing reduce hunger.

From U.S. Department of Health and Human Services, Office of Disease Prevention and Health Promotion: *Healthy People 2020,* 2012. Available at http://www.healthypeople.gov/2020.

Generally, older adults need fewer calories because they may not be as active and metabolic rates decline. However, they still require the same or higher levels of nutrients for optimal health outcomes. The recommendations may need modification for individuals who have illnesses. The Dietary Approaches to Stop Hypertension (DASH) eating plan is a recommended eating plan to assist with maintenance of optimal weight and management of hypertension. This plan consists of fruits, vegetables, whole grains, low-fat dairy products, poultry, and fish, as well as restriction of salt intake.

In recent studies the Mediterranean diet has also been associated both with a lower incidence of chronic illness, weight gain, and impaired physical function and with improved cognition (Martinez-Lapiscina et al., 2013; Samieri et al., 2013a,b; Slomski, 2014; Yang et al., 2014). This diet is characterized by a greater intake of fruits, vegetables, legumes, whole grains, and fish; a lower intake of red and processed meats; higher amounts of monosaturated fats, mostly provided by olive oil from Mediterranean countries; and lower amounts of saturated fats (Box 10.2).

Other Dietary Recommendations

Fats

Similar to other age groups, older adults should limit intake of saturated fat and trans fatty acids. High-fat diets cause obesity and increase the risk of heart disease and cancer. Recommendations are that 20% to 35% of total calories should be from fat, 45% to 65% from carbohydrates, and 10% to 35% from proteins. Monounsaturated fats, such as olive oil, are the best type of fat because they lower low-density lipoprotein (LDL)

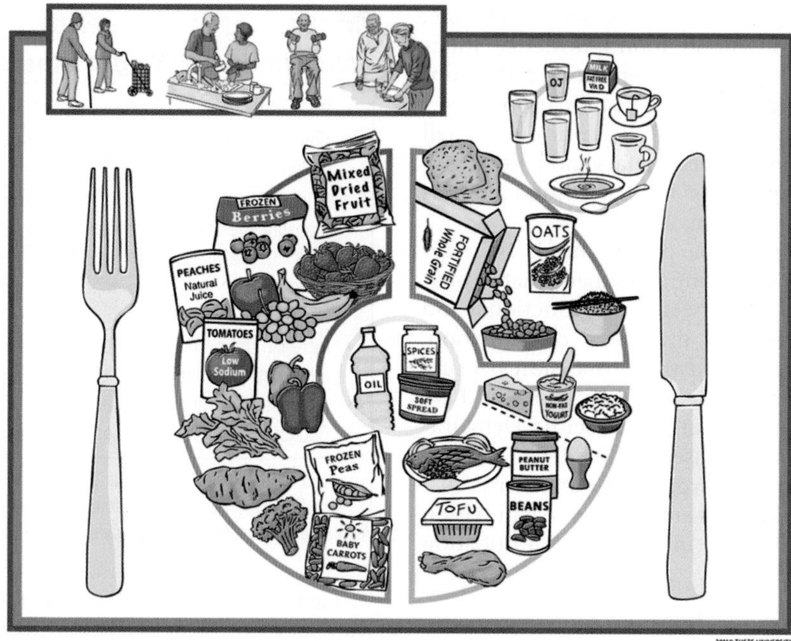

FIGURE 10.1 *MyPlate for Older Adults.* (From the Jean Mayer USDA Human Nutrition Research Center on Aging, Tufts University: *MyPlate for Older Adults,* 2011. Available at http://hnrca.tufts.edu/my-plate-for-older-adults.)

BOX 10.2 Resources for Best Practice

American Heart Association: DASH diet, Mediterranean diet.

Capezuti E, Zwicker D, Mezey M, et al., editors: *Evidence-based geriatric nursing protocols for best practice,* ed 4, New York, 2012, Springer.

HelpGuide.com: Eating well after 50. Nutrition and diet tips for healthy eating as you age.

National Institute on Aging: What's on your plate? Smart food choices for healthy aging.

Pioneer Network: New Dining Practice Standards (LTC).

The American Geriatrics Society: Position statement: Feeding tubes in advanced dementia.

The Hartford Foundation for Geriatric Nursing: Assessing nutrition in older adults (includes a video of administration of MNA), Mealtime difficulties, Preventing aspiration in older adults with dysphagia (includes video).

level but leave the high-density lipoprotein (HDL) level intact or even slightly raise it.

Protein

There has been discussion that the Institute of Medicine's Recommended Dietary Allowance (RDA) for protein of 0.8 g/kg per day, based primarily on studies in younger men, may be inadequate for older adults. Protein intake of 1.5 g/kg per day, or 20% to 25% of total calorie intake, may be associated with a decline in risk of frailty in older adults (Beasley et al., 2010; Imai et al., 2014). Older people who are ill are the most likely segment of society to experience protein deficiency. Those with limitations affecting their ability to shop, cook, and consume food are also at risk for protein deficiency and malnutrition.

Fiber

Fiber is an important dietary component that some older people do not consume in sufficient quantities. A daily intake of 25 g of fiber is recommended and must be combined with adequate amounts of fluid. Insufficient amounts of fiber in the diet, as well as insufficient fluids, contribute to constipation. Fiber is the indigestible material that gives plants their structure. It is abundant in raw fruits and vegetables and in unrefined grains and cereals.

Vitamins and Minerals

Older people who consume five servings of fruits and vegetables daily will obtain adequate intake of vitamins

A, C, and E and also potassium. Americans of all ages eat less than half of the recommended amounts of fruits and vegetables (Haber, 2010). After age 50, the stomach produces less gastric acid, which makes vitamin B_{12} absorption less efficient. Vitamin B_{12} deficiency is a common and underrecognized condition that is estimated to occur in 12% to 14% of community-dwelling older adults and in up to 25% of those residing in institutional settings (Ahmed & Haboubi, 2010).

Although intake of this vitamin is generally adequate, older adults should increase their intake of the crystalline form of vitamin B_{12} from fortified foods such as whole-grain breakfast cereals. Use of proton pump inhibitors for more than 1 year, as well as histamine H_2-receptor blockers, can lead to lower serum vitamin B_{12} levels by impairing absorption of the vitamin from food. Metformin, colchicine, and antibiotic and anticonvulsant agents may also increase the risk of vitamin B_{12} deficiency (Cadogan, 2010). Calcium and vitamin D are essential for bone health and may prevent osteoporosis and decrease the risk of fracture (see Chapter 21).

OBESITY (OVERNUTRITION)

The World Health Organization (WHO, 2003) noted that an escalating global epidemic of overweight and obesity—"globesity"—is a major public health concern in both developed and developing countries. The number of obese adults worldwide is 300 million, with estimates that 115 million people in developing countries suffer from obesity-related problems. The WHO has developed the Global Action Plan to address the issue. Overweight and obesity are associated with increased health care costs, functional impairments, disability, chronic disease, and nursing home admission. It is important to remember that overweight/obese individuals are also at risk for malnutrition as a result of chronic illness or diets inadequate in appropriate nutrients.

The prevalence of obesity is higher among middle-aged (40.2%) and older (37.0%) adults than younger adults (32.3%). The prevalence of obesity was lowest among non-Hispanic Asian adults (11.7%), followed by non-Hispanic white (34.5%), Hispanic (42.5%), and non-Hispanic black (48.1%) adults. Since 2008, Americans aged 65 and older have seen the sharpest rise in obesity and the proportion of older adults who are obese has doubled in the past 30 years (Flicker et al., 2010; Rettner, 2015). Socioeconomic deprivation and lower levels of education have been linked to obesity (Ogden et al., 2014).

Although there is strong evidence that obesity in younger people decreases life expectancy and has a negative effect on functionality and morbidity, it remains unclear whether overweight and obesity are predictors of mortality in older adults. In what has been termed the *obesity paradox,* some research has found that for people who have survived to 70 years of age, mortality risk is lowest in those with a body mass index (BMI) classified as overweight (Felix, 2008; Tobias et al., 2014). For nursing home residents with severely decreased functional status, obesity may be regarded as a protective factor with regard to functionality and mortality (Kaiser et al., 2010).

Further research is needed to understand how long-term intentional weight loss and associated shifts in body composition affect the onset of chronic disease. Weight loss recommendations for older people should be carefully considered on an individualized basis with attention to the weight history and medical conditions. The most effective weight loss program combines nutrition education, diet, and exercise with behavioral strategies (Mathew & Jacobs, 2014). Maintaining a healthy weight throughout life can prevent many illnesses and functional limitations as a person grows older.

MALNUTRITION (UNDERNUTRITION)

Malnutrition is a recognized geriatric syndrome. The rising incidence of malnutrition among older adults has been documented in acute care, long-term care, and the community. Malnutrition is estimated to occur in 1% to 15% of ambulatory outpatients, 25% to 60% of institutionalized patients, 35% to 65% of hospitalized patients, and 49% of patients discharged from the hospital (Buys et al., 2013; Mathew & Jacobs, 2014). These figures are expected to rise dramatically in the next 30 years (Ahmed & Haboubi, 2010). Malnutrition among older people is clearly a serious challenge for health professionals in all settings.

Consequences

Malnutrition is a precursor to frailty and has serious consequences, including infections, pressure ulcers, anemia, hypotension, impaired cognition, hip fractures, prolonged hospital stay, institutionalization, and increased morbidity and mortality (DiMaria-Ghalili, 2012; White et al., 2012). "Malnourished older adults take 40% longer to recover from illness, have two to three times as many complications, and have hospital stays that are 90% longer" (Haber, 2010, p. 211). Many factors contribute to the occurrence of malnutrition in older adults (Fig. 10.2).

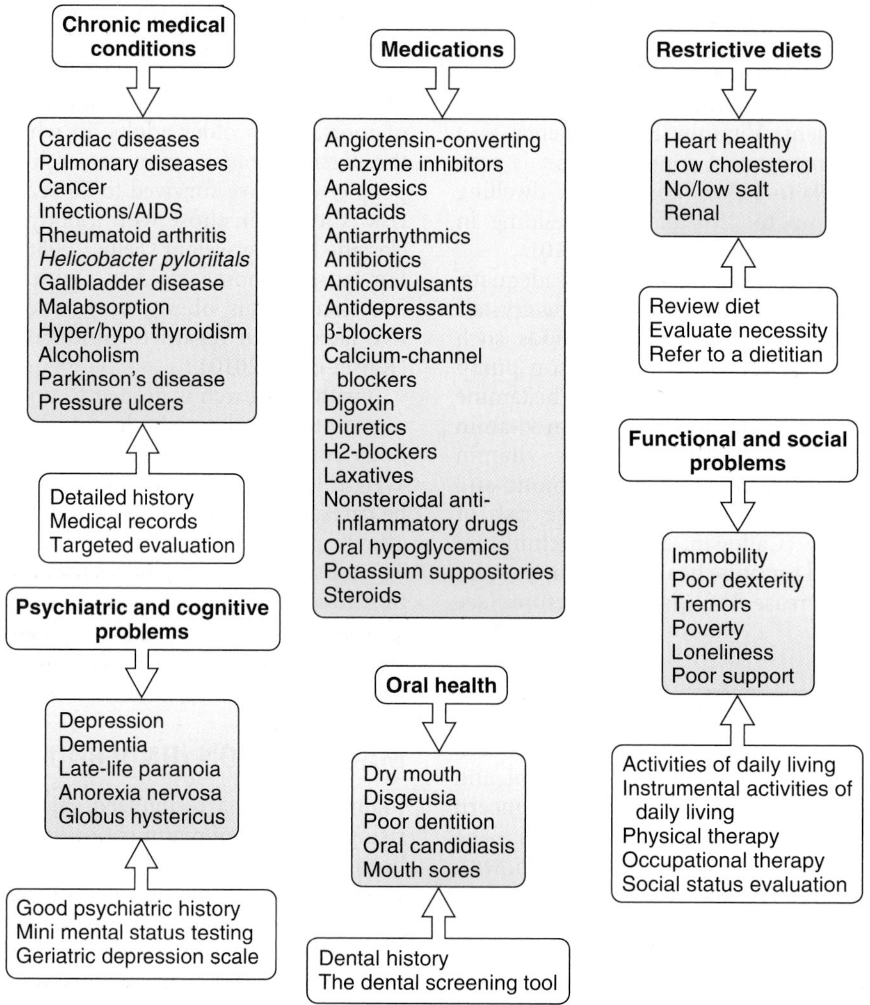

FIGURE 10.2 Risk factors for undernutrition illustrated by clinical approach. (From Omran M, Salem P: Diagnosing undernutrition, *Clin Geriatr Med* 18:719–736, 2002.)

Characteristics

The understanding of malnutrition is evolving, and research is ongoing. "Malnutrition is a complex syndrome that develops following two primary trajectories. It can occur when the individual does not consume sufficient amounts of micronutrients (i.e., vitamins, minerals, phytochemicals) and macronutrients (i.e., protein, carbohydrates, fat, water) required to maintain organ function and healthy tissues. This type of malnutrition can occur from prolonged undernutrition or overnutrition. In contrast, inflammation-related malnutrition develops as a consequence of injury, surgery, or disease states that trigger inflammatory mediators that contribute to increased metabolic rate and impaired nutrient utilization" (Litchford, 2013, p. 38). Inflammation is increasingly identified as an important underlying factor that increases risk for malnutrition and a contributing factor to suboptimal responses to nutritional intervention and increased risk of mortality (DiMaria-Ghalili, 2012). Weight loss frequently occurs in both trajectories (White et al., 2012).

FACTORS AFFECTING FULFILLMENT OF NUTRITIONAL NEEDS

Fulfillment of the older person's nutritional needs is affected by numerous factors including changes associated with aging (see Chapter 3), lifelong eating habits, acute and chronic illness, medication regimens, ethnicity and culture, ability to obtain and prepare food, mood, socialization, socioeconomic deprivation, transportation, housing, and food knowledge.

Lifelong Eating Habits

The nutritional state of a person reflects the individual's dietary history and present food practices. Lifelong habits of dieting or eating fad foods also echo through the later years. Individuals may fall prey to advertisements that claim specific foods can reverse aging or rid one of chronic conditions. Following the *MyPlate for Older Adults* (Fig. 10.1) is best for an ideal diet, with changes based on particular problems, such as hypercholesterolemia. Individuals should be counseled to base their dietary decisions on valid research and consultation with their primary care provider. For the healthy individual, essential nutrients should be obtained from food sources rather than relying on dietary supplements.

Socialization

The fundamentally social aspect of eating has to do with sharing and the feeling of belonging that it provides. All of us use food as a means of giving and receiving love, friendship, or belonging. The presence of others during meals is a significant predictor of caloric intake (Locher et al., 2008). The meaning and enjoyment of eating can often be challenged as one ages, requires hospitalization or nursing home residence, or experiences chronic illnesses, depression, isolation, and functional limitations. Disinterest in food may also result from the effects of medication or disease processes. Misuse and abuse of alcohol are prevalent among older adults and are growing public health concerns. Excessive drinking interferes with nutrition. Drinking alcohol depletes the body of necessary nutrients and often replaces meals, thus making an individual susceptible to malnutrition (see Chapter 24).

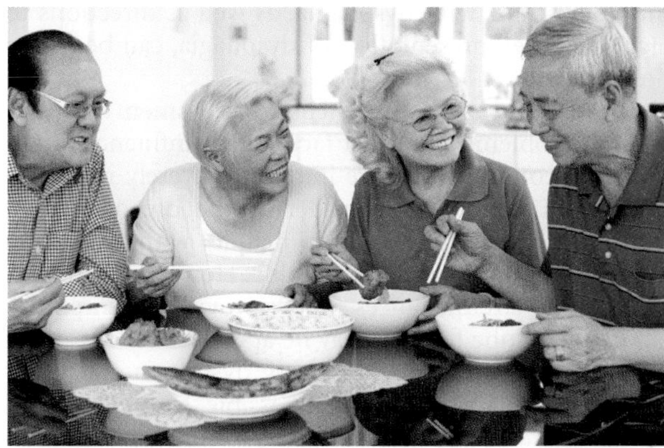

Older adults enjoying a meal together. (© iStock.com/monkeybusinessimages.)

The elderly nutrition program, authorized under Title III of the Older Americans Act (OAA), is the largest national food and nutrition program specifically for older adults. Programs and services include congregate nutrition programs, home-delivered nutrition services (Meals-on-Wheels), and nutrition screening and education. The program is not means tested, and participants may make voluntary confidential contributions for meals. With the emphasis on community-based care rather than institutional care, expansion of nutrition services should be a priority.

Chronic Diseases and Conditions

Many chronic diseases and their sequelae pose nutritional challenges for older adults. Functional and cognitive impairments associated with chronic disease interfere with the individual's ability to shop, cook, and eat independently. More detailed information on chronic illness can be found in Chapters 17–24. The side effects of medications prescribed for chronic conditions may further impair nutritional status (Fig. 10.2). There are clinically significant drug-nutrient interactions that result in nutrient loss, and evidence is accumulating that shows the use of nutritional supplements may counteract these possible drug-induced nutrient depletions. A thorough medication review is an essential component of nutritional assessment, and individuals should receive education about the effects of prescription medications, as well as herbals and supplements, on nutritional status (see Chapter 9).

Dysphagia

Dysphagia, or difficulty swallowing, is a common problem in older adults. The prevalence of swallowing disorders is 16% to 22% in adults older than 50 years of age, and up to 60% of nursing home residents have clinical evidence of dysphagia (Aslam & Vaezi, 2013). Dysphagia can be the result of behavioral, sensory, or motor problems and is common in individuals with neurological disease and dementia (Box 10.3) (see Chapters 22 and 23). Dysphagia is a serious problem and has negative consequences, including weight loss, malnutrition, dehydration, aspiration pneumonia, and even death. Aspiration (the misdirection of oropharyngeal secretions or gastric contents into the larynx and lower respiratory tract) is common in older adults.

❖ IMPLICATIONS FOR GERONTOLOGICAL NURSING AND HEALTHY AGING

◆ Assessment

It is important to obtain a careful history of the older adult's response to dysphagia and to observe the person

BOX 10.3 Risk Factors for Dysphagia

- Cerebrovascular accident
- Parkinson's disease
- Neuromuscular disorders (ALS, MS, myasthenia gravis)
- Dementia
- Head and neck cancer
- Traumatic brain injury
- Aspiration pneumonia
- Inadequate feeding technique
- Poor dentition

ALS, Amyotrophic lateral sclerosis; *MS,* multiple sclerosis.

BOX 10.4 Symptoms of Dysphagia or Possible Aspiration

- Difficult, labored swallowing
- Drooling
- Copious oral secretions
- Coughing, choking at meals
- Holding or pocketing of food/medications in the mouth
- Difficulty moving food or liquid from mouth to throat
- Difficulty chewing
- Nasal voice or hoarseness
- Wet or gurgling voice
- Excessive throat clearing
- Food or liquid leaking from the nose
- Prolonged eating time
- Pain with swallowing
- Unusual head or neck posturing while swallowing
- Sensation of something stuck in the throat during swallowing; sensation of a lump in the throat
- Heartburn
- Chest pain
- Hiccups
- Weight loss
- Frequent respiratory tract infections, pneumonia

during mealtime. Symptoms that alert the nurse to possible swallowing problems are presented in Box 10.4. Patients referred for a dysphagia evaluation ("swallowing study") must be assumed to be dysphagic and at risk for aspiration. Nothing-by-mouth (NPO) status should be maintained until the swallowing evaluation is completed. During this period, if necessary, nutrition and hydration needs can be met by intravenous, nasogastric, or gastric tubes. A comprehensive evaluation by a speech-language pathologist (SLP), usually including a video fluoroscopic recording of a modified barium swallow, should be considered when dysphagia is suspected.

◆ Interventions

After the swallowing evaluation, a decision must be made about the potential for functional improvement of the swallowing disorder and the safety in swallowing liquid and solid food. The goal is safe oral intake to maintain optimal nutrition and caloric needs. Nurses work closely with speech-language pathologists and the dietitian to implement interventions to prevent aspiration. Compensatory interventions include postural changes, such as chin tucks or head turns while swallowing, and modification of bolus volume, consistency, temperature, and rate of presentation. Diets may be modified in texture from pudding-like to nearly normal-textured solids. Liquids may range from spoon-thick to honey-like, nectar-like, and thin. Commercial thickeners and thickened products are also available (Mathew & Jacobs, 2014).

Neuromuscular electrical stimulation has received clearance by the U.S. Food and Drug Administration for treatment of dysphagia. This therapy involves the administration of small electrical impulses to the swallowing muscles in the throat and is used in combination with traditional swallowing exercises (Shune & Moon, 2012).

Aspiration is the most profound and dangerous problem for older adults experiencing dysphagia. It is important to have a suction machine available at the bedside or in the dining room in the institutional setting. Suggested interventions helpful in preventing aspiration during hand feeding are presented in Box 10.5. Research on the appropriate management of swallowing disorders in older people, particularly during acute illness and in long-term care facilities, is very limited, and additional study is essential. A protocol for preventing aspiration in older adults with dysphagia, as well as directions to access a video presentation of dysphagia, can be found in Box 10.2.

◆ ***Feeding tubes.*** Comprehensive assessment of swallowing problems and other factors that influence intake must be conducted before initiating severely restricted diet modifications or considering the use of feeding tubes, particularly in older people with end-stage dementia or those at the end of life. However, there may be certain circumstances when providing temporary short-term tube feeding may be appropriate (e.g., individuals with stroke and resulting dysphagia and other conditions when it may be possible to resume oral nutrition at some point).

◆ **Tube feeding in end-stage dementia.** Currently, there is no scientific study that demonstrates improved

BOX 10.5 Tips for Best Practice

Preventing Aspiration in Patients With Dysphagia: Hand Feeding

- Provide a 30-minute rest period before meal consumption; a rested person will likely have less difficulty swallowing.
- The person should sit at 90 degrees during all oral (PO) intake and remain in this position for at least 1 hour after intake.
- Adjust rate of feeding and size of bites to the person's tolerance; avoid rushed or forced feeding.
- Alternate solid and liquid boluses.
- Have the person swallow twice before the next mouthful.
- Stroke under chin downward to initiate swallowing.
- Follow speech therapist's recommendation for safe swallowing techniques and modified food consistency (may need thickened liquids, pureed foods).
- If facial weakness is present, place food on the nonimpaired side of the mouth.
- Avoid sedatives and hypnotics that may impair cough reflex and swallowing ability.
- Keep suction equipment ready at all times.
- Supervise all meals.
- Monitor temperature.
- Observe color of phlegm.
- Visually check the mouth for pocketing of food in cheeks.
- Check for food under dentures.
- Provide mouth care every 4 hours and before and after meals, including denture cleaning.

Adapted from Metheny N, Boltz M, Greenberg S: Preventing aspiration in older adults with dysphagia, *Am J Nurs* 108(2):45–46, 2008.

BOX 10.6 Myths and Facts About Percutaneous Endoscopic Gastrostomy (PEG) Tubes in Advanced Dementia and End-of-Life Care

Myths

- PEGs prevent death from inadequate intake.
- PEGs reduce aspiration pneumonia.
- PEGs improve albumin levels and nutritional status.
- PEGs assist in healing pressure ulcers.
- PEGs provide enhanced comfort for people at the end of life.
- Not feeding people is a form of euthanasia, and we cannot let people starve to death.

Facts

- PEGs do not improve quality of life.
- PEGs do not reduce risk of aspiration and increase the rate of pneumonia development. In one study, the use of feeding tubes was associated with an increased risk of pressure ulcers among nursing home residents with advanced cognitive impairment (Teno et al., 2012).
- PEGs do not prolong survival in dementia.
- Nearly 50% of patients die within 6 months following PEG tube insertion.
- PEGs cause increased discomfort from both the tube presence and the use of restraints.
- PEGs are associated with infections, gastrointestinal symptoms, and abscesses.
- PEG tube feeding deprives people of the taste of food and contact with caregivers during feeding.
- PEGs are popular because they are convenient and labor beneficial.

Data from Aparanji K, Dharmarajan T: Pause before a PEG: A feeding tube may not be necessary in every candidate, *J Am Med Dir Assoc* 11:453–456, 2010; Teno J, Gozalo P, Mitchell S, et al: Feeding tubes and the prevention or healing of pressure ulcers, *Arch Intern Med* 172(9):697–701, 2012; Vitale C, Monteleoni C, Burke L, et al: Strategies for improving care for patients with advanced dementia and eating problems: Optimizing care through physician and speech pathologist collaboration, *Ann Longterm Care* 17:32–39, 2009.

survival, reduced incidence of pneumonia or other infections, improved function, or fewer pressure ulcers with the use of feeding tubes in older people with advanced dementia who have poor nutritional intake (Teno et al., 2011, 2012) (Box 10.6). However, there is a continued need for randomized controlled trials to determine the benefits and risks (Glick & Jolkowitz, 2013). An estimated 5% to 30% of nursing home residents with dementia in the United States and Europe have percutaneous endoscopic gastrostomy (PEG) tubes inserted (Glick & Jolkowitz, 2013).

The American Geriatrics Society (AGS) (2013) does not recommend feeding tubes for older adults with advanced dementia (Box 10.2). The AGS guidelines suggest that careful hand feeding for patients with severe dementia is at least as good as tube feeding for the outcomes of death, aspiration pneumonia, functional status, and patient comfort (Box 10.5). Further, tube feeding is associated with agitation, increased use of physical and chemical restraints, and worsening of pressure ulcers (Teno et al., 2012).

Decisions about feeding tube placement are challenging and require thoughtful discussion with patients and caregivers, who should be free to make decisions without duress and with careful consideration of the patient's advance directives, if available. Individuals have the right to use or not use a feeding tube but should be given information about the risks and benefits of enteral feeding, particularly in late-stage dementia. In difficult situations, an ethics committee may be consulted to help make decisions. It is important that everyone involved in the care of the patient be knowledgeable about the evidence related to the risks and benefits of tube feeding. The decision should never be understood as a question of tube feeding versus no feeding. No family member should be made to feel that he or she is starving his or her loved one to death if a decision is made not to institute enteral feeding. Efforts to provide nutrition should continue, and patients should be able to take any type of nutrition they desire any time they desire.

Regardless of the decision, an important nursing role is to journey with the patient's loved ones, providing support and encouraging expression of feelings. Making these decisions is very difficult and loved ones "have to make peace with their decisions" (Teno et al., 2011).

Socioeconomic Deprivation

There is a strong relationship between poor nutrition and socioeconomic deprivation. About 1 in 10 individuals ages 65 and older has an income below the poverty level in the United States. Rates are closer to 15% when the supplemental poverty measure is used rather than the official poverty measure (Levinson et al., 2013). Poverty rates among older African Americans and Hispanics, as well as older single women, are higher than for other groups.

The Supplemental Nutrition Assistance Program (SNAP), a program of the United States Department of Agriculture (UDSA), Food and Nutrition Services, offers nutrition assistance to eligible, low-income individuals and families; however, older adults are less likely than any other age group to use food assistance programs. This is likely because of the stigma attached to food stamps, the low benefit amounts, the belief that they are ineligible, and the cumbersome application process (Berg, 2015; Fuller-Thomson & Redmond, 2008).

Free food programs, such as donated commodities, are also available at distribution centers (food banks) for those with limited incomes. Although this is another valuable option, use of such programs is not always feasible. One takes a chance on the types of food available on any particular day or week; quantities distributed are frequently too large for the single older person or the older couple to use or even carry from the distribution site; the site may be too far away or difficult to reach; and the time of food distribution may be inconvenient.

There are cafeterias and restaurants that provide special meal prices for older people, but costs have risen with increases in food costs. The previous advantages of eating out have diminished. Yet many single elders eat out for most meals. More elders are eating at fast food restaurants that typically do not offer low-fat/low-salt menu items. Providing education about the nutritional content of fast food and other convenient ways to enhance healthy nutritional intake is important.

Transportation

Available and easily accessible transportation may be limited for older people. Many small, long-standing neighborhood food stores have been closed in the wake of the expansion of larger supermarkets, which are located in areas that serve a greater segment of the population. It may become difficult to walk to the market, to reach it by public transportation, or to carry a bag of groceries while using a cane or walker. Despite reduced senior citizen bus fares, many older people remain very fearful of attack when using public transportation. Functional impairments also make the use of public transportation difficult for others.

Senior citizen organizations in many parts of the United States have been helpful in providing older adults with van service to shopping areas. In housing complexes, it may be possible to schedule group trips to the supermarket. Many urban communities have multiple sources of transportation available, but the individual may be unaware of them. Resources in rural areas are more limited. It is important for nurses to be knowledgeable about transportation resources in the community.

In addition, many older adults, particularly widowed men, may have never learned to shop and prepare food. Often, individuals have to rely on others to shop for them, and this may be a cause of concern depending on the availability of support and the reluctance to be dependent on someone else, particularly family. For those who own a computer, shopping over the Internet and having groceries delivered offers advantages, although prices may be higher than those in the stores.

❖ IMPLICATIONS FOR GERONTOLOGICAL NURSING AND HEALTHY AGING

Comprehensive nutritional screening and assessment are essential in identifying older adults at risk for nutrition problems or who are malnourished. Older people are less likely than younger people to show signs of malnutrition and nutrient malabsorption. Evaluation of nutritional health can be difficult in the absence of severe malnutrition, but a comprehensive assessment can reveal deficits. Screening and assessment of concerns identified should be conducted on admission to hospital, home health, or long-term care. Nutritional status changes as health status changes, and ongoing assessment is also important. The role of nursing in nutrition assessment and intervention should be comprehensive and include increased attention to the process of eating and the entire ritual of meals, as well as the assessment of nutritional status within the interprofessional team (Amella & Aselage, 2012).

◆ Nutritional Screening

Nutritional screening is the first step in identifying individuals who are at risk for malnutrition, or have undetected malnutrition, and determines the need for a more comprehensive assessment and nutritional interventions. There are several screening tools specific to older individuals, and screening can be completed in any setting. The Nutrition Screening Initiative Checklist (Fig. 10.3) can be self-administered or completed by a family member or any member of the health care team.

The Mini Nutritional Assessment (MNA) is both a screening tool and a detailed assessment. Developed by Nestle of Geneva, Switzerland, the MNA is only validated for individuals older than age 65 and intended for use by professionals. If an individual scores less than 12 on the screen, then the assessment section should be completed (DiMaria-Ghalili, 2012). The MNA is recommended by the Hartford Institute for Geriatric Nursing, and a video of administration of the tool is provided on their website (Box 10.2).

The Minimum Data Set 3.0 (MDS 3.0) (see Chapter 8), used in long-term care facilities, includes assessment information that can be used to identify potential nutritional problems, risk factors, and the likelihood for improved function. Triggers for more thorough investigation of problems include weight loss, alterations in taste, medical therapies, prescription medications, hunger, parenteral or intravenous feedings, mechanically altered or therapeutic diets, percentage of food left uneaten, pressure ulcers, and edema.

◆ Nutritional Assessment

When risk for undernutrition or malnutrition is detected, a comprehensive nutritional assessment is indicated and will provide the most conclusive data about a person's actual nutritional state. Interprofessional approaches are paramount to appropriate assessment and intervention and should involve staff from medicine; nursing; dietary, physical, occupational, and speech therapy; and social work. The collective results provide the data needed to identify the immediate and the potential nutritional problems so that plans for supervision, assistance, and education in the attainment of adequate nutrition can be implemented. Components of a nutrition assessment include interview, history, physical examination, anthropomorphic data, laboratory data, food/nutrient intake, and functional assessment. Explanations of several components are discussed in the following sections.

◆ Interview

◆ Food/Nutrient Intake

Frequently a 24-hour diet recall compared with the *MyPlate for Older Adults* can provide an estimate of nutritional adequacy. When the individual cannot

Read the statements below. Circle the number in the Yes column for those that apply to you or someone you know. For each "yes" answer, score the number listed. Total your nutritional score.

	YES
I have an illness or condition that made me change the kind or amount of food I eat.	2
I eat fewer than two meals per day.	3
I eat few fruits, vegetables, or milk products.	2
I have three or more drinks of beer, liquor, or wine almost every day.	2
I have tooth or mouth problems that make it hard for me to eat.	2
I don't always have enough money to buy the food I need.	4
I eat alone most of the time.	1
I take three or more different prescriptions or over-the-counter drugs each day.	1
Without wanting to, I have lost or gained 10 pounds in the past 6 months.	2
I am not always physically able to shop, cook, and/or feed myself.	2
Total Nutritional Score	______

0-2 indicates good nutrition
3-5 moderate risk
6+ high nutritional risk

FIGURE 10.3 Nutrition screening initiative. (Courtesy The Nutrition Screening Initiative, Washington, DC.)

supply all of the requested information, it may be possible to obtain data from a family member or another source such as a shopping receipt. There will be times, however, when information will not be as complete as one would like, or the individual, too proud to admit that he or she is not eating, will furnish erroneous information. Even so, the nurse will be able to obtain additional data from the other three areas of the nutritional assessment.

A 3-day dietary record, completed by the individual or the caregivers, is another assessment tool. What foods were eaten, when food was eaten, and the amounts eaten must be carefully recorded. Computer analysis of the dietary records provides information on energy and vitamin and mineral intake. Printouts can provide the older person and the health care provider with a visual graph of the intake. Accurate completion of 3-day dietary records in hospitals and nursing homes can be problematic, and intake may be either underestimated or overestimated. Standardized observational protocols should be developed to ensure accuracy of oral intake documentation, as well as the adequacy and quality of feeding assistance during mealtimes. Nurses should ensure that direct caregivers are educated on the proper observation and documentation of intake and should closely monitor performance in this area.

◆ Anthropomorphic Measurements

Anthropomorphic measurements include height, weight, midarm circumference, and triceps skinfold thickness. These measurements offer information about the status of the older person's muscle mass and body fat in relation to height and weight. Muscle mass measurements are obtained by measuring the arm circumference of the nondominant upper arm. The arm hangs freely at the side, and a measuring tape is placed around the midpoint of the upper arm, between the acromion of the scapula and the olecranon of the ulna. The centimeter circumference is recorded and compared with standard values.

Body fat and lean muscle mass are assessed by measuring specific skinfolds with Lange or Harpenden calipers. The midpoint of the upper arm, the triceps area, is used to obtain arm circumference. The nondominant arm is again used. Lift the skin with the thumb and forefinger so that it is parallel to the humerus. The calipers are placed around the skinfold, 1 cm below where the fingers are grasping the skin. Two readings are averaged to the nearest 0.5 cm. If there is a neuropathological condition or hemiplegia following a stroke, the unaffected arm should be used for obtaining measurements (DiMaria-Ghalili, 2012).

◆ Weight/Height Considerations

A detailed weight history should be obtained along with current weight. Weight loss is a key indicator of malnutrition, even in overweight older adults. History should include a history of weight loss, if the weight loss was intentional or unintentional, and during what period it occurred. A history of anorexia is also important, and many older people, especially women, have limited their weight throughout life. Although weight alone does not indicate the adequacy of diet, unplanned fluctuations in weight are significant and should be evaluated.

Accurate weight patterns are sometimes difficult to obtain in long-term care settings. Procedures for weighing people should be established and followed consistently to obtain an accurate representation of weight changes. Weighing procedure should be supervised by licensed personnel, and changes should be reported immediately to the provider. One might meet correct weight values for height, but weight changes may be the result of fluid retention, edema, or ascites and merit investigation. An unintentional weight loss of more than 5% of body weight in 1 month, more than 7.5% in 3 months, or more than 10% in 6 months is considered a significant indicator of poor nutrition, as well as an MDS trigger.

Height should always be measured and never estimated or given by self-report. If the person cannot stand, an alternative way of determining standing height is knee-height measurement using special calipers. An alternative to knee-height measurements is a demi-span measurement, which is half the total arm span (DiMaria-Ghalili, 2012). BMI should be calculated to determine if weight for height is within the normal range of 22 to 27. Individuals at either extreme of BMI may be at increased risk of poor nutritional status (White et al., 2012).

◆ Biochemical Analysis/Measures of Visceral Protein

There is no single biochemical marker of malnutrition, and unintentional weight loss remains the most important indicator of a potential nutritional deficit (Ahmed & Haboubi, 2010). The relevance of laboratory tests of serum albumin and prealbumin, as indicators of malnutrition, is limited. These acute phase proteins do not consistently or predictability change with weight loss, calorie restriction, or negative nitrogen balance. They appear to better reflect severity of inflammatory response rather than poor nutritional status (White et al., 2012).

Further investigation of the significance of low protein levels is needed. Serum albumin level has been noted as a "strong prognostic marker for morbidity and mortality in the older hospitalized patient" and remains a recommendation in evaluation of nutritional status

(DiMaria-Ghalili, 2012, p. 442). With continued research on biomarkers of inflammation, these may be included in future diagnostic recommendations for malnutrition.

◆ Interventions

Interventions are formulated around the identified nutritional problem or problems. Nursing interventions are centered on techniques to increase food intake and enhance and manage the environment to promote increased food intake (DiMaria-Ghalili, 2012). Jefferies and colleagues (2011) suggest that nurturing and nourishing describe the nurses' role in nutritional care. Nurses hold a pivotal role in ensuring adequate nutrition to promote healthy aging (Box 10.7). Collaboration with the interprofessional team (dietitian, pharmacist, social worker, occupational therapist, speech therapist) is important in planning interventions.

For the community-dwelling elder, nutrition education and problem solving with the elder and family members or caregivers on how to best resolve the potential or actual nutritional deficit is important. Causes of poor nutrition are complex, and all of the factors emphasized in this chapter are important to assess when planning individualized interventions to ensure adequate nutrition for older people.

Older adults in hospitals and long-term care are more likely to enter the settings with malnutrition, be at high risk for malnutrition, and have disease conditions that contribute to malnutrition. Severely restricted diets, long periods of nothing-by-mouth (NPO) status, and insufficient time and staff for feeding assistance also contribute to inadequate nutrition. Older adults with dementia are particularly at risk for weight loss and inadequate nutrition (see Chapter 25).

◆ Feeding Assistance

The incidence of eating disability in long-term care is high, with estimates that 50% of all residents cannot eat independently (Burger et al., 2000). Inadequate staffing in long-term care facilities is associated with poor nutrition and hydration. In response to concerns about the lack of adequate assistance during mealtime in long-term care facilities, the Centers for Medicare and Medicaid Services (CMS) implemented a rule that allows feeding assistants with 8 hours of approved training to help residents with eating. Feeding assistants must be supervised by a registered nurse (RN) or licensed practical/licensed vocational nurse (LPN/LVN). Family members may also be willing and able to assist at mealtimes and also provide a familiar social context for the patient.

Assistance with meals in hospitals is also a concern. An innovative volunteer program to address the unique needs of older hospitalized patients was reported by Buys and colleagues (2013). Support for and Promotion of Optimal Nutritional Status (SPOONS) focused on three important factors of the mealtime experience: socialization, functional assistance, and staffing challenges. Further research is needed on the effectiveness of feeding assistance programs in hospital settings.

BOX 10.7 Tips for Best Practice

Nutritional Care

- Assessment of the individual for issues related to performance at mealtimes
- Modification of the environment to be pleasurable for eating
- Supervision of eating
- Provision of guidance and support to staff on feeding techniques that enhance intake and preserve dignity and independence
- Evaluation of outcomes

From Amella E, Aselage M: Mealtime difficulties. In Boltz M, Capezuti E, Fulmer T, et al, editors: *Evidence-based geriatric nursing protocols for best practice,* ed 4, pp 453–468, New York, 2012, Springer.

◆ Approaches to Enhancing Intake in Long-Term Care

In addition to adequate staff, many innovative and evidence-based ideas can improve nutritional intake in institutions. Many suggestions are found in the literature: homelike dining rooms; cafeteria-style service; refreshment stations with easy access to juices, water, and healthy snacks; kitchens on the nursing units; choice of mealtimes; finger foods; visually appealing pureed foods with texture and shape; music; touch (see Chapter 25).

◆ Restrictive Diets and Caloric Supplements

The use of restrictive therapeutic diets for frail elders in long-term care (low cholesterol, low salt, no concentrated sweets) often reduces food intake without significantly helping the clinical status of the individual (Pioneer Network and Rothschild Foundation, 2011). If caloric supplements are used, they should be administered at least 1 hour before meals or they interfere with meal intake. These products are widely used and can be costly. Often, they are not dispensed or consumed as ordered. Powdered breakfast drinks added to milk are an adequate substitute (Duffy, 2010).

Dispensing a small amount of calorically dense oral nutritional supplement (2 calories/mL) during the routine medication pass may have a greater effect on weight gain than a traditional supplement (1.06 calories/mL) with or between meals. Small volumes of nutrient-dense supplement may have less of an effect on appetite and will enhance food intake during meals and snacks.

This delivery method allows nurses to observe and document consumption.

◆ Pharmacological Therapy

The American Geriatrics Society (2014) does not recommend drugs that stimulate appetite (orexigenic drugs) to treat anorexia or malnutrition in older people. Use of drugs, such as megestrol acetate, results in minimal improvement in appetite and weight gain, no improvement in quality of life or survival, and increased risk of thrombotic events, fluid retention, and death. The antidepressant drug mirtazapine (Remeron) is likely to cause weight gain or increased appetite when used to treat depression, but there is little evidence to support its use to promote appetite and weight gain in the absence of depression. Optimizing social supports, providing feeding assistance, and clarifying patient goals and expectations are recommended interventions.

◆ Patient Education

Education should be provided on nutritional requirements for health, special diet modifications for chronic illness management, the effect of age-associated changes and medication on nutrition, and community resources to assist in maintaining adequate nutrition. Medicare covers nutrition therapy for select diseases, such as diabetes and kidney disease.

❖ IMPLICATIONS FOR GERONTOLOGICAL NURSING AND HEALTHY AGING

Maintenance of adequate nutritional health as a person ages is extremely complex. Knowledge of nutritional needs in later years and of the many factors contributing to inadequate nutrition is essential for the gerontological nurse and should be a part of every assessment of an older person. Working with members of the interprofessional team in appropriate assessment and development of therapeutic interventions is a major role in community, hospital, and long-term care settings. Use of evidence-based practice protocols is important in determining nursing interventions to support and enhance nutritional status.

Prevention of undernutrition and malnutrition and the maintenance of dietary needs and food are also ethical responsibilities. No older person should be hungry or thirsty because he or she cannot shop, cook, buy and prepare food, or eat independently. Nor should any older person have to suffer because of a lack of assistance with these activities in whatever setting the person may reside.

KEY CONCEPTS

- Diet can affect longevity and, when combined with lifestyle changes, reduce disease risk.
- Many factors affect adequate nutrition in late life, including lifelong eating habits, income, chronic illness, dentition, mood disorders, capacity for food preparation, and cognitive and functional limitations.
- Overweight and obesity are major public health concerns around the globe. The proportion of older adults who are obese has doubled in the past 30 years.
- A rising incidence of malnutrition among older adults has been documented in acute care, long-term care, and the community and is expected to rise dramatically in the next 30 years.
- Malnutrition is a precursor to frailty and has serious consequences, including infections, pressure ulcers, anemia, hypotension, impaired cognition, hip fractures, prolonged hospital stay, institutionalization, and increased morbidity and mortality.
- A comprehensive nutritional assessment is an essential component of the assessment of older adults.
- Making mealtime pleasant and attractive for the older adult who is unable to eat unassisted is a nursing challenge; mealtime must be made enjoyable, and adequate assistance must be provided.
- Dysphagia is a serious problem and contributes to weight loss, malnutrition, dehydration, aspiration pneumonia, and death. Careful assessment of risk factors, observation for signs and symptoms, and collaboration with speech-language pathologists on interventions are essential.

ACTIVITIES AND DISCUSSION QUESTIONS

1. What are the factors affecting the nutrition of the older adult?
2. How can the nurse intervene to provide better nutrition for elders in the community, in acute care, and in long-term care settings?
3. What are the causes of malnutrition?
4. What is included in the nutritional assessment of an older person?
5. How is dysphagia assessed, and what interventions may be helpful in preventing aspiration?

REFERENCES

Ahmed T, Haboubi N: Assessment and management of nutrition in older people and its importance to health, *Clin Interv Aging* 5:207, 2010.

Amella E, Aselage M: Mealtime difficulties. In Boltz M, Capezuti E, Fulmer T, et al, editors: *Evidence-based geriatric nursing protocols for best practice*, ed 4, New York, 2012, Springer, pp 453–468.

American Dietetic Association (ADA), American Society for Nutrition (ASN), and Society for Nutrition Education (SNE): Position of the American Dietetic Association, American Society for Nutrition and Society for Nutrition Education: Food and nutrition programs for community-residing older adults, *J Am Diet Assoc* 110:463, 2010.

American Geriatrics Society: *Feeding tubes in advanced dementia position statement*, May 2013. Available at http://www.americangeriatrics.org/health_care_professionals/clinical_practice/clinical_guidelines_recommendations. Accessed November 2015.

American Geriatrics Society: *Choosing wisely: Five things physicians and patients should question*, 2014. Available at http://www.choosingwisely.org/clinician-lists/american-geriatrics-society-prescription-appetite-stimulants-to-treat-anorexia-cachexia-in-elderly/. Accessed November 2015.

Aslam M, Vaezi M: Dysphagia in the elderly, *Gastroenterol Hepatol* 9(12):784–795, 2013.

Beasley J, LaCroix A, Neuhouser M, et al: Protein intake and incident frailty in the women's health initiative observational study, *J Am Geriatr Soc* 58:1063, 2010.

Berg J: The hunger-obesity paradox in older Americans, *Aging Today*. 2015. Available at http://www.asaging.org/blog/hunger-obesity-paradox-older-americans. Accessed November 2015.

Burger S, Kayser-Jones J, Bell J: *Malnutrition and dehydration in nursing homes: Key issues in prevention and treatment*, 2000. Available at http://www.commonwealthfund.org/usr_doc/burger_mal_386.pdf.

Buys D, Flood K, Real K, et al: Mealtime assistance for hospitalized older adults: A report on the SPOONS volunteer program, *J Gerontol Nurs* 39(9):18–22, 2013.

Cadogan M: Clinical concepts: Functional consequences of vitamin B12 deficiency, *J Gerontol Nurs* 36:18, 2010.

DiMaria-Ghalili R: Nutrition. In Boltz M, Capezuti E, Fulmer T, et al, editors: *Evidence-based geriatric nursing protocols for best practice*, New York, 2012, Springer.

Duffy E: *Malnutrition in older adults, ADVANCE for NPs and PAs*, 2010. Available at http://nurse-practitioners-and-physician-assistants.advanceweb.com/article/malnutrition-in-older-adults.aspx.

Ervin R: Healthy eating index—2005 total component scores for adults age 20 and over: National Health and Nutrition Examination Survey, 2003–2004, *National Health Statistics Reports*, No. 44, 2011. Available at http://www.cdc.gov/nchs/data/nhsr/nhsr044.pdf. Accessed November 2015.

Felix H: Obesity, disability and nursing home admission, *Ann Longterm Care* 16:33, 2008.

Flicker L, McCaul K, Hankey G, et al: Body mass index and survival in men and women aged 70 to 75, *J Am Geriatr Soc* 58:234–241, 2010.

Fuller-Thomson E, Redmond M: Falling through the social safety net: Food stamp use and nonuse among older impoverished Americans, *Gerontologist* 48:235–244, 2008.

Glick S, Jolkowitz A: Feeding dementia patients via percutaneous endoscopic gastrostomy, *Ann Longterm Care* 21(1):32–34, 2013.

Haber D: *Health promotion and aging*, ed 5, New York, 2010, Springer.

Imai E, Tsubota-Utsugi M, Kikuya M, et al: Animal protein intake is associated with higher-level functional capacity in elderly adults: The Ohasama study, *J Am Geriatr Soc* 62:426–434, 2014.

Jefferies D, Johnson M, Ravens J: Nurturing and nourishing: The nurses' role in nutritional care, *J Clin Nurs* 20:317–330, 2011.

Kaiser R, Winning K, Uter W, et al: Functionality and mortality in obese nursing home residents: An example of "risk factor paradox?" *J Am Med Dir Assoc* 11:428, 2010.

Levinson Z, Damico A, Cubanski J: *A state-by-state snapshot of poverty among seniors: Findings from analysis of the supplemental poverty measure* (Issue brief), May 20, 2013. http://kff.org/medicare/issue-brief/a-state-by-state-snapshot-of-poverty-among-seniors. Accessed August 2016.

Litchford M: Putting the nutrition-focused physical assessment into practice in long-term care, *Ann Longterm Care* 21(11):38–41, 2013.

Locher J, Ritchie C, Robinson C, et al: A multidimensional approach to understanding under-eating in homebound older adults: The importance of social factors, *Gerontologist* 48(2):223–234, 2008.

Lustbader W: Thoughts on the meaning of frailty, *Generations* 13(4):21–22, 1999.

Martinez-Lapiscina E, Clavero P, Toledo E, et al: Mediterranean diet improves cognition: The PREDIMEN-NAVARRA randomised trial, *J Neurol Neurosurg Psychiatry* 84(12):1318–1325, 2013.

Mathew M, Jacobs M: Malnutrition and feeding problems. In Ham R, Sloane P, Warshaw G, et al, editors: *Primary care geriatrics*, ed 6, Philadelphia, 2014, Elsevier, pp 315–322.

Metheny M, Boltz M, Greenberg S: Preventing aspiration in older adults with dysphagia, *Am J Nurs* 108(2):45–46, 2008.

Ogden C, Carroll M, Kit B, et al: Prevalence of childhood and adult obesity in the United States, 2011-2012, *JAMA* 311(8):806–814, 2014.

Pioneer Network and Rothschild Foundation: *New dining practice standards*, 2011. Available at http://www.pioneernetwork.net/Providers/DiningPracticeStandards/.

Rettner R: *US obesity rates have risen most in older adults*, 2015. Available at http://www.livescience.com/49587-obesity-rates-older-adults.html. Accessed November 2015.

Samieri C, Grodstein F, Rosner B, et al: Mediterranean diet and cognitive function in older age, *Epidemiology* 24(4):490–499, 2013a.

Samieri C, Sun Q, Townsend M, et al: The association between dietary patterns in midlife and health in aging: An observational study, *Ann Intern Med* 159(9):584–591, 2013b.

Shune S, Moon J: Neuromuscular electrical stimulation in dysphagia management: Clinician use and perceived barriers, *Contemp Issues Commun Sci Disord* 39:55–68, 2012.

Slomski A: Mediterranean diet may reduce diabetes risk in older people, *JAMA* 311(8):790, 2014.

Teno J, Gozalo F, Mitchell S, et al: Feeding tubes and the prevention or healing of pressure ulcers, *Arch Intern Med* 172(9):697–701, 2012.

Teno J, Mitchell S, Kuo S, et al: Decision-making and outcomes of feeding tube insertion: A five-state study, *J Am Geriatr Soc* 59(5):881–886, 2011.

Tobias D, Pan A, Jackson C, et al: Body-mass index and mortality among older adults with incident type 2 diabetes, *N Engl J Med* 370(3):233–244, 2014.

U.S. Department of Health and Human Services (USDHHS), U.S. Department of Agriculture (USDA): *2015-2020 Dietary guidelines for Americans, ed 8*, 2015. Available at http://health.gov/dietaryguidelines/2015/guidelines.

White J, Guenter P, Jensen G, et al: Consensus statement of the Academy of Nutrition and Dietetics/American Society for Parenteral and Enteral Nutrition: Characteristics recommended for the identification and documentation of adult malnutrition (undernutrition), *J Acad Nutr Diet* 112: 730–738, 2012.

World Health Organization (WHO): *Nutrition: Controlling the global obesity epidemic*, 2003. Available at http://www.who.int/nutrition/topics/obesity/en. Accessed November 2015.

Yang J, Farioli A, Korre M, et al: Modified Mediterranean diet score and cardiovascular risk in a North American working population, *PLoS ONE* 9(2):e87539, 2014. doi: 10.1371/journal.pone.0087539.

11

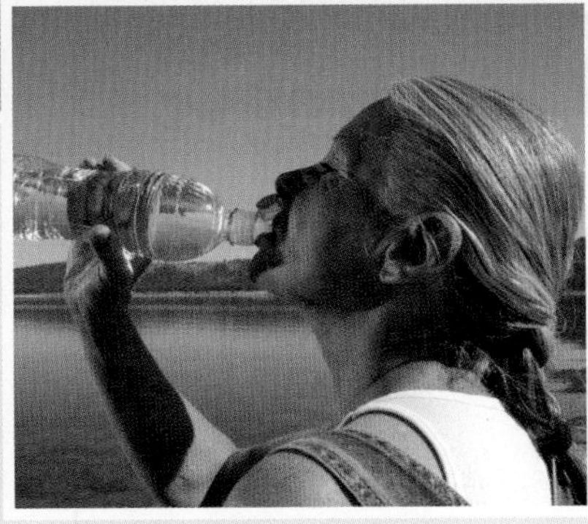

Hydration and Oral Care

Theris A. Touhy

evolve.elsevier.com/Touhy/gerontological

LEARNING OBJECTIVES

Upon completion of this chapter, the reader will be able to:

- Identify factors that influence hydration management in older adults.
- Identify the components of hydration assessment.
- Describe interventions for prevention and treatment of dehydration.
- Demonstrate understanding of the relationship between oral health and disease.
- Discuss common oral problems that can occur with aging and appropriate assessment and interventions.
- Discuss interventions that promote good oral hygiene for older people in a variety of settings.

THE LIVED EXPERIENCE

I know I don't drink enough water—coffee, yes; water, no. It's hard when you are in a wheelchair and only have one arm that works. This smart little student nurse really fixed me up. She gave me a plastic water bottle and attached it to my chair on my good side. Now wherever I go, the water goes.

Jack, age 84

HYDRATION MANAGEMENT

Hydration management is the promotion of an adequate fluid balance, which prevents complications resulting from abnormal or undesirable fluid levels. Daily needs for water can usually be met by functionally independent older adults through intake of fluids with meals and social drinks. However, a significant number of older adults (up to 85% of those 85 years of age and older) drink less than 1 liter of fluid per day. Older adults, with the exception of those requiring fluid restrictions, should consume at least 1500 mL of fluid per day. Maintenance of fluid balance (fluid intake equals fluid output) is essential to health, regardless of a person's age (Mentes, 2006). Age-related changes (see Chapter 3), medication use, functional impairments, and comorbid medical and emotional illnesses place some older adults at risk for changes in fluid balance, especially dehydration (Mentes, 2012).

DEHYDRATION

Dehydration is defined clinically as "a complex condition resulting in a reduction in total body water. In older people, dehydration most often develops as a result of disease, age-related changes, and/or the effects of medication and not primarily due to lack of access to water" (Thomas et al., 2008, p. 293). Dehydration is considered a geriatric syndrome that is frequently associated with common diseases (e.g., diabetes, respiratory illness, heart failure) and frailty. It is often an unappreciated comorbid condition that exacerbates an underlying condition such as a urinary tract infection, respiratory tract infection, or worsening depression. Dehydration is a significant risk factor for delirium, thromboembolic complications, infections, kidney stones, constipation and obstipation, falls, medication toxicity, renal failure, seizure, electrolyte imbalance, hyperthermia, and delayed wound healing (Faes et al., 2007; Mentes, 2012).

SAFETY ALERT

Dehydration is a problem prevalent among older adults in all settings. If not treated adequately, mortality from dehydration can be as high as 50% (Faes et al., 2007).

Thomas and colleagues (2008) comment that there are few diagnoses that generate as much concern about causes and consequences as does dehydration. Because of a lack of understanding of the pathogenesis and consequences of dehydration in older adults, the condition is often attributed to poor care by nursing home staff and/or primary care providers. However, the majority of older people develop dehydration as a result of increased fluid losses combined with decreased fluid intake, related to decreased thirst (Riberio & Morley, 2014). The condition is rarely attributable to neglect.

Risk Factors for Dehydration

The presence of physical or emotional illness, surgery, trauma, or conditions of higher physiological demands increases the risk of dehydration. Individuals older than age 85 who have experienced volume deficits, weight loss, malnutrition, or infection, and those with neurocognitive disorders and functional impairments are at high risk for dehydration. When the fluid balance of older adults is at risk, the limited capacity of homeostatic mechanisms becomes significant. Chapter 3 discusses age-related changes in the amount of body water, and Box 11.1 presents risk factors for dehydration.

BOX 11.1 Risk Factors for Dehydration

Age-related changes
Medications: diuretics, laxatives, angiotensin-converting enzyme (ACE) inhibitors, psychotropics
Use of four or more medications
Functional deficits
Communication and comprehension problems
Oral problems
Dysphagia
Delirium
Dementia
Hospitalization
Low body weight
Diagnostic procedures requiring fasting
Inadequate assistance with fluid/food intake
Diarrhea
Fever
Vomiting
Infections
Bleeding
Draining wounds
Artificial ventilation
Fluid restrictions
High environmental temperatures
Multiple comorbidities

BOX 11.2 Simple Screen for Dehydration

Drugs (e.g., diuretics)	**T**achycardia
End of life	**I**ncontinence (fear of)
High fever	**O**ral problems/sippers
Yellow urine turns dark	**N**eurological impairment (confusion)
Dizziness (orthostasis)	**S**unken eyes
Reduced oral intake	
Axilla dry	

From Thomas D, Cote T, Lawhorne L, et al: Understanding clinical dehydration and its treatment, *J Am Med Dir Assoc* 9(5):292–301, 2008.

❖ IMPLICATIONS FOR GERONTOLOGICAL NURSING AND HEALTHY AGING

◆ Assessment

Prevention of dehydration is essential, but assessment is complex in older people. Clinical signs may not appear until dehydration is advanced. Attention to risk factors for dehydration using a screening tool (Box 11.2) is very important. Additionally, older patients should be formally assessed for dehydration at admission to the hospital and throughout their hospital stay (McCrow et al., 2016). In addition, the MDS 3.0 (see Chapter 8) assesses for dehydration/fluid maintenance. Education should be provided to older people and their caregivers about the need for fluids and the signs and symptoms of dehydration. Acute situations such as vomiting, diarrhea, or febrile episodes should be identified quickly and treated.

◆ Signs/Symptoms of Dehydration

Typical signs of dehydration may not always be present in older people and symptoms are often atypical. Skin turgor, assessed at the sternum and commonly included in the assessment of dehydration, is an unreliable marker in older adults because of the loss of subcutaneous tissue with aging. Dry mucous membranes in the mouth and nose, longitudinal furrows on the tongue, orthostasis, speech incoherence, rapid pulse rate, decreased urine output, extremity weakness, dry axilla, and sunken eyes may indicate dehydration. However, the diagnosis of dehydration is biochemically proven (Thomas et al., 2008).

◆ Laboratory Tests

If dehydration is suspected, laboratory tests include blood urea nitrogen (BUN)/creatinine ratio, serum sodium level, serum and urine osmolarity, and specific gravity (Mentes, 2012). Although most cases of dehydration have an elevated BUN measurement, there are many other causes of an elevated BUN/creatinine ratio, so this test cannot be used alone to diagnose dehydration in older adults (Thomas et al., 2008). Attention to risk factors is important to identify possible dehydration and to intervene early. Body weight changes should also be assessed as indicators of changes in hydration (Faes et al., 2007).

◆ Urine Color

Urine color, which is measured using a urine color chart, has been suggested as helpful in assessing hydration status (not dehydration) in individuals in nursing homes with adequate renal function (Mentes, 2012). The urine color chart has eight standardized colors, ranging from pale straw (number 1) to greenish brown (number 8), approximating urine specific gravities of 1.003 to 1.029, respectively. Urine color should be assessed and charted over several days. Pale straw–colored urine usually indicates normal hydration status, and as urine darkens, poor hydration may be indicated (after taking into account discoloration by food or medications). For older adults, a reading of 4 or less is preferred (Mentes, 2006). If a person's urine becomes darker than his or her usual color, fluid intake assessment is indicated, and fluids can be increased before dehydration occurs (Mentes, 2012).

◆ Interventions

Interventions are derived from a comprehensive assessment and consist of risk identification and hydration management (Box 11.3). Any individual who develops fever, diarrhea, vomiting, or a nonfebrile infection should be monitored closely by implementing intake and output records and providing additional fluids. NPO (nothing-by-mouth) requirements for diagnostic tests and surgical procedures should be as short as possible for older adults, and adequate fluids should be given once tests and procedures are completed. A 2-hour suspension of fluid intake is recommended for many procedures (Mentes, 2012).

Hydration management involves both acute and ongoing management of oral intake. Oral hydration is the first treatment approach for dehydration. Individuals with mild to moderate dehydration who can drink and do not have significant mental or physical compromise attributable to fluid loss may be able to replenish fluids orally. Water is considered the best fluid to offer, but other clear fluids may also be useful depending on the person's preference.

◆ Rehydration Methods

Rehydration methods depend on the severity and the type of dehydration and may include intravenous or hypodermoclysis (HDC) approaches. A general rule is to replace 50% of the loss within the first 12 hours (or 1 L/day in afebrile elders) or a sufficient quantity to relieve tachycardia and hypotension. Further fluid replacement can be administered more slowly over a longer period of time. It is important to monitor for symptoms of overhydration (unexplained weight gain, pedal edema, neck vein distention, shortness of breath), especially in individuals with heart failure or renal disease. Individuals taking selective serotonin reuptake inhibitors (SSRIs) should have serum sodium levels and hydration status closely monitored because of risk for hyponatremia (see Chapter 9). Increasing fluid intake may aggravate an evolving hyponatremia (Mentes, 2012).

◆ Hypodermoclysis

HDC is an infusion of isotonic fluids into the subcutaneous space. HDC is safe, easy to administer, and a useful alternative to intravenous administration for persons with mild to moderate dehydration, particularly those patients with altered mental status. HDC cannot be used in severe dehydration or for any situation requiring more than 3 L over 24 hours. Common sites of infusion are the lateral abdominal wall; the anterior or lateral aspects of the thighs; the infraclavicular region; and the back, usually the interscapular or subscapular regions with a fat fold at least 1 inch thick (Gabriel, 2014; Mei & Auerhahn, 2009). Normal saline (0.9%), half normal saline (0.45%), 5% glucose in water infusion (D5W), or Ringer's solution can be used (Thomas et al., 2008). Between 1.5 and 3 L a day can be given subcutaneously (Riberio & Morley, 2014). Hypodermoclysis can be administered in almost any setting, so hospital admissions may be avoided. Hypodermoclysis is "an evidence-based low-cost therapy in geriatrics" (Faes et al., 2007). Other resources on hydration can be found in Box 11.4.

BOX 11.3 Tips for Best Practice

Hydration Management

1. Calculate a daily fluid goal.
   - All older adults should have an individualized fluid goal determined by a documented standard for daily fluid intake. At least 1500 mL of fluid/day should be provided.
2. Compare current intake to fluid goal to evaluate hydration status.
3. Provide fluids consistently throughout the day.
   - Provide 75% to 80% of fluids at mealtimes and the remainder during non-mealtimes such as medication times.
   - Offer a variety of fluids and fluids that the person prefers.
   - Standardize the amount of fluid that is offered with medication administration (e.g., at least 6 oz).
4. Plan for at-risk individuals.
   - Have fluid rounds midmorning and midafternoon.
   - Provide two 8-oz glasses of fluid in the morning and evening.
   - Offer a "happy hour" or "tea time," when residents can gather for additional fluids and socialization.
   - Provide modified fluid containers based on resident's abilities—for example, lighter cups and glasses, weighted cups and glasses, plastic water bottles with straws (attach to wheelchairs, deliver with meals).
   - Make fluids accessible at all times and be sure residents can access them—for example, filled water pitchers, fluid stations, or beverage carts in congregate areas.
   - Allow adequate time and staff for eating or feeding. Meals can provide two-thirds of daily fluids.
   - Encourage family members to participate in feeding and offering fluids.
5. Perform fluid regulation and documentation.
   - Teach individuals, if possible, to use a urine color chart to monitor hydration status.
   - Document complete intake including hydration habits.
   - Know volumes of fluid containers to accurately calculate fluid consumption.
   - Frequency of documentation of fluid intake will vary among settings and is dependent on the individual's condition. In most settings, at least one accurate intake and output recording should be documented, including amount of fluid consumed, difficulties with consumption, and urine specific gravity and color.
   - For individuals who are not continent, teach caregivers to observe incontinent pads or briefs for amount and frequency of urine, color changes, and odor, and report variations from individual's normal pattern.

Adapted from Mentes JC: Managing oral hydration. In Boltz M, Capezuti E, Fulmer T, et al, editors: *Evidence-based geriatric nursing protocols for best practice,* ed 4, pp. 419–438, New York, 2012, Springer.

BOX 11.4 Resources for Best Practice

Hydration and Oral Care

Administration on Aging: Older adults and oral health.

American Medical Directors Association: Oral Healthcare Toolkit.

Mentes J: Hydration management. In Boltz M, Capezuti E, Fulmer T, et al., editors: *Evidence-based geriatric nursing protocols for best practice,* ed 4, New York, 2012, Springer.

O'Connor L: Oral health care. In Boltz M, Capezuti E, Fulmer T, et al., editors: *Evidence-based geriatric nursing protocols for best practice,* ed 4, New York, 2012, Springer.

Oral Health America: Educational materials, resources, affordable dental care.

The Hartford Institute for Geriatric Nursing: Nursing Standard of Practice Protocols: Oral health care in aging, hydration management.

Oral Health Assessment of Older Adults: The Kayser-Jones Brief Oral Health Status Examination (BOHSE).

ORAL HEALTH

Orodental health is integral to general health. Orodental health is a basic need that is increasingly neglected with advanced age, debilitation, and limited mobility. Age-related changes in the oral cavity (see Chapter 3), the presence of medical conditions, the practice of poor dental hygiene, and lack of dental care contribute to poor oral health. Poor oral health is recognized as a risk factor for dehydration and malnutrition, as well as a number of systemic diseases, including pneumonia, joint infections, cardiovascular disease, and poor glycemic control in type 1 and type 2 diabetes (Jablonski, 2010; O'Connor, 2012; Stein et al., 2014).

In frail older adults at the end of life, poor oral hygiene facilitates the colonization of respiratory pathogens on the surfaces of the teeth and dentures and increases the risk of life-threatening respiratory tract infections. Pain from infected teeth, ill-fitting dentures, or oral candidiasis can limit eating ability and compromise comfort and quality of life (Chen & Kistler, 2015). Tips for promotion of oral health are presented in Box 11.5. *Healthy People 2020* addresses dental health goals for older adults (Box 11.6).

Common Oral Problems

Xerostomia (Mouth Dryness)

Xerostomia and hyposalivation are present in approximately 30% of older adults and can affect eating, swallowing, and speaking and contribute to dental caries and periodontal disease. Dry mouth especially affects seriously ill individuals, including more than 90% of individuals with cancer in hospice (Chen & Kistler, 2015). Adequate saliva is necessary for the beginning stage of digestion, helping to break down starches and fats. It also functions to clear the mouth of food debris and prevent overgrowth of oral microbes. The flow of saliva does not decrease with age, but medical conditions and medications affect salivary flow (Stein et al., 2014). More than 500 medications have a side effect of hyposalivation, including antihypertensives, antidepressants, antihistamines, antipsychotics, diuretics, and antiparkinson agents.

BOX 11.5 Tips for Best Practice

Promoting Oral Health

- Encourage annual dental exams, including individuals with dentures.
- Brush and floss twice daily; use a fluoride dentrifice and mouthwash.
- Ensure dentures fit well and are cleaned regularly.
- Maintain adequate daily fluid intake (1500 mL).
- Avoid tobacco.
- Limit alcohol.
- Eat a well-balanced diet.
- Use an ultrasonic toothbrush (more effective in removing plaque).
- Use a commercial floss handle for easier flossing.
- Adapt toothbrush if manual dexterity is impaired. Use a child's toothbrush or enlarge the handle of an adult-sized toothbrush by adding a foam grip or wrapping it with gauze or rubber bands to increase handle size.
- If medications cause a dry mouth, ask your health care provider if there are other drugs that can be substituted. If dry mouth cannot be avoided, drink plenty of water, chew sugarless gum, and avoid alcohol and tobacco.

BOX 11.6 *Healthy People 2020*

Dental Health Goals for Older Adults

- Prevent and control oral and craniofacial diseases, conditions, and injuries, and improve access to preventive services and dental care.
- Reduce the proportion of adults with untreated dental decay.
- Reduce the proportion of older adults with untreated caries.
- Reduce the proportion of adults who have ever had a permanent tooth extracted because of dental caries or periodontal disease.
- Reduce the proportion of older adults 65 to 74 years of age who have lost all of their natural teeth.
- Reduce the proportion of adults 45 to 74 years of age with moderate or severe periodontitis.
- Increase the proportion of oral and pharyngeal cancers detected at the earliest stages.

Data from U.S. Department of Health and Human Services, Office of Disease Prevention and Health Promotion: *Healthy People 2020*, 2012. Available at http://www.healthypeople.gov/2020.

Treatment of xerostomia. A review of all medications is important, and if medication side effects are contributing to dry mouth, medications may be changed or altered. Affected individuals should practice good oral hygiene practices and have regular dental care to screen for decay. Consumption of adequate water intake and avoidance of alcohol and caffeine are recommended. Over-the-counter saliva substitutes (Oral Balance Gel, MouthKote) and salivary stimulants such as Biotene xylitol gum and sugarless candy can be helpful (Stein et al., 2014).

Oral Cancer

Oral cancers occur more with age. The median age at diagnosis is 61 years; men are affected twice as often as women. Oral cancer occurs more frequently in black men, and the incidence of oral cancer varies in different countries. It is much more common in Hungary and France than in the United States and much less common in Mexico and Japan (American Geriatrics Society, 2006). The 5-year survival rate is 50% and has not changed significantly in the past 50 years.

Early detection is essential, but more than 60% of oral cancers are not diagnosed until an advanced stage. Early signs and symptoms may be subtle and not recognized by the individual or health care provider (Stein et al., 2014). Oral examinations can assist in early identification and treatment. All persons, especially those older than 50 years of age, with or without dentures, should have oral examinations on a regular basis. Box 11.7 presents common signs and symptoms of oral cancer, and Box 11.8 lists risk factors. Once diagnosed, therapy options are based on diagnosis and staging and include surgery, radiation, and chemotherapy. If detected early, these cancers can almost always be treated successfully.

Oral Care

Nearly one-third of individuals older than age 65 have untreated tooth decay. About one-fourth of persons age

BOX 11.7 Signs and Symptoms of Oral and Throat Cancer

- Swelling or thickening, lumps or bumps, or rough spots or eroded areas on the lips, gums, or other areas inside the mouth
- Velvety white, red, or speckled patches in the mouth
- Persistent sores on the face, neck, or mouth that bleed easily
- Unexplained bleeding in the mouth
- Unexplained numbness or pain or tenderness in any area of the face, mouth, neck, or tongue
- Soreness in the back of the throat; a persistent feeling that something is caught in the throat
- Difficulty chewing or swallowing, speaking, or moving the jaw or tongue
- Hoarseness, chronic sore throat, or changes in the voice
- Dramatic weight loss
- Lump or swelling in the neck
- Severe pain in one ear—with a normal eardrum
- Pain around the teeth; loosening of the teeth
- Swelling or pain in the jaw; difficulty moving the jaw

BOX 11.8 Risk Factors for Oral Cancer

Tobacco, including smokeless tobacco
Alcohol
Oncogenic viruses (especially human papillomavirus)
Genetic susceptibility

From Stein P, Miller C, Fowler C: Oral disorders. In Ham R, Sloane P, Warshaw G, et al, editors: *Primary care geriatrics: A case-based approach*, ed 6, Philadelphia, 2014, Elsevier.

65 and older have no remaining teeth (edentulous), primarily as a result of periodontitis, which occurs in about 95% of those in this age group (U.S. Department of Health and Human Services [USDHHS], 2014). There has been a dramatic reduction in the prevalence of tooth loss as knowledge increases and more people use fluorides, improve nutrition, engage in new oral hygiene practices, and take advantage of improved dental health care. Half of all Americans were edentulous in the 1950s, but today the rate has decreased to 18% (Stein et al., 2014). However, many individuals may not have had the advantages of new preventive treatment, and those with functional and cognitive limitations may be unable to perform oral hygiene.

Access to dental care for older people may be limited and cost prohibitive. In the existing health care system, dental care is a low priority. If a seriously ill or institutionalized individual needs dental care, they have to be transferred to dental offices. This can be physically challenging and stressful and many dental offices are not equipped to handle this type of patient (Chen & Kistler, 2015). Medicare does not provide any coverage for oral health care services, and few Americans 75 years of age or older have private dental insurance. Medicaid coverage for dental care varies from state to state, but funding has decreased and coverage can be limited. Elders have fewer dentist visits than any other age group, and dental care utilization among low-income adults has declined or remained constant in almost every state from 2000 to 2010 (Vujicic, 2013). Older Americans with the poorest oral health are those who are economically disadvantaged and lack insurance. Being disabled, homebound, or institutionalized increases the risk of poor oral health.

❖ IMPLICATIONS FOR GERONTOLOGICAL NURSING AND HEALTHY AGING

◆ Assessment

Good oral hygiene and timely assessment of oral health are essentials of nursing care. "Mouth care is oral infection control" (Jablonski-Jaudon et al., 2016, p. 15). In addition to identifying oral health problems, examination of the mouth can serve as an early warning system for some diseases and lead to early diagnosis and treatment. Assessment of the mouth, teeth, and oral cavity is an essential part of health assessment (see Chapter 8) and especially important when an individual is hospitalized or in a long-term care facility. The MDS 3.0 requires information obtained from an oral assessment. Federal regulations mandate an annual examination for residents of long-term care facilities. Although the oral examination is best performed by a dentist, nurses in health care settings can provide oral health screenings using an instrument such as the Kayser-Jones Brief Oral Health Status Examination (BOHSE) (see Box 11.4).

◆ Interventions

Nurses may be involved in promoting oral health through teaching individuals or caregivers recommended interventions, screening for oral disease, and making dental referrals, or by providing, supervising, and evaluating oral care in hospitals and long-term care facilities. Box 11.9 presents information on providing oral hygiene.

◆ Dentures

Older adults and those who may care for them should be taught proper care of dentures and oral tissue to prevent odor, stain, plaque buildup, and oral infections. All nursing staff should be knowledgeable about care of

BOX 11.9 Tips for Best Practice

Provision of Oral Care

1. Explain all actions to the individual; use gestures and demonstration as needed; cue and prompt to encourage as much self-care performance as possible.
2. If the individual is in bed, elevate his or her head by raising the bed or propping the head with pillows, and have the individual turn his or her head to face you. Place a clean towel across the chest and under the chin, and place a basin under the chin.
3. If the individual is sitting in a stationary chair or wheelchair, stand behind the individual and stabilize his or her head by placing one hand under the chin and resting the head against your body. Place a towel across the chest and over the shoulders.
4. The basin can be kept handy in the individual's lap or on a table placed in front of or at the side of the patient. A wheelchair may be positioned in front of the sink.
5. If the individual's lips are dry or cracked, apply a light coating of petroleum jelly or use lip balm.
6. Inspect the oral cavity to identify teeth in ill repair, pain, lesions, or inflammation.
7. Brush and floss the individual's teeth (use an electric toothbrush if possible, with sulcular brushing). It may be helpful to retract the lips and cheek with a tongue blade or fingers in order to see the area that is being cleaned. Use a mouth prop as needed if the individual cannot hold his or her mouth open. If manual flossing is too difficult, use a floss holder or interproximal brush to clean the proximal surfaces between the teeth. Use a dentifrice containing fluoride.
8. Provide the conscious individual with fluoride rinses or other rinses as indicated by the dentist or hygienist.

BOX 11.10 Tips for Best Practice

Providing Denture Care

1. Remove dentures or ask individual to remove dentures. Observe ability to remove dentures.
2. Inspect oral cavity.
3. Rinse denture or dentures after each meal to remove soft debris. Do not use toothpaste on dentures because it abrades denture surfaces.
4. Once each day, preferably before retiring, remove denture and brush thoroughly.
   a. Although an ordinary soft toothbrush is adequate, a specially designed denture brush may clean more effectively. (**CAUTION:** Acrylic denture material is softer than natural teeth and may be damaged by being brushed with very firm bristles.)
   b. Brush denture over a sink lined with a facecloth and half-filled with water. This will prevent breakage if the denture is dropped.
   c. Hold the denture securely in one hand, but do not squeeze. Hold the brush in the other hand. Never use a commercial tooth powder because it is abrasive and may damage the denture materials. Plain water, mild soap, or sodium bicarbonate may be used.
   d. When cleaning a removable partial denture, great care must be taken to remove plaque from the curved metal clasps that hook around the teeth. This can be done with a regular toothbrush or with a specially designed clasp brush.
5. After brushing, rinse denture thoroughly; then place it in a denture-cleaning solution and allow it to soak overnight or for at least a few hours. (**NOTE:** Acrylic denture material must be kept wet at all times to prevent cracking or warping.) In the morning, remove denture from the cleaning solution and rinse it thoroughly before inserting it into the mouth. Use denture paste if necessary to secure dentures.
6. Dentures should be worn constantly except at night (to allow relief of compression on the gums) and replaced in the mouth in the morning.

dentures (Box 11.10). Dentures are very personal and expensive possessions and the utmost care should be taken when handling, cleaning, and storing dentures, especially in hospitals and long-term care facilities. It is not uncommon to hear that dentures were lost, broken, or mixed up with those of others, or not removed and cleaned during a hospital or nursing home stay. Dentures should be marked, and many states require all newly made dentures to contain the client's identification. A commercial denture marking system called iDenture, produced by the 3M Company, provides a simple, efficient, and permanent means of marking dentures.

Broken or damaged dentures and dentures that no longer fit because of weight loss or changes in the oral cavity are a common problem for older adults. Many elders believe that there is no longer a need for oral care once they have dentures, but regular professional attention is important. "Only 13% of denture wearers seek annual dental care, and nearly half have not seen a dentist in 5 years" (Stein et al., 2014, p. 566). Rebasing of dentures is a technique to improve the fit of dentures. Ill-fitting dentures or dentures that are not cleaned contribute to oral problems (lesions, stomatitis), as well as to poor nutrition and reduced enjoyment of food.

◆ Oral Hygiene in Hospitals and Long-Term Care

Oral care is an often neglected part of daily nursing care and should receive the same priority as other kinds of care. When the person is unable to carry out his or her dental/oral regimen, it is the responsibility of the caregiver to provide oral care. Lack of attention to oral hygiene contributes significantly to poor nutrition and other negative outcomes such as aspiration pneumonia. There is evidence that cleaning the person's teeth with a toothbrush after meals lowers the risk of developing aspiration pneumonia (van der Maarel-Wierink et al., 2013).

In the acute care setting, good oral care is crucial to the prevention of ventilator-associated pneumonia (VAP), one of the most common hospital-acquired infections and a leading cause of morbidity and mortality in intensive care units (ICUs). Oral care practices among critical care nurses are not consistently implemented and mouth care may be perceived as a comfort measure rather than a critical component of infection control (Booker et al., 2013). Booker and colleagues (2013) provide a comprehensive protocol for provision of oral care to ventilator-dependent patients.

Illness, acute care situations, and functional and cognitive impairments make the provision of oral care difficult. Factors contributing to less than adequate oral care include inadequate knowledge of how to provide care, lack of appropriate supplies, inadequate training and staffing, and lack of oral care protocols. Individuals residing in long-term care facilities are particularly vulnerable to problems with oral care as a result of functional and cognitive impairments. A large number are dependent on staff for the provision of oral hygiene.

Individuals with cognitive impairment may be resistive to mouth care, and this is one of the reasons caregivers may neglect oral care. Nursing home residents with dementia are three times more likely to have more tooth decay than those who allow mouth care. Jablonski-Jaudon and colleagues (2016) describe the MOUTh (Managing Oral Hygiene Using Threat Reduction Strategies) intervention to deliver oral hygiene and decrease care-resistant behavior within the context of person-centered, relationship-based care. Strategies include placing yourself at eye level, establishing rapport, using touch judiciously, explaining all actions in step-by-step instructions with cues and gestures, and using distractions. Even with individuals who need help, caregivers should encourage as much self-care as possible. Caregivers can have the person hold the toothbrush but place their hand over the person's hand (hand-over-hand technique).

The use of therapeutic rinses (e.g., chlorhexidine) that are broad-spectrum antimicrobial agents has been shown to help control plaque. These can be used in conjunction with brushing or in place of brushing in those unable to tolerate brushing. Xylitol products (gum, mints, toothpaste) have also been evaluated as an effective method of reducing oral pathogens (Gulkowski, 2013).

Many long-term care institutions have implemented programs, such as special training of nursing assistants for dental care teams, providing visits from mobile dentistry units on a routine basis, or using dental students to perform oral screening and cleaning of teeth. An important nursing role is to assist in the development of oral care protocols and staff education in all health care settings.

◆ Tube Feeding and Oral Hygiene

Tube feeding is associated with significant pathologic colonization of the mouth, greater than that observed in people who received oral feeding. Oral care should be provided every 4 hours for patients with gastrostomy tubes, and teeth should be brushed with a toothbrush after each feeding to decrease the risk of aspiration pneumonia (Metheny et al., 2008; O'Connor, 2012). Foam swabs are available to provide oral hygiene but do not remove plaque as well as toothbrushes. Foam swabs may be used to clean the oral mucosa of an edentulous older adult.

SAFETY ALERT

Lemon glycerin swabs should never be used for oral care. In combination with decreased salivary flow and xerostomia, they inhibit salivary production, causing dry mouth and promoting bacterial growth (Booker et al., 2013).

KEY CONCEPTS

- Age-related changes, medication use, functional impairments, and comorbid medical and emotional illnesses place some older adults at risk for changes in fluid balance, especially dehydration.
- Dehydration is considered a geriatric syndrome that is frequently associated with common diseases (e.g., diabetes, respiratory illness, heart failure) and declining stages of the frail elderly.
- In older people, dehydration most often develops as a result of disease, age-related changes, and/or the

effects of medication; dehydration is not primarily due to lack of access to water.

- Prevention of dehydration is essential, but assessment is complex in older people. Clinical signs may not appear until dehydration is advanced and signs and symptoms may be nonspecific, making prevention and early identification important.
- Age-related changes in the oral cavity, the presence of medical conditions, the practice of poor dental hygiene, and lack of dental care contribute to poor oral health. Poor oral health is a risk factor for dehydration and malnutrition, as well as a number of systemic diseases, including pneumonia, joint infections, cardiovascular disease, and poor glycemic control in type 1 and type 2 diabetes.
- Good oral hygiene and timely assessment of oral health are essentials of nursing care.
- Nurses may be involved in promoting oral health by teaching individuals or caregivers recommended interventions, by screening for oral disease and making dental referrals, or by providing, supervising, and evaluating oral care in hospitals and long-term care facilities.

ACTIVITIES AND DISCUSSION QUESTIONS

1. What are some of the risk factors for dehydration in an older adult who is hospitalized for pneumonia?
2. What are your suggestions for enhancing fluid intake for individuals with dementia residing in skilled nursing facilities?
3. What factors influence adequate dental care among older adults?
4. What are suggestions to encourage better oral care in hospitalized older adults and residents of long-term care facilities?

REFERENCES

American Geriatrics Society: *Geriatric review syllabus*, ed 6, New York, 2006, American Geriatrics Society.

Booker S, Murff S, Kitko L, et al: Mouth care to reduce ventilator-associated pneumonia, *Am J Nurs* 113(10): 24–30, 2013.

Chen X, Kistler C: Oral health care for older adults with serious illness: When and how?, *J Am Geriatr Soc* 63(2):375–378, 2015.

Faes MC, Spift MG, Olde MG, et al: Dehydration in geriatrics, *Geriatr Aging* 10:590, 2007.

Gabriel J: Subcutaneous fluid administration and the hydration of older people, *Br J Nurs* 23(Suppl 14):S10–S14, 2014.

Gulkowski S: Using Xylitol products and MI paste to reduce oral biofilm in long-term care residents, *Ann Longterm Care* 21(12):26–28, 2013.

Jablonski R: Examining oral health in nursing home residents and overcoming mouth-care resistive behaviors, *Ann Longterm Care* 18:21, 2010.

Jablonski-Jaudon R, Kolanowski A, Winstead V, et al: Maturation of the MOUTh Interventions, *J Gerontol Nurs* 42(3):15–23, 2016.

Mei A, Auerhahn C: Hypodermoclysis: Maintaining hydration in the frail older adult, *Ann Longterm Care* 17:28, 2009.

Mentes JC: Oral hydration in older adults: Greater awareness is needed in preventing, recognizing, and treating dehydration, *Am J Nurs* 106(6):40–49, 2006.

Mentes JC: Managing oral hydration. In Boltz M, Capezuti E, Fulmer T, et al, editors: *Evidence-based geriatric nursing protocols for best practice*, ed 4, New York, 2012, Springer, pp 419–438.

McCrow J, Morton M, Traver C, et al: Associations between dehydration, cognitive impairment, and frailty in older hospitalized patients: An exploratory study, *J Gerontol Nurs* 42(5):19–27, 2016.

Metheny M, Boltz M, Greenberg S: Preventing aspiration in older adults with dysphagia, *Am J Nurs* 108(2):45–46, 2008.

O'Connor L: Oral health care. In Boltz M, Capezuti E, Fulmer T, et al, editors: *Evidence-based geriatric nursing protocols for best practice*, New York, 2012, Springer.

Riberio S, Morley J: Dehydration is difficult to detect and prevent in nursing homes, *JAMDA* 16(3):175–176, 2014.

Stein P, Miller C, Fowler C: Oral disorders. In Ham R, Sloane P, Warshaw G, et al, editors: *Primary care geriatrics: A case-based approach*, ed 6, Philadelphia, 2014, Elsevier.

Thomas D, Cote T, Lawhorne L, et al: Understanding clinical dehydration and its treatment, *J Am Med Dir Assoc* 9(5):292–301, 2008.

U.S. Department of Health and Human Services: *Oral health, 2014*. Available at http://www.aoa.gov/AoA_Programs/HPW/Oral_Health/index.aspx. Accessed November 2015.

van der Maarel-Wierink C, Vanobbergen J, Bronkhorst E, et al: Oral health care and aspiration pneumonia in frail older people: A systematic literature review, *Gerodontology* 30(1):3–9, 2013.

Vujicic M: *Dental care utilization declined among low-income adults, increased among low-income children in most states from 2000-2010*, Health Policy Resources Center Research Brief, Feb 2013. Available at http://www.ada.org/~/media/ADA/Science%20and%20Research/HPI/Files/HPIBrief_0213_3.ashx. Accessed November 2015.

12

Elimination

Theris A. Touhy

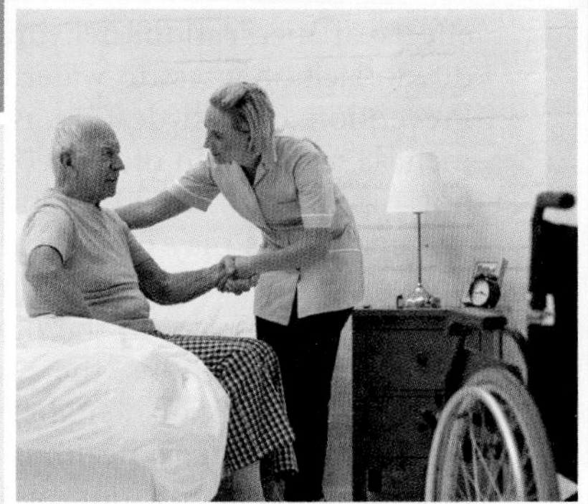

evolve.elsevier.com/Touhy/gerontological

LEARNING OBJECTIVES

Upon completion of this chapter, the reader will be able to:

- Identify appropriate assessment of bowel and bladder elimination.
- Explain the types of urinary incontinence and their causes.
- Identify risk factors for accidental bowel leakage and describe appropriate nursing interventions.
- Use evidence-based protocols in assessment and development of interventions to promote bowel and bladder health.

THE LIVED EXPERIENCE

"UI (urinary incontinence) is like being a bad kid or a big baby."

"There's nothing that can be done. Well, I don't think there is anything else but a diaper."

"Sometimes I have to wet my bed before they get here, you know, and they are all busy and I have to wait for somebody, then I can't control it."

"I do something that is very wrong. I try not to drink too much but that's so wrong. So how can you drink a lot, you would be soaked all the time."

Comments from participants in a study of living with urinary incontinence in long-term care (MacDonald & Butler, 2007).

UI is a preventable and treatable condition and yet, "continence remains undervalued and UI remains underassessed. Even though UI is a basic nursing issue, nurses are not claiming it as one."

Comment from nurses in expert continence care (Mason et al., 2003, p. 3).

The body must remove waste products of metabolism to sustain healthy function, but bladder activity and bowel activity are fraught with social implications. Bladder and bowel function in later life, although normally only slightly altered by the physiological changes of aging, can contribute to problems severe enough to interfere with the ability to continue independent living and can seriously threaten the body's capacity to function and to survive. The effects of uncontrolled bladder and bowel action are a threat to the person's independence and well-being. Elimination is a private matter, not publicized socially. In most cultures, children are

BOX 12.1 Promotion of a Healthy Bladder

- Drink 8 to 10 glasses of water a day before 8 PM.
- Eliminate or reduce the use of coffee, tea, brown cola, and alcohol, particularly before bedtime.
- Empty bladder completely before and after meals and at bedtime.
- Urinate whenever the urge arises; never ignore it.
- Limit the use of sleeping pills, sedatives, and alcohol because they decrease sensation to urinate.
- Make sure toilet is nearby with a clear path to it and good lighting, especially at night. Consider a grab bar or a raised toilet seat if there is difficulty getting on and off the toilet.
- Maintain ideal body weight.
- Get regular physical exercise.
- Avoid smoking.
- Seek professional treatment for complaints of burning, urgency, pain, blood in urine, or difficulties maintaining continence.

taught early to deal with their own body waste. Deviations from this are socially unacceptable and can lead to chastisement, ostracism, and social withdrawal.

Nurses are in a key position to implement evidence-based assessment and interventions to enhance continence and improve function, independence, and quality of life for older people. Additionally, teaching about bladder health is an important nursing intervention for individuals of all ages (Box 12.1).

URINARY INCONTINENCE

Urinary incontinence (UI) is the involuntary loss of urine sufficient to be a problem (Dowling-Castronovo & Bradway, 2012). UI is a geriatric syndrome that is a stigmatized, underreported, underdiagnosed, and undertreated condition erroneously thought to be part of normal aging.

Two-thirds of men and women ages 30 to 70 years have never discussed bladder health with their health care providers, and only one in eight persons who have experienced bladder control problems has been diagnosed. On average, women wait 6.5 years from the first time they experience symptoms until they obtain a diagnosis for their bladder control problems (National Association for Continence, 2014). Men may be unlikely to report UI to their primary care provider because they feel it is a woman's disease.

Individuals may not seek treatment for UI because they are embarrassed to talk about the problem or think that it is a normal part of aging. They may be unaware that successful treatments are available. Instead, they try to cope with the condition on their own, with variable success (Wilde et al., 2014). Older individuals are less likely to receive evidence-based care for UI complaints than younger people (Gibson & Wagg, 2014). Older people want more information about bladder control, and nurses must take the lead in implementing approaches to continence promotion and public health education about UI (Palmer & Newman, 2006).

Health care providers in all settings view UI as an inconvenience rather than a condition requiring assessment and treatment. In comparison with nurses in other health care settings, nurses in hospitals view incontinent patients more negatively (Dowling-Castronovo & Bradway, 2012). In nursing facilities, physicians, geriatric nurse practitioners, and directors of nursing evaluated and managed UI significantly less often than five other geriatric syndromes (falls, dementia, unintended weight loss, pain, and delirium). Nursing assistants were more likely to be involved in care provision for UI than any other syndrome and rated UI second only to pain with respect to its effect on quality of life (Lawhorne et al., 2008).

Without an adequate knowledge base of continence care and use of evidence-based practice guidelines, nursing care will continue to consist of just containment strategies, such as the use of pads and briefs, to manage UI. Nurses in all practice settings who care for older adults should be prepared to assess data that relate to urine control and implement nursing interventions that promote continence. There is a growing role for nurses in continence care, and advanced training and certification are available through specialty organizations such as the Society of Urologic Nurses and Associates and the Wound, Ostomy and Continence Nurses Society.

UI Facts and Figures

Because of the high prevalence and chronic but preventable nature of UI, it is most appropriately considered a public health problem. UI affects millions of adults worldwide. As a result of the aging population, estimates are that UI will increase 22% between 2008 and 2018, affecting an estimated 546 million people (Castronovo & Bradway, 2012; Seshan & Muliira, 2013).

UI is more common in women, with the peak incidence around the time of menopause. In men, there is a steady increase in prevalence with age (Gibson & Wagg, 2014). Twenty-five percent of young women, 44% to 57% of middle-aged and postmenopausal women, and 75% of older women in nursing homes have some involuntary urine loss (Agency for Healthcare Research and Quality, 2012). UI is more prevalent than diabetes, Alzheimer's disease, and many other chronic conditions that have prompted more attention and treatment. Incontinence is also costly; the indirect costs are estimated at more than $16 billion annually in the United States. UI costs exceed those of coronary artery bypass surgery and renal dialysis combined (Dowling-Castronovo & Bradway, 2008).

Risk Factors for UI

Many of the risk factors associated with UI are unrelated to changes in the urinary tract (see Chapter 3) (Box 12.2). "The maintenance of continence is dependent not only on a functional lower urinary tract and pelvic floor, but also on sufficient cognition to interpret the desire to void and locate a toilet, adequate mobility and dexterity to manipulate clothing and allow safe and effective walking to the toilet, and an appropriate environment in which to allow this" (Gibson & Wagg, 2014, p. 168). Older people with dementia are at high risk for UI.

Dementia does not cause urinary incontinence but affects the ability of the person to find a bathroom and recognize the urge to void. Mobility problems and dependency in transfers are better predictors of continence status than dementia, suggesting that persons with dementia may have the potential to remain continent as long as they are mobile. Drugs that increase urinary output and sedatives, tranquilizers, and hypnotics, which produce drowsiness, confusion, or limited mobility, promote incontinence by dulling the transmission of the desire to urinate.

BOX 12.2 Risk Factors for UI

- Age
- Immobility, functional limitations
- Diminished cognitive capacity (dementia, delirium)
- Medications (those with anticholinergic properties, diuretics)
- Smoking
- High caffeine intake
- Low fluid intake
- Obesity
- Constipation, fecal impaction
- Pregnancy, vaginal delivery, episiotomy, forceps birth, large baby
- Environmental barriers
- High-impact physical exercise
- Diabetes, stroke, Parkinson's disease, multiple sclerosis, spinal cord injury
- Hysterectomy
- Pelvic muscle weakness, pelvic organ prolapse
- Childhood nocturnal enuresis
- Prostate surgery
- Estrogen deficiency
- Arthritis and/or back problems
- Malnutrition
- Depression
- Hearing or visual impairments

Adapted from Dowling-Castronovo A, Bradway C: Urinary incontinence. In Boltz M, Capzuti E, Fulmer T, et al, editors: *Evidence-based geriatric nursing protocols for best practice,* ed 4, pp 363–387, New York, 2012, Springer.

Consequences of UI

UI affects quality of life and has physical, psychosocial, and economic consequences. UI is identified as a marker of frailty in community-dwelling older adults. UI is more common and more severe in older people and associated with sequelae not seen in younger people, such as increased risk of falls, fractures, and hospitalization.

UI affects self-esteem and increases the risk for depression, anxiety, loss of dignity and autonomy, social isolation, falls, skin breakdown, and avoidance of sexual activity (Wilson et al., 2015; Xu & Kane, 2013). UI also increases the risk of admission to a nursing home in individuals older than 65 years of age. Older adults with UI experience a loss of independence and self-confidence, as well as feelings of shame and embarrassment (Dowling-Castronovo & Bradway, 2012; Wilde et al., 2014). The psychosocial impact of UI affects the individual and the family caregivers.

Types of UI

Incontinence is classified as either *transient* (acute) or *established* (chronic). *Transient* incontinence has a sudden onset, is present for 6 months or less, and is usually caused by treatable factors such as urinary tract infections (UTIs), delirium, constipation and stool impaction, and increased urine production caused by metabolic conditions such as hyperglycemia and hypercalcemia. Hospitalized older adults are at risk of developing transient UI and may also be at risk of being discharged without resolution of the condition. Use of medications such as diuretics, anticholinergic agents, antidepressants, sedatives, hypnotics, calcium channel blockers, and alpha-adrenergic agonists and blockers can also lead to transient UI (Dowling-Castronovo & Bradway, 2012).

Established UI may have either a sudden or a gradual onset and is categorized into the following types: (1) stress; (2) urge; (3) urge, mixed, or stress UI with high postvoid residual (PVR) (originally termed overflow UI); (4) functional UI; and (5) mixed UI (Table 12.1).

❖ IMPLICATIONS FOR GERONTOLOGICAL NURSING AND HEALTHY AGING

◆ Assessment

Continence must be routinely addressed in the initial assessment of every older person. Health care personnel

TABLE 12.1 Types and Symptoms of UI

Type	Symptoms
Stress	Loss of small amount of urine with activities that increase intra-abdominal pressure (coughing, sneezing, exercising, lifting, bending) More common in women but can occur in men after prostate surgery/treatment PVR low
Urge	Loss of moderate to large amount of urine before getting to toilet; inability to suppress need to urinate Frequency and nocturia may be present PVR low May be associated with overactive bladder (OAB) characterized by urinary frequency (>8 voids/24 hr), nocturia, urgency, with or without UI
Urge, mixed, or stress with high residuals (formerly called overflow)	Nearly constant urine loss (dribbling), hesitancy in starting urine, slow urine stream, passing small volumes of urine, feeling of incomplete bladder emptying PVR high
Functional	Lower urinary tract intact but individual unable to reach toilet because of environmental barriers; physical limitations; cognitive impairment; lack of assistance; difficulty managing belts and zippers or getting a dress up and undergarments down; or difficulty sitting on a toilet
	May occur with other types of UI; more common in individuals who are institutionalized or cognitively impaired
Mixed	Combination of more than one UI problem; usually stress and urge

must begin to change their thinking about incontinence and acknowledge that incontinence can be cured in about 80% of individuals (Wound, Ostomy and Continence Nurses Society, 2009). If it cannot be cured, it can be treated to minimize its detrimental effects. Nurses are often the ones to identify urinary incontinence, but neither nurses nor physicians have been particularly aggressive in its management. Nurses in all settings are expected to be able to collect and organize data about urine control, report findings to the interprofessional team, and implement evidence-based intrventions to promote continence. It is essential that nurses play a leading role in assessing and managing UI.

Assessment of UI is multidimensional and targeted to identify continence patterns, alterations in continence, and contributing factors. If the individual is being admitted to a hospital, home care agency, or skilled nursing facility, it is important to document the presence or absence of UI, past continence patterns, the presence or absence of a urinary catheter, and the reasons for the catheter if present. An environmental assessment including the accessibility of bathrooms, the adequacy of room lighting, the availability of assistance, and the use of aids such as raised toilet seats or commodes is also important.

In the nursing home, the Minimum Data Set 3.0 (MDS 3.0) (see Chapter 8) provides an evidence-based overview of the assessment, treatment, and evaluation of bladder continence based on the Centers for Medicare and Medicaid Services (CMS) guidelines. Continence programs in nursing homes are required by CMS regulations. Monitoring and documentation of continence status in relation to implemented continence care is a *quality of care indicator* for nursing homes. Residents should be assessed on admission and whenever there is a change in cognition, physical ability, or urinary tract function.

For individuals with UI, the nurse collaborates with the interprofessional team to (1) determine if UI is transient or established (or both); (2) determine the type of UI; and (3) identify and document possible etiologies of the UI, including a review of risk factors (Dowling-Castronovo & Bradway, 2012). Additional areas of assessment for UI are presented in Box 12.3, and Box 12.4 provides information on a video of a nurse conducting an assessment for transient UI. More extensive examinations are considered after the initial findings are assessed. Individuals who do not fit a simple pattern for UI should be referred promptly for urodynamic assessment (DeBeau, 2014).

◆ Interventions

◆ Behavioral

Most of the evidence on the efficacy of behavioral treatments has been among community living and institutionalized older individuals, and there are a number of

BOX 12.3 Tips for Best Practice

Continence Assessment

Bladder (Voiding) Diary
Kept for 3 to 7 days by the individual or caregiver (Fig. 12.1)
Voiding record for even 1 day can be helpful

Patterns of Fluid Intake
Usual fluid intake in 24 hours
Types of fluids and time consumed
Decreased or increased urine output

Bowel Patterns
Frequency, consistency, straining
Use of laxatives

Exploration of Symptoms of UI
"When did UI start?"
"What have you done to manage the problem?"
"How often does it occur?"
"What things make it better or worse?"
"How severe is it?"

Focused History (Medical, Neurological, Gynecological, Genitourinary)
Review past health history: possible contributing factors to UI, pertinent diagnoses (heart failure, stroke, diabetes mellitus, multiple sclerosis, Parkinson's disease)

Medication Review
Review all medications including OTC with focus on diuretics, anticholinergics, psychotropics, alpha-adrenergic blockers, alpha-adrenergic agonists, calcium channel blockers
Review use of alcohol

Focused Assessment
Screen for depression
Cognitive, functional

Observe Individual Using the Toilet
Ability to reach a toilet and use it; time it takes to reach the toilet; finger dexterity for clothing manipulation; character of the urine (color, odor, sediment); difficulty starting or stopping urinary stream.

Physical Examination
Abdominal, rectal, genital: Assess for suprapubic distention indicative of urinary retention
Observe for signs of perineal irritation, itching, burning, lesions, discharge, tenderness, thin and pale genital tissues (atrophic vaginitis), dyspareunia, pelvic organ prolapse
Check for fecal impaction, tenderness

Other Tests That May Be Ordered
Urinalysis; culture and sensitivity if clinically significant systemic or urinary symptoms
If indicated, PVR (bladder sonography or catheterization) 16 minutes or less post-void

Adapted from Dowling-Castronovo A, Bradway C: Urinary incontinence. In Boltz M, Capzuti E, Fulmer T, et al, editors: *Evidence-based geriatric nursing protocols for best practice,* ed 4, pp 363–387, New York, 2012, Springer; Ham R, Sloane P, Warshaw G, et al, editors: *Primary care geriatrics,* ed 6, Philadelphia, 2014, Elsevier.

behavioral interventions that have a good basis in research and can be implemented by nurses without extensive and expensive evaluation (Talley et al., 2011). Selection of a modality and interventions will depend on a comprehensive assessment, the type of incontinence and its underlying cause, and the goal of treatment (i.e., whether the outcome is to cure or to minimize the extent and complications of the incontinence).

Behavioral techniques, such as scheduled voiding, prompted voiding, bladder training, biofeedback, and pelvic floor muscle exercises (PFMEs), are recommended as first-line treatment of UI. Because UI in older adults can have multiple precipitating factors, a single intervention may not be adequate, and more complex, multicomponent interventions may be required (Gibson & Wagg, 2014).

Nursing interventions focus primarily on the appropriate assessment of continence, education about treatments, and implementation and evaluation of supportive and therapeutic modalities to promote and restore continence and to prevent incontinence-related complications, such as skin breakdown. The nurse should share appropriate resources and explain clinical information and differences in treatment choices (Box 12.5).

◆ ***Scheduled (timed) voiding.*** Scheduled (timed) voiding is used to treat urge and functional UI in both cognitively

BOX 12.4 Resources for Best Practice

Centers for Disease Control and Prevention: Guideline for prevention of catheter-associated urinary tract infections, 2009

Catheterout.org: Protocols, Educational tools, Toolkit

Di Rico N: NICHE Solution 27, 2012: A nurse-driven urinary catheter removal protocol: http://www.nicheprogram.org

Dowling-Castronovo A, Bradway C: Urinary incontinence. In Boltz M, Capezuti E, Fulmer T, et al, editors: *Evidence-based geriatric nursing protocols for best practice,* ed 4, pp 363–387, New York, 2012, Springer

Hartford Institute for Geriatric Nursing (consultgerirn.org)**:** *Try This: Series:* Urinary incontinence assessment in older adults. Part 1: Transient Incontinence (includes link to video of assessment). Part 2: Persistent Incontinence (includes UI assessment tools—Urogenital Distress Inventory and Incontinence Impact Questionnaire)

Hartford Institute for Geriatric Nursing: Want to know more: Urinary tract infection prevention, geriatric nursing protocol: prevention of catheter-associated urinary tract infection

International Continence Society: Educational materials, product guide, research, advocacy

National Association for Continence (NAC): Educational materials, product guide, advocacy

National Institute of Diabetes and Digestive and Kidney Disease: The NIDDK Bowel Control Awareness Campaign

Safe Care Campaign: Preventing health care and community associated infections: urinary tract infections

Simon Foundation for Continence: Educational materials, resources, and products; stool diary and Bristol Form Stool Scale

U.S. National Library of Medicine: Pelvic floor muscle training exercises, available at https://www.nlm.nih.gov/medlineplus/ency/article/003975.htm

intact and cognitively impaired older adults. The schedule or timing of voiding is based on the person's bladder diary (Fig. 12.1) or common voiding patterns (voiding on arising, before and after meals, midmorning, midafternoon, and bedtime). Many persons with UI have a very short time between voiding and leaking urine. With a program of timed voiding the goal is to slowly increase the time between voids without increasing the number, or even reducing the number, of incontinent episodes or reaching continence altogether. The person is encouraged to NOT void at an unscheduled time, thus achieving "mind over bladder."

◆ ***Bladder training.*** Bladder training aims to increase the time interval between the urge to void and voiding. This method is appropriate for people with urge UI who are cognitively intact and independent in toileting or after removal of an indwelling catheter. Bladder training involves frequent voluntary voiding to keep bladder volume low and suppression of the urge to void using pelvic muscle contractions, distraction, or relaxation techniques. When the individual feels the urge to urinate, the person uses the urge control techniques. After the urge subsides, the person walks at a normal pace to the toilet. The initial toileting frequency is every 2 hours and it is progressively lengthened to 4 hours, depending on tolerance, over the course of days or weeks (DeBeau, 2014; Wilde et al., 2014).

BOX 12.5 Tips for Best Practice

Teaching About UI Interventions

- Use therapeutic communication skills and a positive and supportive attitude to help individuals overcome any embarrassment about UI.
- Teach about the range of interventions available for management of UI.
- Share helpful resources for continence management.
- Share techniques found useful by others.
- Collaborate with the individual to help him or her choose the most appropriate and acceptable intervention based on needs.
- Assist individual to develop a detailed, realistic action plan and set goals.
- Determine an evaluation plan to assess the effectiveness of interventions.
- Review progress, identify any barriers to implementation, set alternative goals, or select alternate treatments if indicated.
- Reinforce effort and persistence.

From Wilde M, Bliss D, Booth J, et al: Self-management of urinary and fecal incontinence, *Am J Nurs* 114(2):38–45, 2014.

◆ ***Pelvic floor muscle exercises.*** Pelvic floor muscle exercises (PFMEs), also called Kegel exercises, involve repeated voluntary pelvic floor muscle contraction. The targeted muscle is the pubococcygeal muscle, which forms the support for the pelvis and surrounds the vagina, the urethra, and the rectum. The goal of the repetitive contractions is to strengthen the muscle and decrease UI episodes (Box 12.4).

PFMEs are recommended for stress, urge, and mixed UI in older women and have also been shown to be helpful for men who have undergone prostatectomy. In community-dwelling older adults, PFMEs are at least as effective as medications in treating stress and urge UI (Dowling-Castronovo & Bradway, 2012). Biofeedback may improve PFME teaching and outcomes, but further research is needed. Medicare covers biofeedback for individuals who do not improve after 4 weeks of a trial of PFMEs (DeBeau, 2014).

Bladder Diary ("Uro-Log")

Complete one form for each day for 4 days before your appointment with a health care provider. In order to keep the most accurate diary possible, you'll want to keep it with you at all times and write down the events as they happen. Take the completed forms with you to your appointment.

Your Name: ______________________

Date: ______________________

Time	Fluids		Foods		Did you urinate?		Accidents			
							Leakage	Did you feel an urge to urinate?		What were you doing at the time?
	What kind?	How much?	What kind?	How much?	How many times?	How much? (sm, med, lg)	How much? (sm, med, lg)			Sneezing, exercising, etc.
Sample	*Coffee*	*1 cup*	*Toast*	*1 slice*	✓✓	*med*	*sm*	Yes	(No)	*Running*
6-7 a.m.								Yes	No	
7-8 a.m.								Yes	No	
8-9 a.m.								Yes	No	
9-10 a.m.								Yes	No	
10-11 a.m.								Yes	No	
11-12 noon								Yes	No	
12-1 p.m.								Yes	No	
1-2 p.m.								Yes	No	
2-3 p.m.								Yes	No	
3-4 p.m.								Yes	No	
4-5 p.m.								Yes	No	
5-6 p.m.								Yes	No	
6-7 p.m.								Yes	No	
7-8 p.m.								Yes	No	
8-9 p.m.								Yes	No	

FIGURE 12.1 Bladder diary. (Provided by the National Association for Continence; 1-800-BLADDER; available at http://www.nafc.org.)

- ***Prompted voiding.*** Prompted voiding (PV) is a technique used in the nursing home that combines scheduled voiding with monitoring, prompting, and verbal reinforcement. The objective of PV is to increase self-initiated voiding and decrease the number of episodes of UI. Newly admitted nursing home residents who are incontinent (and able to use the toilet) should receive a 3- to 5-day trial of prompted voiding or other toileting programs. The trial can be helpful in demonstrating responsiveness to toileting and determining patterns of and symptoms associated with the incontinence (Box 12.6).
- ***Lifestyle modifications.*** Several lifestyle factors have been associated with either the development or the

BOX 12.6 Prompted Voiding Protocol: Long-Term Care

1. Contact resident every 2 hours from 8 AM to 9 PM (or the resident's usual bedtime).
2. Focus attention on voiding by asking if the resident is wet or dry.
3. Ask a second time if the resident does not respond.
4. Check clothes and bedding to determine if wet or dry. Give feedback on whether response was correct or incorrect.
5. Whether wet or dry, ask if the resident would like to use toilet or urinal.

   If the resident says **YES:**

   Offer assistance.

   Record results on bladder record.

   Praise for appropriate toileting.

   If the resident says **NO:**

   Repeat the question once or twice.

   If wet and declines to use the toilet, change him or her.

   Inform the resident you will be back in 2 hours and request that the resident try to delay voiding until then.

   If there has been no attempt to void in the past 2 to 3 hours, repeat the request to use the toilet at least twice more before leaving.

   1. Offer fluids.
   2. For nighttime management, either use modified prompted voiding schedule or toilet when awake or use padding, depending on individual's sleep pattern and preferences.
   3. If the individual who has been responding well has an increase in incontinence frequency despite adequate staff implementation of the protocol, further evaluation for reversible factors is indicated.

From Joseph Ouslander, MD, personal communication.

exacerbation of UI. These include increased fluid intake, smoking cessation, bowel management, physical activity, and weight reduction. Research has shown that women with stress UI who undergo a 5% to 10% weight loss experience a positive impact on UI symptoms. This is most likely due to the effects of reduced abdominal weight, intra-abdominal pressure, and intravesicular pressure (DeBeau, 2014; Wilde et al., 2014).

◆ Promotion of Continence Friendly Environment

An environmental, functional, and cognitive assessment is important to determine factors that may affect the individual's ability to use the toilet in public settings, at home, and in hospital and institutional settings. Observing the individual using the toilet should be included in any assessment of UI. If the individual is in a hospital or institution, occupational therapists can be helpful in these assessments and provide suggestions and equipment for improved abilities (e.g., elevated toilet seat, grab bars). In all settings, nurses play a key role in arranging the environment to facilitate toilet use and assist the individual to maintain or return to continence.

◆ ***Absorbent products.*** Some individuals prefer to use absorbent products in addition to toileting interventions to maintain "social continence," and a wide variety of products are available (Box 12.4). Disposable types are available in several sizes, determined by hip and waist measurements, or as one size made to fit all. Many of these undergarments now look like regular underwear and you even see them in stylish television commercials.

Nurses should avoid the use of the word *diaper* because it is infantilizing and demeaning to older people; the word *brief* is preferred. It is important that individuals are counseled to purchase proper continence products that will wick moisture away from the skin. These products are costly but they protect skin integrity. Women may tend to use menstrual pads but these do not absorb significant amounts of fluid.

◆ Pharmacological Treatment

Medications are not considered first-line treatment but can be considered in combination with behavioral strategies in some cases. Pharmacological treatment (anticholinergic, antimuscarinic agents) may be indicated for urge UI and overactive bladder (OAB). These include oxybutynin (Oxytrol, Ditropan), tolterodine (Detrol), trospium chloride (Sanctura), darifenacin (Enablex), fesoterodine (Toviaz), and solifenacin (VESIcare). Oxytrol for Women is the first FDA-approved over-the-counter (OTC) treatment for OAB. It is available in patch form, which is applied to the skin every 4 days. All of these medications have similar efficacy in reducing urge UI frequency, and choice of medication depends on avoidance of adverse drug effects, drug-drug and drug-disease interactions, dosing frequency, titration range, and cost (DeBeau, 2014). Beta$_3$-agonists (mirabegron) are a new class of medications for urge UI and OAB.

None of these medications have been evaluated in frail older people. Undesirable side effects of anticholinergic medications such as dry mouth and eyes, constipation, and cognitive impairment are problematic. People with narrow-angle glaucoma cannot use these medications, and they should not be combined with cholinesterase inhibitors. These medications can be especially problematic for those with cognitive impairment (DeBeau, 2014). Dosages of medications for urge UI and overactive bladder should be started low and titrated with careful attention to side effects and drug interactions. A trial of 4 to 8 weeks is adequate and recommended. If one medication is not effective, another may be tried (DeBeau, 2014).

Surgical Treatment

Surgical interventions may be indicated for stress UI and have a high cure rate. The most common procedures are colposuspension (Burch operation) and slings. Surgical suspension of the bladder neck (sling procedure) in women has proved effective in 80% to 95% of those electing to have this surgical corrective procedure. Outcomes in older women are comparable with those in younger women. Outflow obstruction incontinence secondary to prostatic hypertrophy is generally corrected by prostatectomy. Sphincter dysfunction resulting from nerve damage following surgical trauma or radical perineal procedures is 70% to 90% repairable through sphincter implantation. Periurethral injections of collagen are also used and add bulk to the internal sphincter and close the gap that allowed leakage to occur. This is a short-term alternative and usually requires a series of injections (DeBeau, 2014).

Nonsurgical Devices

There are a variety of intravaginal or intraurethral devices to relieve stress UI. These include intravaginal support devices, pessaries, external occlusive devices, and urethral plugs for women. For men, there are foam penile clamps. The pessary, used primarily to prevent uterine prolapse, is a device that is fitted into the vagina and exerts pressure to elevate the urethrovesical junction of the pelvic floor. The patient is taught to insert and remove the pessary, much like inserting and removing a diaphragm used for contraception. The pessary is removed weekly or monthly for cleaning with soap and water and then reinserted. Adverse effects include vaginal infection, low back pain, and vaginal mucosal erosion. Another concern is the danger of forgetting to remove the pessary. An evaluation of the stress UI by the health care provider should be conducted to determine if these devices would be helpful.

Urinary catheters. *Intermittent catheterization* may be used in people with urinary retention related to a weak detrusor muscle (e.g., diabetic neuropathy), those with a blockage of the urethra (e.g., benign prostatic hypertrophy), or those with reflux incontinence related to a spinal cord injury. The goal is to maintain 300 mL or less of urine in the bladder. Most of the research on intermittent catheterization has been conducted with children or young adults with spinal cord injuries, but it may be useful for older adults who are able to self-catheterize. It provides an important alternative to indwelling catheterization.

BOX 12.7 Indications for Indwelling Urinary Catheter Use

- Presence of acute urinary retention or bladder outlet obstruction
- Need for accurate measurements of urinary output in critically ill patients
- Perioperative use for selected surgical procedures: urological or other surgery on contiguous structures of the genitourinary tract; anticipated prolonged surgery duration (should be removed in postanesthesia unit); patients anticipated to receive large-volume infusions or diuretics during surgery; need for intraoperative monitoring of urinary output
- Assistance in healing of open sacral or perineal wounds in incontinent patients
- Requirement for prolonged patient immobilization (e.g., potentially unstable thoracic or lumbar spine, multiple traumatic injuries such as pelvic fractures)
- Improvement in comfort for end-of-life care if needed

From catheterout.org: *Indications for indwelling catheter use,* available at http://catheterout.org/?q=Indications-for-indwelling-urinary-catheter-use; Meddings J, Krein SL, Fakih MG, et al: Reducing unnecessary urinary catheter use and other strategies to prevent catheter-associated urinary tract infections: Brief update review. In *Making health care safer II: An updated critical analysis of the evidence for patient safety practices* (Evidence Reports/Technology Assessments no. 211), Rockville, MD, 2013, Agency for Healthcare Research and Quality. Available at http://www.ncbi.nlm.nih.gov/books/NBK133354. Accessed November 2015.

Indwelling catheter use is not appropriate for long-term management (more than 30 days) except in certain clinical conditions (Box 12.7). Regulatory standards in nursing homes follow these same guidelines, and the use of indwelling catheters must be justified on the basis of medical conditions and failure of other efforts to maintain continence. In hospitals, the use of indwelling catheters is often unjustified, and they are used inappropriately or left in place too long. Between 14% and 25% of patients in the hospital setting will have an indwelling catheter, up to half of which can be inappropriate (So et al., 2014). Reasons for this include (1) convenience to manage UI; (2) lack of knowledge of risks associated with use and alternative treatments; (3) failure of providers to track continued use; and (4) lack of valid continence assessment tools for older adults (DiRico, 2012).

Misuse of catheterization should be considered a medical error. Cognitive impairment and the presence of pressure ulcers almost double the risk of receiving a catheter, and severe functional decline is associated with a fourfold risk of catheter placement (Inelmen et al., 2007).

SAFETY ALERT

Long-term catheter use increases the risk of recurrent urinary tract infections leading to urosepsis, urethral damage in men, urethritis, or fistula formation. Catheter-associated urinary tract infection is the most frequent health care–associated infection in the United States. Indwelling catheters should be inserted only for appropriate conditions and must be removed as soon as possible. A comprehensive evaluation of continence status should be performed to determine the most appropriate interventions to maintain bladder health.

External catheters (condom catheters) are sometimes used in male patients who are incontinent and cannot be toileted. Long-term use of external catheters can lead to fungal skin infections, penile skin maceration, edema, fissures, contact burns from urea, phimosis, UTIs, and septicemia. The catheter should be removed and replaced daily and the penis cleaned, dried, and aired to prevent irritation, maceration, and the development of skin breakdown. If the catheter is not sized appropriately and applied and monitored correctly, strangulation of the penile shaft can occur.

URINARY TRACT INFECTIONS

Urinary tract infections (UTIs) are the most common cause of bacterial sepsis in older adults and are 10 times more common in women than in men. The clinical spectrum of UTIs ranges from asymptomatic and recurrent UTIs to sepsis associated with UTI requiring hospitalization. Assessment and appropriate treatment of UTIs in older people, particularly nursing home residents, is complex. Cognitively impaired residents may not recall or report symptoms, and older people frequently do not present with classic symptoms (fever, dysuria, flank pain) (Mody & Juthani-Mehta, 2014).

Asymptomatic bacteriuria is transient and considered benign in older women. It should not be treated with antibiotics and often resolves without treatment. Antimicrobials should not be used to treat bacteriuria in older adults unless specific urinary tract symptoms are present (American Geriatrics Society, 2014). Screening urine cultures should also not be performed in patients who are asymptomatic. The diagnosis of symptomatic UTI is made when the patient has both clinical features (painful urination, lower abdominal pain/tenderness, blood in urine, new or worsening urinary urgency or frequency, incontinence, and fever) and laboratory evidence of a urinary tract infection. Treatment is with antibiotics selected by identifying the pathogen, knowing local resistance rates, and considering adverse effects.

BOX 12.8 Tips for Best Practice

Prevention of CAUTI: ABCDE

Adherence to general infection control principles (hand hygiene, surveillance, aseptic catheter insertion, education, and proper maintenance of a sterile, closed, unobstructed drainage system)

Bladder ultrasound may aid indwelling catheterization

Condom catheters or other alternatives to an indwelling catheter such as intermittent catheterization should be considered in appropriate patients

Do not use the indwelling catheter unless you must. **D**o not use antimicrobial catheters. **D**o not irrigate catheters unless obstruction is anticipated (e.g., as might occur with bleeding after prostatic or bladder surgery). **D**o not clean the periurethral area with antiseptics (cleansing of the metal surface during daily bathing or showering is appropriate)

Early removal of the catheter using a reminder or nurse-initiated removal protocol

From Centers for Disease Control and Prevention: *Guideline for prevention of catheter-associated urinary tract infections*, 2009, available at http://www.cdc.gov/hicpac/cauti/001_cauti.htm, accessed November 2015; Meddings J, Krein SL, Fakih MG, et al: Reducing unnecessary urinary catheter use and other strategies to prevent catheter-associated urinary tract infections: Brief update review. In *Making health care safer II: An updated critical analysis of the evidence for patient safety practices* (Evidence Reports/Technology Assessments no. 211), Rockville, MD, 2013, Agency for Healthcare Research and Quality. Available at http://www.ncbi.nlm.nih.gov/books/NBK133354. Accessed November 2015.

Catheter-Associated Urinary Tract Infections

Catheter-associated urinary tract infections (CAUTIs) refer to urinary tract infections that occur in a patient with an indwelling catheter or within 48 hours of catheter removal (Andreessen et al., 2012). CAUTIs are the most common hospital-acquired infection worldwide (So et al., 2014). One of the goals of *Healthy People 2020* is to prevent, reduce, and ultimately eliminate health care–associated infections. Implementation of evidence-based guidelines, catheter reminders, stop orders, nurse-initiated removal protocols, and a urinary catheter bundle can decrease CAUTIs in acute care (Andreesen et al., 2012; Leis et al., 2015; Shekelle et al., 2013) (Box 12.8).

BOWEL ELIMINATION

Bowel function of the older adult, although normally only slightly altered by the physiological changes of age (see Chapter 3), can be a source of concern and a potentially serious problem, especially for the older person who is functionally impaired. Normal elimination

BOX 12.9 Rome III Criteria for Defining Chronic Functional Constipation in Adults

Two or more of the following for at least 12 weeks in the preceding 12 months:

- Straining with defecation more than 25% of the time
- Lumpy or hard stools more than 25% of the time
- Sensation of incomplete emptying more than 25% of the time
- Manual maneuvers used to facilitate emptying in more than 25% of defecations (digital evacuation or support of the pelvic floor)
- Fewer than 3 bowel movements per week

should be an easy passage of feces, without undue straining or a feeling of incomplete evacuation or defecation.

Constipation

Constipation is defined as a reduction in the frequency of stool or difficulty in formation or passage of stool (McKay et al., 2012). The Rome Criteria outline the operational definitions of constipation and should be used as a guide to diagnosis (Box 12.9). Constipation is one of the most common gastrointestinal complaints encountered in clinical practice in all settings. Approximately 40% of people 65 years of age and older experience constipation. Women have two to three times more constipation than men, and black women also exhibit increased risk (Alayne et al., 2013; Markland, 2014). Constipation is seen more frequently among nursing home residents, with 50% to 74% of this patient population using laxatives on a daily basis (Foxx-Orstein & Gallegos-Orozco, 2012).

Many individuals, both the lay public and health care professionals, may view constipation as a minor problem or nuisance. However, it is associated with impaired quality of life, significant health care costs, and a large economic burden. Constipation can also have very serious consequences including fecal impaction, bowel obstruction, cognitive dysfunction, delirium, falls, and increased morbidity and mortality (Osei-Boamah et al., 2012). Individuals with chronic constipation are also at greater risk for developing colorectal cancer and benign colorectal neoplasms (Guerin et al., 2014).

Constipation is a symptom, not a disease. It is a reflection of poor habits, delayed response to the colonic reflex, and many chronic illnesses—both physical and psychological—as well as a common side effect of medication. Diet and activity level play a significant role in constipation. Constipation and other changes in bowel habits can also signal more serious underlying problems, such as colonic dysmotility or colon cancer. Thorough assessment is important, and these complaints should not be blamed on age alone. It is important to note that alterations in cognitive status, incontinence, increased temperature, poor appetite, or unexplained falls may be the only clinical symptoms of constipation in the cognitively impaired or frail older person. Numerous precipitating factors or conditions can cause or worsen constipation.

Fecal Impaction

Fecal impaction (FI) is a major complication of constipation. Unrecognized, unattended, or neglected constipation eventually leads to fecal impaction. It is especially common in incapacitated and institutionalized older people and in those who require narcotic medications (e.g., for chronic pain). FI is reported to occur in more than 40% of older adults admitted to the hospital (Roach & Christie, 2008). Symptoms of fecal impaction include malaise, urinary retention, elevated temperature, incontinence of bladder or bowel, alterations in cognitive status, fissures, hemorrhoids, and intestinal obstruction.

Paradoxical diarrhea, caused by leakage of fecal material around the impacted mass, may occur. Digital rectal examination for impacted stool and abdominal x-rays will confirm the presence of impacted stool. Continued obstruction by a fecal mass may eventually impair sensation, leading to the need for larger stool volume to stimulate the urge to defecate, which contributes to megacolon.

Removal of a fecal impaction is at times worse than the misery of the condition. Management of fecal impaction requires the digital removal of the hard, compacted stool from the rectum with use of lubrication containing lidocaine jelly. In general, this is preceded by an oil-retention enema to soften the feces in preparation for manual removal. Use of suppositories is not effective because their action is blocked by the amount and size of the stool in the rectum. Suppositories do not facilitate the removal of stool in the sigmoid, which may continue to ooze once the rectum is emptied.

Several sessions or days may be necessary to totally cleanse the sigmoid colon and rectum of impacted feces. Once this is achieved, attention should be directed to planning a regimen that includes adequate fluid intake, increased dietary fiber, administration of medications if needed, and many of the suggestions presented later in this chapter for prevention of constipation.

For patients who are hospitalized or residing in long-term care settings, accurate bowel records are essential; unfortunately, they are often overlooked or inaccurately completed. This is especially important for frail or cognitively impaired elders. Education about the importance of bowel function and the accurate reporting of size, consistency, and frequency of bowel movements should be provided to all direct care providers.

❖ IMPLICATIONS FOR GERONTOLOGICAL NURSING AND HEALTHY AGING

◆ Assessment

Assessment and management of bowel function is an important nursing responsibility. The precipitants and causes of constipation must be included in the evaluation of the individual. A review of these factors will also determine whether the patient is at risk for altered bowel function and if any of the known risks are modifiable. Recognizing constipation can be a challenge because there may be a significant disconnect between patient definitions of constipation and those of clinicians (Box 12.9).

Constipation has different meanings to different people. Assessment begins with clarification of what the person means by constipation. Of persons who consider themselves to be constipated, nearly half actually have a bowel movement on a daily basis but a high percentage report persistent straining and passage of hard stools on a regular basis (Foxx-Orstein & Gallegos-Orozco, 2012).

It is important to obtain a bowel history including description of usual patterns; frequency of bowel movements; size, consistency, or any changes in bowel movements; and occurrence of straining and hard stools. However, recall of bowel frequency has been shown to be unreliable in establishing the presence of constipation. Having the patient keep a bowel diary and using the Bristol Stool Form Scale, which provides a visual description of stool appearance, will be more accurate (Lewis & Heaton, 1997; McKay et al., 2012). Box 12.4 provides a resource for a bowel diary and the Bristol Stool Form Scale. Assessment data are presented in Box 12.10.

BOX 12.10 Tips for Best Practice

Assessment of Constipation

Sample Questions
- What is your usual bowel pattern?
- How many minutes did you sit on the bedpan or toilet before you had your bowel movement?
- How much did you have to strain before you had your bowel movement?
- Do you think you are constipated? If yes, why do you think so?
- Have you had any abdominal pain, nausea, vomiting, weight loss, blood in your bowel movement, or rectal pain?
- Have you had any bowel or rectal surgery?
- What type of physical activity do you engage in and how often?

Review of Food and Fluid Intake

Medication Review (Include OTC, Herbal Preparations, Supplements)

Psychosocial History With Attention to Depression, Anxiety, Stress Management

Review of Concurrent Medical Conditions

Other Measures
- Bowel diary
- Bristol Stool Form Survey

Focused Physical Examination
- Abdominal exam to detect masses, distention, tenderness, high-pitched or absent bowel sounds
- If these abnormalities are present, primary care provider should be contacted
- Rectal exam, following institutional policy, to identify painful anal disorders such as hemorrhoids or fissures, rectal prolapse, stool presence in the vault, strictures, masses, anal reflex

Other Tests as Indicated
- Complete blood count, fasting glucose level, chemistry panel, thyroid studies
- Flexible sigmoidoscopy, colonoscopy, CT scan, abdominal x-ray

Adapted from McKay S, Fravel M, Scanlon C: Management of constipation, *J Gerontol Nurs* 38(7):9–16, 2012.

◆ Interventions

◆ Nonpharmacological Treatment

The first intervention is to examine the medications the person is taking and eliminate those that produce constipation, preferably changing to medications that do not carry that side effect. Medications are the leading cause of constipation, and almost any drug can cause it. Other interventions that have been implemented and evaluated are as follows: (1) fluid and diet related, (2) physical activity, (3) environmental manipulation, (4) toileting regimen, and (5) a combination of these.

Fluid intake of at least 1.5 L per day, unless contraindicated, is the cornerstone of constipation therapy, with fluids coming mainly from water. A gradual increase in fiber intake, either taken as supplements or incorporated into the diet, is generally recommended. Fiber helps stools become bulkier and softer and move through the body more quickly. This will produce easier and more regular bowel movements. The importance of dietary fiber to adequate nutrition and bowel function is discussed in Chapter 10.

◆ ***Physical activity.*** Physical activity is important as an intervention to stimulate colon motility and bowel evacuation. Daily walking for 20 to 30 minutes, if tolerated, is helpful, especially after a meal. Pelvic tilt exercises and range-of-motion (passive or active) exercises are beneficial for those who are less mobile or who are bedridden. Exercise and physical activity are discussed in Chapter 13.

- ***Positioning.*** The squatting or sitting position, if the patient is able to assume it, facilitates bowel function. A similar position may be obtained by leaning forward and applying firm pressure to the lower abdomen or by placing the feet on a stool. Rocking back and forth while sitting solidly on the toilet may facilitate stool movement. Massaging the abdomen or rectum may also help stimulate the bowel.
- ***Toileting regimen.*** Establishing a routine for toileting promotes or normalizes bowel function (bowel retraining). The gastrocolic reflex occurs after breakfast or supper and may be enhanced by a warm drink. Given privacy and ample time (a minimum of 10 minutes), many will have a daily bowel movement. However, any urge to defecate should be followed by a trip to the bathroom. Older people dependent on others to meet toileting needs should be assisted to maintain normal routines and provided opportunities for routine toilet use. Box 12.11 presents a bowel training program.

Pharmacological Treatment

When changes in diet and lifestyle are not effective, the use of laxatives can be considered. Use of these medications, both prescribed and OTC, is high. The extensive use of laxatives among older adults in the United States can be considered a cultural habit. During earlier times, weekly doses of rhubarb, cascara, castor oil, and other types of laxatives were consumed and believed by many to promote health. The belief that cleaning out the colon and having a daily bowel movement is paramount to maintaining good health still persists in some groups. Providing information about normal bowel function, definition of constipation, and lifestyle modifications can assist in promoting healthy bowel habits without the use of laxatives.

If laxatives are indicated, those commonly used in chronic constipation include the following:

- Bulking agents (e.g., psyllium, methylcellulose)
- Stool softeners (surfactants) (e.g., docusate sodium)
- Osmotic laxatives (e.g., lactulose, sorbitol)
- Stimulant laxatives (e.g., senna, bisacodyl)
- Saline laxatives (e.g., magnesium hydroxide [Milk of Magnesia])

Bulk laxatives are often the first prescribed because of their safety. Bulk laxatives absorb water from the intestinal lumen and increase stool mass. Adequate fluid intake is essential, and use of these laxatives is contraindicated in the presence of obstruction or compromised peristaltic activity. They should be used with caution in frail older people, bed-bound individuals, and those with swallowing problems. Bulk-forming agents can decrease absorption of other medications, particularly aspirin, warfarin, and carbamazepine, and may also affect blood glucose levels. A saline or osmotic laxative

BOX 12.11 Tips for Best Practice

Bowel Training Program

1. Obtain a bowel history and establish a schedule for the bowel training program that is normal and comfortable for the patient and conforms to his or her lifestyle.
2. Ensure adequate fiber and fluid intake (normalize stool consistency).
   a. Fiber
      i. Add high-fiber foods to diet (dried fruit, dried beans, vegetables, and wheat products).
      ii. Suggest adding one to three tablespoons of bran or Metamucil to the diet once or twice each day. (Titrate dosage on the basis of response.)
   b. Fluid
      i. Consume 2 to 3 L daily (unless contraindicated).
      ii. Four ounces of prune, fig, or pear juice (or a warm fluid) may be given daily as a stimulus (e.g., 30 to 60 min before the established time for defecation).
3. Encourage an exercise program.
   a. Pelvic tilt, modified sit-ups for abdominal strength
   b. Walking for general muscle tone and cardiovascular system
   c. More vigorous program if appropriate
4. Establish a regular time for the bowel movement.
   a. Established time depends on patient's schedule.
   b. Best times are 20 to 40 minutes after regularly scheduled meals, when the gastrocolic reflex is active.
   c. Attempts at evacuation should be made daily within 15 minutes of the established time and whenever the patient senses rectal distention.
   d. Instruct patient about normal posture for defecation. (The patient normally sits on the toilet or bedside commode; for the patient who is unable to get out of bed, the left side–lying position is best.)
   e. Instruct the patient to contract the abdominal muscles and "bear down."
   f. Have the patient lean forward to increase the intra-abdominal pressure by use of compression against the thighs.
   g. Stimulate the anorectal reflex and rectal emptying if necessary.
5. Insert a rectal suppository or mini-enema into the rectum 15 to 30 minutes before the scheduled bowel movement, placing the suppository against the bowel wall; or insert a gloved, lubricated finger into the anal canal and gently dilate the anal sphincter.

can be added if the bulk laxative is not effective. Use of saline laxatives should be avoided in patients with poor renal function or congestive heart failure because they may cause electrolyte imbalances.

Stimulant laxatives should be used when other laxatives are ineffective but are indicated for opioid-induced constipation. The emollient laxative mineral oil should be avoided because of the risk of lipoid aspiration pneumonia. Stool softeners (surfactants) are frequently used as laxatives. They are poorly absorbed and have a detergent-like effect of reducing the water-oil interface in the stool. Studies of surfactants, such as docusate, have reported minimal effectiveness, particularly in older adults with limited mobility. Because stool softeners do not increase bowel activity, their use may result in certain individuals having a bowel filled with soft stool (Osei-Boamah et al., 2012). Use should be limited to patients in whom excessive straining or painful defecation occurs, or for individuals at high risk for developing constipation, in combination with other types of laxatives and bowel programs (McKay et al., 2012).

◆ ***Enemas.*** Enemas of any type should be reserved for situations in which other methods produce no response or when it is known that there is an impaction. Enemas should not be used on a regular basis. A normal saline or tap water enema (500 to 1000 mL) at a temperature of 105°F is the best choice. Sodium citrate enemas are another safe choice. Soapsuds and phosphate enemas irritate the rectal mucosa and should not be used. Oil retention enemas are used for refractory constipation and in the treatment of fecal impaction.

SAFETY ALERT

Sodium phosphate enemas (e.g., Fleet) should not be used in older adults because they may lead to severe metabolic disorders associated with high mortality and morbidity (Ori et al., 2012).

◆ Alternative Treatments

Combinations of natural fiber, fruit juices, and natural laxative mixtures are often recommended in clinical practice, and some studies have found an increase in bowel frequency and a decrease in laxative use when these mixtures are used (Box 12.12). Although research is still limited, many modalities of complementary and alternative medicine, such as probiotic bacteria, traditional herbal medicines, biofeedback, and massage, are also used to treat constipation. Further study is needed but probiotic bacteria might be easiest to use, and supermarkets in several countries carry brands of yogurt labeled probiotic (Cherniack, 2013).

BOX 12.12 Natural Laxative Recipe

Power Pudding

Ingredients

1 cup wheat bran
1 cup applesauce
1 cup prune juice

Directions

Mix and store in refrigerator. Start with administration of 1 tablespoon/day. Increase slowly until desired effect is achieved and no disagreeable symptoms occur.

ACCIDENTAL BOWEL LEAKAGE/FECAL INCONTINENCE

Fecal incontinence (FI) is defined by the International Continence Society as the involuntary loss of liquid or solid stool that is a social and hygienic problem (Markland, 2014). Prevalence of FI varies with the study population: 2% to 17% in community-dwelling older people; 50% to 65% in older adults in nursing homes; and 33% in hospitalized older adults. Higher prevalence rates are found among patients with diabetes, irritable bowel syndrome, stroke (new onset, 30%; 16% at 3 years poststroke), multiple sclerosis, and spinal cord injury (Grover et al., 2010; Roach & Christie, 2008).

A lack of consistency in the definitions used for FI and differences in populations studied and methodology affect statistics. Additionally, accurate estimates are difficult to obtain because many people are reluctant to discuss this disorder and many primary care providers do not ask about it.

Often FI is associated with urinary incontinence, and up to 50% to 70% of patients with UI also carry the diagnosis of FI. FI can be transient (episodes of diarrhea, acute illness, fecal impaction) or persistent. Fecal incontinence, like urinary incontinence, has devastating social ramifications for the individuals and families who experience it. UI and FI share similar contributing factors, including damage to the pelvic floor as a result of surgery or trauma, neurological disorders, functional impairment, immobility, and dementia.

Bowel continence and defecation depend on coordination of sensory and motor innervation of the rectum and anal sphincters. Impairment of the anorectal unit, such as weakness from prolonged straining secondary to constipation, or overt anal tears seen after vaginal delivery in women (35%) are common causes of FI. Injury from obstetrical trauma is often delayed in onset, and many women do not manifest symptoms until after the age of 50 years (Roach & Christie, 2008).

❖ IMPLICATIONS FOR GERONTOLOGICAL NURSING AND HEALTHY AGING

◆ Assessment

An important point in assessment is the term that is chosen to describe FI. Brown and colleagues (2012) reported that the term accidental bowel leakage was preferred over FI. Assessment should include a complete client history, as in urinary incontinence, and investigation into stool consistency and frequency, laxative or enema use, surgical and obstetrical history, medications taken, effect of FI on quality of life, focused physical examination with attention to the gastrointestinal system, and a bowel record. A digital rectal examination should be performed to identify any presence of a mass, impaction, or occult blood.

◆ Interventions

Nursing interventions are aimed at managing and/or restoring bowel continence. Therapies similar to those used to treat urinary incontinence are effective, such as environmental manipulation (access to toilet), dietary alterations, habit training schedules, PFMEs, improvements in transfer and ambulation ability, sphincter training exercises, biofeedback, medications, and/or surgery to correct underlying defects. Providing resources and educational information are important and will help in self-management (Box 12.4).

Pharmacological interventions may include the use of antidiarrheal medications and fiber therapy. Dextranomer in stabilized sodium hyaluronate (Solesta) is an FDA-approved treatment that may be helpful for those who do not find relief with conservative therapies. Solesta is a sterile, injectable gel that is thought to work by thickening anal tissue. It is an outpatient procedure that is well tolerated for up to 18 months following treatment (Hoy, 2012).

Biofeedback may also be recommended and there are some surgical options. The InterStim Therapy System, also used for UI and approved by the FDA, is a surgically implanted device that applies a small electrical stimulation to the sacral nerve that controls the anal sphincter. It is used in individuals who have failed or could not tolerate more conservative measures (U.S. Food and Drug Administration, 2013).

The effectiveness of interventions in fecal incontinence will be self-evident but will take time. As in the treatment of urinary incontinence, goals must be realistic. It cannot be stated too often or too strongly that the nurse must always provide immaculate skin care to persons with incontinence, because self-esteem and skin integrity depend on it.

KEY CONCEPTS

- Urinary incontinence is not a part of normal aging. UI is a symptom of an underlying problem and requires thorough assessment.
- Urinary incontinence can be minimized or cured, and there are many therapeutic modalities available for treatment of UI that nurses can implement.
- Health promotion teaching, identification of risk factors, comprehensive assessments of UI, education of informal and formal caregivers, and use of evidence-based interventions are basic continence competencies for nurses.
- A number of interventions for urinary incontinence are applicable to the management of bowel incontinence.

ACTIVITIES AND DISCUSSION QUESTIONS

1. Discuss risk factors for UI in older adults.
2. What health teaching would you provide to a 70-year-old woman who asks you if it is normal to leak urine when coughing or sneezing? What suggestions could you give her to deal with this concern?
3. When you are at your clinical site, ask the nurses what concerns they have with the bowel elimination of their patients.
4. Develop a nursing care plan for an older adult with urinary or fecal incontinence.

REFERENCES

Agency for Healthcare Research and Quality: *Experts seek better diagnosis and treatment for women's urinary incontinence and chronic pelvic pain, AHRQ Res Activities* no. 383, 2012.

Alayne D, Markland D, Palsson O, et al: Association of low dietary intake of fiber and liquids with constipation, *Am J Gastroenterol* 8(5):796–803, 2013.

American Geriatrics Society Choosing Wisely Workgroup: American Geriatrics Society identifies another five things that healthcare providers and patients should question, *J Am Geriatr Soc* 62(5):950–960, 2014.

Andreessen L, Wilde M, Herrendeen P: Preventing catheter-associated urinary tract infection in acute care: the bundle approach, *J Nurs Care Qual* 27(3):209–217, 2012.

Brown H, Wexner M, Segall K, et al: Accidental bowel leakage in the mature women's health study, *Int J Clin Pract* 66(11):1101–1108, 2012.

Cherniack P: Use of complementary and alternative medicine to treat constipation in the elderly, *Geriatr Gerontol Int* 13(3):533–538, 2013.

DeBeau C: Urinary incontinence. In Ham R, Sloane R, Warshaw G, et al, editors: *Primary care geriatrics*, ed 6, Philadelphia, 2014, Elsevier, pp 269–280.

DiRico N: *A nurse driven urinary catheter removal protocol* (NICHE solution no. 27), 2012. Available at https://s3.amazonaws.com/Resources2014/NICHESolutions_Dirico_27.pdf. Accessed November 2015.

Dowling-Castronovo A, Bradway C: Urinary incontinence (UI) in older adults admitted to acute care. In Capezuti E, Zwicker D, Mezey M, et al, editors: *Evidence-based geriatric nursing protocols for best practice*, ed 3, New York, 2008, Springer, pp 309–336.

Dowling-Castronovo A, Bradway C: Urinary incontinence. In Boltz M, Capezuti E, Fulmer T, et al, editors: *Evidence-based geriatric nursing protocols for best practice*, ed 4, New York, 2012, Springer, pp 363–387.

Foxx-Orstein A, Gallegos-Orozco J: *Chronic constipation in the elderly: Impact, classification, mechanisms, and common contributing factors, a special 2012 WDHD supplement*, 2012. Available at http://www.wgofoundation.org/assets/docs/pdf/wdhd12-supplement-HI.pdf?utm_source=wdhd2012&utm_medium=download&utm_campaign=2012supplement. Accessed November 2015.

Gibson W, Wagg A: New horizons: Urinary incontinence in older people, *Age Ageing* 43:157–163, 2014.

Grover M, Busby-Whitehead J, Palmer MH, et al: Survey of geriatricians on the effect of fecal incontinence on nursing home referral, *J Am Geriatr Soc* 58:1058, 2010.

Guerin A, Mody R, Lasch K, et al: Risk of developing colorectal cancer and benign colorectal neoplasm in patients with chronic constipation, *Aliment Pharmacol Ther* 40(1):83–92, 2014.

Hoy S: Dextranomer in stabilized sodium hyaluronate (Solesta) in adults with faecal incontinence, *Drugs* 72(12):1671–1678, 2012.

Inelmen E, Giuseppe S, Giuliano E: When are indwelling catheters appropriate in elderly patients? *Geriatrics* 62(10):18–22, 2007.

Lawhorne L, Ouslander J, Parmelee P, et al: Urinary incontinence: A neglected geriatric syndrome in nursing facilities, *J Am Med Dir Assoc* 9(1):9–35, 2008.

Leis J, Corpus C, Rahmani A, et al: *Medical directive for urinary catheter removal by nurses on general medical wards, JAMA Intern Med*, published online November 16, 2015. doi: 10.1001/jamainternmed.2015.6319.

Lewis SJ, Heaton KW: Stool Form Scale as a useful guide to intestinal transit time, *Scand J Gastroenterol* 32:920, 1997.

MacDonald C, Butler L: Silent no more: Elderly women's stories of living with urinary incontinence in long-term care, *J Gerontol Nurs* 33(1):14–20, 2007.

Markland A: Constipation and fecal incontinence. In Ham R, Sloane R, Warshaw G, et al, editors: *Primary care geriatrics*, ed 6, Philadelphia, 2014, Elsevier, pp 281–291.

Mason DJ, Newman DK, Palmer MH: Changing UI practice, *Am J Nurs* 3(Suppl):2–3, 2003.

McKay S, Fravel M, Scanlon C: Management of constipation, *J Gerontol Nurs* 38(7):9–16, 2012.

Meddings J, Krein SL, Fakih MG, et al: Reducing unnecessary urinary catheter use and other strategies to prevent catheter-associated urinary tract infections: Brief update review. In *Making health care safer II: An updated critical analysis of the evidence for patient safety practices* (Evidence Reports/Technology Assessments no. 211), Rockville, MD, 2013, Agency for Healthcare Research and Quality. Available at http://www.ncbi.nlm.nih.gov/books/NBK133354. Accessed March 2014.

Mody L, Juthani-Mehta M: Urinary tract infections in older women, *JAMA* 311(8):844–854, 2014.

National Association for Continence: 2014. Available at http://www.nafc.org.

Osei-Boamah E, Chui J, Diaz C, et al: Constipation in the hospitalized older patient, *Clin Geriatr* 20(10):20–26, 2012.

Ori Y, Rozen B, Herman M, et al: Fatalities and severe metabolic distress associated with the use of sodium phosphate enema: A single center's experience, *Arch Intern Med* 172(3):263–265, 2012.

Palmer MH, Newman D: Bladder control educational needs of older adults, *J Gerontol Nurs* 32(10):28–32, 2006.

Roach M, Christie J: Fecal incontinence in the elderly, *Geriatrics* 63(2):13–22, 2008.

Seshan V, Muliira J: Self-reported urinary incontinence and factors associated with symptom severity in community dwelling older women: Implications for women's health promotion, *BMC Womens Health* 13:16, 2013.

Shekelle P, Wachter R, Pronovost P, et al: *Making healthcare safer II: An updated critical analysis of the evidence for patient safety practices* (AHRQ publication no. 13-E001-EF), Rockville, MD, 2013, Agency for Healthcare Research and Quality.

So K, Habashy D, Doyle B, et al: Indwelling urinary catheters: Pattern of use in a public tertiary-level Australian hospital, *Urol Nurs* 34(2):69–73, 2014.

Talley K, Wyman J, Shamliyan T: State of the science: conservative interventions for urinary incontinence in community-dwelling older adults, *Nurs Outlook* 50(4):215–220, 2011.

U.S. Food and Drug Administration: *Medical devices: Medtronic Inter-Stim therapy system*, 2013. http://www.fda.gov/MedicalDevices/ProductsandMedicalProcedures/DeviceApprovalsandClearances/Recently-ApprovedDevices/ucm249208.htm. Accessed November 2015.

Wilde M, Bliss D, Booth J, et al: Self-management of urinary and fecal incontinence, *Am J Nurs* 114(2):38–45, 2014.

Wilson A, Dugger R, Ehlman K, et al: Implementation science in nursing homes: A case study of the integration of bladder ultrasound scanners, *Ann Longterm Care Aging* 23(6):21–26, 2015.

Wound, Ostomy and Continence Nurses Society: Position statement: Role of the wound, ostomy, continence nurse or continence care nurse in continence care, *J Wound Ostomy Continence Nurs* 36:529–531, 2009.

Xu D, Kane R: Effect of urinary incontinence on older nursing home residents' self-reported quality of life, *J Am Geriatr Soc* 61(9):1473–1481, 2013.

13

Rest, Sleep, and Activity

Theris A. Touhy

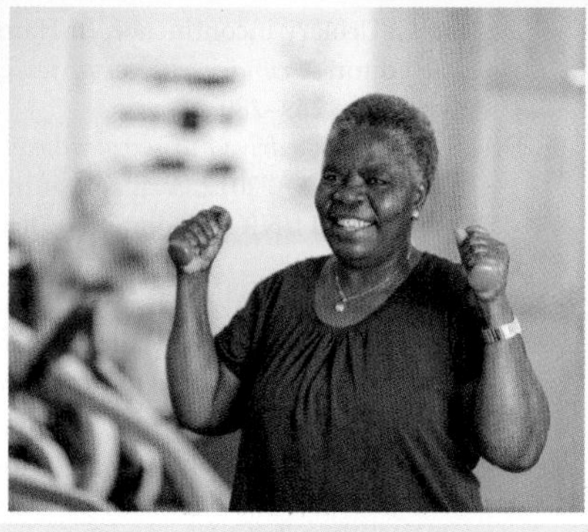

evolve.elsevier.com/Touhy/gerontological

LEARNING OBJECTIVES

Upon completion of this chapter, the reader will be able to:

- Identify factors that affect rest, sleep, and activity as we age.
- Discuss the importance of sleep and activity to the health and well-being of older adults.
- Describe the beneficial effects of exercise and appropriate exercise regimens for older adults.
- Use evidence-based protocols in assessment and development of interventions for rest, sleep, and promotion of activity.

THE LIVED EXPERIENCE

You know, I never get a decent night's sleep. I wake up at least 4 times every night, and I just know I won't get back to sleep. I really don't want to keep taking pills for sleep, but when I lie there awake, I just think of all the difficult times and situations I can't manage. After a while, I'm really in a stew about everything.

Richard, a 67-year-old recent retiree

This is really beginning to tire me out. Richard keeps waking me at night because he can't sleep. I try to tell him to get up and read or something. I really need my sleep if I'm going to get to work on time. I wonder if Richard needs to see a doctor. Maybe he is depressed about being retired and alone while I'm at work. I'll talk to him about it.

Clara, Richard's wife

Rest, sleep, and activity depend on one another. Inadequacy of rest and sleep affects any activity, whether it is considered strenuous exertion or performance of activities of daily living (ADLs). Activity, in turn, is necessary to maintain physical and physiological integrity (e.g., cardiopulmonary endurance and function; musculoskeletal strength, agility, and structure) and it helps a person obtain adequate sleep. Rest, sleep, and activity contribute greatly to overall physical and mental well-being.

REST AND SLEEP

The human organism needs rest and sleep to conserve energy, prevent fatigue, provide organ respite, and relieve tension. Sleep is an extension of rest, and both are physiological and mental necessities for survival. Sleep is a basic need. Rest occurs with sleep in sustained unbroken periods. Sleep occupies one-third of our lives and is a vital function that affects cognition and performance. The restorative function of sleep may be a consequence of the enhanced removal of potentially neurotoxic waste products that accumulate in the conscious central nervous system (Xie et al., 2013).

Sleep is a barometer of health, and sleep assessment and interventions for sleep concerns should receive as much attention as other vital signs. There is increasing awareness of the relationship between sleep problems and health outcomes, including premature mortality, osteoporosis, cardiovascular disease, diabetes, metabolic disease, impaired cognition and physical function, anxiety and depression, pain, and decreased quality of life (Chen et al., 2014; Ferrie et al., 2011; McBeth et al., 2014; Schmid et al., 2014).

Insufficient sleep is a public health epidemic and the Centers for Disease Control and Prevention (CDC, 2014a) has called for continued public health surveillance of sleep quality, duration, behaviors, and disorders to monitor for sleep difficulties and their health impact. Sleep problems are more common in women and older adults (Stranges et al., 2012; World Association of Sleep Medicine, 2014). Because of the public health burden of chronic sleep loss and sleep disorders, and the low awareness of poor sleep health, *Healthy People 2020* includes sleep health as a special topic area. Goals for adults are presented in Box 13.1.

Biorhythm and Sleep

Our lives proceed in a series of rhythms that influence and regulate physiological function, chemical concentrations, performance, behavioral responses, moods, and the ability to adapt. Body temperature, pulse rate, blood pressure, and hormonal levels change significantly and predictably in a circadian rhythm. Circadian rhythms are linked to the 24-hour day by time cues (zeitgebers), the most important of which is the light-dark cycle. Biorhythms vary between individuals, and age-related changes in biorhythms (circadian rhythms) are relevant to health and the process of aging. With aging, there is a reduction in the amplitude of all circadian endogenous responses (e.g., body temperature, pulse rate, blood pressure, hormonal levels).

The most important biorhythm is the circadian sleep-wake rhythm. As people age, the natural circadian rhythm may become less responsive to external stimuli, such as changes in light during the course of the day. In addition, the endogenous changes in the production of melatonin are diminished, resulting in less sleep efficacy and further disruption of restorative sleep (Saccomano, 2014). Genetic research is investigating pathways linking sleep, circadian rhythm, metabolism, functioning, and disease, as well as genome-wide determinants of sleep duration (Ferrie et al., 2011).

Sleep and Aging

The predictable pattern of normal sleep is called sleep architecture. The body progresses through the stages of the normal sleep pattern consisting of rapid eye movement (REM) sleep and non–rapid eye movement (NREM) sleep. Most of the changes in sleep architecture in healthy adults begin between the ages of 40 and 60 years. Changes include less time spent in stages 3 and 4 sleep (slow-wave sleep) and more time spent awake or in stage 1 sleep. Time spent in REM sleep also declines with age, and transitions between stages 1 and 2 are more common.

The most notable changes in sleep with aging are an increase in the number of nighttime awakenings and lower sleep efficiency (ratio of time in bed asleep to time in bed) (Teodorescu, 2014) (Box 13.2). Sleep complaints are usually linked to other health problems and sleep

BOX 13.1 *Healthy People 2020*

Sleep Health

Goals:

- Increase public knowledge of how adequate sleep and treatment of sleep disorders improve health, productivity, wellness, quality of life, and safety on roads and in the workplace.
- Increase the proportion of persons with symptoms of obstructive sleep apnea who seek medical evaluation.
- Increase the proportion of adults who get sufficient sleep.

From U.S. Department of Health and Human Services, Office of Disease Prevention and Health Promotion: *Healthy People 2020*, 2012. Available at http://www.healthypeople.gov/2020.

BOX 13.2 Changes in Sleep With Age

- More time spent in bed awake before falling asleep
- Total sleep time and sleep efficiency are reduced
- Awakenings are frequent, increasing after age 50 years (>30 min of wakefulness after sleep onset in >50% of older subjects)
- Daytime napping
- Changes in circadian rhythm (early to bed, early to rise)
- Sleep is subjectively and objectively lighter (more stage 1, little stage 4, more disruptions)
- Rapid eye movement (REM) sleep is short, less intense, and more evenly distributed
- Frequency of abnormal breathing events is increased
- Frequency of leg movements during sleep is increased

Adapted from Teodorescu M, Husain N: Nonpharmacological approaches to insomnia in older adults, *Ann Longterm Care* 18:36–42, 2010.

disorders. Older adults with good general health, positive moods, and engagement in more active lifestyles and meaningful activities report better sleep and fewer sleep complaints.

SAFETY ALERT

Poor sleep is not an inevitable consequence of aging but rather an indicator of health status and necessitates investigation (Grandner et al., 2012).

Sleep Disorders

Insomnia

Insomnia is the most common sleep disorder worldwide (Ferrie et al., 2011; Sexton-Radek, 2013). Insomnia is "a condition that interferes with sleep quality and quantity and is associated with subjective complaints of sleep disturbance that are generally characterized as (a) difficulty initiating sleep, (b) difficulty maintaining sleep, (c) premature morning awakening, and/or (d) nonrestorative sleep" (Deratnay, 2013, p. 22). The diagnosis of insomnia requires that the person has difficulty falling asleep for at least 1 month and that impairment in daytime functioning results from difficulty sleeping.

According to epidemiological data, the prevalence of chronic late-life insomnia ranges from 20% to nearly 50%, and is generally higher in women than in men (Haimov & Shatil, 2013). Chronic insomnia is a significant risk factor for cognitive decline in men and a strong predictor of both mortality and long-term care placement (Teodorescu, 2014). There are many influencing factors, both physiological and behavioral (Box 13.3).

Prescription and nonprescription medications also create sleep disturbances. Drugs and alcohol are thought to account for 10% to 15% of cases of insomnia (Martin & Alessi, 2014) (Box 13.4). The times of day that medications are given can also contribute to sleep problems—for example, a diuretic given before bedtime or sedating medication given in the morning.

Insomnia and Alzheimer's disease. About half of individuals with dementia experience sleep dysregulation, which may be associated with agitation, wandering, comorbid illnesses, primary sleep disorders, or the medications used to treat dementia (Teodorescu, 2014). Some research suggests that sleep decline in aging may be the result of the deterioration of a cluster of neurons associated with regulating sleep patterns, the ventrolateral preoptic nucleus. The more neurons lost, the more difficult it is for the person to sleep. For individuals with Alzheimer's disease (AD), the link between the loss of neurons is greater and causes more problems with sleep (Lim et al., 2014). Caregivers of individuals with dementia also experience poor sleep quality, and this influences caregiver stress, as well as health problems (Rowe et al., 2010) (see Chapter 27). Behavioral techniques to enhance sleep for individuals with AD include sleep hygiene education, daily walking, and increased light exposure (McCurry et al., 2009).

BOX 13.3 Risk Factors for Sleep Disturbances in Older Adults

Internal
- Age-related changes in sleep architecture
- Chronic illness
- Sleep disorders (SDB, OSA, RL/WED, RBD, CRSD)
- Pain
- Worry, anxiety
- Depression, delirium, dementia, psychosis
- Sleep-related beliefs

External
- Medications
- Life stressors/response to stress
- Loss of spouse
- Relocation to new environment
- Sleep habits (daily sleep/activity cycle, napping)
- Poor sleep hygiene
- Lack of exercise
- Lack of socialization/stimulation
- Excessive napping
- Caregiving for a dependent elder
- Environmental noise, institutional routines
- Limited exposure to sunlight
- Alcohol
- Smoking

BOX 13.4 Medications Affecting Sleep

Selective serotonin reuptake inhibitors (SSRIs)
Antihypertensives (clonidine, beta blockers, reserpine, methyldopa)
Anticholinergics
Sympathomimetic amines
Diuretics
Opiates
Cough and cold medications
Thyroid preparations
Phenytoin
Cortisone
Levodopa

❖ IMPLICATIONS FOR GERONTOLOGICAL NURSING AND HEALTHY AGING

◆ Assessment

Sleep habits should be reviewed with older adults in all settings. Many people do not seek treatment for insomnia and may blame poor sleep on the aging process. Nurses are in an excellent position to assess sleep and suggest interventions to improve the quality of the older person's sleep. "No other group of health care providers watch more people sleep than nurses, and sleep disorders can affect all aspects of health and illness" (Chasens & Umlauf, 2012, p. 83).

Assessment for sleep disorders and awareness of contributing factors to poor sleep (pain, chronic illness, medications, alcohol use, depression, anxiety) are important. Assess for significant lifestyle changes such as loss of spouse and relocation, especially to long-term care where the individual may have to share a room. Loneliness and lack of affective touch and socialization can influence sleep as well. The nurse should learn how well the person sleeps at home, how many times the person is awakened at night, what time the person retires, and what rituals occur at bedtime. Rituals include eating bedtime snacks, watching television, listening to music, or reading—activities whose execution is crucial to the individual's ability to fall asleep.

The sleep diary or log is also an important part of assessment (Box 13.5). This information will provide an accurate account of the person's sleep problem and help identify the sleep disturbance. A period of 2 to 4 weeks is needed to obtain a clear picture of the sleep problem. A self-rating scale, the Pittsburgh Sleep Quality Index (PSQI), can be used to measure the quality and patterns of sleep in the older adult, and daytime sleepiness can be assessed with the Epworth Sleepiness Scale, both recommended by the Hartford Institute for Geriatric Nursing (Box 13.6). Objective measures include polysomnography conducted in sleep laboratories, including electroencephalograms (EEGs), electromyograms (EMGs), wrist actigraphy, and direct observations.

BOX 13.5 Sleep Diary

Instructions: Record the following for 2 to 4 weeks. Should be completed by the person or the caregiver if the person is unable. Record when you:

- Go to bed
- Go to sleep
- Wake up
- Get out of bed
- Take naps
- Exercise
- Consume alcohol
- Consume caffeinated beverages

From Centers for Disease Control and Prevention: *What should I do if I can't sleep?* 2013. Available at http://www.cdc.gov/sleep/about_sleep/cant_sleep.htm. Accessed November 2015.

◆ Interventions

◆ Nonpharmacological Treatment

Interventions begin after a thorough sleep history has been recorded and, if possible, a sleep log obtained. Management is directed at identifiable causes. Nonpharmacological interventions are considered first-line treatment for insomnia (Sexton-Radek, 2013). Education should be provided on changes in sleep architecture with aging and the importance of attention to sleep hygiene principles to promote good sleep habits.

Cognitive behavioral therapy for insomnia is a multidimensional approach combining psychological and behavioral therapies that include sleep hygiene, sleep restriction, stimulus control, relaxation techniques, circadian interventions, and cognitive therapy (Box 13.7). A combination of approaches is most effective and these interventions have been reported to be an effective and practical treatment for chronic insomnia in older adults (Buysse et al., 2011; Sexton-Radek, 2013; Teodorescu, 2014). Cognitive training programs (see Chapter 4) may improve sleep quality and cognitive performance (Haimov & Shatil, 2013).

BOX 13.6 Resources for Best Practice

Sleep

Chasen E, Umlauf M: Excessive sleepiness. In Boltz M, Capezuti E, Fulmer T, et al, editors: *Evidence-based geriatric nursing protocols for best practice,* ed 4, pp 74–88, New York, 2012, Springer.

Hartford Institute for Geriatric Nursing: *Try This:* General Assessment Series: Epworth Sleepiness Scale and Pittsburg Sleep Quality Index; Want to know more: Sleep: Nursing Standard Practice Protocol, Excessive Sleepiness.

Qaseem A, Owens D, Dallas P, et al: *Management of obstructive sleep apnea in adults: A clinical practice guideline from the American College of Physicians.* Available at http://www.hhs.gov. Accessed March 2014.

Willis-Ekbom Foundation: *Symptom diary.* Available at http://www.willis-ekbom.org/about-rls-wed/publications? Accessed March 2014.

BOX 13.7 Interventions for Insomnia

Sleep Hygiene

- Develop a regular physical exercise regimen for those who are able; regular exercise can deepen sleep, increase daytime arousal, and decrease depression.
- Avoid exercise before bedtime.
- Limit computer use before bedtime.
- Limit tobacco, caffeine, and alcohol use before bedtime.
- Avoid heavy meals before bedtime. If waking caused by hunger, eat light carbohydrate snack.
- If you have reflux, eat the evening meal 3–4 hours before bedtime.
- Reduce or eliminate fluids in the evening (reduce nocturia).
- Ensure bed and bed coverings are comfortable, not too restrictive.
- Keep bedroom temperature comfortable, not too warm and well ventilated.
- Minimize light exposure in bedroom.
- Remove hearing aids/use earplugs to reduce noise.
- Limit sleeping partner's disruptive nighttime activities and pets from bedroom.
- Review all medications with health care provider; evaluate administration times, review side effects/interactions/effect on sleep.

Relaxation Techniques

- Diaphragmatic breathing
- Progressive relaxation
- White noise or music
- Guided imagery
- Stretching
- Yoga or tai chi

Sleep Restriction Measures

- Limit or avoid daytime napping; napping should not exceed 2 hours.
- Limit opportunities for unplanned napping or dozing, particularly in the evening.
- Limit time in bed to more closely match the number of hours of actual sleep.

Stimulus Control

- Create bedtime sleep rituals, such as taking a warm bath and eating a small snack.
- Go to bed only when sleepy.
- Avoid falling asleep in places other than own bed (e.g., couch, recliner).
- If unable to fall asleep in a reasonable time (15–20 min), get out of bed and pursue relaxing activities (e.g., reading) and return to bed only when sleepy.
- Use the bedroom for sleep and sex only; do not watch television from bed or work in bed.

Circadian Interventions

- Reestablish connection with various environmental signals to cue the circadian rhythm (light exposure, meals, physical activity, social interactions).
- Establish a regular bedtime and waking time.
- Maintain stable daytime routines in regard to meals, activity, medications.
- Increase duration and intensity (2500–5000 lux) of bright light or sunlight exposure during the day. In patients with dementia, evening bright light may help with advanced sleep phase disorder.
- Melatonin 1–2 hours before bedtime may be helpful.

Adapted from Teodorescu M: Sleep disruptions and insomnia in older adults, *Consultant* 54(3):166–173, 2014; Saccomano S: Sleep disorders in older adults, *J Gerontol Nurs* 40(3):38–45, 2014.

Tai chi can be considered a useful nonpharmacological approach for sleep complaints (Lo & Lee, 2014; Raman et al., 2013). Aromatherapy has also been noted as beneficial in sleep promotion but further research is needed. Some individuals may be sensitive or allergic to essential oils that come into contact with the skin or are inhaled, particularly patients with pulmonary disease. Essential oils mentioned as beneficial in sleep promotion include true lavender, Roman chamomile, Clary sage, sandalwood, and rose. The person can place a cotton ball with a few drops of oil under the pillowcase when going to bed, pin a handkerchief with oil to the pajamas, drop oil in a diffuser, or add a few drops to a before-bedtime bath (Hwang & Shin, 2015; Welhbrecht, 2015).

◆ ***Sleep in hospitals and nursing homes.*** In hospital and institutional settings, promotion of a good sleep environment is important. Studies have shown that as many as 22% to 61% of hospitalized patients experience impaired sleep (Chasens & Umlauf, 2012). In addition to physical causes, noise, light, and staff interactions interfere with sleep. Sleep deprivation attributable to noise can potentially exacerbate delirium (see Chapter 23), and noise from monitoring equipment alarms and infusion devices and the ringing of telephones cause an elevation of heart rate (Buxton et al., 2012). The Joint

Commission (2013) has approved a National Patient Safety Goal (NPSG) to establish alarm safety and management of alarms as a critical access hospital priority. Efforts to allow sufficient time for a person to complete a full sleep cycle of 90 minutes are important and can have a positive influence on sleep effectiveness (Missildine, 2008; Missildine et al., 2010). This may mean limiting awakenings or routine rounds and scheduling necessary care when the patient is awake or has completed a full sleep cycle (Box 13.8).

◆ Pharmacological Treatment

The use of over-the-counter (OTC) sleep aids, as well as the use of prescription sedative and hypnotic medications, is increasing in the United States (Priedt, 2014). Use of narcotic pain medications and sedatives and the consumption of alcohol, in combination with these medications and other prescribed medications, is a growing concern (Substance Abuse and Mental Health Services Administration [SAMSHA], 2013) (see Chapter 24). Individuals who received prescriptions for narcotic painkillers were 4.2 times more likely to also have sedative prescriptions, which place them at high risk for adverse effects, including death (Kao et al., 2014). Patients should be educated on the proper use of medications, their side effects, and their interactions with alcohol and other prescription drugs.

Pharmacological treatments for sleep disorders may be used in combination with behavioral interventions but must be managed with caution in the older population (Teodorescu, 2014; Townsend-Roccichelli et al., 2010). Medications must be chosen carefully, started at the lowest possible dose, and monitored closely for untoward effects. Individuals should be educated on the proper use of medications and their side effects. Sedatives and hypnotics, including benzodiazepines and barbiturates, should be avoided. In long-term care settings, there are specific regulatory guidelines on the use of hypnotics, including appropriate prescribing and tapering and discontinuation of use.

BOX 13.8 Tips for Best Practice

Promoting Sleep in Health Care Facilities

- Allow individual to stay out of bed and out of the room for as long as possible before bedtime.
- Provide 30 minutes or more of sunlight exposure in a comfortable outdoor location.
- Provide low-level physical activity three times a day.
- Keep noise level at a minimum, speak in hushed tones, do no use overhead paging, reduce light in hallways and resident rooms.
- Institute a sleep improvement protocol—"do not disturb" times, soft music, relaxation, massage, aromatherapy, sleep masks, headphones, allowing patients to shut doors. Consider having a kit that can be taken to bedside with music, aromatherapy.
- Perform necessary care (e.g., turning, changing) when the individual is awake rather than awakening the individual between the hours of 10:00 PM and 6:00 AM.
- Limit intake of caffeine and other fluids in excess before bedtime.
- Provide a light snack or warm beverage before bedtime.
- Discontinue invasive treatments when possible (Foley catheters, percutaneous gastrostomy tubes, intravenous lines).
- Encourage and assist to the bathroom before bed and as needed.
- Give pain medication before bedtime for patients with pain.
- Institute the same time for resident to arise and get out of bed every morning.
- Maintain comfortable temperature in room; provide blankets as needed.
- Provide meaningful activities (individualized and group) during the daytime.

SAFETY ALERT

Benzodiazepines or other sedative-hypnotics should not be used in older adults as a first choice of treatment for insomnia (American Geriatrics Society, 2014).

Over-the-counter (OTC) drugs such as diphenhydramine are found in many OTC sleep products, such as Tylenol PM. These OTC medications are often thought to be relatively harmless but should be avoided because of antihistaminic and anticholinergic side effects. Other OTC sleep aid preparations contain ingredients such as kava kava, valerian root, melatonin, chamomile, and tryptophan. Because these ingredients are not regulated, information and outcomes of efficacy may not be known. Endogenous nocturnal melatonin, a major loop for circadian rhythm, may have decreased levels in older adults. Melatonin, available OTC, taken 1 to 2 hours before bedtime, may replicate the natural secretion pattern of melatonin and lead to improvements in the circadian regulation of the sleep-wake cycle (Teodorescu, 2014). Melatonin is also available in a dissolving tablet, which works faster.

Routine use of OTC medications for sleep may delay appropriate assessment and treatment of contributing medical or psychological conditions, identification of sleep disorders, and initiation of appropriate counseling and treatment. The individual should report use of all OTC drugs to his or her health care provider because they may interact with other medications.

Benzodiazepine receptor agonists, such as zolpidem (Ambien), eszopiclone (Lunesta), and zaleplon (Sonata), are considered benzodiazepine-like in their action because they induce sleep easily. They can have detrimental effects, causing changes in mental status (delirium), falls and fractures, daytime drowsiness, and increased risk for motor vehicle accidents, with only minimal improvement in sleep latency and duration (American Geriatrics Society, 2014). Doses of these medications should be cut in half for older adults and individuals should be cautioned about next-day impairment and monitored closely for untoward effects (FDA, 2013; Hampton et al., 2014).

SAFETY ALERT

Assessment of sleep problems should be conducted before medication use. Nonpharmacological interventions are first-line treatment. If sleeping medications are used, they should be taken immediately before bedtime because of their rapid action. Short-term use (2 to 3 weeks, never more than 90 days) is recommended.

Sleep Disordered Breathing and Sleep Apnea

Sleep disordered breathing (SDB) affects approximately 25% of older individuals (more men than women), and the most common form is obstructive sleep apnea (OSA). In long-term care facilities, the prevalence of OSA has been estimated to be as high as 70% to 80% (Rose & Lorenz, 2010). Age-related decline in the activity of the upper airway muscles, resulting in compromised pharyngeal patency, predisposes older adults to OSA. A high body mass index (BMI) and large neck circumference have been identified as risk factors for OSA but are not as significant in older adults (Martin & Alessi, 2014). Other risk factors are presented in Box 13.9.

The individual with sleep apnea stops breathing while asleep. Apneas (complete cessation of respiration) and hypopneas (partial decrease in respiration) result in hypoxemia and changes in autonomic nervous system activity. This results in increased systemic and pulmonary arterial pressures and changes in cerebral blood flow. The episodes are generally terminated by an arousal (brief awakening), which results in fragmented sleep and excessive daytime sleepiness. Other symptoms of sleep apnea include loud periodic snoring, gasping and choking on awakenings, unusual nighttime activity such as sitting upright or falling out of bed, morning headache, poor memory and intellectual functioning, and irritability and personality change. If the person has a sleeping partner, it is often the partner who reports the nighttime symptoms. If there is a sleeping partner, he or she may move to another room to sleep because of the disturbance to his or her own rest.

BOX 13.9 Risk Factors for Obstructive Sleep Apnea

- Increasing age
- Increased neck circumference (not as significant in older people)
- Male gender
- Anatomical abnormalities of the upper airway
- Upper airway resistance and/or obstruction
- Family history
- Excess weight
- Use of alcohol, sedatives, or tranquilizers
- Smoking
- Hypertension

❖ IMPLICATIONS FOR GERONTOLOGICAL NURSING AND HEALTHY AGING

◆ Assessment

The individual with SDB may present with complaints of insomnia or daytime sleepiness and assessment should include review of sleep complaints as discussed previously, including the use of screening instruments such as the Epworth Sleepiness Scale (Box 13.6). Assessment of symptoms of OSA and information from the sleeping partner, if present, are obtained. Recognition of OSA in older adults may be more difficult because there may not be a sleeping partner to report symptoms. If presenting symptoms suggest the disorder, a tape recorder can be placed at the bedside to record snoring and breathing sounds during the night.

A medication review is always indicated when investigating sleep complaints. The upper airway, including the nasal and pharyngeal airways, should be examined for anatomical obstruction, tumors, or cysts. Comorbid conditions such as heart failure and diabetes should be assessed and managed appropriately.

If OSA is suspected, a referral for a sleep study should be made. A sleep study or polysomnogram is a multiple-component test that electronically transmits and records specific physical activities during sleep. The data obtained are analyzed by a qualified physician to determine whether or not the person has a sleep disorder. In most cases, sleep studies take place in a sleep lab specially prepared for the test and are monitored by a technician, but they can also be conducted at home.

◆ Interventions

Therapy will depend on the severity and type of sleep apnea, as well as the presence of comorbid illnesses.

Treatment of sleep apnea may involve avoidance of alcohol and sedative-hypnotic medications, cessation of smoking, avoidance of supine sleep positions, and a reduction in body weight. The Clinical Practice Guidelines for Management of OSA recommends weight loss for obese individuals but should be combined with another treatment such as continuous positive airway pressure (CPAP) because of the low cure rate with weight loss alone (Qaseem et al., 2013). There should be risk counseling about impaired judgment from sleeplessness and the possibility of accidents when driving.

CPAP is recommended as initial therapy for OSA, with moderate-quality evidence (Qaseem et al., 2013). The CPAP device delivers pressurized air through tubing to a nasal mask or nasal pillows, which are fitted around the head. The pressurized air acts as an airway splint and gently opens the patient's throat and breathing passages, allowing the patient to breathe normally, but only through the nose. Teaching should be provided about the effects of untreated OSA and emphasize the need for treatment.

A stepwise approach during the initiation of therapy and continued monitoring can foster better use of CPAP or prevent discontinuation of therapy. Estimates are that about half of individuals either discontinue the therapy or are nonadherent (use of <4 hours per night) (Dettenmeier et al., 2013; Schwab et al., 2013; Weaver & Sawyer, 2010). Mandibular advancement devices may be used as an alternative treatment but these devices have elicited a weak recommendation with low-quality evidence (Qaseem et al., 2013). These appliances also require a stable dentition and may be problematic for individuals with dentures or extensive tooth loss (Chasens & Umlauf, 2012).

Restless Legs Syndrome/Willis-Ekbom Disease (RLS/WED)

Restless legs syndrome/Willis-Ekbom disease (RLS/WED) is a neurological movement disorder of the limbs that is often associated with a sleep complaint. Individuals with RLS/WED have an uncontrollable need to move the legs, often accompanied by discomfort in the legs. Other symptoms include paresthesias; creeping sensations; crawling sensations; tingling, cramping, and burning sensations; pain; or even indescribable sensations. RLS/WED has a circadian rhythm, with the intensity of the symptoms becoming worse at night and improving toward the morning. Symptoms may be temporarily relieved by movement.

In most cases, RLS/WED is a primary idiopathic disorder but it also can be associated with underlying medical disorders including iron deficiency, end-stage renal disease (especially in patients requiring dialysis), diabetes, and pregnancy. Antidepressants, antihypertensives, and neuroleptic medications can aggravate RLS/WED symptoms. Increased body mass index, caffeine use, alcohol or tobacco use, sleep deprivation, and sedentary lifestyle may also be contributing factors. Other contributing factors under study include iron metabolism and neurotransmitter dysfunctions involving dopamine and glutamate (National Institute of Neurological Disorders and Stroke [NINDS], 2010; Willis-Ekbom Disease Foundation, 2014).

Diagnosis of RLS/WED is based on symptoms and a sleep study may be indicated. Possible contributing conditions should be evaluated and all individuals with symptoms should be tested for iron deficiency with a complete iron panel (Tarsy, 2014). If iron stores are low, iron replacement is needed. Medication choice depends on the frequency of symptoms and the response to medication. Medications used include levodopa, benzodiazepines, or low-potency opioids. The chronic persistent form of the disorder may be treated with non-ergot dopamine agonists (pramipexole, ropinirole, rotigotine patch) or with gabapentin, gabapentin enacarbil, and pregabalin (Silber et al., 2013).

Nonpharmacological therapy includes stretching of the lower extremities, mild to moderate physical activity, hot baths, massage, acupressure, relaxation techniques, and avoidance of caffeine, alcohol, and tobacco. Individuals should be encouraged to keep a symptom diary for 7 to 14 days to identify triggers and aid in diagnosis (Box 13.6).

Rapid Eye Movement Sleep Behavior Disorder

The mean age at emergence of rapid eye movement sleep behavior disorder (RBD) is 60 years and it is more common in males. Characteristics are loss of normal voluntary muscle atonia during REM sleep associated with complex behavior while dreaming. Patients report elaborate enactment of their dreams, often with violent content, during sleep. This may include violent behaviors, such as punching and kicking, with the potential for injury of both the patient and the bed partner (National Sleep Foundation, 2014).

The chronic form is usually idiopathic or associated with Parkinson's disease and dementia with Lewy bodies. The acute form of the disorder can be caused by toxic-metabolic abnormalities, drug or alcohol withdrawal, and medications (tricyclic antidepressants, monoamine oxidase inhibitors, cholinergic agents, and selective serotonin reuptake inhibitors [SSRIs]). Diagnosis is based on history, symptoms, and a sleep study to test for the key features of the disorder. Clonazepam curtails or eliminates the disorder about 90% of the time. If clonazepam is not effective, some antidepressants or melatonin may reduce the behaviors. A safe environment in the bedroom should be provided (Martin &

Alessi, 2014; Murray et al., 2013; National Sleep Foundation, 2014).

Circadian Rhythm Sleep Disorders

In circadian rhythm sleep disorders (CRSDs) relatively normal sleep occurs at abnormal times. Two clinical presentations are seen: advanced sleep phase disorder (ASPD) and irregular sleep-wake disorder (ISWD). In ASPD, the individual begins and ends sleep at unusually early times (e.g., going to bed as early as 6 or 7 PM and waking up between 2 and 5 AM). Not all individuals with an advanced sleep phase have ASPD. If they are not bothered by their sleep phases and have no functional impairment, we may just consider them "morning" people. In irregular sleep-wake disorder, sleep is dispersed across the 24-hour day in bouts of irregular length. Factors contributing to these disorders are age-related changes in sleep and circadian rhythm regulation combined with decreased levels of light exposure and activity.

A combination of good sleep hygiene practices and methods to delay the timing of sleep and wake times is recommended as treatment for ASPD. Bright light therapy (2500 to 10,000 lux) for 1 to 2 hours at about 7 to 8 PM can help normalize or delay circadian rhythm patterns (Bloom et al., 2009).

In ISWD, the individual may obtain enough sleep over the 24-hour period, but time asleep is broken into at least three different periods of variable length. Erratic napping occurs during the day, and nighttime sleep is severely fragmented and shortened. Chronic insomnia and/or daytime sleepiness are present. ISWD is most commonly encountered in individuals with dementia, particularly those who are institutionalized. Sleep disturbances of individuals with dementia are often among the reasons for nursing home placement. Increasing exposure to bright light or sunlight during the day and evening bright light exposure may be helpful. For individuals with dementia, evening bright light may help with APSD. Structured activity during the day and a quiet sleeping environment may also improve the condition (Teodorescu, 2014).

ACTIVITY

Few factors contribute as much to health in aging as being physically active. The adage "Use it or lose it" certainly applies to muscles and physical fitness. Regular physical activity throughout life is essential for healthy aging. Physical activity enhances health and functional status while also decreasing the number of chronic illnesses and functional limitations often assumed to be a part of growing older. Physical activity is also a protective factor for depression (Lee et al., 2014) (Box 13.10). The frail health and loss of function we associate with aging are, in large part, due to physical inactivity.

> **BOX 13.10 Health Benefits of Physical Activity**
>
> - Reduced risk of hypertension, coronary artery disease, heart attack, stroke, diabetes, colon and breast cancers, metabolic syndrome, depression
> - Reduced adverse blood lipid profile
> - Prevention of weight gain
> - Improved cardiorespiratory and muscular fitness
> - Reduced risk of falls and hip fracture
> - Improved sleep quality
> - Improved bone and functional health
> - Decreased risk of early death (life expectancy increased even in persons who do not begin exercising regularly until age 75)
> - Improved functional independence
> - Improvement in walking speed, strength, functional ability of frail nursing home residents with diagnoses ranging from arthritis to lung disease and dementia

Physical activity is defined as any bodily movement produced by skeletal muscle that requires energy expenditure. This includes exercise and other activities such as playing, working, active transportation (walking, running, biking), household chores, and recreational activities. Exercise is a subcategory of physical fitness that is planned, structured, repetitive, and purposeful in the sense that improvement or maintenance of one or more components of physical fitness is the objective (World Health Organization [WHO], 2010).

Physical Activity and Aging

Despite a large body of evidence about the benefits of physical activity to maintain and improve function, more than 60% of American adults aged 50 and older fail to achieve the recommended activity levels. The levels of physical activity among older adults have not improved over the past decade in the United States. With advancing age (75 years and older), participation is even lower, with only 9% of men and 6% of women meeting the recommended guidelines (Taylor, 2014).

Older women are sedentary for approximately two-thirds of their waking hours (Shiroma et al., 2013). For women, patterns of physical activity have been reported to decline between ages 55 and 64, and again at age 75 and older (Fan et al., 2013). These may be prime times to enhance education on the benefits of physical activity for women as they age. There are a number of global and national guidelines for physical activity, although physical activity among older adults has attracted less

BOX 13.11 Resources for Best Practice

Physical Activity

Centers for Disease Control and Prevention: *Making physical activity a part of an older adult's life*—Includes exercise program information, videos, success stories, ways to overcome barriers (Growing Stronger Program and resources for strength training including pictures/videos).

EASY: *Exercise and Screening for You:* http://easyforyou.info/. Accessed April 2014.

National Center on Health, Physical Activity and Disability: *14 Weeks to a healthier you:* http://www.ncpad.org/14weeks. Accessed April 2104.

National Institute on Aging: *Exercise & physical activity: Your everyday guide from the National Institute on Aging.*

Resnick B: *Restorative care nursing for older adults: A guide for all settings,* ed 2, New York, 2011, Springer.

World Health Organization: *Global strategy on diet, physical activity and health: Global recommendations on physical activity for health,* Document 1.

BOX 13.12 *Healthy People 2020*

Physical Activity

- Reduce the proportion of adults who engage in no leisure-time physical activity.
- Increase the proportion of adults who engage in aerobic physical activity or at least moderate intensity for at least 150 minutes/week, or 75 minutes/week of vigorous intensity, or an equivalent combination.

From U.S. Department of Health and Human Services, Office of Disease Prevention and Health Promotion: *Healthy People 2020,* 2012. Available at http://www.healthypeople.gov/2020.

interest and research (Sun et al., 2013) (Box 13.11). Box 13.12 provides *Healthy People 2020* goals for physical activity.

Physical activity is important for all older people, not just active healthy elders. Even a small amount of time (at least 30 minutes of moderate activity several days a week) can improve health. Studies have found that increasing physical activity improves health outcomes in persons with chronic illnesses (regardless of severity) and in those with functional impairment. Strength training interventions seem most important for functional improvement, but further research is needed to determine the type of exercise necessary to maintain or improve functional ability in adults with disabilities and frail older adults (Taylor, 2014). Walking may be a particularly beneficial activity for frail elders.

❖ IMPLICATIONS FOR GERONTOLOGICAL NURSING AND HEALTHY AGING

◆ Assessment

Assessment of function and mobility is a component of a health assessment for older adults. Exercise counseling should be provided as a part of assessment. For individuals 65 years of age and older, if they are relatively fit and have no limiting health conditions, initiation of a moderate intensity exercise program is safe and does not require any type of cardiac screening. Individuals with specific health conditions, such as cardiovascular disease and diabetes, may need to take extra precautions and seek medical advice before beginning an exercise program (CDC, 2014b). Frail individuals will need more comprehensive assessment to adapt exercise recommendations to their abilities and ensure benefit without compromising safety.

◆ Screening

The Exercise and Screening for You (EASY) (Box 13.11) tool is a screening tool that can be used to determine a safe exercise program for older adults on the basis of underlying physical problems. EASY is an interactive web-based tool that can be completed by the individual or the health care provider. The tool also provides suggestions for the types of exercises that are appropriate for individuals with underlying health concerns. Resources are provided on types of exercise and programs that have all been reviewed and endorsed by national organizations such as the National Institute on Aging (Bethesda, MD) and can be printed and given to the person.

◆ Interventions

The nurse should be knowledgeable about recommended physical activity guidelines, educate individuals about the importance of exercise and physical activity, and provide suggestions on ways to incorporate exercise into daily routines (CDC, 2014b). Many older people mistakenly believe that they are too old to begin a fitness program. Research has noted that health care providers value the benefits of physical activity but have inadequate knowledge of specific recommendations. Giving specific advice about the type and frequency of exercise is important (CDC, 2014b; Taylor, 2014). Nurses can also design and lead exercise and physical activity programs for groups of older adults in the community or in long-term care (see Box 13.11).

BOX 13.13 Exercise Guidelines

Older adults need at least:

- 2 hours and 30 minutes (150 minutes) of moderate-intensity aerobic activity (e.g., brisk walking, swimming, bicycling) every week ***and***
- Muscle-strengthening activities on 2 or more days that work all major muscle groups (legs, hips, abdomen, chest, shoulders, and arms)

Additionally: Stretching (flexibility) and balance exercises (particularly for older people at risk of falls) are also recommended. Yoga and tai chi exercises have been shown to be of benefit to older people in terms of improving flexibility and balance, as well as reducing pain and enhancing psychological well-being (Miller and Taylor-Piliae, 2014). Tai chi can be adapted for level of function and mobility status. Home-based balance-training exercise programs are also available.

From Centers for Disease Control and Prevention: *How much physical activity do older adults need?* 2014. Available at http://www.cdc.gov/physicalactivity/everyone/guidelines/olderadults.html. Accessed April 2014.

◆ Physical Activity Guidelines

Guidelines for physical activity for adults 65 years of age or older who are generally fit and have no limiting health conditions are presented in Box 13.13. Recommendations for all adults include participation in 30 minutes of moderate-intensity physical activity for 5 or more days of the week. People do not have to be active for 30 minutes at a time but can accumulate 30 minutes over 24 hours. As little as 10 minutes of exercise has health benefits and three 10-minute bouts of activity have the same fitness effects as one 30-minute bout. Extremely frail individuals may not be able to engage in aerobic activities and should begin with strength and balance training before participating in as little as 5 minutes of aerobic training.

◆ Incorporating Physical Activity Into Lifestyle

One does not have to invest in expensive gym equipment or gym memberships to incorporate the recommended physical activity guidelines into his or her daily routine. Hand weights (or use cans of food as weights), a chair, and an exercise mat can easily get the individual started (Fig. 13.1). The benefits of group exercise in terms of social and emotional health have been reported, and the socialization provided may be important for individuals who live alone or do not have social networks. Adhering to a program of physical activity can be problematic for some individuals. Adherence may be improved if the individual can integrate activity into daily life rather than doing a specific exercise. Examples include walking, golfing, tennis, biking, raking leaves, yard work/gardening, dancing, washing windows or floors, washing and waxing the car, and swimming and water-based exercises. If the individual is engaging in activities he or she enjoys, adherence is improved (Miranda et al., 2014). Swimming is a low-risk activity that provides aerobic benefit, and water-based exercises are particularly beneficial for individuals with arthritis or other mobility limitations.

Many senior living communities, as well as assisted living facilities (ALFs) and skilled nursing facilities (SNFs), provide gym equipment for residents. The SilverSneakers program, the nation's leading exercise program for active community-dwelling older adults, is a membership benefit through some of the Medicare health plans. Local community centers often provide exercise programs for older adults, and many gyms in the United States have reduced-cost memberships for individuals older than age 65. Some have trainers on staff with expertise in exercises appropriate for older individuals. The nurse can share resources in the community, and communities should be encouraged to provide accessible and affordable options for physical activity.

◆ Special Considerations

The benefits of physical activity extend to the more physically frail older adult, those who are nonambulatory or experience cognitive impairment, and those residing in ALFs or SNFs. In fact, these individuals may benefit most from an exercise program in terms of function and quality of life (Resnick et al., 2006). There are many creative and enjoyable ideas for enhancing physical activity such as using lower extremity cycling equipment, marching in place, tossing a ball, stretching, performing range-of-motion exercises, using resistive bands (Chen et al., 2013), and doing chair yoga. The Wii game system offers other possibilities for exercise at all levels and is increasingly being used by older people in their own homes and in senior living residences to encourage physical activity, improve balance, and provide enjoyable entertainment (Bieryla & Dold, 2013; Chao et al., 2013).

Results of research suggest that older adults with cognitive impairment who participate in exercise programs may improve strength and endurance, cognitive function, and ability to perform activities of daily living (Forbes et al., 2013; Schwenk et al., 2014; Taylor, 2014). A growing body of research suggests that exercise programs are likely to be more successful if they are individualized, are enjoyable, and involve caregivers (Yao et al., 2013). Strength-training interventions and one-component exercises seem to be more effective in

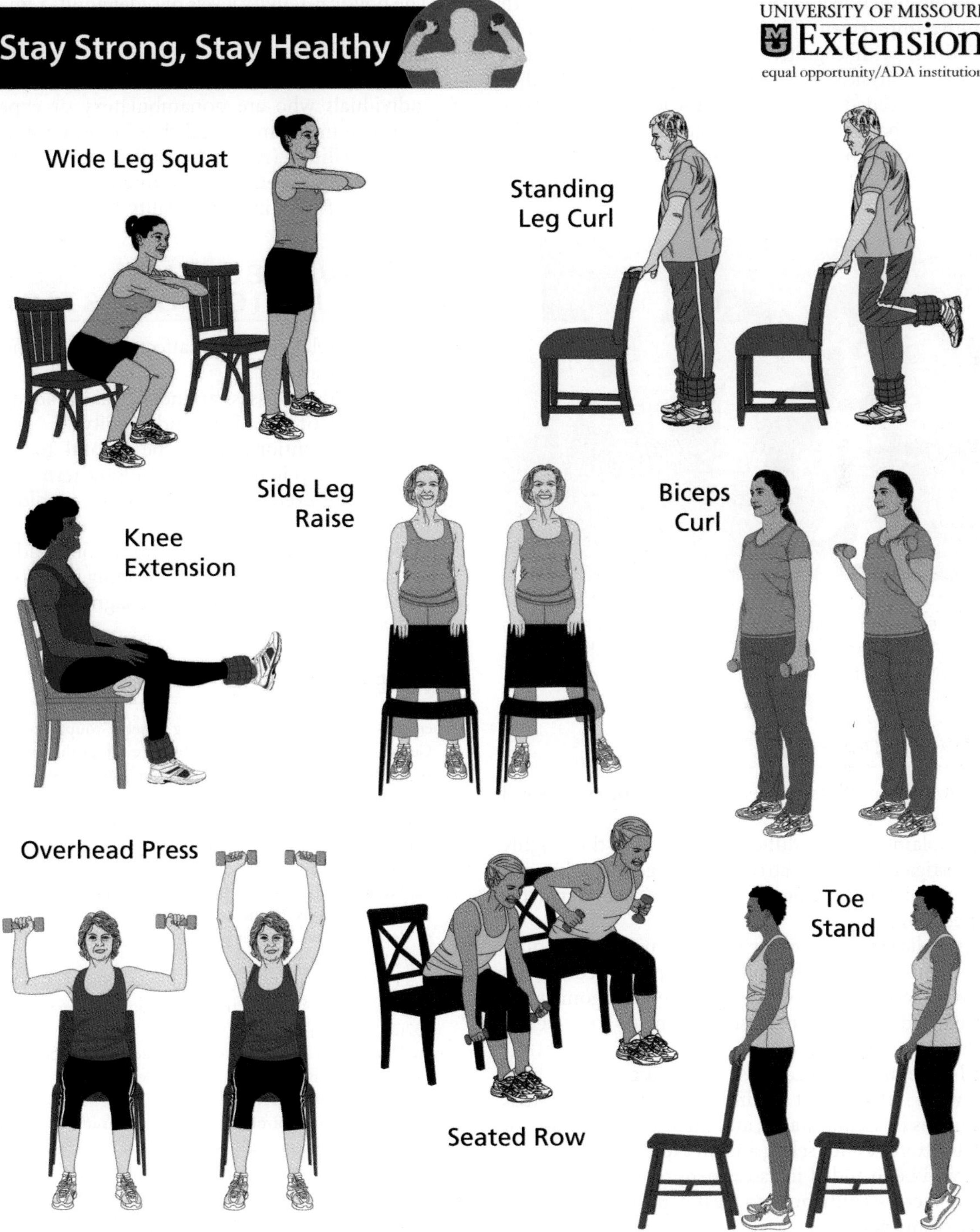

FIGURE 13.1 Stay Strong, Stay Healthy. (Adapted from The Strong Women Program, A National Fitness Program for Women, John Hancock Center for Physical Activity and Nutrition, Friedman School of Nutrition Science and Policy, © 2008 Tufts University, Boston, Massachusetts. Illustrations by J. Bintzer, University of Missouri Extension.)

increasing functional improvement in individuals with cognitive impairment (Taylor, 2014; Tseng et al., 2011). Individuals with cognitive impairment are often not included in physical activity programs. Although further research is needed to understand the level and intensity of exercise that is beneficial for each type of dementia, exercise should be a component of the plan of care (Forbes et al., 2013).

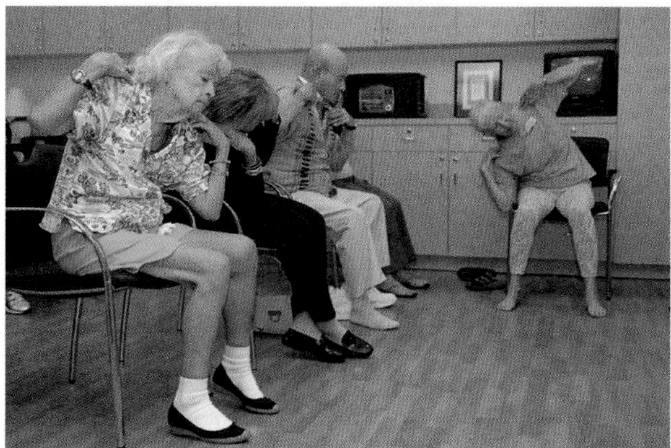

Age is not a barrier to fitness and exercise. 95-year-old Vera Paley leads yoga class. (Courtesy Louis and Anne Green Memory and Wellness Center of the Christine E. Lynn College of Nursing at Florida Atlantic University.)

KEY CONCEPTS

- Sleep is a barometer of health and can be considered one of the vital signs.
- Complaints of sleep difficulties should be thoroughly investigated and not attributed to age. Nonpharmacological interventions are first-line treatments for sleep problems.
- Benzodiazepines or other sedative-hypnotics should not be used in older adults. If sleeping medications are prescribed, benzodiazepine receptor agonists are preferred and used only short-term (2 to 3 weeks, never more than 90 days).
- All sleeping medications, including OTC, have adverse effects that include daytime drowsiness, changes in mental status, and increased likelihood of falls. Exercise counseling and an exercise prescription should be included in assessment of all older adults.
- Few factors contribute to health in aging as being physically active.
- Physical activity enhances health and functional status while also decreasing the number of chronic illnesses and functional limitations often assumed to be part of growing older.
- The physical activity levels of older adults remain low and have not improved over the past decade.
- Exercise counseling should be provided as part of the assessment of the older individual.
- Individuals who are nonambulatory or experience cognitive impairment and those residing in assisted living facilities (ALFs) or skilled nursing facilities (SNFs) may benefit most from an exercise program in terms of function and quality of life.

ACTIVITIES AND DISCUSSION QUESTIONS

1. What age-related changes affect rest, sleep, and activity in older adults?
2. How would you assess an individual for adequacy or inadequacy of rest, sleep, and activity?
3. What interventions would be helpful to promote adequate sleep in acute care? In long-term care?
4. Develop an exercise prescription for an older adult residing in the community.
5. Develop a nursing care plan for an older adult who is complaining of difficulty sleeping using wellness and North American Nursing Diagnosis Association (NANDA) diagnoses.

REFERENCES

American Geriatrics Society Choosing Wisely Group: American Geriatrics Society identifies another five things that healthcare providers and patients should question, *J Am Geriatr Soc* 62(5):950–960, 2014.

Bieryla K, Dold N: Feasibility of Wii Fit training to improve clinical measures of balance in older adults, *Clin Interv Aging* 8:775–781, 2013.

Bloom H, Ahmed I, Alessi C, et al: Evidence-based recommendations for the assessment and management of sleep disorders in older persons, *J Am Geriatr Soc* 57:761, 2009.

Buxton O, Ellenbogen J, Wang W, et al: Sleep disturbances due to hospital noises: A prospective evaluation, *Ann Intern Med* 157(3):170–179, 2012.

Buysse D, Germain A, Moul D, et al: Efficacy of brief behavioral treatment for chronic insomnia in older adults, *Arch Intern Med* 171(10):887–895, 2011.

Centers for Disease Control and Prevention: *Insufficient sleep is a public health epidemic*, 2014a. Available at http://www.cdc.gov/features/dssleep. Accessed November 2015.

Centers for Disease Control and Prevention: *How much physical activity do older adults need?* 2014b. Available at http://www.cdc.gov/physicalactivity/everyone/guidelines/olderadults.html. Accessed November 2015.

Chao Y, Scherer Y, Wu Y, et al: The feasibility of an intervention combining self-efficacy theory and Wii Fit exergames in assisted living residents: A pilot study, *Geriatr Nurs* 34(5):377–382, 2013.

Chasens E, Umlauf M: Excessive sleepiness. In Boltz M, Capezuti E, Fulmer T, et al, editors: *Evidence-based geriatric nursing protocols for best practice*, ed 4, New York, 2012, Springer, pp 74–88.

Chen K, Tseng WS, Chang YH, et al: Feasibility appraisal of an elastic band exercise program for older adults in wheelchairs, *Geriatr Nurs* 34(5):373–376, 2013.

Chen Y, Weng S, Shen Y, et al: Obstructive sleep apnea and risk of osteoporosis: A population-based cohort study in Taiwan, *J Clin Endocrinol Metab* 99(7):2441–2447, 2014.

Deratnay P: The effect of insomnia on functional status of community-dwelling older adults, *J Gerontol Nurs* 39(10):22–30, 2013.

Dettenmeier P, Ordoz E, Espiritu J: Evaluation of a continuous positive airway pressure desensitization protocol for CPAP-intolerant patients: A pilot study, *Chest* 144:979A, 2013.

Fan J, Kowaleski-Jones L, Wen M: Walking or dancing: Patterns of physical activity by cross-sectional age among U.S. women, *J Aging Health* 25:1182–1203, 2013.

Federal Drug Administration: *FDA safety communication: FDA approves new label changes and dosing for zolpidem products and a recommendation to avoid driving the day after using Ambien CR*, 2013. Available at http://www.fda.gov/drugs/drugsafety/ucm352085.htm. Accessed August 21, 2016.

Ferrie J, Kumari M, Salo P, et al: Sleep epidemiology—A rapidly growing field, *Int J Epidemiol* 40:1431–1437, 2011.

Forbes D, Thiessen EJ, Blake CM, et al: Exercise programs for people with dementia, *Cochrane Database Syst Rev* (12):CD006489, 2013. doi: 10.1002/14651858.CD006489.pub3.

Grandner M, Martin J, Patel N, et al: Age and sleep disturbances among American men and women: Data from the U.S. behavioral risk factor surveillance system, *Sleep* 35(3):396–406, 2012. http://doi.org/10.5665/sleep.1704.

Haimov I, Shatil E: Cognitive training improves sleep quality and cognitive function among older adults with insomnia, *PLoS ONE* 8(4):e61390, 2013. doi: 10.1371/journalpone.0061390.

Hampton L, Daubresse M, Chang H-Y, et al: Emergency department visits by adults for psychiatric medication adverse effects, *JAMA Psychiatry* 79(9):1006–1014, 2014. doi: 10.1001/jamapsychiatry.2014.436.

Hwang E, Shin S: The effects of aromatherapy on sleep improvement: A systematic literature review and meta-analysis, *J Altern Complement Med* 00(0):1–8, 2015.

Kao M-C, Zheng P, Mackey S: *Trends in benzodiazepine prescription and co-prescription with opioids in the United States, 2002–2009*, 2014. Available at http://www.painmed.org/2014posters/abstract-109. Accessed November 2015.

Lee H, Lee K, Brar J, et al: Physical activity and depressive symptoms in older adults, *Geriatr Nurs* 35(1):37–41, 2014.

Lim A, Ellison B, Wang J, et al: Sleep is related to neuron numbers in the ventrolateral preoptic/intermediate nucleus in older adults with and without Alzheimer's disease, *Brain* 137:2847–2861, 2014. doi: 10.1093/brain/awu222.

Lo C, Lee P: Feasibility and effects of TAI CHI for the promotion of sleep quality and quality of life: A single-group study in a sample of older Chinese individuals in Hong Kong, *J Gerontol Nurs* 49(3):46–52, 2014.

Martin J, Alessi C: Sleep disorders. In Ham R, Sloane P, Warshaw G, et al, editors: *Primary care geriatrics*, ed 6, Philadelphia, 2014, Elsevier, pp 343–352.

McBeth J, Lacey R, Wilkie R: Predictors of new-onset widespread pain in older adults: Results from a population-based prospective cohort study in the UK, *Arthritis Rheumatol* 66(3):757–767, 2014.

McCurry S, LaFazia D, Pike K, et al: Managing sleep disturbances in adult family homes: Recruitment and implementation of a behavioral treatment program, *Geriatr Nurs* 30:36–44, 2009.

Miller S, Taylor-Piliae R: Effects of Tai Chi on cognitive function in community-dwelling older adults, *Geriatr Nurs* 35:9–19, 2014.

Miranda A, Picorelli A, Pereira D, et al: Adherence of older women with strength training and aerobic exercise, *Clin Interv Aging* 9:323–331, 2014.

Missildine K: Sleep and the sleep environment of older adults in acute care settings, *J Gerontol Nurs* 34(6):15–21, 2008.

Missildine K, Bergstrom N, Meininger J, et al: Sleep in hospitalized elders: A pilot study, *Geriatr Nurs* 31:263–271, 2010.

Murray M, Ferman T, Boeve B, et al: *REM sleep behavior disorder is associated with reduced Alzheimer's pathology, hippocampal and parietotemporal atrophy in dementia with Lewy bodies* (Abstract no. S44.006), Program and Abstracts of the American Academy of Neurology 65th Annual Meeting, March 16–23, 2013, San Diego, CA.

National Institute of Neurological Disorders and Stroke: *Restless legs syndrome (Fact sheet)*, 2010. Available at http://www.ninds.nih.gov/disorders/restless_legs/detail_restless_legs.htm. Accessed November 2015.

National Sleep Foundation: *REM behavior disorder and sleep*, 2014. Available at http://sleepfoundation.org/sleep-disorders-problems/abnormal-sleep-behaviors/rem-behavior-disorder/page/0%2C3. Accessed November 2015.

Priedt R: *Study finds doctors prescribing more sedatives, Medline Plus*, 2014. Available at http://www.nlm.nih.giv/medlineplus/news/fullstory_144996.html. Accessed March 2014.

Qaseem A, Holty J-E, Owens D, et al: Management of obstructive sleep apnea in adults: A clinical practice guidelines from the American College of Physicians, *Ann Intern Med* 159:471–483, 2013.

Raman G, Zhang Y, Minichiello V, et al: Tai Chi improves sleep quality in healthy adults and patients with chronic conditions: A systematic review and meta-analysis, *J Sleep Disord Ther* 2(6):141, 2013. Available at http://www.omicsgroup.org/journals/tai-chi-improves-sleep-quality-in-healthy-adults-and-patients-with-chronic-conditions-a-systematic-review-and-metaanalysis-2167-0277-2-141.pdf. Accessed November 2015.

Resnick B, Ory M, Rogers M, et al: Screening for and prescribing exercise for older adults, *Geriatr Aging* 9:174–182, 2006.

Rose K, Lorenz R: Sleep disturbances in dementia: What they are and what to do, *J Gerontol Nurs* 36:9–14, 2010.

Rowe M, Kairalla J, McCrae C: Sleep in dementia caregivers and the effects of a nighttime monitoring system, *J Nurs Scholarsh* 42:338–347, 2010.

Saccomano S: Sleep disorders in older adults, *J Gerontol Nurs* 40(3):38–45, 2014.

Schmid S, Hallschmid M, Schultes B: The metabolic burden of sleep loss, *Lancet Diabetes Endocrinol* 2014. doi: 10.1016/S2213-8587(14)70012-9. [Epub ahead of print].

Schwab R, Badr S, Epstein L, et al: An official American Thoracic Society statement: Continuous positive airway pressure adherence tracking systems, *Am J Respir Crit Care Med* 184(5):613–620, 2013.

Schwenk M, Dutzi I, Englert S, et al: An intensive exercise program improves motor performance in patients with dementia: Translational model of geriatric rehabilitation, *J Alzheimers Dis* 39(3):487–498, 2014.

Sexton-Radek K: A look at worldwide sleep disturbance, *J Sleep Disord Ther* 2:115, 2013.

Shiroma E, Freedson P, Stewart G, et al: Patterns of acceleromotor-assessed sedentary behavior in older women, *JAMA* 310(23):2562–2563, 2013.

Silber M, Becker P, Earley C, et al: Willis-Ekbom Disease Foundation revised consensus statement on the management of restless legs syndrome, *Mayo Clin Proc* 88(9):977–986, 2013.

Stranges S, Tigbe W, Gomez-Olive F, et al: Sleep problems: An emerging global epidemic? Findings from the INDEPTH WHO-SAGE study among more than 40,000 older adults from 8 countries across Africa and Asia, *Sleep* 35(8):1173–1181, 2012.

Substance Abuse and Mental Health Services Administration: *Emergency department visits for adverse reactions involving the insomnia medication zolpidem, The Dawn Report*, May 1, 2013. Available at http://www.samhsa.gov/data/2k13/DAWN079/sr079-Zolpidem.htm. Accessed November 2015.

Sun F, Norman I, White A: Physical activity in older people: A systematic review, *BMC Public Health* 13:449, 2013.

Tarsy D: Clinical manifestation and diagnosis of restless legs syndrome in adults, *UpToDate* 2014.

Taylor D: Physical activity is medicine for older adults, *Postgrad Med J* 90:26–32, 2014.

Teodorescu M: Sleep disruptions and insomnia in older adults, *Consultant* 54(3):166–173, 2014.

The Joint Commission: *Joint Commission perspectives: National patient safety goal on alarm management* 33(7), July 2013.

Townsend-Roccichelli J, Sanford J, VandeWaa E: Managing sleep disorders in the elderly, *Nurse Pract* 35(5):31–37, 2010.

Tseng C, Gau B, Lou M: The effectiveness of exercise on improving cognition functions in older people: A systematic review, *J Nurs Res* 19(2):119–131, 2011.

Weaver T, Sawyer A: Adherence to continuous positive airway pressure treatment for obstructive sleep apnea, *Indian J Med Res* 131:245–258, 2010.

Welhbrecht L: Clinical aromatherapy, *Today's Geriatr Med* 7(4): 30, 2015.

Willis-Ekbom Disease Foundation: *What is WED/RLS?* 2014. Available at http://www.willis-ekbom.org/about-wed-rls. Accessed November 2015.

World Association of Sleep Medicine: *World Sleep Day*, 2014. Available at http://worldsleepday.org. Accessed November 2015.

World Health Organization: *Global recommendations on physical activity for health*, 2010. http://www.who.int/dietphysicalactivity/publications/9789241599979/en. http://www.who.int.or. Accessed April 2014.

Xie L, Kang H, Xu Q, et al: Sleep drives metabolite clearance from the adult brain, *Science* 342(6156):373–377, 2013.

Yao L, Giordani B, Algase D, et al: Fall risk-relevant functional mobility outcomes in dementia following dyadic Tai Chi exercise, *West J Nurs Res* 35(3):281–296, 2013.

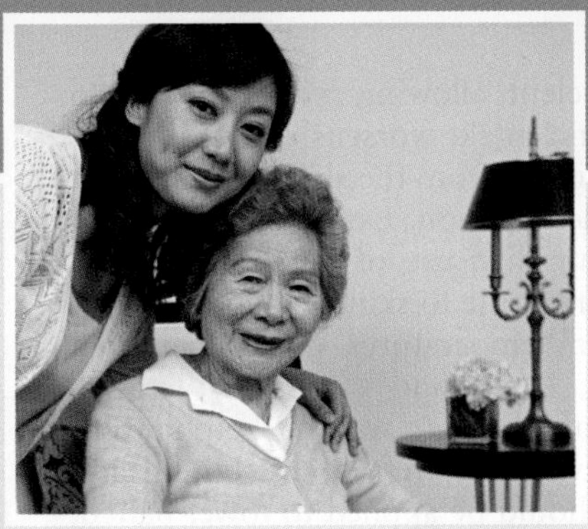

14

Promoting Healthy Skin

Theris A. Touhy

evolve.elsevier.com/Touhy/gerontological

LEARNING OBJECTIVES

Upon completion of this chapter, the reader will be able to:

- Identify skin conditions commonly found in later life.
- Identify preventive, maintenance, and restorative measures for skin health.
- Identify risk factors for pressure injuries and describe evidence-based interventions for prevention and treatment.

THE LIVED EXPERIENCE

An elderly woman and her little grandson, whose face was sprinkled with bright freckles, spent the day at the zoo. Lots of children were waiting in line to get their cheeks painted by a local artist who was decorating them with tiger paws.

"You've got so many freckles, there's no place to paint!" a girl in the line said to the little fellow.

Embarrassed, the little boy dropped his head. His grandmother knelt down next to him.

"I love your freckles. When I was a little girl I always wanted freckles," she said, while tracing her finger across the child's cheek. "Freckles are beautiful."

The boy looked up, "Really?"

"Of course," said the grandmother. "Why just name me one thing that's prettier than freckles?"

The little boy thought for a moment, peered intensely into his grandma's face, and softly whispered, "Wrinkles."

Anonymous

Gerontological nurses have an instrumental role in promoting the health of the skin of individuals who seek their care. Care of the skin may be often overlooked when the focus is on management of chronic illness or acute problems. However, skin conditions can be challenging concerns, affecting health and compromising quality of life. Thorough assessment and intervention based on age-related evidence-based protocols is important to healthy aging and best practice gerontological nursing.

SKIN

The skin is the largest organ of the body. Exposure to heat, cold, water, trauma, friction, and pressure notwithstanding, the skin's function is to maintain a homeostatic environment. Healthy skin is durable, pliable, and strong enough to protect the body by absorbing, reflecting, cushioning, and restricting various substances and forces that might enter and alter its function; yet it is sensitive enough to relay subtle messages to the brain. When the integument malfunctions or is overwhelmed, discomfort, disfigurement, or death may ensue. However, the nurse can both promptly recognize and help to prevent many of the sources of danger to a person's skin in the promotion of the best possible health.

Many age-related changes in the skin are visible; similar changes in other organs of the body are not so readily observed. Although there are some changes related to the aging process (see Chapter 3), genetics and environmental factors (ultraviolet [UV] radiation, tobacco smoke, inflammatory responses, and gravity) contribute to these changes (McCance & Huether, 2014). The most common skin problems of aging are xerosis (dry skin), pruritus, seborrheic keratosis, herpes zoster, and cancer. Those who are immobilized or medically fragile are at risk for fungal infections and pressure injuries, both major threats to wellness.

COMMON SKIN PROBLEMS

Xerosis

Xerosis is extremely dry, cracked, and itchy skin. Xerosis is the most common skin problem experienced and may be linked to a dramatic age-associated decrease in the amount of epidermal filaggrin, a protein required for binding keratin filaments into macrofibrils. This leads to separation of dermal and epidermal surfaces, which compromises the nutrient transfer between the two layers of the skin. Xerosis occurs primarily in the extremities, especially the legs, but can affect the face and the trunk as well. The thinner epidermis of older skin makes it less efficient, allowing more moisture to escape. Inadequate fluid intake worsens xerosis because the body will pull moisture from the skin in an attempt to combat systemic dehydration. Exposure to artificial heat or decreased humidity, use of harsh soaps, and frequent hot baths contribute to skin dryness.

Using tepid water temperatures and superfatted soaps (e.g., Cetaphil, Dove, and Caress; or Jergens, Neutrogena, and Oil of Olay bath washes) help prevent the loss of the protective lipid film from the skin surface. Lotions and creams should be applied to towel-patted, damp skin immediately after showering or bathing.

Pruritus

One of the consequences of xerosis is *pruritus,* that is, itchy skin. It is a symptom, not a diagnosis or disease, and is a threat to skin integrity because of the attempts to relieve it by scratching. It is aggravated by perfumed detergents, fabric softeners, heat, sudden temperature changes, pressure, vibration, electrical stimuli, sweating, restrictive clothing, fatigue, exercise, and anxiety. Medication side effects are another common cause of pruritus. Pruritus also may accompany systemic disorders such as chronic renal failure and biliary or hepatic disease. Subacute to chronic, generalized pruritus that awakens the individual is an indication to look for secondary causes (especially lymphoma or hematological conditions) (Endo & Norman, 2014).

The gerontological nurse should always listen carefully to the patient's ideas of why the pruritus is occurring, as well as the patient's description of aggravating and relieving factors. If rehydration of the stratum corneum (outer layer of the skin) and other measures to prevent and treat xerosis are not sufficient to control itching, cool compresses or oatmeal or Epsom salt baths may be helpful. Failure to control the itching increases the risk for eczema, excoriations, cracks in the skin, inflammation, and infection arising from the usually linear excoriations resulting from scratching. The nurse should be alert to signs of infection.

Scabies

Scabies is a skin condition that causes intense itching, particularly at night. Scabies is caused by a tiny burrowing mite called *Sarcoptes scabiei.* Scabies is contagious and can be passed easily by an infested person to his or her household members, caregivers, or sexual partners. Scabies can spread easily through close physical contact in a family, childcare group, or school class. Scabies outbreaks have occurred among patients, visitors, and staff in institutions such as nursing homes and hospitals. These types of outbreaks are frequently the result of delayed diagnosis and treatment of crusted (Norwegian) scabies. Some immunocompromised, disabled, or debilitated persons are at risk for this form of scabies.

In addition, individuals with crusted scabies have thick crusts of skin that contain large numbers of scabies mites and eggs. In addition to spreading through skin-to-skin contact, crusted scabies can transmit indirectly through contamination of clothing, linen, and furniture. Because the characteristic itching and rash of scabies can be absent in crusted scabies, there may be misdiagnosis and delayed or inadequate treatment and continued transmission. To diagnose scabies, a close skin examination is conducted to look for signs of mites, including their characteristic burrows. A scraping may be taken from an area of skin for microscopic examination to determine the presence of mites or their eggs.

Scabies treatment involves eliminating the infestation with prescribed lotions and creams. Two or more applications, about 1 week apart, may be necessary, especially for crusted scabies. Treatment is usually provided to family members and other close contacts even if they show no signs of scabies infestation. Medication kills the mites, but itching may not stop for several weeks. Oral medications may be prescribed for individuals with altered immune systems, for those with crusted scabies, or for those who do not respond to prescription lotions and creams. All clothes and linen used at least three times before treatment should be washed in hot, soapy water and dried with high heat. Rooms used by the person with crusted scabies should be thoroughly cleaned and vacuumed (Centers for Disease Control and Prevention [CDC], 2010).

Purpura

Thinning of the dermis leads to increased fragility of the dermal capillaries and to easy rupture of blood vessels with minimal trauma. Extravasation of the blood into the surrounding tissue, commonly seen on the dorsal forearm and hands, is called *purpura*. Most cases are not related to a pathological condition. The incidence of purpura increases with age because of the normal changes in the skin. Persons who take blood thinners are especially prone to easily acquiring purpura. For those who find that they are prone to purpura, it is advisable to use protective garments—such as long-sleeved pants and shirts. Health care personnel must be advised to be gentle while providing care to persons with sensitive or easily traumatized skin.

Skin Tears

Skin tears occur commonly in persons with thin and fragile skin, and they occur to persons in all settings, from persons in long-term care to active persons in the community. They are painful, acute, accidental wounds, perhaps more prevalent than pressure injuries, and are largely preventable. The top causes of skin tears are equipment injury, patient transfers, activities of daily living, and treatment and dressing removal. Care must be taken with patient transfers; bed rails, wheelchair arms, leg supports, and furniture edges can be padded; and at-risk individuals should wear long sleeves or pants to protect extremities. Avoid adhesive products and use nonadherent dressings and paper tape only as needed. Education on prevention and management of skin tears should be provided to patients and staff.

Skin tears should be classified using the Payne-Martin classification system: category 1—a skin tear without tissue loss; category 2—a skin tear with partial tissue loss; and category 3—a skin tear with complete tissue loss where the epidermal flap is absent (Ayello & Sibbald, 2012). Management of skin tears includes proper assessment of skin tear category, control of bleeding, cleansing with nontoxic solutions (normal saline or nonionic surfactant cleaners) at safe pressures, use of appropriate dressings that provide moist wound healing, protection of periwound skin, management of exudate, prevention of infection, and implementation of prevention protocols and education. Skin flaps, if present, should not be removed but instead rolled back over the open, cleaned area. Steri-Strips can be very useful; suturing is not recommended. Dressing recommendations can be found in the Skin Tear Tool Kit (LeBlanc & Baranoski, 2013) or online at http://www.skintears.org (Box 14.1).

Keratoses

There are two types of keratosis: seborrheic and actinic. *Actinic keratosis* is a precancerous lesion, and *seborrheic keratosis* is a benign growth that appears mainly on the trunk, the face, the neck, and the scalp as single or multiple lesions. One or more lesions are present on nearly all adults older than 65 years and are more common in men. An individual may have dozens of these benign lesions. Seborrheic keratosis is a waxy, raised lesion, flesh colored or pigmented in various sizes. The lesions have a "stuck-on" appearance, as if they could be scraped off. Seborrheic keratoses may be removed by a dermatologist for cosmetic reasons (Fig. 14.1). A variant seen in darkly pigmented persons occurs mostly on the face and appears as numerous small, dark, possibly taglike lesions.

Actinic keratosis is a precancerous lesion that is thought to be in the middle of the spectrum between photoaging changes and squamous cell carcinoma (Endo & Norman, 2014). It is directly related to years of overexposure to UV light. Risk factors are older age and fair complexion. It is found on the face, the lips, and the hands and forearms—areas of chronic sun exposure in

BOX 14.1 Resources for Best Practice

Pressure Injury Prevention and Treatment

Agency for Healthcare Research and Quality: Preventing pressure ulcers in hospitals: a toolkit for improving quality of care; On-time pressure ulcer healing project: http://www.ahrq.gov/professionals/systems/long-term-care/resources/ontime/pruhealing/index.html

Ayello E, Sibbald G: Preventing pressure ulcers and skin tears. In Boltz M, Capezuti E, Fulmer T, et al, editors: *Evidence-based geriatric nursing protocols for best practice,* ed 4, pp 298–323, New York, 2012, Springer. Also available at Hartford Institute for Geriatric Nursing: *Want to know more: Nursing standard of practice protocol: pressure ulcer prevention and skin tear prevention,* consultgerirn.org

Hartford Institute for Geriatric Nursing: Braden Scale; Nursing Standard of Practice Protocol: Pressure ulcer preventions and skin tear prevention

National Pressure Ulcer Advisory Panel (NPUAP): International Pressure Ulcer Prevention Guidelines (available in 17 languages); Pressure ulcer scale for healing (PUSH): PUSH Tool 3.0, Pressure Ulcer Healing Chart, Pressure Ulcer Prevention Points, Support Surface Standards Initiative, Pressure Ulcer Photos, and other educational materials on prevention and treatment also available online and via an application for iPhones, iPads, and Android devices

Perry D, Borchert K, Burke S, et al: Institute for Clinical Systems Improvement, Pressure Ulcer Prevention and Treatment Protocol. Available from Institute for Clinical Systems Improvement: http://www.icsi.org

SkinTears.org: Skin Tears Tool Kit, State of the Science Consensus Statements, educational materials

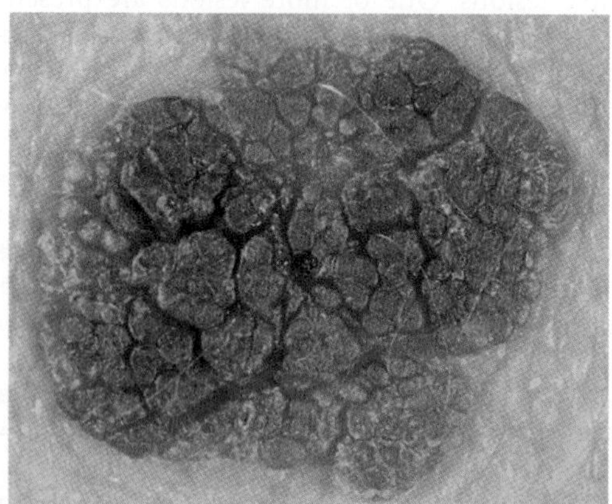

FIGURE 14.1 Seborrheic keratosis in the older adult. (From Habif TP: *Clinical dermatology: A color guide to diagnosis and therapy,* ed 5, St Louis, 2010, Mosby.)

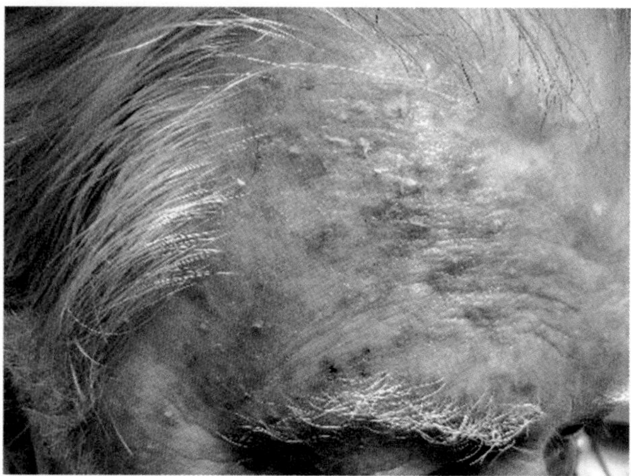

FIGURE 14.2 Actinic keratosis. (Courtesy Dr. Robert Norman.)

everyday life. Actinic keratosis is characterized by rough, scaly, sandpaper-like patches, pink to reddish brown on an erythematous base (Fig. 14.2). Lesions may be single or multiple; they may be painless or mildly tender. The person with actinic keratoses should be monitored by a dermatologist every 6 to 12 months for any change in appearance of the lesions. Early recognition, treatment, and removal of these lesions are easy and important removal may be combined with topical field therapy (Endo & Norman, 2014).

Herpes Zoster

Herpes zoster (HZ), or shingles, is a viral infection frequently seen in adults older than age 50, those who have medical conditions that compromise the immune system, or people who receive immunosuppressive drugs. HZ is caused by reactivation of latent varicella-zoster virus (VZV) (chicken pox) within the sensory neurons of the dorsal root ganglion decades after the initial VZV infection is established. More than 90% of the world's population is infected with this virus, and by the age of 85, about 50% of the population has reactivated the virus as manifested by a rash (Langana et al., 2014).

HZ always occurs along a nerve pathway, or *dermatome.* The more dermatomes involved, the more serious the infection, especially if it involves the head. When the eye is affected it is always a medical emergency. Most HZ occurs in the thoracic region, but it can also occur in the trigeminal area and cervical, lumbar, and sacral areas. HZ vesicles never cross the midline. In most cases, the severity of the infection increases with age.

The onset may be preceded by itching, tingling, or pain in the affected dermatome several days before the outbreak of the rash. It is important to differentiate HZ from herpes simplex. Herpes simplex does not occur in a dermatome pattern and is recurrent. During the healing process of HZ, clusters of papulovesicles develop along a nerve pathway. The lesions themselves eventually rupture, crust over, and resolve. Scarring may result, especially if scratching or poor hygiene leads to a secondary bacterial infection. HZ is infectious until it becomes crusty. HZ may be very painful and pruritic. Prompt treatment with the oral antiviral agents acyclovir, valacyclovir, and famciclovir may shorten the length and severity of the illness; however, to be effective, the medications must be started as soon as possible after the rash appears. Analgesics may help relieve pain. Wet compresses, calamine lotion, and colloidal oatmeal baths may help relieve itching.

Zoster vaccine (Zostavax) is recommended for all persons aged 60 years and older who have no contraindications, including persons who report a previous episode of zoster or who have chronic medical conditions (CDC, 2014). Older adults who are vaccinated may reduce their risk of acquiring HZ in half; and if they do get it, they are likely to have a milder case. HZ vaccination rates are low overall: 2% of blacks and 14% of whites have been vaccinated. More public awareness and education is needed to increase vaccination rates (Lee et al., 2013). *Healthy People 2020* includes a goal of increasing the percentage of adults who are vaccinated against zoster (shingles) in the overall goal of reducing or eliminating cases of vaccine-preventable diseases.

A common complication of HZ that is minimized for those who are immunized is postherpetic neuralgia (PHN), a chronic, often debilitating painful condition that can last months or even years. Older adults are more likely to have PHN and to have longer lasting and more severe pain. Another complication of HZ is eye involvement, which occurs in 10% to 25% of zoster episodes and can result in prolonged or permanent pain, facial scarring, and loss of vision.

The pain of PHN has been difficult to control and can significantly affect one's quality of life. Treatment should include medical, psychological, and complementary and alternative medicine options, as well as rehabilitation. The best evidence studies for medications indicate that the most effective are the tricyclic antidepressants, gabapentin and pregabalin, carbamazepine (for trigeminal neuralgia), opioids, tramadol, topical lidocaine patch, and duloxetine or venlafaxine. Relatively newer treatments for PHN include a high-concentration (8%) topical capsaicin patch, gastroretentive gabapentin, gabapentin enacarbil, and pregabalin in combination with lidocaine plaster, oxycodone, or transcutaneous electrical nerve stimulation (TENS) (Endo & Norman, 2014; Harden et al., 2013). Assessment and management of pain are discussed in Chapter 18.

Candidiasis *(Candida albicans)*

The fungus *Candida albicans* (referred to as "yeast") is present on the skin of healthy persons of any age. However, under certain circumstances and in the right environment, a fungal infection can develop. Persons who are obese or malnourished, are receiving antibiotic or steroid therapy, or have diabetes are at increased risk. *Candida* grows especially well in areas that are moist, warm, and dark, such as in skinfolds, in the axilla, in the groin area, and under pendulous breasts. It can also be found in the corners of the mouth associated with the chronic moisture of angular cheilitis. In the vagina it is also called a "yeast infection." If this is found in an older woman, it may mean that her diabetes either has not yet been diagnosed or is in poor control.

Inside the mouth a *Candida* infection is referred to as "thrush" and is associated with poor hygiene and immunocompromised individuals, such as those who have a history of long-term steroid use, who are receiving chemotherapy, or who test positive for or are infected with human immunodeficiency virus (HIV) or have acquired immunodeficiency syndrome (AIDS). In the mouth, candidiasis appears as irregular, white, flat to slightly raised patches on an erythematous base that cannot be removed by scraping. The infection can extend down into the throat and cause swallowing to be painful. In severely immunocompromised persons the infection can extend down the entire gastrointestinal tract.

On the skin, *Candida* is usually maculopapular, glazed, and dark pink in persons with less pigmentation and grayish in persons with more pigmentation. If it is advanced, the central area may be completely red and/or dark, and weeping with characteristic bright red and/or dark satellite lesions (distinct lesions a short distance from the center). At this point the skin may be edematous, itching, and burning.

The best approach to managing fungal infections is to prevent them, and the key to prevention is limiting the conditions that encourage fungal growth. Prevention is prioritized for persons who are obese, bedridden, incontinent, or diaphoretic. Attention is given to the adequate drying of bodily target areas after bathing, the prompt management of incontinence episodes, the use of loose-fitting cotton clothing and underwear, the changing of clothing when damp, and the avoidance of incontinence products that are tight or have plastic that touches the skin. One of the best ways to dry hard-to-reach vulnerable areas is with a hair dryer set on low. A folded, dry washcloth or cotton sanitary pad can be placed under pendulous breasts or between skinfolds to promote exposure to air and light. Optimizing nutrition and glycemic control is important. Antifungal medications are also used to treat *Candida*.

Photo Damage of the Skin

Although exposure to sunlight is necessary for the production of vitamin D, the sun is also the most common cause of skin damage and skin cancer. More than 90% of the visible changes commonly attributed to skin aging are caused by the sun (Skin Cancer Foundation, 2014). With aging one accumulates years of sun exposure and the epidermis is thinner, significantly increasing the risk of skin cancer for older adults. The damage (photo or solar damage) comes from prolonged exposure to UV light from the environment or in tanning booths. Although the amount of sun-induced damage varies with skin type, genetics, and geographical location, much of the associated damage is preventable. Ideally, preventive measures begin in childhood, but clinical evidence has shown that some improvement can be achieved at any time by limiting sun exposure and using sunscreens regularly regardless of skin tones.

SKIN CANCERS

Facts and Figures

Currently, between 2 and 3 million nonmelanoma skin cancers and 132,000 melanoma skin cancers occur globally each year. Cancer of the skin (including melanoma and nonmelanoma skin cancer) is the most common of all cancers. Skin cancer is a major public health problem, and the occurrence of skin cancer in the United States, unlike many other cancers, continues to rise (U.S. Department of Health and Human Services [USDHHS], 2014). One in five Americans will develop skin cancer in the course of a lifetime (World Health Organization [WHO], 2014).

Caucasian populations generally have a much higher risk of getting nonmelanoma or melanoma skin cancers than dark-skinned populations, but individuals of all skin colors should minimize sun exposure. Individuals with pale or freckled skin, fair or red hair, and blue eyes belong to the highest risk group. However, excessive exposure to intense sunlight can damage all skin types, and the risk of eye damage and heat stroke is the same for everyone (WHO, 2014).

Basal Cell Carcinoma

Basal cell carcinoma is the most common malignant skin cancer. It occurs mainly in older age groups but is found more and more in younger persons. It is slow growing, and metastasis is rare. A basal cell lesion can be triggered by extensive sun exposure, especially burns, chronic irritation, and chronic ulceration of the skin. It is more prevalent in light-skinned persons. It usually begins as a pearly papule with prominent telangiectasias (blood vessels) or as a scarlike area with no history of trauma (Fig. 14.3). Basal cell carcinoma is also known to ulcerate. It may be indistinguishable from squamous cell carcinoma and is diagnosed by biopsy. Early detection and treatment are necessary to minimize disfigurement. Treatment is usually surgical with either simple excision or Mohs micrographic surgery (Endo & Norman, 2014).

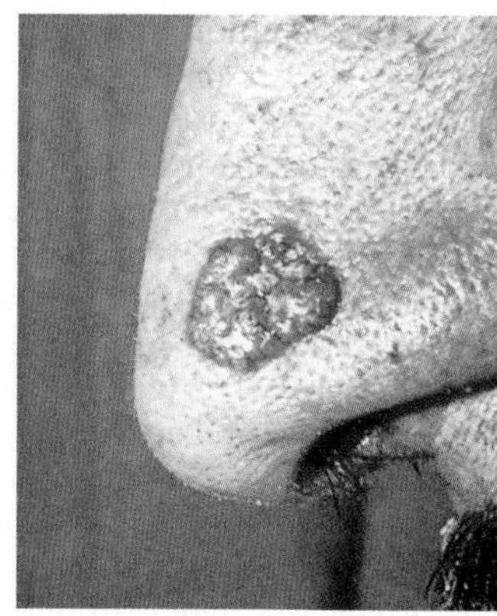

FIGURE 14.3 Basal cell carcinoma. (Courtesy Gary Monheit, MD, University of Alabama at Birmingham School of Medicine.)

Squamous Cell Carcinoma

Squamous cell carcinoma is the second most common skin cancer. However, it is aggressive and has a high incidence of metastasis if not identified and treated promptly. Major risk factors include sun exposure, fair skin, and immunosuppression. Individuals in their middle sixties who have been or are chronically exposed to the sun (e.g., persons who work out of doors or are athletes) are prime candidates for this type of cancer. Less common causes include chronic stasis ulcers, scars from injury, and exposure to chemical carcinogens, such as topical hydrocarbons, arsenic, and radiation (especially for individuals who received treatments for acne in the mid-twentieth century) (Endo & Norman, 2014).

The lesion begins as a firm, irregular, fleshy, pink-colored nodule that becomes reddened and scaly, much like actinic keratosis, but it may increase rapidly in size. It may also be hard and wartlike with a gray top and horny texture, or it may be ulcerated and indurated with raised, defined borders. Because it can appear so differently, it is often overlooked or thought to be insignificant. All persons, especially those who live in sunny climates, should be regularly screened by a dermatologist. Treatment depends on the size, histological features, and patient preference and may include electrodesiccation and curettage, Mohs micrographic surgery, aggressive cryotherapy, or topical 5-fluorouracil (Endo & Norman, 2014). Once a person has been diagnosed with a squamous cell carcinoma, he or she needs to be routinely followed because the majority of recurrences are within the first few years.

Melanoma

Melanoma, a neoplasm of the melanocytes, affects the skin or, less commonly, the retina. Melanoma has a classical multicolor, raised appearance with an asymmetrical, irregular border. It may appear to be of any size, but the surface diameter is not necessarily reflective of the size beneath the surface, similar in concept to an iceberg. It is treatable if diagnosed early, before it has a chance to invade surrounding tissue. Melanoma accounts for less than 2% of skin cancer cases, but it causes most skin cancer deaths. Melanoma is highly curable if the cancer is detected in its earliest stages and treated promptly (Garrett et al., 2014).

Incidence and Prevalence

The number of new cases of melanoma in the United States has been increasing for at least 30 years. Overall, the lifetime risk of being diagnosed with melanoma is about 1 in 50 for the white population, 1 in 1000 for black individuals, and 1 in 200 for the Hispanic population. Melanoma rates among middle-aged adults, especially women, have increased in the past 4 decades (American Cancer Society, 2014; Garrett et al., 2014). Men have a higher rate of melanoma than women and a person who has already had a melanoma has a higher risk of developing another one. The risk of melanoma is more than 10 times higher for white Americans than for black Americans.

Risk Factors

Risk factors for melanoma include a personal history of melanoma; the presence of atypical, large, or numerous (more than 50) moles; sensitivity to the sun; history of excessive sun exposure and severe sunburns; use of tanning booths; presence of natural blonde or red hair color; history of diseases or treatments that suppress the immune system; and a history of skin cancer. Increasing age along with a history of sun exposure increases one's risk even further. The legs and backs of women and the backs of men are the most common sites of melanoma. Many studies have linked melanoma on the trunk, legs, and arms to frequent sunburns, especially in childhood. Blistering sunburns before the age of 18 years are thought to damage Langerhans cells, which affect the immune response of the skin and increase the risk for a later melanoma. Two-thirds of melanomas develop from preexisting moles; only one-third arise alone.

Indoor tanning. Although melanoma occurs more often in older people, it is one of the most common cancers in people younger than 30 years. Exposure to indoor tanning, common in Western countries, is thought to be contributing to the increasing rates of melanoma and other skin cancers among younger individuals. Indoor tanning increases the risk of melanoma by 75% when started before age 35 years. Indoor tanners are 2.5 times more likely to develop squamous cell cancer and 1.5 times more likely to develop basal cell cancer.

In the United States, 35% of adults and 55% of college students have used indoor tanning devices. Worldwide, there are more skin cancer cases attributable to indoor tanning than there are lung cancer cases caused by smoking (Wehner et al., 2013). This is considered a major public health issue with many states limiting minors' access to tanning salons. The U.S. Food and Drug Administration (USFDA) has issued a final order reclassifying sunlamp products (including tanning beds and booths) and UV lamps from low-risk to moderate-risk and requiring black-box warnings on the devices, cautioning against use by anyone younger than 18 years of age (USFDA, 2014). *Healthy People 2020* includes objectives to reduce the proportion of adolescents and adults using indoor tanning devices.

❖ IMPLICATIONS FOR GERONTOLOGICAL NURSING AND HEALTHY AGING

Age-related skin changes, such as thinning and diminished numbers of melanocytes, significantly increase the risk for solar damage and subsequent skin cancer. The nurse has an active role in the prevention and early recognition of skin cancers. This role may include working with community awareness and education programs, as well as participating in screening clinics and providing direct care. By far the most important preventive nursing intervention is to provide education regarding skin cancer risk factors and adequate lifelong protective measures (Box 14.2).

Careful skin inspection is essential, and the nurse is vigilant in observing skin for changes that require further evaluation. Patient education also includes teaching the individual how to examine his or her skin once a month to look for warning signs or any suspicious lesions. If the individual has a partner, partners can perform regular "checks" of each other's skin, watching for signs of change and the need to contact a primary care provider or dermatologist promptly. For the person with keratosis and multiple freckles (nevi), photographing the body parts may be a useful reference.

BOX 14.2 Promoting Healthy Skin

Sun Protection

- Seek the shade.
- Do not burn.
- Avoid indoor tanning booths and sunlamps.
- Wear hats with a brim wide enough to shade face, ears, and neck, as well as clothing that adequately covers the arms, legs, and torso. Cover up with clothing, including a broad-brimmed hat and UV-blocking sunglasses.
- Use a broad-spectrum (UVA/UVB) sunscreen with an SPF of 30 or higher every day.
- Apply 1 ounce (2 tablespoons) of sunscreen to your entire body 30 minutes before going outdoors. Reapply every 2 hours or immediately after swimming or excessive sweating.
- Examine your skin head-to-toe every month.
- See your health care provider every year for a professional skin exam.

Modified from Skin Cancer Foundation: *Prevention guidelines.* Available at http://www.skincancer.org/prevention/sun-protection/prevention-guidelines. Accessed May 5, 2015.

BOX 14.3 Danger Signs: Remember ABCDE

Asymmetry of a mole (one that is not regularly round or oval)
Border is irregular
Color variation (areas of black, brown, tan, blue, red, white, or a combination)
Diameter greater than the size of a pencil eraser (although early stages may be smaller)
Elevation and **E**nlargement*

*Lesions that change, itch, bleed, or do not heal are also alarm signals.
From Skin Cancer Foundation: *Do you know your ABCDEs?* Available at http://www.skincancer.org/skin-cancer-information/melanoma/melanoma-warning-signs-and-images/do-you-know-your-abcdes. Accessed March 7, 2014.

The adage "when in doubt, get it checked" is an important one and regular screenings should be a part of the health care of all older adults. The "ABCDE" approach to assessing such potential lesions is used (Box 14.3).

PRESSURE INJURIES

Aging carries a high risk for the development of pressure injuries; 70% of pressure injuries (PIs) occur in older adults (Jamshed & Schneider, 2010). Pressure injuries are recognized as one of the geriatric syndromes (see Chapter 8), and *Healthy People 2020* has addressed this issue with a goal of reducing the rate of pressure injury–related hospitalizations among older adults. Nurses play a key role in the prevention of pressure injuries and the selection of evidence-based treatment strategies.

Definition

The National Pressure Ulcer Advisory Panel (NPUAP) and the European Pressure Ulcer Advisory Panel (EPUAP) constitute an international collaboration convened to develop evidence-based recommendations to be used throughout the world to prevent and treat pressure-related injuries. In 2016 the NPUAP began using the term pressure injury to replace pressure ulcer to more accurately describe pressure injuries to both intact and ulcerated skin. A pressure injury is "localized damage to the skin and/or underlying soft tissue usually over a bony prominence or related to a medical or other device. The injury can present as intact skin or an open ulcer and may be painful. The injury occurs as a result of intense pressure and/or prolonged pressure or pressure in combination with shear. The tolerance of soft tissue for pressure and sear may also be affected by microclimate, nutrition, perfusion, co-morbidities and condition of the soft tissue" (NPUAP, 2016).

In addition to the change in terminology, Arabic numbers are now used in the names of the stages instead of Roman numerals. Stages have been more fully described and two additional pressure injury definitions have been added.

Scope of the Problem

Pressure injuries are a major challenge worldwide and a major cause of morbidity, mortality, and health care burden globally (Wounds International, 2009). The epidemiology of pressure injuries varies by clinical setting. Critically ill patients in the intensive care unit (ICU) are considered to be at the greatest risk for pressure injury development as a result of high acuity and the multiple interventions and therapies they receive. In ICUs, prevalence ranges from 49% across Western Europe, 22% in North America, 50% in Australia, and 29% in Jordan (Tayyib et al., 2013). Although overall prevalence rates have dropped some in the United States in acute care settings, multiple studies have shown that the incidence of facility-acquired pressure injuries remains high in ICUs (10% to 41%) (Cooper, 2013).

Data from the United States and Europe suggest that pressure injury rates have failed to respond to prevention strategies, with many countries continuing to report double-figure percentage results (Phillips & Buttery, 2009). Concern over the global problem of pressure injuries led the NPUAP to establish a Pressure Ulcer Registry, the first database of its type to allow clinicians to input cases of pressure injuries in an effort to provide statistically significant rigorous analysis of the variables associated with the development of unavoidable pressure injuries (NPUAP, 2014).

Cost and Regulatory Requirements

Treatment of pressure injuries is costly in terms of both health care expenditure and patient suffering. In 2008 the Centers for Medicare and Medicaid Services (CMS) included hospital-acquired pressure injuries as one of the preventable adverse events (health care–acquired conditions [HACs]). The development of a stage/category 3 or 4 pressure injury is considered a "never event" (serious medical errors or adverse events that should never happen to a patient). Hospitals no longer receive additional reimbursement to care for a patient who has acquired pressure injuries under the hospital's care, and this has the potential to greatly increase the financial strain for facilities that fail to rise to this challenge (Armstrong et al., 2008; Cooper, 2013; Gray-Siracusa & Schrier, 2011).

Characteristics

Pressure injuries can develop anywhere on the body but are seen most frequently on the posterior aspects, especially the sacrum, the heels, and the greater trochanters. Secondary areas of breakdown include the lateral condyles of the knees and the ankles. The pinna of the ears, occiput, elbows, and scapulae are other areas subject to breakdown. Heels are particularly prone to the development of pressure injuries because there is little soft tissue; 25% to 30% of pressure injuries are on the heels, and individuals with peripheral arterial disease are at high risk for pressure injuries on heels (McGinnis et al., 2013).

SAFETY ALERT

Approximately 25% to 35% of pressure injuries are on heels. Those with peripheral vascular disease (PVD) are at high risk. Keep heels elevated off the bed with a pillow under each calf or use heel suspension boots.

Classification

The new EPUAP and NPUAP classification of pressure injuries is presented in Box 14.4. The following two additional pressure injury definitions have also been added:

Medical Device–Related Pressure Injury: Medical device–related pressure injuries result from the use of devices designed and applied for diagnostic

BOX 14.4 Pressure Injury Stages

Deep Tissue Pressure Injury (DTPI): Persistent Nonblanchable Deep Red, Maroon, or Purple Discoloration

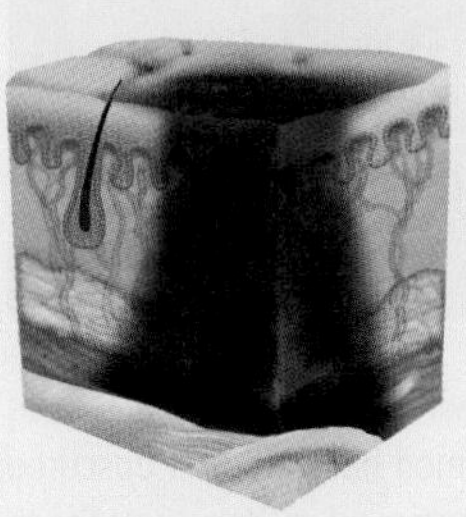

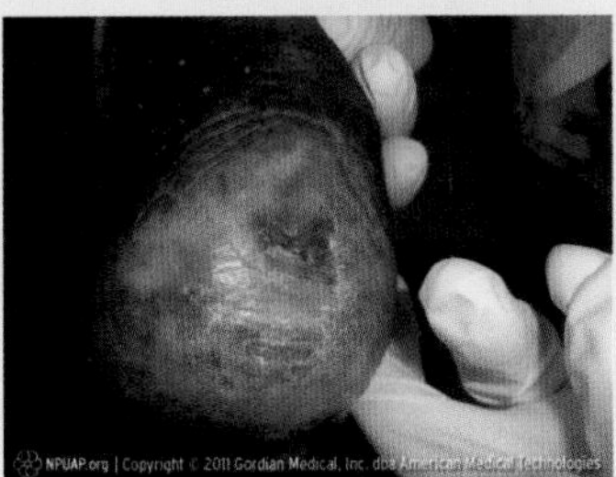

Heel, ethnic skin

Intact or nonintact skin with localized area of persistent nonblanchable deep red, maroon, or purple discoloration or epidermal separation revealing a dark wound bed or blood-filled blister. Pain and temperature change often precede skin color changes. Discoloration may appear differently in darkly pigmented skin. This injury results from intense and/or prolonged pressure and shear forces at the bone-muscle interface. The wound may evolve rapidly to reveal the actual extent of tissue injury, or may resolve without tissue loss. If necrotic tissue, subcutaneous tissue, granulation tissue, fascia, muscle, or other underlying structures are visible, this indicates a full-thickness pressure injury (Unstageable, Stage 3, or Stage 4). Do not use DTPI to describe vascular, traumatic, neuropathic, or dermatological conditions.

Stage 1 Pressure Injury: Nonblanchable Erythema of Intact Skin

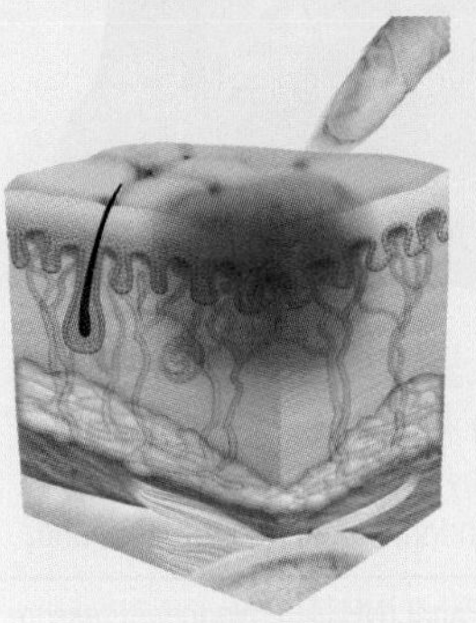

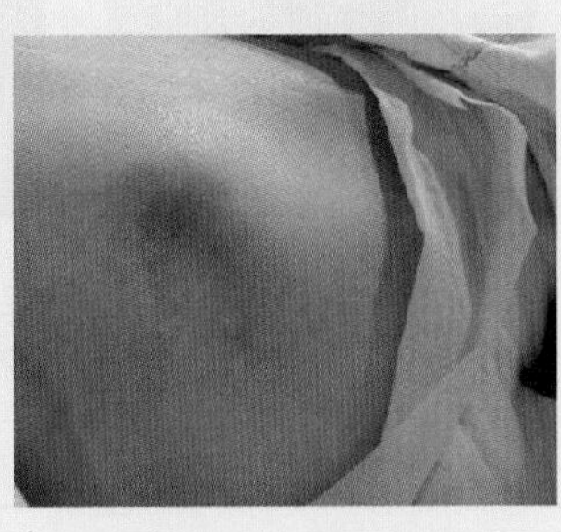

Intact skin with a localized area of nonblanchable erythema, which may appear differently in darkly pigmented skin. Presence of blanchable erythema or changes in sensation, temperature, or firmness may precede visual changes. Color changes do not include purple or maroon discoloration; these may indicate deep tissue pressure injury.

Continued

BOX 14.4 Pressure Injury Stages—cont'd

Stage 2 Pressure Injury: Partial-Thickness Skin Loss With Exposed Dermis

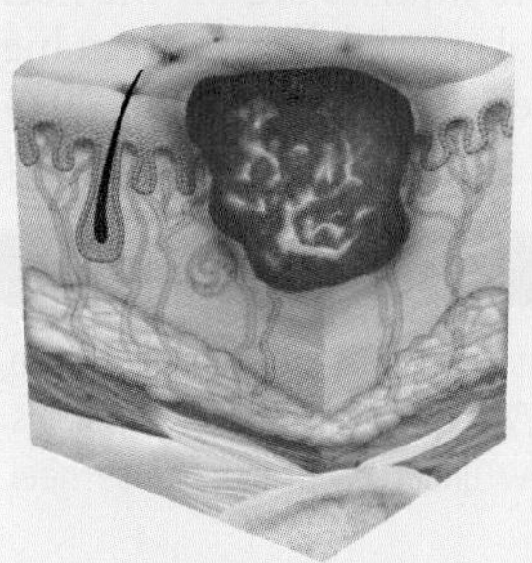

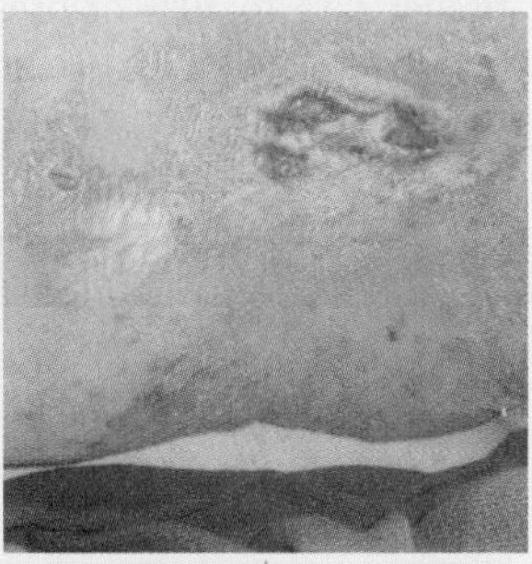

Partial-thickness loss of skin with exposed dermis. The wound bed is viable, pink or red, and moist, and may also present as an intact or ruptured serum-filled blister. Adipose (fat) is not visible and deeper tissues are not visible. Granulation tissue, slough, and eschar are not present. These injuries commonly result from adverse microclimate and shear in the skin over the pelvis and shear in the heels. This stage should not be used to describe moisture-associated skin damage (MASD) including incontinence-associated dermatitis (IAD), intertriginous dermatitis (ITD), medical adhesive–related skin injury (MARS), or traumatic wounds (skin tears, burns, abrasions).

Stage 3 Pressure Injury: Full-Thickness Skin Loss

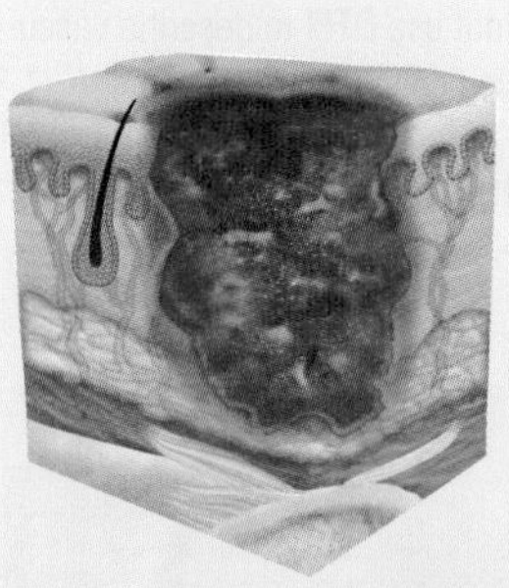

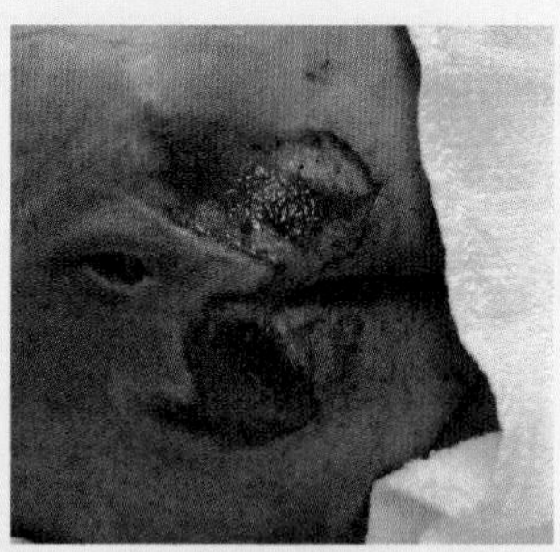

Full-thickness loss of skin, in which adipose (fat) is visible in the ulcer and granulation tissue and epibole (rolled wound edges) are often present. Slough and/or eschar may be visible. Undermining and tunneling may occur. Fascia, muscle, tendon, ligament, cartilage, and/or bone are not exposed. If slough or eschar obscures the extent of tissue loss this is an Unstageable Pressure Injury.

Stage 4 Pressure Injury: Full-Thickness Skin and Tissue Loss

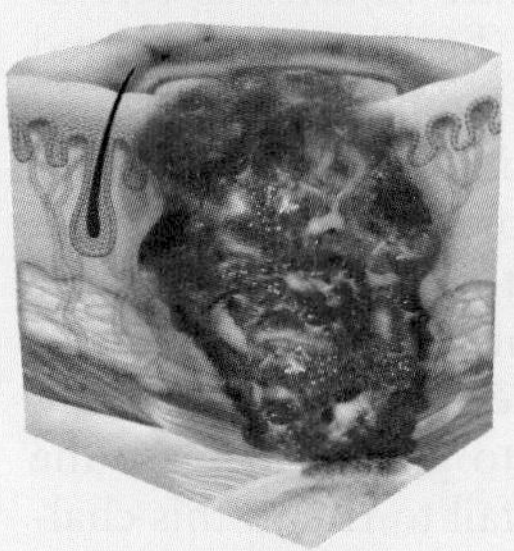

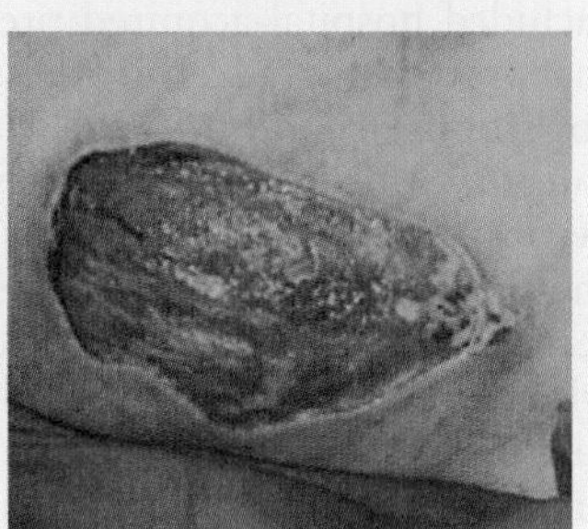

Full-thickness skin and tissue loss with exposed or directly palpable fascia, muscle, tendon, ligament, cartilage, or bone in the ulcer. Slough and/or eschar may be visible. Epibole (rolled edges), undermining, and/or tunneling often occur. Depth varies by anatomical location. If slough or eschar obscures the extent of tissue loss, this is an Unstageable Pressure Injury.

Unstageable Pressure Injury: Obscured Full-Thickness Skin and Tissue Loss

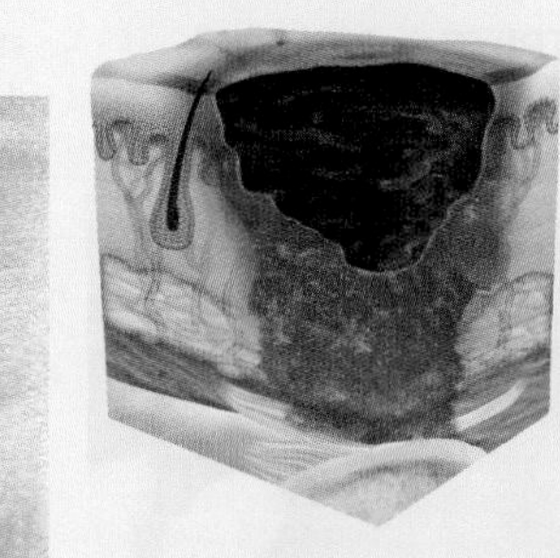

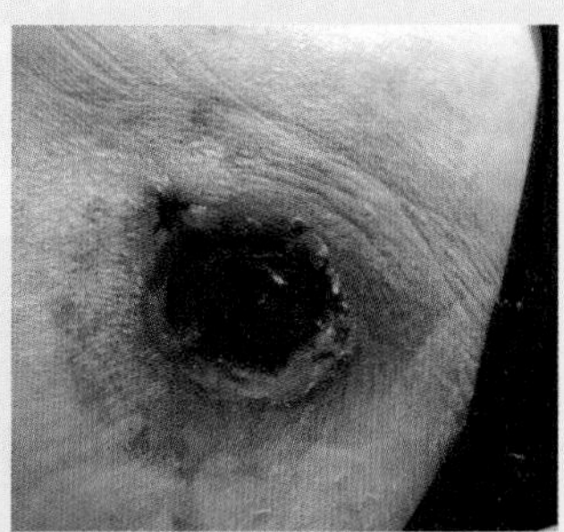

Full-thickness skin and tissue loss in which the extent of tissue damage within the ulcer cannot be confirmed because it is obscured by slough or eschar. If slough or eschar is removed, a Stage 3 or Stage 4 pressure ulcer will be revealed. Stable eschar (e.g., dry, adherent, intact without erythema or fluctuance) on an ischemic limb or the heels should not be removed.

From the National Pressure Ulcer Advisory Panel (NPUAP): *National Pressure Ulcer Advisory Panel (NPUAP) announces a change in terminology from pressure ulcer to pressure injury and updates the stages of pressure injury,* 2016. Reprinted with permission of the NPUAP, 2016. DTPI photo: From NPUAP. Stages 1–4 photos: From Cameron MH, Monroe L, editors: *Physical rehabilitation for the physical therapist assistant,* St Louis, MO, 2011, Saunders. Unstageable photo: From Ham RJ, Sloane PD, Warshaw GA, et al, editors: *Primary care geriatrics,* ed 6, Philadelphia, 2014, Elsevier.

or therapeutic purposes. The resultant pressure injury generally conforms to the pattern or shape of the device. The injury should not be staged using the staging system.

Mucosal Membrane Pressure Injury: Mucosal membrane pressure injury is found on mucous membranes with a history of a medical device in use at the location of the injury. Because of the anatomy of the tissue, these injuries cannot be staged.

Pressure injuries are always classified by the highest stage "achieved," and reverse staging is never used. This means that the wound is documented as the stage representing the maximal damage and depth that has occurred. As the wound heals, it fills with granulation tissue composed of endothelial cells, fibroblasts, collagen, and an extracellular matrix. Muscle, subcutaneous fat, and dermis are not replaced. A stage 4 pressure injury that is healing does not revert to stage 3 and then stage 2. It remains defined as a healing stage 4 pressure injury.

Skin Changes at Life's End (SCALE)

Skin failure is defined as "an event in which the skin and underlying tissue die due to hypoperfusion that occurs concurrent with severe dysfunction or failure of other organ systems" (White-Chu & Langemo, 2012, p. 28). Skin failure is identified as a real condition that can occur in the last days or weeks of life and can occur in both acute and chronic conditions. Skin failure is a documentable condition and not the same as a pressure injury (Black et al., 2011).

In 2009 an interdisciplinary panel of experts in wound healing developed a consensus statement on the changes that occur to the skin at the end of life (SCALE) (European Pressure Ulcer Advisory Panel, 2014; Sibbald et al., 2010). Knowledge of this condition is limited, and further research is required. The Kennedy Terminal Ulcer, first described in 1989 and now explained as an unavoidable skin breakdown that occurs during the dying process, presents as a red, yellow, or purple lesion shaped like a pear, butterfly, or horseshoe on the coccyx or sacrum. The lesion will darken deeply and progress to a full-thickness ulcer in a few days, and usually indicates that death is imminent (Sibbald et al., 2010; White-Chu & Langemo, 2012). The consensus statement concludes that these changes can be an unavoidable part of the dying process and may occur even with appropriate evidence-based interventions (Sibbald et al., 2010).

Treatment decisions are made after careful assessment of the skin and underlying physical factors such as diminished tissue perfusion, suboptimal nutrition, weakness and progressive limitation of mobility, and impaired immune function. Determination should be made if the injury is (1) healable within an individual's lifetime; (2) maintained; or (3) nonhealable or palliative.

Risk Factors

Many factors increase the risk of pressure injuries, including changes in the skin, comorbid illnesses, nutritional status, frailty, surgical procedures (especially orthopedic/cardiac), cognitive deficits, incontinence, and reduced mobility (Box 14.5). A major risk factor is the combination of intensity and duration of pressure and tissue tolerance (Ayello & Sibbald, 2012). Individuals confined to a bed or chair and who are unable to shift weight or reposition themselves at regular intervals are at high risk. Tissue tolerance, in addition to unrelieved pressure, contributes to the risk of a pressure injury. Tissue tolerance is related to the ability of the tissue to distribute and compensate for pressure exerted over bony prominences. Factors that affect tissue tolerance

BOX 14.5 Pressure Injury Risk Factors

Prolonged Pressure/Immobilization

- Lying in bed or sitting in a chair or wheelchair without changing position or relieving pressure over an extended period
- Lying for hours on hard x-ray and operating tables
- Neurological disorders (coma, spinal cord injuries, cognitive impairment, or cerebrovascular disease)
- Fractures or contractures
- Debilitation: elderly persons in hospitals and nursing homes
- Pain
- Sedation
- Shearing forces (moving by dragging on coarse bed sheets)

Disease/Tissue Factors

- Impaired perfusion; ischemia
- Fecal or urinary incontinence; prolonged exposure to moisture
- Malnutrition, dehydration
- Chronic diseases accompanied by anemia, edema, renal failure, malnutrition, peripheral vascular disease, or sepsis
- Previous history of pressure injuries

Additional Risk Factors for the Critically Ill

- Norepinephrine infusion
- Acute Physiology and Chronic Health Evaluation (APACHE II) score
- Anemia
- Age older than 40 years
- Multiple organ system disease or comorbid complications
- Length of hospital stay

From McCance KL, Huether SE, editors: *Pathophysiology*, ed 7, St Louis, MO, 2014, Elsevier.

include moisture, friction, shear force, nutritional status, age, sensory perception, and arterial pressure.

In darker-pigmented persons, redness and blanching may not be observed as early signs of skin damage. In dark skin, early signs of skin damage can manifest as a purplish color or appear like a bruise. It is important to observe for induration, darkening, change in color from surrounding skin, or a shadowed appearance of the skin. The affected skin area, when compared with adjacent tissues, may be firm, warmer, cooler, or painful (Garcia & White-Chu, 2014). Several studies have reported a higher prevalence and incidence of pressure injuries among black individuals in nursing homes than other race groups (Baumgarten et al., 2009; Harms et al., 2014; Howard & Taylor, 2009). Improved assessment of dark skin for early signs of damage and increased attention to prevention of pressure injuries before admission and during nursing home stays are important (Harms et al., 2014).

Prevention of Pressure Injuries

The importance of prevention of pressure injuries has been frequently emphasized and is the key to treatment. A consensus paper from the International Expert Wound Care Advisory Panel (Armstrong et al., 2008) provides recommendations for prevention of pressure injuries that include patient education, clinician training for all members of the health care team, strategies in developing communication and terminology materials, implementation of toolkits and protocols (prevention bundles), documentation checklists, outcome evaluation, quality improvement efforts, evidence-based treatment protocols, and appropriate products.

A comprehensive pressure injury program that includes multiple interventions (care bundle) appears to be related to better outcomes. A bundle is composed of a set of evidence-based practices that when performed collectively and reliably have been shown to improve patient outcomes (Gray-Siracusa & Schrier, 2011). Involvement of the patient and family may enhance the effectiveness of care bundles (Gillespie et al., 2014). Core preventive strategies include risk assessment, skin assessment, nutritional assessment, repositioning, and appropriate support surfaces. Interventions that addressed limited mobility, compromised skin integrity, and nutritional support have been associated with significant improvements in pressure injury rates (Gillespie et al., 2014; Gray-Siracusa & Schrier, 2011).

Systematic prevention programs have been shown to decrease hospital-acquired pressure injuries by 34% to 50% (Armstrong et al., 2008). Olsho and colleagues (2014) reported a 59% reduction in the monthly incidence of pressure injuries in a nursing home with the use of the Agency for Healthcare Research and Quality [AHRQ] On-Time Pressure Ulcer Prevention Program (AHRQ, 2009) (see Box 14.1). However, "despite a number of national prevention initiatives and existing evidence-based protocols, pressure injury frequency has not declined in recent years and pressure injuries continue to have a negative impact on patient outcomes and health care costs in a variety of care settings" (Baumgarten et al., 2009, p. 253). Several studies have reported that compliance with evidence-based protocol recommendations is a concern and less than half of at-risk patients actually receive core preventive strategies (Baumgarten et al., 2009; Gillespie et al., 2014; Spillsbury et al., 2007).

The prevention and treatment of pressure injuries is complex and does not belong to any one specialty; a team approach that involves primary care providers, nursing staff, physical therapists, nutritionists, and other clinicians is most effective (Armstrong et al., 2008).

Consequences of Pressure Injuries

Pressure injuries are costly to treat and prolong recovery and extend rehabilitation. Complications include the need for grafting or amputation, sepsis, or even death and may lead to legal action by the individual or his or her representative against the caregiver. The personal impact of a pressure injury on health and quality of life is also significant and not well understood or researched. Findings from a study exploring patients' perceptions of the impact of a pressure injury and its treatment on health and quality of life suggest that pressure injuries cause suffering, pain, discomfort, and distress that are not always recognized or adequately treated by nursing staff. Pressure injuries had a profound impact on the patients' lives—physically, socially, emotionally, and mentally (Spillsbury et al., 2007).

❖ IMPLICATIONS FOR GERONTOLOGICAL NURSING AND HEALTHY AGING

Nursing staff, as direct caregivers, are key team members who perform skin assessment, identify risk factors, and implement numerous preventive interventions. The nurse alerts the health care provider of the need for prescribed treatments, recommends treatments, and administers and evaluates the changing status of the wound(s) and adequacy of treatments.

◆ Assessment of Pressure Injury Risk

Skin assessments are performed on admission and whenever there is a change in the status of the patient (Box 14.6). In the nursing home, the MDS 3.0 provides an evidence-based assessment of skin integrity and

BOX 14.6 Guidelines for Skin Assessment

Acute care: On admission, reassess at least every 24 hours or sooner if patient's condition changes
Long-term care: On admission, weekly for 4 weeks, then quarterly and whenever resident's condition changes
Home care: On admission and at every nurse visit

Data from NPUAP: *Pressure ulcer prevention points,* 2007. Available at http://www.npuap.org/wp-content/uploads/2012/03/PU_Prev_Points.pdf. Accessed March 11, 2014.

pressure injuries with accompanying care guidelines (see Chapter 8). Assessment begins with a history, detailed head-to-toe skin examination, nutritional evaluation, and analysis of laboratory findings. Laboratory values that have been correlated with risk for the development and the poor healing of pressure injuries include those that reflect anemia and poor nutritional status. Visual and tactile inspection of the entire skin surface with special attention to bony prominences is essential. The nurse looks for any interruption of skin integrity or other changes, including redness or *hyperemia*. Special attention must be given to the assessment of dark skin because tissue injury will appear differently. Assessment of pain related to the pressure injury (dressing changes, turning) is important so that appropriate treatment can be given to relieve pain (see Chapter 18).

If pressure is present, it should be relieved and the area reassessed in 1 hour. Pressure areas and surrounding tissue should be palpated for changes in temperature and tissue resilience. Blisters or pimples with or without hyperemia and scabs over weight-bearing areas in the absence of trauma should be considered suspect. Inspection is best accomplished in nonglare daylight or, if that is not possible, with focused lighting. Special attention should be directed to affected areas when an individual uses orthotic devices such as corsets, braces, prostheses, postural supports, splints, slings, or casts and to areas of skin around other devices such as endotracheal and tracheostomy tubes as well.

Early identification of risk status is critical so that timely interventions can be designed to address specific risk factors. The Braden Scale for Predicting Pressure Sore Risk, developed by nurses Barbara Braden and Nancy Bergstrom, is widely used and clinically validated (see Box 14.1). This scale assesses the risk of pressure injuries on the basis of a numerical scoring system of six risk factors: sensory perception, moisture, activity, mobility, nutrition, and friction/shear. Because the Braden Scale does not include all of the risk factors for pressure injuries, it is recommended that it be used as an adjunct rather than in place of clinical judgment. A thorough patient history to assess other risk factors such as age, medications, comorbidities (diabetes, peripheral vascular disease [PVD]), history of pressure injuries, and other factors is important to fully address the risk of pressure injury development so that appropriate preventive interventions can be developed (Jull & Griffiths, 2010; Warner-Maron, 2015).

Most institutions have special forms or screens on their computer software for recording skin assessments. The AHRQ provides the On-Time Pressure Ulcer Healing Project (Olsho et al., 2014) (Box 14.1). The focus of this project is on prevention and timely treatment of pressure injuries in long-term care. Tools to document pressure injury healing and treatments and reports to monitor the healing process are available. The reader is referred to the NPUAP website (http://www.npuap.org) for more information.

◆ Interventions

The goal of nurses is to help maintain skin integrity against the various environmental, mechanical, and chemical assaults that are potential causes of breakdown. Nursing actions include eliminating friction and irritation to the skin, such as from shearing; reducing moisture so that tissues do not macerate; managing incontinence; and displacing body weight from prominent areas to facilitate circulation to the skin. The nurse should be familiar with the types of supportive surfaces so that the most effective products are used. Use lifting devices to move the person rather than dragging the person during transfers and position changes. Use pillows or foam wedges so that skin surfaces do not touch and use devices that eliminate pressure on heels. Bed-bound and chair-bound patients should be repositioned at least every 2 hours.

Repositioning guidelines must be followed when the patient is on a pressure-redistributing mattress as well. Maintain the head of the bed at 30 degrees or less and avoid positioning directly on the trochanter when using a side-lying position; use the 30-degree lateral inclined position. Ensuring adequate fluid and food intake is important. Pressure injury prevention education programs should be provided to all levels of health care providers, patients, families, and caregivers.

SAFETY ALERT

Individuals placed on pressure redistribution mattresses continue to need turning and repositioning according to an established schedule.

Consultation with the nutritional team is important. Nutritional intake should be monitored, as well as the serum albumin, hematocrit, and hemoglobin levels. Caloric, protein, vitamin, and/or mineral supplementation can be considered if there is evidence of deficiencies of these nutrients. Routine use of higher than the recommended daily allowance of vitamin C and zinc for the prevention and/or treatment of pressure injuries is not supported by evidence (Jamshed & Schneider, 2010). The nurse promotes nutritional health by ensuring that the person receives adequate assistance with eating and that dining time is a pleasant experience for the person.

Pressure Injury Assessment

Pressure injuries are assessed with each dressing change and repeated on a weekly, biweekly, and as-needed basis. The purpose is to specifically and carefully evaluate the effectiveness of treatment. The PUSH tool (Pressure Ulcer Scale for Healing) (see Box 14.1) provides a detailed form that covers all aspects of assessment but contains only three items and takes a short time to complete (NPUAP, 2014). Photographic documentation is highly recommended both at the onset of the problem and at intervals during treatment (Ahn & Salicido, 2008; Garcia & White-Chu, 2014).

If there are no signs of healing from week to week or worsening of the wound is seen, then either the treatment is insufficient or the wound has become infected; in both cases, treatment must be changed. Determining the cause of the pressure injury is important so that appropriate preventive measures can be implemented. The care team, in consultation with the individual and family, reviews the assessment and care plan and determines, if possible, if the underlying cause is reversible so that appropriate treatment decisions can be made to ensure patient comfort. Consultation with a wound care specialist is advisable for wounds that are extensive or nonhealing. Specialized nurses such as enterostomal therapists or nurse practitioners, who may work with wound centers or surgeons, provide consultation in nursing homes, offices, or clinics.

Pressure Injury Dressings

The type of dressing selected is based on careful assessment of the condition of the pressure injury; the presence of granulation, necrotic tissue, and slough; the amount of drainage; the microbial status; and the quality of the surrounding skin. If the wound has necrotic tissue, it must be debrided. Debridement methods include mechanical (whirlpool, wet-to-dry); sharp (scalpel, scissors); enzymatic (collagenase); and autolytic (hydrocolloid, hydrogel). Wound cleansing should be done with nontoxic preparations; normal saline is recommended. Other principles are presented in Box 14.7. The NPUAP *Prevention and Treatment of Pressure Ulcers Clinical Practice Guidelines* (2014) provides guidance on selection of appropriate wound dressings based on wound characteristics. Box 14.8 presents general guidelines for pressure injury dressings.

Provision of education to patients, families, and professional staff must also be included in any skin care program. Teach the individual and his or her family about the normal healing process and keep them informed about progress (or lack of progress) toward healing, including signs and symptoms that should be brought to the professional's attention.

BOX 14.7 Mnemonic for Pressure Injury Treatment: DIPAMOPI

Debride
Identify and treat infection
Pack dead space lightly
Absorb excess exudate
Maintain moist wound surface
Open or excise closed wound edges
Protect healing wound from infection/trauma
Insulate to maintain normal temperature

BOX 14.8 Factors to Consider in Selecting Pressure Injury Dressing

- Shallow, dry wounds with no/minimal exudate need hydrating dressings that add or trap moisture; very shallow wounds require cover dressing only (gels/transparent adhesive dressings, thin hydrocolloid, thin polyurethane foam).
- Shallow wounds with moderate to large exudate need dressings that absorb exudate, maintain moist surface, support autolysis if necrotic tissue present, protect and insulate, and protect surrounding tissue (hydrocolloids, semipermeable polyurethane foam, calcium alginates, gauze). Cover with an absorptive cover dressing.
- Deep wounds with moderate to large exudate require filling of dead space, absorption of exudate, maintenance of moist environment, support of autolysis if necrotic tissue present, protection, and insulation (copolymer starch, dextranomer beads, calcium alginates, foam cavity). Cover with gauze pad, ABD, transparent thin film, or polyurethane foam.

KEY CONCEPTS

- The skin is the largest and most visible organ of the body; it has multiple roles in maintaining one's health.

- Maintaining adequate oral hydration and skin lubrication will reduce the incidence of xerosis and other skin problems.
- The best way to minimize the risk of skin cancer is to avoid prolonged sun exposure.
- The primary risk factors for pressure injury development are immobility and reduced activity. Individuals at greatest risk include those who are confined to bed or chair and unable to shift weight or reposition themselves.
- Structured protocols and prevention bundles should be present in all facilities and have been shown to reduce pressure injury development.
- A pressure injury is documented by stage, which reflects the greatest degree of tissue damage; and as the pressure injury heals, reverse staging is not appropriate.
- A pressure injury that is covered in dead tissue (eschar or slough) cannot be staged until it has been debrided.
- Darkly pigmented persons will not display the "typical" erythema of a stage 1 pressure injury or early PVD; therefore, closer vigilance is necessary.

ACTIVITIES AND DISCUSSION QUESTIONS

1. Describe the common skin conditions an older adult is more likely to experience.
2. What is the nurse's responsibility in health promotion related to maintaining skin integrity?
3. How does skin color affect the presentation of deep tissue injury?
4. What evidence-based protocols can the nurse utilize for prevention of pressure injuries?
5. Develop a nursing care plan for an older adult at risk for pressure injury using wellness and North American Nursing Diagnosis Association (NANDA) diagnoses.

REFERENCES

Agency for Healthcare Research and Quality: *On-time pressure ulcer healing project*, 2009. Available at http://www.ahrq.gov/professionals/systems/long-term-care/resources/pressure-ulcers/pressureulcerhealing/index.html. Accessed August 2016.

Ahn C, Salicido R: Advances in wound photography and assessment methods, *Adv Skin Wound Care* 21(2):94–95, 2008.

American Cancer Society: *Cancer facts and figures 2014*, 2014. Available at http://www.cancer.org/research/cancerfactsstatistics/cancerfactsfigures2014. Accessed March 7, 2014.

Armstrong D, Ayello E, Capitulo K, et al: New opportunities to improve pressure ulcer prevention and treatment: Implementations of the CMS inpatient hospital care present on admission (POA) indicators/hospital acquired conditions (HAC) policy, *Wounds* 20:A14, 2008.

Ayello E, Sibbald R: Preventing skin ulcers and skin tears. In Boltz M, Capezuti E, Fulmer T, et al, editors: *Evidence-based geriatric nursing protocols for best practice*, ed 4, New York, 2012, Springer, pp 298–319.

Baumgarten N, Margolis D, Orwig D, et al: Use of pressure-redistributing support surfaces among elderly hip fracture patients across the continuum of care: Adherence to pressure ulcer prevention guidelines, *Gerontologist* 50:253–262, 2009.

Black J, Edsberg L, Baharestani M, et al: Pressure ulcers: Avoidable or unavoidable? Results of the National Pressure Ulcer Advisory Panel Consensus Conference, *Ostomy Wound Manage* 57(2):24–37, 2011.

Centers for Disease Control and Prevention: *Parasites-scabies*, 2010. Available at http://www.cdc.gov/parasites/scabies/. Accessed November 2015.

Centers for Disease Control and Prevention: *Shingles (herpes zoster)*, 2014. Available at http://www.cdc.gov/shingles. Accessed November 2015.

Cooper K: Evidence-based prevention of pressure ulcers in the intensive care unit, *Crit Care Nurse* 33(6):57–66, 2013.

Endo J, Norman R: Skin problems. In Ham R, Sloane P, Warshaw G, et al, editors: *Primary care geriatrics*, ed 6, Philadelphia, 2014, Elsevier, pp 573–587.

European Pressure Ulcer Advisory Panel: *SCALE—Skin changes at life's end*, 2009. Available at http://www.epuap.org/scale-skin-hanges-at-lifes-end/. Accessed March 11, 2014.

Garcia A, White-Chu E: Pressure ulcers. In Ham R, Sloane P, Warshaw G, et al, editors: *Primary care geriatrics*, ed 6, Philadelphia, 2014, Elsevier, pp 333–343.

Garrett C, Saavedra A, Reed K, et al: Increasing incidence of melanoma among middle-aged adults: An epidemiological study in Olmsted County, Minnesota, *Mayo Clin Proc* 89(1):52–59, 2014.

Gillespie B, Chaboyer W, Sykes M, et al: Development and pilot testing of a patient-participatory pressure ulcer prevention bundle, *J Nurs Care Qual* 29(1):74–82, 2014.

Gray-Siracusa K, Schrier L: Use of an intervention bundle to eliminate pressure ulcers in critical care, *J Nurs Care Qual* 26(3):216–225, 2011.

Harden R, Kaye A, Kintanar T, et al: Evidence-based guideline for the management of postherpetic neuralgia in primary care, *Postgrad Med* 125(4):191–202, 2013.

Harms S, Bliss D, Garrad J, et al: Prevalence of pressure ulcers by race and ethnicity for older adults admitted to nursing homes, *J Gerontol Nurs* 40(3):20–26, 2014.

Howard D, Taylor Y: Racial and gender differences in pressure development among nursing home residents in the southeastern United States, *J Women Aging* 21:266–278, 2009.

Jamshed N, Schneider E: Is the use of supplemental vitamin C and zinc for the prevention and treatment of pressure ulcers evidence-based? *Ann Longterm Care* 18:28–32, 2010.

Jull A, Griffiths P: Is pressure ulcer prevention a sensitive indicator of the quality of nursing care? A cautionary note, *Int J Nurs Stud* 47:531–533, 2010.

Langana S, Minassiana C, Smeeth L, et al: Risk of stroke following herpes zoster: A self-controlled case-series study, *Clin Infect Dis*

Apr 2, 2014. doi: 10.1093/cid/ciu098. http://cid.oxfordjournals.org/content/early/2014/03/25/cid.ciu098.abstract. Accessed August 2016. [Epub ahead of print].

LeBlanc K, Baranoski S: International skin tear advisory panel: A tool kit to aid in the prevention, assessment, and treatment of skin tears using a simplified classification system, *Adv Skin Wound Care* 26:459–476, 2013.

Lee J, Cummings H, Carpenter C, et al: Herpes zoster knowledge, prevalence, and vaccination rate by race, *J Am Board Fam Med* 26(1):45–51, 2013.

McCance S, Huether S: Structure, function, and disorders of the integument. In McCance K, Huether S, editors: *Pathophysiology*, ed 7, St Louis, MO, 2014, Elsevier, pp 1616–1651.

McGinnis E, Greenwood D, Nelson A, et al: A prospective cohort study of prognostic factors for the healing of heel pressure ulcers, *Age Ageing* 43:267–271, 2013.

National Pressure Ulcer Advisory Panel: *New 2014 Prevention and Treatment of Pressure Ulcers Clinical Practice Guideline*, 2014. Available at http://www.npuap.org/resources/educational-and-clinical-resources/prevention-and-treatment-of-pressure-ulcers-clinical-practice-guideline/. Accessed August 2016.

National Pressure Ulcer Advisory Panel: *NPUAP announces a change in terminology from pressure ulcer to pressure injury and updates the stages of pressure injury*, April 13, 2016. Available at http://www.npuap.org/national-pressure-ulcer-advisory-panel-npuap-announces-a-change-in-terminology-from-pressure-ulcer-to-pressure-injury-and-updates-the-stages-of-pressure-injury/. Accessed August 2016.

Olsho L, Spector W, Williams C, et al: Evaluation of AHRQ's on-time pressure ulcer prevention program: A facilitator-assisted clinical decision support intervention for nursing homes, *Med Care* 52(3):258–266, 2014.

Phillips L, Buttery J: Exploring pressure ulcer prevalence and preventative care, *Nurs Times* 105(16):34–36, 2009.

Sibbald R, Krasner D, Lutz J, et al: SCALE: Skin changes at life's end: Final consensus statement: October 1, 2009, *Adv Skin Wound Care* 23(5):225–236, 2010.

Skin Cancer Foundation: *Skin cancer facts*, 2014. Available at http://www.skincancer.org/skin-cancer-information. Accessed March 7, 2014.

Spillsbury K, Nelson A, Cullum N, et al: Pressure ulcers and their treatment and effects on quality of life: Hospital inpatient perspectives, *J Adv Nurs* 57:494–504, 2007.

Tayyib N, Coyer F, Lewis P: Pressure ulcers in the adult intensive care unit: A literature review of patient risk factors and risk assessment scales, *J Nurs Educ Pract* 3(11):28–42, 2013.

U.S. Department of Health and Human Services: *Surgeon General calls for action to prevent skin cancer*, 2014. Available at http://www.surgeongeneral.gov/library/calls/prevent-skin-cancer. Accessed August 2014.

U.S. Food and Drug Administration: *FDA to require warnings on sunlamp products*, May 29, 2014. Available at http://www.fda.gov/NewsEvents/Newsroom/PressAnnouncements/ucm399222.htm. Accessed November 2015.

Warner-Maron I: The risk of risk assessment: Pressure ulcer assessment and the Braden Scale, *Ann Longterm Care Clin Care Aging* 23(5):23–27, 2015.

Wehner M, Chren C, Nameth D, et al: International prevalence of indoor tanning: A systematic review and meta-analysis, *JAMA Dermatol* Jan 29, 2013. doi: 10.1001/jamadermatol.2013.6896. [Epub ahead of print].

White-Chu F, Langemo D: Skin failure: Identifying and managing an underrecognized condition, *Ann Longterm Care* 20(7):28–32, 2012.

World Health Organization: *Ultraviolet radiation and the INTERSUN Programme: Skin cancers*, 2014. Available at http://www.who.int/uv/faq/skincancer/en/index2.html. Accessed March 23, 2014.

Wounds International: *International guidelines. Pressure ulcer prevention: Prevalence and incidence in context. A consensus document,* London, 2009, Medical Education Partnership (MEP) Ltd. Available at http://www.woundsinternational.com/clinical-guidelines/international-guidelines-pressure-ulcer-prevention-prevalence-and-incidence-in-context-a-consensus-document. Accessed March 10, 2014.

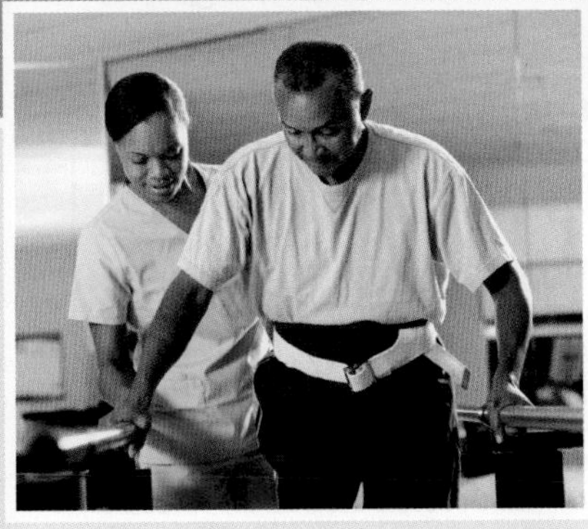

15

Falls and Fall Risk Reduction

Theris A. Touhy

evolve.elsevier.com/Touhy/gerontological

LEARNING OBJECTIVES

Upon completion of this chapter, the reader will be able to:

- Identify factors that increase vulnerability to falls.
- Discuss the components of comprehensive assessment of fall risk.
- List several interventions to reduce fall risks and identify those at high risk.
- Describe the effects of physical restraints and identify alternative safety interventions.

THE LIVED EXPERIENCE

After that fall last year when I slipped on the urine in the bathroom, I feel so insecure. I find myself taking small, shuffling steps to avoid falling again, but it makes me feel awkward and clumsy. When I was younger, I never worried about falling, but now I'm so afraid I will break a bone or something.

Betty, age 75

FALLS

Falls are one of the most important geriatric syndromes and the leading cause of morbidity and mortality for people older than 65 years of age. In the United States, falls occur in one-third of adults 65 and older. Among older adults, falls are the leading cause of both fatal and nonfatal injuries and the most common cause of hospital admissions for trauma. Approximately 20% to 30% of people who fall suffer moderate to severe injuries (lacerations, hip fracture, traumatic brain injury [TBI]) (Centers for Disease Control and Prevention [CDC], 2015a; Gray-Micelli & Quigley, 2012). Estimates are that up to two-thirds of falls may be preventable (Lach, 2010). Box 15.1 presents further data on falls.

Falls are considered a nursing-sensitive quality indicator. In acute care hospitals, patient falls are the most common incidents reported (Zhao & Kim, 2015). All falls in skilled nursing facilities are considered sentinel events and must be reported to the Centers for Medicare and Medicaid Services (CMS). The Joint Commission (TJC) has established national patient safety goals (NPSG) for fall reduction in all TJC-approved institutions across the health care continuum. CMS implemented a new policy in 2008 that eliminated the reimbursement to hospitals for treatment of injuries

BOX 15.1 Statistics on Falls and Fall-Related Concerns

- Up to 50% of hospitalized patients are at risk for falls and almost half of those who fall suffer an injury. Between 50% and 75% of nursing home residents fall annually, twice the rate of community-dwelling older adults.
- The death rate from falls is 40% higher for men than women.
- Rates of fall-related fractures among older adults are more than twice as high for women as for men.
- More than 95% of hip fractures among older adults are caused by falls. White women have significantly higher hip fracture rates than black women.
- Up to 25% of adults who lived independently before their hip fracture have to stay in a nursing home for at least 1 year after their injury.
- The direct medical costs of fall injuries are $31 billion annually. Hospital costs account for two-thirds of the total costs.
- Falls are considered a nursing-sensitive quality indicator.

Data from Centers for Disease Control and Prevention: *Important facts about falls.* Available at http://www.cdc.gov/homeandrecreationalsafety/falls/adultfalls.html. Accessed September 2016.

resulting from falls occurring during hospitalization (Zhao & Kim, 2015). *Healthy People 2020* includes several goals related to falls (Box 15.2).

SAFETY ALERT

Education on falls and fall risk reduction is an important consideration in the Quality and Safety Education for Nurses (QSEN) safety competency, which addresses the need to minimize risk of harm to patients and providers through both system effectiveness and individual performance. Safe and effective transfer techniques are an important component of safety measures.

Consequences of Falls

Hip Fractures

More than 95% of hip fractures among older adults are caused by falls. Hip fracture is the second leading cause of hospitalization for older people, occurring predominantly in older adults with underlying osteoporosis. Hip fractures are associated with considerable morbidity and mortality. Recovery from hip fractures is complicated by the presence of multiple comorbid conditions and potentially avoidable problems such as weight loss, delirium, pain, falls, and incontinence (Popejoy et al., 2012). Only 50% to 60% of patients with hip fractures will recover their prefracture ambulation abilities in the first year postfracture. Older adults who fracture a hip have a five to eight times increased risk of mortality

BOX 15.2 *Healthy People 2020*

Falls, Fall Prevention, Injury

- Reduce the rate of emergency department visits due to falls among older adults.
- Reduce fatal and nonfatal injuries.
- Reduce hospitalizations for nonfatal injuries.
- Reduce emergency department visits for nonfatal injuries.
- Reduce fatal and nonfatal traumatic brain injuries.

From U.S. Department of Health and Human Services, Office of Disease Prevention and Health Promotion: *Healthy People 2020,* 2012. Available at http://www.healthypeople.gov/2020.

during the first 3 months after hip fracture. This excess mortality persists for 10 years after the fracture and is higher in men. Most research on hip fractures has been conducted with older women, and further studies of both men and racially and culturally diverse older adults are necessary.

Traumatic Brain Injury

Older adults (75 years of age and older) have the highest rates of traumatic brain injury (TBI)-related hospitalization and death. Falls are the leading cause of TBI for older adults. Advancing age negatively affects the outcome after TBI, even with relatively minor head injuries. A CDC initiative, *Help Seniors Live Better Longer: Prevent Brain Injury,* provides educational resource materials on TBI for older adults, caregivers, and health care professionals in both Spanish and English (CDC, 2015b) (Box 15.3).

Factors that place the older adult at greater risk for TBI include the presence of comorbid conditions, use of aspirin and anticoagulants, and changes in the brain with age. Brain changes with age, although clinically insignificant, do increase the risk of TBIs and especially subdural hematomas, which are much more common in older adults. There is a decreased adherence of the dura mater to the skull, increased fragility of bridging cerebral veins, and increased subarachnoid space and atrophy of the brain, which results in more space within the cranial vault for blood to accumulate before symptoms appear (Timmons & Menaker, 2010). While most TBIs occur from falls, older people may experience TBI with seemingly more minor incidents (e.g., sharp turns or jarring movement of the head). Some patients may not even remember the incident.

In cases of moderate to severe TBI, there will be cognitive and physical sequelae obvious at the time of injury or shortly afterward that will require emergency treatment. However, older adults who experience a minor incident with seemingly lesser trauma to the head

BOX 15.3 Resources for Best Practice

Fall Prevention and Restraint Alternatives

Advancing Excellence in America's Nursing Homes: Fast Facts: Physical Restraints

AHRQ: Preventing falls in hospitals: a toolkit for improving quality of care

American Geriatrics Society/British Geriatrics Society: *Clinical Practice Guideline for Prevention of Falls in Older Persons*

American Nurses Association: *Safe patient handling and mobility: Interprofessional national standards across the care continuum,* 2013

Bradas C, Sandhu S, Mion L: Physical restraints and side rails in acute and critical care settings. In Boltz M, Capezuti E, Fulmer T, et al, editors: *Evidence-based geriatric nursing protocols for best practice,* ed 4, pp 1229–1245, New York, 2012, Springer

CDC: STEADI (Stopping Elderly Accidents, Deaths & Injuries): Educational materials for patients and providers; Check for safety: a home fall prevention checklist for older adults; Safe patient handling for schools of nursing (curricular materials)

Gericareonline: Story of Your Falls

Gray-Micelli D, Quigley P: Fall prevention, assessment, diagnoses, and intervention strategies. In Boltz M, Capezuti E, Fulmer T, et al, editors: *Evidence-based geriatric nursing protocols for best practice,* ed 4, pp 268–297, New York, 2012, Springer

HELP (Hospital Elder Life Program): http://www.hospitalelderlifeprogram.org/public/public-main.php

Hartford Institute for Geriatric Nursing (consultgerirn.org): Fall prevention: assessment, diagnosis, intervention strategies; Avoiding restraints in hospitalized older adults with dementia; Dementia series

Institute for Clinical Systems Improvement: Health care protocol: Prevention of falls (acute care)

NIH Senior Health: Falls and Older Adults—Fall Proofing Your Home

The GROW Program: Getting Residents Out of Wheelchairs

TMF Health Quality Institute: Restraints: Side Rail Utilization Assessment

VA National Center for Patient Safety: Falls Toolkit; Morse Fall Scale

often present with more insidious and delayed symptom onset. Because of changes in the aging brain, there is an increased risk for slowly expanding subdural hematomas. Health professionals should have a high suspicion of TBI in an older adult who falls and strikes the head or experiences even a more minor event, such as sudden twisting of the head.

For older adults who are receiving anticoagulant therapy and experience minor head injury with a negative computed tomography (CT) scan, a protocol of 24-hour observation followed by a second CT scan is recommended (Mendito et al., 2012). Manifestations of TBI are often misinterpreted as signs of dementia, which can lead to inaccurate prognoses and limit implementation of appropriate treatment. Box 15.4 presents signs and symptoms of TBI.

BOX 15.4 Signs and Symptoms of Traumatic Brain Injury (TBI) in Older Adults

Symptoms of Mild TBI

- Low-grade headache that will not dissipate
- Having more trouble than usual remembering things, paying attention or concentrating, organizing daily tasks, or making decisions and solving problems
- Slowness in thinking, speaking, acting, or reading
- Getting lost or easily confused
- Feeling tired all of the time, lack of energy or motivation
- Change in sleep pattern (sleeping much longer than usual, having trouble sleeping)
- Loss of balance, feeling light-headed or dizzy
- Increased sensitivity to sounds, lights, distractions
- Blurred vision or eyes that tire easily
- Loss of sense of taste or smell
- Ringing in the ears
- Change in sex drive
- Mood changes (feeling sad, anxious, listless, or becoming easily irritated or angry for little or no reason)

Symptoms of Moderate to Severe TBI

- Severe headache that gets worse or does not disappear
- Repeated vomiting or nausea
- Seizures
- Inability to wake from sleep
- Dilation of one or both pupils
- Slurred speech
- Weakness or numbness in the arms or legs
- Loss of coordination
- Increased confusion, restlessness, or agitation

NOTE: Older adults taking blood thinners should be seen immediately by a health care provider if they have a bump or blow to the head, even if they do not have any of the symptoms listed here.

From Centers for Disease Control and Prevention: *Help seniors live better, longer: prevent brain injury,* 2014. Available at http://www.cdc.gov/traumaticbraininjury/seniors.html. Accessed April 2014.

Fallophobia

Even if a fall does not result in injury, falls contribute to a loss of confidence that leads to reduced physical activity, increased dependency, and social withdrawal. Fear of falling (fallophobia) may cause a person to restrict his or her physical and social activities, leading to further functional decline, depression, social isolation, and decreased quality of life (Zhao & Kim, 2015). Fear of falling is an important predictor of general functional decline and a risk factor for future falls (Hill et al., 2010; Rubenstein et al., 2003).

Nursing staff may also contribute to fear of falling in their patients by telling them not to get up by themselves or by using restrictive devices to keep them from independently moving. More appropriate nursing responses include assessing fall risk and designing individual interventions and safety plans that will enhance mobility and independence, as well as reduce fall risk.

Fall Risk Factors

Falls are a symptom of a problem and are rarely benign in older people. The etiology of falls is multifactorial; falls may indicate neurological, sensory, cardiac, cognitive, medication, or musculoskeletal problems or impending illness. Episodes of acute illness, infection, or exacerbations of chronic illness are times of high fall risk (Fig. 15.1).

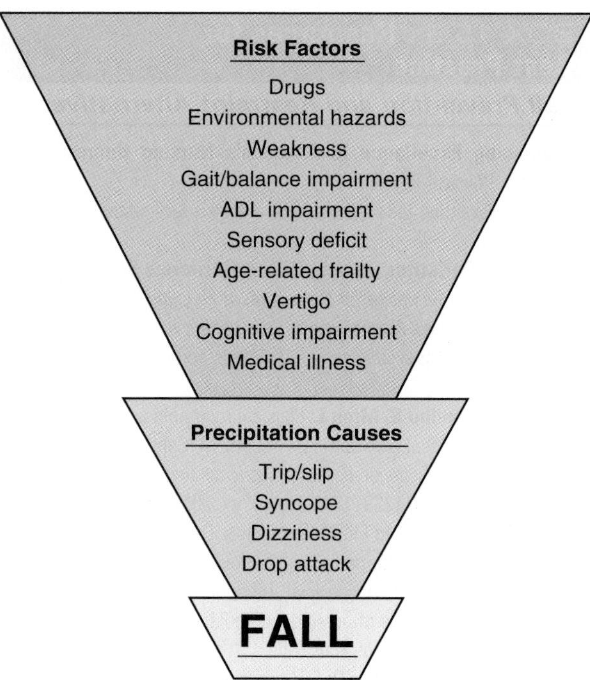

FIGURE 15.1 Multifactorial nature of falls. (From Ham RJ, Sloane PD, Warshaw GA, et al: *Primary care geriatrics,* ed 6, Philadelphia, 2014, Elsevier.)

SAFETY ALERT

A history of falls is an important risk factor and individuals who have fallen have three times the risk of falling again compared with persons who did not fall in the past year. Recurrent falls are often the result of the same underlying cause but can also be an indication of disease progression (e.g., heart failure, Parkinson's disease) or a new acute problem (e.g., infection, dehydration) (Rubenstein & Dillard, 2014).

Risk factors can be categorized as either intrinsic or extrinsic. Intrinsic risk factors are unique to each individual and are associated with factors such as reduced vision and hearing, unsteady gait, cognitive impairment, acute and chronic illnesses, and effects of medications. Extrinsic risk factors are external to the individual and related to the physical environment and include lack of support equipment for bathtubs and toilets, height of beds, condition of floors, poor lighting, inappropriate footwear, and improper use of assistive devices.

Falls in the young-old and the more healthy old occur more frequently because of external reasons; however, with increasing age and comorbid conditions, internal and locomotor reasons become increasingly prevalent as factors contributing to falls. The risk of falling increases as the number of risk factors increases, and the majority of falls occur from a combination of intrinsic and extrinsic factors that combine at a certain point in time. "Most falls in hospitals result from interactions between person-specific risk factors, the physical environment, the riskiness of a person's behavior, and the interactions between the patient and the hospital staff" (Basic & Hartwell, 2015, p. 1637).

In institutional settings, extrinsic factors such as limited staffing, the lack of toileting programs, and the use of restraints and side rails also interact to increase fall risk. In hospitals, inadequate staff communication and training, incomplete patient assessments and reassessments, environmental issues, incomplete care planning or delayed care provision, and an inadequate organizational culture of safety have been reported as factors contributing to falls.

Gait Disturbances

Gait disturbances affect between 20% and 50% of people older than 65 years, and are associated with a threefold increase in fall risk (Alexander, 2014). Marked gait disorders are not normally a consequence of aging alone but are more likely indicative of an underlying pathological condition. Arthritis of the knee may result in ligamentous weakness and instability, causing the legs to give way or collapse. Diabetes, dementia, Parkinson's disease, stroke, alcoholism, and vitamin B deficiencies may cause neurological damage and resultant gait problems.

The Hendrich II Fall Risk Model (Mathias et al., 1986) (Fig. 15.2) includes the Get-Up-and-Go Test, which can be used to assess mobility, gait, and gait speed. This test is useful in fall risk assessment as well. It is a practical assessment tool that can be adapted to any setting. The client is asked to rise from a straight-backed chair, stand briefly, walk forward about 10 feet, turn, walk back to the chair, turn around, and sit down. The test can be timed as well, and gait speed has been found to be a predictor of mobility. On the basis of the results of initial screening, older adults may need further evaluation.

Foot Deformities

Foot deformities and ill-fitting footwear also contribute to gait problems and potential for falls. Care of the feet is an important aspect of mobility, comfort, and a stable gait and is often neglected. Little attention is given to

Hendrich II Fall Risk Model™

Confusion Disorientation Impulsivity		4	
Symptomatic Depression		2	
Altered Elimination		1	
Dizziness Vertigo		1	
Male Gender		1	
Any Administered Antiepileptics		2	
Any Administered Benzodiazepines		1	
Get Up & Go Test			
Able to rise in a single movement – No loss of balance with steps		0	
Pushes up, successful in one attempt		1	
Multiple attempts, but successful		3	
Unable to rise without assistance during test (OR if a medical order states the same and/or complete bed rest is ordered) * If unable to assess, document this on the patient chart with the date and time		4	
A Score of 5 or Greater = High Risk	**Total Score**		

FIGURE 15.2 The Hendrich II Fall Risk Model is a fall risk assessment tool recommended by the Hartford Institute for Geriatric Nursing. (© 2013 AHI of Indiana Inc. All rights reserved. U.S. patent numbers 7,282,031 and 7,682,308.)

one's feet until they interfere with walking and moving and ultimately the ability to remain independent. Foot problems are often unrecognized and untreated, leading to considerable dysfunction.

As we age, feet are subjected to a lifetime of stress and may not be able to continue to adapt, and inflammatory changes in bone and soft tissue can occur. Many individuals are limited by foot problems; approximately 90% of adults 65 and older have some form of altered foot integrity such as nail fungus, dry skin, and corns and calluses (Andersen et al., 2010). Some older persons are unable to walk comfortably, or at all, because of neglect of corns, bunions, and overgrown nails. The ability to perform self care of the feet may be difficult for elders with functional or cognitive impairments or vision problems.

Other causes of problems may be traced to loss of fat cushioning and resilience with aging, diabetes, ill-fitting shoes, poor arch support, excessively repetitious weight-bearing activities, obesity, or uneven distribution of weight on the feet. Both diabetes and peripheral vascular disease (PVD) commonly cause problems in the lower extremities that can quickly become life-threatening. Estimates are that 20% of individuals with diabetes are admitted to hospitals because of foot problems and more than 60% of nontraumatic lower-limb amputations are performed in people with diabetes (Tewary et al., 2013).

BOX 15.5 Tips for Best Practice

Foot Assessment

Observation of Mobility
- Gait
- Use of assistive devices
- Footwear type and pattern of wear

Past Medical History
- Neuropathies
- Musculoskeletal limitations
- Peripheral vascular disease (PVD)
- Vision problems
- History of falls
- Pain affecting movement

Bilateral Assessment
- Color
- Circulation and warmth
- Pulses
- Structural deformities
- Skin lesions
- Lower-extremity edema
- Evidence of scratching
- Abrasions and other lesions
- Rash or excessive dryness
- Condition and color of toenails

❖ IMPLICATIONS FOR GERONTOLOGICAL NURSING AND HEALTHY AGING

Care of the foot takes a team approach, including the person, the nurse, the podiatrist, and the primary health care provider. Nursing care of the person with foot problems should be directed toward providing optimal comfort and function, removing possible mechanical irritants, and decreasing the likelihood of infection. The nurse has the important function of assessing the feet for clues of functional ability and their owner's well-being (Box 15.5). Nurses can identify potential and actual problems and make referrals or seek assistance as needed from the primary care provider or podiatrist for any changes in the feet.

Orthostatic and Postprandial Hypotension

Declines in depth perception, proprioception, and normotensive response to postural changes are important factors that contribute to falls. Clinically significant orthostatic hypotension (OH) is a common clinical finding in frail older adults. Among cognitively impaired individuals who reside in skilled nursing facilities, estimates are that 50% to 60% experience OH (Momeyer, 2014). Asymptomatic OH is common. Gray-Micelli and colleagues (2012) reported that loss of balance may be predictive of OH and should trigger assessment.

Orthostatic hypotension is considered a decrease of 20 mm Hg (or more) in systolic pressure or a decrease of 10 mm Hg (or more) in diastolic pressure with position change from lying or sitting to standing. However, these criteria may be too restrictive for some older adults (Gray-Micelli et al., 2012). The detection of orthostatic hypotension (OH) is of clinical importance to fall prevention because OH is treatable. Evidence-based standards of care for fall prevention require OH blood pressure assessment among older adults.

Postprandial hypotension (PPH) occurs after ingestion of a carbohydrate meal and may be related to the release of a vasodilatory peptide. PPH is more common in people with diabetes and Parkinson's disease but has been found in approximately 25% of persons who fall. Lifestyle modifications such as increasing water intake before eating or substituting six smaller meals daily for three larger meals may be effective, but further research is needed (Luciano et al., 2010). All older persons should be cautioned against sudden rising from sitting or supine positions, particularly after eating.

Cognitive Impairment

The presence of neurocognitive disorders, such as dementia and delirium, increases risk for falls twofold, and individuals with dementia are also at increased risk of major injuries (fracture) related to falls. Fall risk assessments may need to include more specific cognitive risk factors, and cognitive assessment measures, especially for delirium, may need to be more frequently scheduled for at-risk individuals (Eshkoor et al., 2014; Gray-Micelli et al., 2010).

Vision and Hearing

Formal vision assessment is also an important intervention to identify remediable visual problems. Although a significant relationship exists between visual problems and falls and fractures, little research has been conducted on interventions for visual problems as part of fall risk–reduction programs. Poor visual acuity, reduced contrast sensitivity, decreased visual field, cataracts, and use of nonmiotic glaucoma medications have all been associated with falls. Hearing ability is also directly related to fall risk. For someone with only a mild hearing loss, there is a threefold increased chance of having falls (Lin & Ferrucci, 2012).

Medications

Medications implicated in increasing fall risk include those causing potentially dangerous side effects including drowsiness, mental confusion, problems with balance, loss of urinary control, and sudden drops in blood pressure with standing. These include psychotropics (benzodiazepines, sedative-hypnotics, antidepressants, neuroleptics), opioids, antiarrhythmics, digoxin, antihypertensives, and diuretics (Gray-Micelli & Quigley, 2012; Tinetti et al., 2014). All medications, including over-the-counter (OTC) and herbal medications, should be reviewed and limited to those that are absolutely essential. Patient teaching should be provided related to fall risk, appropriate dosing, and drug-drug and drug-alcohol interactions.

❖ IMPLICATIONS FOR GERONTOLOGICAL NURSING AND HEALTHY AGING

◆ Screening and Assessment

The American Geriatrics Society/British Geriatrics Society *Clinical Practice Guideline: Prevention of Falls in Older Persons* (2010) recommends that fall risk assessment be an integral part of primary health care for the older person. All older individuals should be asked whether they have fallen in the past year and whether they experience difficulties with walking or balance. In addition, ask about falls that did not result in an injury and the circumstances of a near-fall, mishap, or misstep because this may provide important information for prevention of future falls. Older people may be reluctant to share information about falls for fear of losing independence, so the nurse must use judgment and empathy in eliciting information about falls, assuring the person that there are many modifiable factors to increase safety and help maintain independence.

Comprehensive fall assessments include the following components: cognitive, nutrition, environment, medications, pathological conditions, functional assessment, gait, feet and footwear, home safety, and a complete physical examination (including vision and hearing, as well as musculoskeletal and cardiovascular status).

◆ Screening and Assessment in Hospital/Long-Term Care

Individuals admitted to acute or long-term care settings should have an initial fall assessment on admission, after any change in condition, and at regular intervals during their stay. Assessment is an ongoing process that includes multiple and continual types of assessment, reassessment, and evaluation following a fall or intervention to reduce the risk of a fall. "Assessment includes: (1) assessment of the older adult at risk; (2) nursing assessment of the patient following a fall; (3) assessment of the environment and other situational circumstances upon admission to a health care facility; (4) assessment of the older adult's knowledge of falls and their prevention, including willingness to change behavior, if necessary, to prevent falls" (Gray-Micelli, 2008, p. 164) (Table 15.1).

An interprofessional team (physician or nurse practitioner, nurse, risk manager, physical and occupational therapists, and other designated staff) should be involved in planning care on the basis of findings from an individualized assessment. Nurses bring expert knowledge of patient activities, abilities, and needs from a 24-hours-per-day, 7-days-per week perspective to help the team implement the most appropriate interventions and evaluate outcomes.

Fall Risk Assessment Instruments

Fall risk is formally assessed through administration of fall risk tools. However, current literature (Degelau et al., 2012) supports using the following three questions to determine fall risk: (1) Has the patient fallen in the past year? (2) Does the patient look like he or she is going to fall (does the patient have clinically detected gait/balance abnormalities)? (3) Does the patient have

TABLE 15.1 Nursing Assessment to Identify Underlying Causes of Unsafe Behavior

Assessment	Strategy
Behavior history	Obtain background about unsafe behavior from patient, family, and prior caregivers (e.g., nursing home staff).
Physiological factors	Assess for sedation levels; pain; electrolyte disturbances; infection; orthostatic hypotension; syncope; urinary symptoms or urinary or fecal retention; inadequate sleep; and difficulties with walking, balance, or mobility.
Psychological concerns	Assess communication ability (i.e., in regard to stroke, dementia, and different primary language); depression; anxiety; impulsivity; agitation; fear; grief; posttraumatic stress disorder; substance abuse, including drugs, alcohol, or nicotine; and stressors, support systems, and coping strategies.
Medications	Identify medications that may contribute to confusion, delirium, movement disorders, and falls, such as reaction to a new medication or adverse reaction or drug interaction.
Environment	Examine bed appropriateness and safety, medical devices and necessity of use (e.g., ventilator tube, IV, urinary catheter), equipment and furniture (e.g., IV pole, bedside commode, bedside chair, tables, trapeze), lighting, noise levels, room temperature, and floor surface.

From Lach HW, Leach KM, Butcher HK: Changing the practice of physical restraint use in acute care, *J Gerontol Nurs* 42(2):17–26, 2016.

additional risk factors for injurious falls (e.g., osteoporosis, anticoagulant therapy)?

Fall risk assessment instruments are still commonly included in fall prevention interventions; instruments that are utilized need to be reliable and valid and nurses need to use them judiciously (Gray-Micelli & Quigley, 2012). Often, these instruments are completed in a routine manner and risk factors are not identified or may not be known because of lack of assessment and knowledge of the individual's history. Additionally, so many patients are identified as high risk that nurses may become desensitized and have difficulty prioritizing interventions (Harrison et al., 2010; Lach, 2010).

The National Center for Patient Safety recommends the Morse Falls Scale, but not for use in long-term care (Box 15.3). The Performance-Oriented Mobility Assessment (Tinetti, 1986) is a well-validated tool. The Hendrich II Fall Risk Model (Hendrich et al., 2003) (see Fig. 15.2) is recommended by the Hartford Foundation for Geriatric Nursing. This instrument has been validated with skilled nursing and rehabilitation populations and is also easy to use in the outpatient setting. In the skilled nursing facility, the Minimum Data Set (MDS 3.0) includes information about history of falls and hip fractures, as well as an assessment of balance during transitions and walking (moving from seated to standing, walking, turning around, moving on and off toilet, and transfers between bed and chair or wheelchair) (see Chapter 8).

Fall risk assessments provide first-level assessment data as the basis for comprehensive assessment, but comprehensive postfall assessments (PFAs) (Box 15.6) must be used to identify multifactorial risk factors as well as complex fall and injury risk factors in those who have fallen (Gray-Micelli & Quigley, 2012). It is very important that all assessment data reported concerning an individual's risk for falls be tailored with individual assessment so that appropriate fall risk–reduction interventions can be developed and modifiable risk factors identified and managed.

Postfall Assessment

Determination of the reason(s) a fall occurred (postfall assessment [PFA]) is vital and provides information on underlying fall etiologies so that appropriate plans of care can be instituted. Incomplete analysis of the reasons for a fall can result in repeated incidents. The purpose of the PFA is to identify the clinical status of the person, verify and treat injuries, identify underlying causes of the fall when possible, and assist in implementing appropriate individualized risk-reduction interventions. For falls that happen outside the hospital or skilled nursing facility, individuals can complete the "Story of Your Falls" (see Box 15.3) to provide postfall assessment information.

Components of the PFA

PFAs include a fall-focused history; fall circumstances; medical problems; medication review; mobility assessment; vision and hearing assessment; neurological examination (including cognitive assessment); and cardiovascular assessment (orthostatic blood pressure [BP], cardiac rhythm irregularities) (Gray-Micelli & Quigley, 2012). If the older adult cannot tell you about

BOX 15.6 Postfall Assessment Suggestions

Initiate emergency measures as indicated.

History

- Description of the fall from the individual or witness
- Individual's opinion of the cause of the fall
- Circumstances of the fall (trip or slip)
- Person's activity at the time of the fall
- Presence of comorbid conditions, such as a previous stroke, Parkinson's disease, osteoporosis, seizure disorder, sensory deficit, joint abnormalities, depression, cardiac disease
- Medication review
- Associated symptoms, such as chest pain, palpitations, lightheadedness, vertigo, loss of balance, fainting, weakness, confusion, incontinence, or dyspnea
- Time of day and location of the fall
- Presence of acute illness

Physical Examination

- Vital signs: postural blood pressure changes, fever, or hypothermia
- Head and neck: visual impairment, hearing impairment, nystagmus, bruit
- Heart: arrhythmias or valvular dysfunction
- Neurological signs: altered mental status, focal deficits, peripheral neuropathy, muscle weakness, rigidity or tremor, impaired balance
- Musculoskeletal signs: arthritic changes, range of motion (ROM) changes, podiatric deformities or problems, swelling, redness or bruises, abrasions, pain on movement, shortening and external rotation of lower extremities

Functional Assessment

- Functional gait and balance: observe resident rising from chair, walking, turning, and sitting
- Balance test, mobility, use of assistive devices or personal assistance, extent of ambulation, restraint use, prosthetic equipment
- Activities of daily living: bathing, dressing, transferring, toileting

Environmental Assessment

- Staffing patterns, unsafe practice in transferring, delay in response to call light
- Faulty equipment
- Use of bed, chair alarm
- Call light within reach
- Wheelchair, bed locked
- Adequate supervision
- Clutter, walking paths not clear
- Dim lighting
- Glare
- Uneven flooring
- Wet, slippery floors
- Poorly fitted seating devices
- Inappropriate footwear
- Inappropriate eyewear

the circumstances of the fall, information should be obtained from staff or witnesses. Because complications of falls may not occur immediately, all patients should be observed for 48 hours after a fall and vital signs and neurological status monitored for 7 days or more, as clinically indicated. Standard "incident report" forms do not provide adequate postfall assessment information. The Department of Veterans Affairs National Center for Patient Safety provides comprehensive information about fall assessment, fall risk reduction, and policies and procedures (Box 15.3).

Interventions

Lach (2010) reminds us that "while there is much that the nurse can do to manage falls, it may be unrealistic to think that they can be eliminated" (p. 151). Fall risk–reduction programs are a shared responsibility of all health care providers caring for older adults. Choosing the most appropriate interventions to reduce the risk of falls depends on appropriate assessment at various intervals depending on the person's changing condition and tailoring interventions to individual cognitive function and language (American Geriatrics Society and British Geriatrics Society, 2010a,b). A one-size-fits-all approach is not effective and further research is needed to determine the type, frequency, and timing of interventions best suited for specific populations.

Education about fall prevention is an important nursing intervention for patients, families, and the community. The CDC's STEADI (Stopping Elderly Accidents, Deaths & Injuries) Tool Kit is a valuable resource for providers and older adults and includes excellent teaching materials and fall prevention information (http://www.cdc.gov/steadi/about.html) (Box 15.3).

Fall Risk–Reduction Programs

There is some evidence to support the effectiveness of multicomponent fall risk–reduction strategies in many settings to reduce fall risks (Alexander, 2014; Cameron et al., 2010; Gillespie et al., 2012; Lee et al., 2013; Miake-Lye et al., 2013; Quigley & White, 2013; Tinetti et al., 2008). Randomized controlled trial evidence also suggests that single targeted interventions (e.g., exercise programs) might be as effective as multifactorial interventions (Campbell & Robertson, 2013). Frick and colleagues (2010) agree and suggest that multifactorial approaches aimed at all older people, or high-risk elders, are not necessarily more cost-effective or more efficacious than focused intervention approaches and further research is needed.

The optimal bundle of interventions is not established, but common components include risk assessment, patient and staff education, bedside signs and wristband alerts, footwear assessment, scheduled and supervised toileting programs, and medication reviews (Miake-Lye et al., 2013). The components most commonly included in efficacious interventions are shown in Box 15.7

Each institution should design strategies to meet organizational needs and to match patient population needs and clinical realities of the staff (Ireland et al., 2010). Programs that utilize a system-level quality improvement approach, including educational programs for staff, realized a decrease in fall rate of 5.8% in hospitals (Box 15.8). Examples of effective programs include Acute Care of the Elderly (ACE) units, Nurses Improving Care for Healthsystem Elders (NICHE), and the Geriatric Resource Nurse (GRN) model (Gray-Micelli & Quigley, 2012) (see Chapter 5). The Hospital Elder Life Program (HELP) is another valuable resource in fall prevention in the hospital (see Box 15.3).

Environmental Modifications

Environmental modifications alone have not been shown to reduce falls, but when included as part of a multifactorial program, they may be of benefit in risk reduction. However, a home safety assessment and modification interventions have been shown to be effective in reducing the rates of falls in community-dwelling older adults, especially for individuals at high risk of falling and those with visual impairments. It is recommended that home safety interventions be delivered by an occupational therapist (American Geriatrics Society/British Geriatrics Society, 2010a,b; Gillespie et al., 2012). The CDC provides a home fall prevention checklist (Box 15.3).

In institutional settings, the patient care environment should be assessed routinely for extrinsic factors that may contribute to falls and corrective action taken. Patient activities that contribute to falls include walking, transferring, and urinary and bowel elimination needs (Zhao & Kim, 2015). The majority of falls in acute care occur in patient rooms followed by bathrooms and hallways. Patients should be able to access the bathroom or be provided with a bedside commode, routine assistance to toilet, and programs such as prompted voiding (see Chapter 12). Shift change periods and evening and night shifts have also been associated with increased inpatient falls and supervision must be available during these times.

Assistive Devices

Research on multifactorial interventions including the use of assistive devices has demonstrated benefits in fall risk reduction. Many devices are available that are designed for specific conditions and limitations. Physical therapists provide training on use of assistive devices, and nurses can supervise correct use. Improper use of these devices can lead to increased fall risk. For the community-dwelling individual, Medicare may cover up to 80% of the cost of assistive devices with a written prescription. New technologies such as canes that "talk" and provide feedback to the user, sensors that detect

BOX 15.7 Suggested Components of Fall Risk–Reduction Interventions

- Adaptation or modification of the home environment
- Withdrawal or minimization of psychoactive medications
- Withdrawal or minimization of other medications
- Management of orthostatic hypotension
- Continence programs such as prompted voiding
- Management of foot problems and footwear
- Exercise, particularly balance, strength, and gait training
- Staff and patient education

From American Geriatrics Society/British Geriatrics Society: *2010 AGS/BGS clinical practice guideline: Prevention of falls in older persons, Summary of recommendations,* 2010. Available at http://www.americangeriatrics.org/files/documents/health_care_pros/Falls.Summary.Guide.pdf. Accessed April 2014.

BOX 15.8 System-Level Interventions for Fall Risk Reduction in Acute Care

- Nurse Champions
- Teach Backs (all patients and families receive education about their fall and injury risks)
- Comfort Care and Safety Rounds
- Safety Huddle Post Fall
- Protective Bundles: Patients with risk factors for serious injury, such as osteoporosis, anticoagulant use, and history of head injury or falls, are automatically placed on high fall risk precautions and interventions to reduce risk of serious injury
- Bundles may include interventions such as bedside mat on floor at side of bed, height-adjustable bed, helmet use, hip protectors, comfort and safety rounds

when falls have occurred or when risk of falling is increasing, and other developing assistive technologies hold the potential to significantly improve functional ability, safety, and independence for older people (Rantz et al., 2008) (see Chapter 16).

Safe Patient Handling

Lifting, transferring, and repositioning patients are the most common tasks that lead to injury for health care staff and patients in hospital and nursing home environments. Handling and moving patients offers multiple challenges because of variations in size, physical abilities, cognitive function, level of cooperation, and changes in condition. Nelson and Baptiste (2004) recommend the following evidence-based practices for safe patient handling: (1) patient handling equipment/devices; (2) patient-care ergonomic assessment protocols; (3) no-lift policies; (4) training on proper use of patient handling equipment/devices; and (5) patient lift teams. Key aspects of patient assessment to improve safety for patients and staff are presented in Box 15.9.

Wheelchairs

Wheelchairs are a necessary adjunct at some level of immobility and for some individuals, but they are overused in nursing homes, with up to 80% of residents spending time sitting in a wheelchair every day. Often, the individual is not assessed for therapeutic treatment and restorative ambulation programs to improve mobility and function. Improperly maintained or ill-fitting wheelchairs can cause pressure ulcers, skin tears, bruises and abrasions, and nerve impingement, and they account for 16% of nursing home falls (Gavin-Dreschnack et al., 2010). It is important that a professional evaluate the wheelchair for proper fit and provide training on proper use, as well as evaluate the resident for more appropriate mobility and seating devices and ambulation programs. There are many new assistive devices that could replace wheelchairs, such as small walkers with wheels and seats. If the person is unable to ambulate without assistance, the person should be seated in a comfortable chair with frequent repositioning and wheelchairs should be used for transport only.

BOX 15.9 Tips for Best Practice

Assessment of Safe Patient Handling

- Ability of the patient to provide assistance
- Ability of the patient to bear weight
- Upper extremity strength of the patient
- Ability of the patient to cooperate and follow instructions
- Patient height and weight
- Special circumstances likely to affect transfer or repositioning tasks, such as abdominal wounds, contractures, pressure ulcers, presence of tubes
- Specific physician orders or physical therapy recommendations that relate to transferring or repositioning patients (e.g., knee or hip replacement precautions)

From Nelson A, Baptiste A: Evidence-based practices for safe patient handling and movement, *Online J Issues Nurs* 9(3), 2004. Available at http://www.seiu1991.org/files/2013/07/Audrey_Nelson_Safe_Patient_Handling.pdf. Accessed April 2014.

Osteoporosis Treatment/Vitamin D Supplementation

Other potential interventions for fall risk reduction include assessment and treatment of osteoporosis to reduce fracture rates (see Chapter 21). Older people with osteoporosis are more likely to experience serious injury from a fall. The American Geriatrics Society recommends vitamin D supplementation of at least 1000 international units, as well as calcium supplementation, to community-dwelling and older adults residing in institutionalized settings to reduce the risk of fractures and falls (AGS, 2014a).

Hip Protectors

The use of hip protectors for prevention of hip fractures in high-risk individuals may be considered; there is some evidence that hip protectors have an overall effect on rates of hip fracture (Quigley et al., 2010), but further research is needed to determine their effectiveness. Compliance has been a concern related to the ease of removing them quickly enough for toileting, but newer designs that are more attractive and practical may assist with compliance issues (Willy & Osterberg, 2014).

Alarms/Motion Sensors

Alarms, either personal or chair/bed, are often used in fall prevention programs. There has been no research to support their effectiveness in prevention of a fall and "at best, it can shorten 'rescue time' " (Willy & Osterberg, 2014, p. 29). Some have suggested that the use of these alarms may increase patient agitation, especially in cognitively impaired individuals, impede functional status, and negatively impact feelings of dignity among older adults in nursing homes. The use of alarms may be more for the needs of the staff rather than the patients (Crogan & Dupler, 2014; Willy & Osterberg, 2014). Silent alarms, visual or auditory monitoring systems, motion detectors, and physical staff presence may be more effective. A recent study reported that use of motion sensors inside patient rooms may be a viable, cost-efficient, unobtrusive solution to prevent and detect falls (Rantz et al., 2014).

RESTRAINTS AND SIDE RAILS

Definition and History

A physical restraint is defined as any manual method, physical or mechanical device, material, or equipment that immobilizes or reduces the ability of a patient to move his or her arms, legs, body, or head freely. A chemical restraint is when a drug or medication is used as a restriction to manage the patient's behavior or restrict the patient's freedom of movement and is not a standard treatment or dosage for the patient's condition. Historically, restraints and side rails have been used for the "protection" of the patient and for the security of the patient and staff. Originally, restraints were used to control the behavior of individuals with mental illness considered to be dangerous to themselves or others (Evans & Strumpf, 1989).

Research over the past 30 years by nurses such as Lois Evans, Neville Strumpf, and Elizabeth Capezuti has shown that the practice of physical restraint is ineffective and hazardous. The use of physical restraints in long-term care settings was effectively addressed almost 25 years ago in these facilities. The Joint Commission and the Centers for Medicare and Medicaid Services (CMS) have focused on restraint reduction strategies in acute care over the past 10 to 15 years but studies continue to document that it is routine practice (Lach & Leach, 2016).

Consequences of Restraints

Physical restraints, intended to prevent injury, do not protect patients from falling, wandering, or removing tubes and other medical devices. Physical restraints may actually exacerbate many of the problems for which they are used and can cause serious injury and death, as well as emotional and physical problems. Physical restraints are associated with higher death rates, injurious falls, nosocomial infections, incontinence, contractures, pressure ulcers, agitation, and depression.

The use of restraints is a great source of physical and psychological distress to older adults and may intensify agitation and contribute to depression. For some older people, especially those with a history of trauma (such as that induced by war, rape, or domestic violence), side rails may cause fear and agitation and a feeling of being jailed or caged (Sullivan-Marx, 1995; Talerico & Capezuti, 2001).

Side Rails

Side rails are no longer viewed as simply attachments to a patient's bed but are considered restraints with all the accompanying concerns just discussed. Side rails are now defined as restraints or restrictive devices when used to impede a person's ability to voluntarily get out of bed and the person cannot lower them by themselves. Restrictive side rail use is defined as two full-length or four half-length raised side rails. If the patient uses a half- or quarter-length upper side rail to assist in getting in and out of bed, it is not considered a restraint (Talerico & Capezuti, 2001). CMS requires nursing homes to conduct individualized assessments of residents, provide alternatives, or clearly describe the need for restrictive side rails (Box 15.3).

Restraint-Free Care

Restraint-free care is now the standard of practice and an indicator of quality care in all health care settings, although transition to that standard is still in progress, particularly in acute care settings. Physical restraint use in acute care is now predominantly in intensive care units (ICUs), particularly for patients with medical devices and those with delirium. Older adults with delirium have higher risks of being restrained than other patients. Both the American Geriatrics Society and the American Board of Internal Medicine recommend that physical restraints should not be used to manage behavioral symptoms of hospitalized older adults with delirium (American Geriatrics Society, 2014b).

Further research is needed in ICU settings to determine the best strategies to manage delirium (see Chapter 25). Daily evaluation of the necessity of medical devices (intravenous lines, nasogastric tubes, catheters, endotracheal tubes), as well as securing or camouflaging (hiding) the device, is important (American Geriatrics Society/British Geriatrics Society, 2010a,b; Bradas et al., 2012). A decision algorithm for promoting restraint-free care in acute care is presented in Fig. 15.3. Evidence-based protocols on physical restraints and other resources on restraint alternatives can be found in Box 15.3.

Flaherty (2004) remarked that a "restraint-free environment should be held as the standard of care and anything less is substandard. The fact that it is done in some European hospitals (Bradas et al., 2012; de Vries et al., 2004) and in some U.S. hospitals, even among delirious patients, and in skilled nursing facilities should be evidence enough that it can be done everywhere" (p. 919). Implementing best practice nursing in fall risk reduction and restraint-free care is a complex clinical decision-making process and calls for recognition, assessment, and intervention for physical and psychosocial concerns contributing to patient safety, knowledge of restraint alternatives, interdisciplinary teamwork, and institutional commitment.

Removing restraints without careful attention to underlying fall risk factors and alternative strategies can

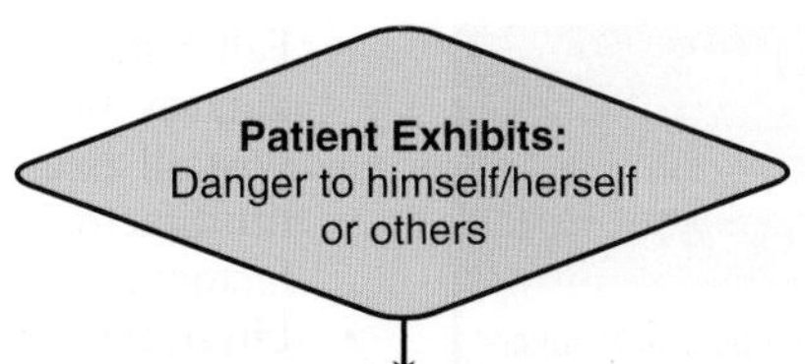

Nursing Assessment: Identify Underlying Factors Related to Unsafe Behavior

Physiological Factors	Psychological Factors	Environmental Factors
Acute illness, infection Medications Discomfort—pain, hunger, sleep deprivation, fatigue Urinary frequency/urgency, need to toilet Mobility problem Orthostasis Electrolyte imbalance	Agitation Delirium/confusion/cognitive impairment Stress/excess demands Grief, fear, anxiety, PTSD Substance abuse/withdrawal Inability to communicate needs Sedation level	Presence of annoying medical devices Bed appropriateness Room arrangement Room location Noise/talking/lighting/temperature Lack of familiar objects

Nursing Interventions:
a) Treat/eliminate the cause b) Meet the patient need c) Collaborate with team members

Physiological Factors	Psychological Factors	Environmental Factors
Early weaning from ventilators or removal of tubes/devices Secure anchoring of devices Appropriate sedation Frequent toileting rounds Pain medication; comfort measures Sleep enhancement Medical management: identify drug effects and interactions	Visitation facilitation, increased family presence Verbal intervention: explain all procedures Emotional support Coping enhancement Communication enhancement Behavior management Stress management	Change in bed to appropriate—low bed; alarms One-on-one observation (staff, family) Environmental management: room consideration, bedside commode Reduce stimuli, quiet environment Medical equipment adjustment, removal, protection (i.e., sleeve) Rest periods

Intervention Effective?

Yes: Needs met/behavior managed

Restraints not needed
- Document interventions
- Continue alternatives

No: Needs unmet/ Behavior continues

Reassess the patient
Try additional interventions
Heightened surveillance
Consult additional team members: MD, APN consultation, PT (exercise, walking aids), OT (seating issues, functional issues)

FIGURE 15.3 Decision algorithm for promoting restraint-free care. (From Lach HW, Leach KM, Butcher HK: Changing the practice of physical restraint use in acute care, *J Gerontol Nurs* 42[2]:17–26, 2016. Adapted from Park M, Tang JHC: Evidence-based practice guideline: Changing the practice of physical restraint use in acute care, *J Gerontol Nurs* 33[2]:9–16, 2007.)

BOX 15.10 Suggestions From Advanced Practice Nursing Consultation on Restraint-Free Fall Prevention Interventions

- Compensating for memory loss (e.g., improving behavior, anticipating needs, providing visual and physical cues)
- Improving impaired mobility; reducing injury potential
- Evaluating nocturia/incontinence; reducing sleep disturbances
- Implementing restraint-free fall prevention interventions based on conducting careful individualized assessments; what works for one individual may not necessarily be effective for another

From Wagner L, Capezuti E, Brush B, et al: Description of an advanced practice nursing consultative model to reduce restrictive siderail use in nursing homes, *Res Nurs Health* 30:131–140, 2007.

jeopardize safety. The use of advanced practice nurse consultation in implementing alternatives to restraints has been most effective (Bourbonniere & Evans, 2002; Capezuti, 2004; Wagner et al., 2007). Important areas of focus derived from research on advanced practice nurse consultation are presented in Box 15.10. Many of the suggestions on safety and fall risk reduction in this chapter can be used to promote a safe and restraint-free environment.

❖ IMPLICATIONS FOR GERONTOLOGICAL NURSING AND HEALTHY AGING

Falls are a significant geriatric syndrome, and nurses need to be knowledgeable about fall risk factors and fall risk–reduction interventions in all settings. Health promotion interventions to maintain fitness and mobility; appropriate assessment of fall risk; teaching older adults, their caregivers, and staff about fall risk factors; fall risk–reduction interventions; and restraint–free care are important nursing responses. Accidents and injuries among older adults in all settings are significant in terms of morbidity and mortality, and using evidence-based practice can ensure improvement of many modifiable and preventable injuries, as well as mobility limitations and functional decline.

KEY CONCEPTS

- Falls are one of the most important geriatric syndromes and the leading cause of morbidity and mortality for people older than 65 years of age.
- The risk of falling increases with the number of risk factors. Most falls occur from a combination of intrinsic and extrinsic factors that unite at a certain point in time.
- Fall risk assessments provide first-level assessment data as the basis for a comprehensive assessment. Postfall assessments (PFAs) must be used to identify multifactorial fall risk factors as well as fall risk factors in those who have previously fallen.
- Physical restraints, intended to prevent injury, do not protect patients from falling, wandering, or removing tubes and other medical devices. Physical restraints may actually exacerbate many of the problems for which they are used and can cause serious injury and death, as well as physical and emotional problems.
- Restraint-appropriate care is the standard of practice in all settings and knowledge of restraint alternatives and safety measures is essential for nurses.

ACTIVITIES AND DISCUSSION QUESTIONS

1. Put your shoes on the wrong feet, and then ask another student to analyze your gait.
2. Borrow a pair of bifocals from someone, and then attempt to go up and down stairs.
3. Discuss falls you have had and their consequences. Consider how it might have been different if you were 80 years old.
4. Obtain a wheelchair and sit in it for 20 minutes with a restraining belt around your waist. Discuss your feelings with a partner. Reverse the process with your partner.
5. Discuss the various reasons why you might need to ensure safety for a hospitalized elder, and identify several alternatives that might be appropriate. Are these alternatives available in the acute care setting where you study?

REFERENCES

Alexander N: Balance, gait and mobility. In Ham R, Sloane R, Warshaw G, et al, editors: *Primary care geriatrics*, ed 6, Philadelphia, 2014, Elsevier, pp 227–234.

American Geriatrics Society: American Geriatrics Society identifies another five things that healthcare providers should question, *J Am Geriatr Soc* 2014a. doi: 10.1111/jgs.12770. [Epub ahead of print].

American Geriatrics Society: Recommendations abstracted from the American Geriatrics Society Consensus Statement on vitamin D for prevention of falls and their consequences, *J Am Geriatr Soc* 62:147–152, 2014b.

American Geriatrics Society/British Geriatrics Society: *AGS/BGS clinical practice guideline: Prevention of falls in older persons*, 2010a. Available at http://www.americangeriatrics.org/health_care_professionals/clinical_practice/clinical_guidelines_recommendations/prevention_of_falls_summary_of_recommendations. Accessed August 2016.

American Geriatrics Society/British Geriatrics Society: *AGS/BGS clinical practice guideline: Prevention of falls in older persons*, 2010b. Available at http://www.americangeriatrics.org/health_care_professionals/clinical_practice/clinical_guidelines_recommendations/prevention_of_falls_summary_of_recommendations. Accessed January 2016.

American Nurses Association: *Safe patient handling and mobility: Interprofessional national standards across the care continuum*, 2013. Available at http://nursingworld.org/DocumentVault/OccupationalEnvironment/SPHM-Standards-Resources/Sample-of-the-SPHM-book.pdf. Accessed January 26, 2014.

Andersen D, Osei-Boamah E, Gambert S: Impact of trauma-related hip fractures on the older adult, *Clin Geriatr* 18:18, 2010.

Basic D, Hartwell T: Falls in hospital and new placement in a nursing home among older people hospitalized with acute illness, *Clin Interv Aging* 10:1637–1643, 2015.

Bourbonniere M, Evans LK: Advanced practice nursing in the care of frail older adults, *J Am Geriatr Soc* 50:2062–2076, 2002.

Bradas C, Sandhu S, Mion L: Physical restraints and side rails in acute and critical care settings. In Boltz M, Capezuti E, Fulmer T, et al, editors: *Evidence-based geriatric nursing protocols for best practice*, ed 4, New York, 2012, Springer, pp 1229–1245.

Cameron I, Murray G, Gillespie L, et al: Interventions for preventing falls in older people in nursing facilities and hospitals, *Cochrane Database Syst Rev* (1):CD005465, 2010.

Campbell A, Robertson M: Fall prevention: Single or multiple interventions? Single interventions for fall prevention, *J Am Geriatr Soc* 61(2):281–284, 2013.

Capezuti E: Building the science of falls-prevention research, *J Am Geriatr Soc* 52:461–462, 2004.

Centers for Disease Control and Prevention: *Falls among older adults: An overview*, 2015a. Available at http://www.cdc.gov/homeandrecreationalsafety/falls/adultfalls.html. Accessed January 2016.

Centers for Disease Control and Prevention: *Preventing traumatic brain injury in older adults*, 2015b. Available at http://www.cdc.gov/features/braininjury. Accessed January 2016.

Crogan N, Dupler A: Quality improvement in nursing homes: Testing of an alarm elimination program, *J Nurs Care Qual* 29(1):60–65, 2014.

de Vries OJ, Ligthart GJ, Nikolaus TL: On behalf of the participants of the European Academy of Medicine of Ageing—Course III: Differences in period prevalence of the use of physical restraints in elderly inpatients of European hospitals and nursing homes [letter], *J Gerontol A Biol Sci Med Sci* 59:M922–M923, 2004.

Degelau J, Belz M, Bungum L, et al: *Prevention of falls (acute care)*, Minneapolis, MN, 2012, Institute for Clinical Systems Improvement. Available at https://www.icsi.org/_asset/dcn15z/Falls-Interactive0412.pdf. Accessed May 2014.

Eshkoor S, Hamid T, Nudin S, et al: A research on functional status, environmental conditions, and risk of falls in dementia, *Int J Alzheimers Dis* 2014. doi: http://dx.doi.org/10.1155/2014/769062.

Evans L, Strumpf N: Tying down the elderly: A review of literature on physical restraint, *J Am Geriatr Soc* 37:65–74, 1989.

Flaherty J: Zero tolerance for physical restraints: Difficult but not impossible, *J Gerontol A Biol Sci Med Sci* 59:M919–M920, 2004.

Frick K, Kung J, Parrish J, et al: Evaluating the cost-effectiveness of fall prevention programs that reduce fall-related hip fractures in older adults, *J Am Geriatr Soc* 58:136–141, 2010.

Gavin-Dreschnack D, Volicer L, Morris C: Prevention of overuse of wheelchairs in nursing homes, *Ann Longterm Care* 18:34, 2010.

Gillespie L, Robertson M, Gillespie W, et al: Interventions for preventing falls in older people living in the community, *Cochrane Database Syst Rev* (9):CD007146, 2012.

Gray-Micelli D: Preventing falls in acute care. In Capezuti E, Zwicker D, Mezey M, et al, editors: *Evidence-based geriatric nursing protocols for best practice*, ed 3, New York, 2008, Springer.

Gray-Micelli D, Quigley P: Fall prevention, assessment, diagnoses, and intervention strategies. In Boltz M, Capezuti E, Fulmer T, et al, editors: *Evidence-based geriatric nursing protocols for best practice*, ed 4, New York, 2012, Springer, pp 268–297.

Gray-Micelli D, Ratcliffe S, Johnson J: Use of a postfall assessment tool to prevent falls, *West J Nurs Res* 32(7):932–948, 2010.

Gray-Micelli D, Ratcliffe S, Liu S, et al: Orthostatic hypotension in older nursing home residents who fall: Are they dizzy? *Clin Nurs Res* 21:64–78, 2012.

Harrison B, Ferrari M, Campbell C, et al: Evaluating the relationship between inattention and impulsivity-related falls in hospitalized older adults, *Geriatr Nurs* 31:8–16, 2010.

Hendrich AL, Bender PS, Nyhuis A: Validation of the Hendrich II fall risk model: A large concurrent case/control study of hospitalized patients, *Appl Nurs Res* 16:9–21, 2003.

Hill K, Womer M, Russell M, et al: Fear of falling in older fallers presenting at emergency departments, *J Adv Nurs* 66:1769–1779, 2010.

Ireland S, Lazar T, Mavrak C, et al: Designing a falls prevention strategy that works, *J Nurs Care Qual* 25:198–207, 2010.

Lach H: The costs and outcomes of falls: What's a nursing administrator to do? *Nurs Adm Q* 34:147–155, 2010.

Lach H, Leach K: Changing the practice of physical restraint use in acute care, *J Gerontol Nurs* 42(2):17–26, 2016.

Lee H, Chang K, Tsauo J, et al: Effects of a multifactorial fall prevention program on fall incidence and physical function in community-dwelling older adults with risk of falls, *Arch Phys Med Rehabil* 94(4):606–615, 2013.

Lin F, Ferrucci L: Hearing loss and falls among older adults in the United States, *Arch Intern Med* 172(4):369–371, 2012.

Luciano G, Brennan M, Rothberg M: Postprandial hypotension, *Am J Med* 123(3):281.e1–e6, 2010.

Mathias S, Nayak US, Isaacs B: Balance in elderly patients: The "get up and go test", *Arch Phys Med Rehabil* 67(6):387–389, 1986.

Mendito V, Lucci M, Polonara S, et al: Management of minor head injury in patients receiving oral anticoagulant therapy: A prospective study of a 24-hour observation protocol, *Ann Emerg Med* 59(6):451–455, 2012.

Miake-Lye I, Hempel S, Ganz D, et al: Inpatient fall prevention programs as a patient safety strategy, *Ann Intern Med* 158(5 Pt 2):390–396, 2013.

Momeyer M: Orthostatic hypotension in older adults with dementia, *J Gerontol Nurs* 40(6):22–29, 2014.

Nelson A, Baptiste A: Evidence-based practices for safe patient handling and movement, *Online J Issues Nurs* 9(3):2004. Available at http://www.seiu1991.org/files/2013/07/Audrey_Nelson_Safe_Patient_Handling.pdf. Accessed January 2016.

Popejoy L, Marek K, Scott-Cawiezell J: Patterns and problems associated with transitions after hip fracture in older adults, *J Gerontol Nurs* 39(9):43–52, 2012.

Quigley P, Bulat T, Kurtzman E, et al: Fall prevention and injury protection for nursing home residents, *J Am Med Dir Assoc* 11:284–293, 2010.

Quigley P, White S: Hospital-based fall program measurement and improvement in high reliability organizations, *Online J Issues Nurs* 18(2):5, 2013.

Rantz M, Aud M, Alexander G, et al: Falls, technology, and stunt actors: New approaches to fall detection and fall risk assessment, *J Nurs Care Qual* 23:195–201, 2008.

Rantz M, Banerjee T, Cattoor E, et al: Automated fall detection with quality improvement "rewind" to reduce falls in hospital rooms, *J Gerontol Nurs* 40(1):13–17, 2014.

Rubenstein T, Alexander N, Hausdorff J: Evaluating fall risk in older adults: Steps and missteps, *Clin Geriatr* 11:52–60, 2003.

Rubenstein L, Dillard D: Falls. In Ham SP, Warshaw G, et al, editors: *Primary care geriatrics*, ed 6, Philadelphia, 2014, Elsevier, pp 235–242.

Sullivan-Marx E: Psychological responses to physical restraint use in older adults, *J Psychosoc Nurs Ment Health Serv* 33:20–25, 1995.

Talerico K, Capezuti E: Myths and facts about side rails, *Am J Nurs* 101:43–48, 2001.

Tewary S, Pandya N, Cook N: Prevention of foot problems in nursing home residents with diabetes stratified by dementia diagnosis, *Ann Longterm Care* 21(8):30–34, 2013.

Timmons T, Menaker J: Traumatic brain injury in the elderly, *Clin Geriatr* 18:20–24, 2010.

Tinetti M: Performance-oriented measurement of mobility problems in elderly patients, *J Am Geriatr Soc* 34(2):119–126, 1986.

Tinetti M, Baker D, King M, et al: Effect of dissemination of evidence in reducing injuries from falls, *N Engl J Med* 359(3):252–261, 2008.

Tinetti M, Han L, Lee D, et al: Antihypertensive medications and serious fall injuries in a nationally representative sample of older adults, *JAMA* 174(4):588–595, 2014.

Wagner L, Capezuti E, Brush B, et al: Description of an advanced practice nursing consultative model to reduce restrictive siderail use in nursing homes, *Res Nurs Health* 30:131–140, 2007.

Willy B, Osterberg C: Strategies for reducing falls in long-term care, *Ann Longterm Care* 22(1):23–32, 2014.

Zhao Y, Kim H: Older adult inpatient falls in acute care hospitals, *J Gerontol Nurs* 41(7):29–42, 2015.

16

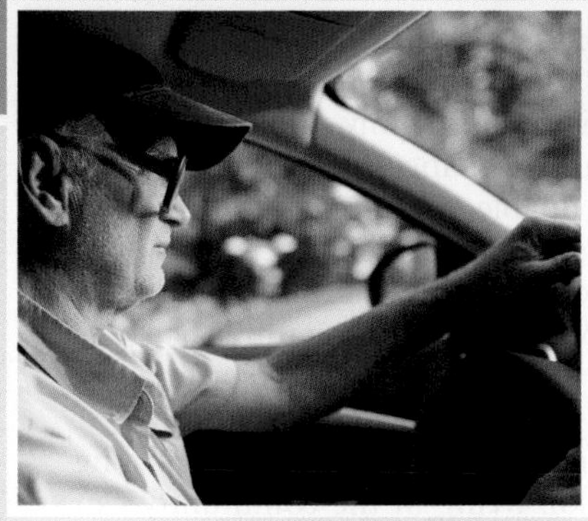

Promoting Safety

Theris A. Touhy

evolve.elsevier.com/Touhy/gerontological

LEARNING OBJECTIVES

Upon completion of this chapter, the reader will be able to:

- Discuss the effects of declining health, reduced mobility, isolation, and unpredictable life situations on the older adult's perception of security.
- Explain the underlying vulnerability of older adults to natural disasters and the effects of extreme temperatures.
- Identify resources for disaster preparedness and actions to prevent and treat hypothermia and hyperthermia.
- Consider the impact of available transportation and driving in relation to independence and safety.
- Discuss the use of assistive technologies to promote self-care, safety, and independence.
- Identify the components of an elder-friendly community to enhance the ability to age in place.

THE LIVED EXPERIENCE

I have been in my home for 50 years and widowed for 25 of those 50. The upkeep on my home is expensive and my resources are limited. I'm hoping I can manage to remain here, but I need some modifications to make it safe and I really don't know how to go about getting assistance to make the necessary changes.

Esther, age 79

HOME SAFETY

Home safety assessments must be multifaceted and individualized to the areas of identified risks. They are particularly important for the older adult who is at risk for falls and are recommended in evidence-based protocols for fall risk reduction. Box 16.1 presents resources for home safety assessments in formats easy for older adults to access and use. A home safety inventory for older adults with dementia can be found on the Hartford Institute for Geriatric Nursing site (https://consultgeri.org/try-this/dementia/issue-d12).

VULNERABILITY TO ENVIRONMENTAL TEMPERATURES

Environmental temperature extremes impose a serious risk to older persons with declining physical health. Preventive measures require attentiveness to impending climate changes, as well as protective alternatives. Many individuals are exposed to temperature extremes in their own dwellings. Early intervention in extreme temperature exposure is crucial because excessively high or low body temperatures further impair thermoregulatory function and can be lethal.

BOX 16.1 Resources for Best Practice

Aging & Technology Research Center: On-line home safety self-assessment
American Association of Retired Persons: CarFit: Helping Mature Drivers Find Their Safety Fit
American Automobile Association: Driver improvement courses, on-line defensive driving course
American Geriatrics Society: Clinician's guide to assessing and counseling older drivers
CDC: STEADI (Stopping Elderly Accidents, Deaths & Injuries): Check for safety: a home fall prevention checklist for older adults; Heat Stress in Older Adults
Cohousing Association of the United States
Dementia Friendly America Initiative: http://www.dfamerica.org
National Crime Prevention Council: Safety in the Golden Years
National Fire Protection Association and the CDC: Remembering When: A Fire and Fall Prevention Program for Older Adults
National Institute on Aging: Age Page: Hyperthermia: Too Hot for Your Health; Hypothermia: A Cold Weather Hazard
National Shared Housing Resource Center
NORC: Aging in Place Initiative
U.S. Department of Health and Human Services, Administration on Aging: Preparing for an Emergency or Disaster, Resources for Individuals, Families, and Caregivers
Village to Village Network (Village Housing Model)
World Health Organization: Global age-friendly cities and communities: A guide; Checklist of Essential Features of Age-Friendly Cities

Thermoregulation

Neurosensory changes in thermoregulation delay or diminish the individual's awareness of temperature changes and may impair behavioral and thermoregulatory response to dangerously high or low environmental temperatures (see Chapter 3). These changes vary widely among individuals and are related more to general health than to age.

Additionally, many drugs influence thermoregulation by affecting the ability of the vascular system to vasoconstrict or vasodilate, both of which are thermoregulatory mechanisms. Other drugs inhibit neuromuscular activity (a significant source of kinetic heat production), suppress metabolic heat generation, or dull awareness (tranquilizers, pain medications). Alcohol is notorious for inhibiting thermoregulatory function by affecting vasomotor responses in either hot or cold weather.

Economic, behavioral, and environmental factors may combine to create a dangerous thermal environment in which older persons are subjected to temperature extremes from which they cannot escape or that they cannot change. Caregivers and family members should be aware that persons are vulnerable to temperature extremes if they are unable to shiver, sweat, control blood supply to the skin, consume sufficient liquids, ambulate, add or remove clothing, adjust bedcovers, or adjust the room temperature. A temperature that may be comfortable for a young and active person may be too cold or too warm for a frail elder.

Economic conditions often play a role in determining whether an older person living in the community can afford air conditioning or adequate heating. Local governments and communities must coordinate response strategies to protect the older person. Strategies may include providing fans and opportunities to spend part of the day in air-conditioned buildings, as well as identification of high-risk individuals.

Temperature Monitoring in Older Adults

Diminished thermoregulatory responses and abnormalities in both the production and the response to endogenous pyrogens may contribute to differences in fever responses to an infection between older and younger individuals. Up to one-third of older people with acute infections may present without a robust febrile response, leading to delays in diagnosis and appropriate treatment, as well as increased morbidity and mortality (Outzen, 2009). Careful attention to temperature monitoring in older adults is very important, and often this technical task is not given adequate consideration by professional nurses.

SAFETY ALERT

Because of thermoregulatory changes, up to one-third of older people with acute infections may present without a febrile response. Additionally, baseline temperatures in frail older people may be lower than the expected 98.6°F. If the baseline temperature is 97°F, a temperature of 98°F is a 1°F elevation and may be significant.

Temperatures reaching or exceeding 100.94°F are very serious in older people and are more likely to be associated with serious bacterial or viral infections. Careful attention to temperature monitoring in older adults is very important and can prevent morbidity and mortality. Accurate measurement and reporting of body temperature require professional nursing supervision.

Hyperthermia

When body temperature increases above normal ranges because of environmental or metabolic heat loads, a clinical condition called heat illness, or *hyperthermia,* develops. Administration of diuretics and low intake of fluids exacerbate fluid loss and can precipitate the onset of hyperthermia in hot weather. Hyperthermia is a temperature-related illness and is classified as a medical emergency. Annually, there are numerous deaths among elders from temperature extremes; therefore prevention and education are very important nursing responsibilities.

Although most of these problems occur in the home among individuals who do not have air conditioning to use during temperature extremes, older adults residing in institutions with multiple physical problems may be especially vulnerable to temperature changes. Individuals with cardiovascular disease, diabetes, or peripheral vascular disease and those taking certain medications (anticholinergics, antihistamines, diuretics, beta blockers, antidepressants, antiparkinsonian drugs) are at risk. Interventions to prevent hyperthermia when ambient temperature exceeds 90°F (32°C) are presented in Box 16.2.

Hypothermia

Nearly 50% of all deaths from hypothermia occur in older adults (University of Maryland Medical Center, 2013). Hypothermia is produced by exposure to cold environmental temperatures and is defined as a core temperature less than 35°C (95°F). Hypothermia is a medical emergency requiring comprehensive assessment of neurological activity, oxygenation, renal function, and fluid and electrolyte balance.

When exposed to cold temperatures, healthy persons conserve heat by vasoconstriction of superficial vessels, shunting circulation away from the skin where most heat is lost. Heat is generated by shivering and increased muscle activity, and a rise in oxygen consumption occurs to meet aerobic muscle requirements. Under normal circumstances, heat is produced in sufficient quantities by cellular metabolism of food, friction produced by contracting muscles, and the flow of blood.

Paralyzed or immobile persons lack the ability to generate significant heat by muscle activity and become cold even at normal room temperatures. Persons who are emaciated and have poor nutrition lack insulation, as well as fuel for metabolic heat-generating processes, so they may be mildly hypothermic (Hogan & Rios-Alba, 2014). Circulatory, cardiac, respiratory, or musculoskeletal impairments affect either the response to or the function of thermoregulatory mechanisms. Other risk factors include excessive alcohol use, exhaustion, poor nutrition, and inadequate housing as well as the use of sedatives, anxiolytics, phenothiazines, and tricyclic antidepressants (Box 16.3).

Older persons with some degree of thermoregulatory impairment, when exposed to cold temperatures, are at high risk for hypothermia if they undergo surgery, are injured in a fall or accident, or are lost or left unattended in a cool place. The more severe the impairment or prolonged the exposure, the less able are thermoregulatory responses to defend against heat loss. Unfortunately, a dulling of awareness accompanies hypothermia, and persons experiencing the condition rarely recognize the problem or seek assistance. For the very old and frail, environmental temperatures less than 65°F (18°C) may cause a serious drop in core body temperature to 95°F (35°C).

Hypothermia is of particular concern for the older adult who undergoes surgery. Almost all anesthetics can inhibit thermoregulatory function, which is exacerbated by the cold operating room environment. Core temperatures should be monitored in surgeries lasting more than 30 minutes. Patient warming with forced air warmers and/or warmed intravenous (IV) fluids should be used in older patients who are undergoing procedures longer than 30 minutes to avoid hypothermia (American College of Surgeons, American Geriatrics Society, 2016).

All body systems are affected by hypothermia, although the most deadly consequences involve cardiac arrhythmias and suppression of respiratory function. Correctly conducted rewarming is the key to good management, and the guiding principle is to warm the core before the periphery and to raise the core temperature 0.5°C to 2°C per hour. Heating blankets and specially designed heating vests are used in addition to warm humidified air by mask, warm intravenous boluses, and other measures depending on the severity of the hypothermia (Hogan & Rios-Alba, 2014).

Detecting hypothermia among community-dwelling older adults is sometimes difficult because, unlike in the

BOX 16.2 Tips for Best Practice

Preventing Hyperthermia

- Drink 2 to 3 L of cool fluid daily.
- Minimize exertion, especially during the warmest times of the day.
- Stay in air-conditioned places, or use fans when possible.
- Wear hats and loose clothing of natural fibers when outside; remove most clothing when indoors.
- Take tepid baths or showers.
- Apply cold wet compresses, or immerse the hands and feet in cool water.
- Evaluate medications for risk of hyperthermia.
- Avoid alcohol.

BOX 16.3 Factors That Increase the Risk of Hypothermia in Older Adults

Thermoregulatory Impairment

Failure to vasoconstrict promptly or sufficiently on exposure to cold
Failure to sense cold
Failure to respond behaviorally to protect oneself against cold
Diminished or absent shivering to generate heat
Failure of metabolic rate to rise in response to cold

Conditions That Decrease Heat Production

Hypothyroidism, hypopituitarism, hypoglycemia, anemia, malnutrition, starvation
Immobility or decreased activity (e.g., stroke, paralysis, parkinsonism, dementia, arthritis, fractured hip, coma)
Thinning hair, baldness
Diabetic ketoacidosis

Conditions That Increase Heat Loss

Open wounds, generalized inflammatory skin conditions, burns

Conditions That Impair Central or Peripheral Control of Thermoregulation

Stroke, brain tumor, Wernicke's encephalopathy, subarachnoid hemorrhage
Uremia, neuropathy (e.g., diabetes, alcoholism)
Acute illnesses (e.g., pneumonia, sepsis, myocardial infarction, congestive heart failure, pulmonary embolism, pancreatitis)
Anesthesia/surgery

Drugs That Interfere With Thermoregulation

Tranquilizers (e.g., phenothiazines); sedative-hypnotics (e.g., barbiturates, benzodiazepines); antidepressants (e.g., tricyclics); vasoactive drugs (e.g., vasodilators); alcohol (causes superficial vasodilation; may interfere with carbohydrate metabolism and judgment); others (e.g., methyldopa, lithium, morphine)

clinical setting, no one is measuring body temperature. For persons exposed to low temperatures in the home or the environment, confusion and disorientation may be the first overt signs. As judgment becomes clouded, a person may remove clothing or fail to seek shelter, and hypothermia can progress to profound levels. For this reason, regular contact with home-dwelling elders during cold weather is crucial. For those with preexisting alterations in thermoregulatory ability, this surveillance should include even mildly cool weather. Because heating costs are high in the United States, the Department of Health and Human Services provides funds to help low-income families pay their heating bills. Specific interventions to prevent hypothermia are shown in Box 16.4.

BOX 16.4 Tips for Best Practice

Preventing Cold Discomfort and Development of Accidental Hypothermia in Frail Elders

- Maintain a comfortably warm ambient temperature no lower than 65°F. Many frail elders will require much higher temperatures.
- Provide generous quantities of clothing and bedcovers. Layer clothing and bedcovers for best insulation. Be careful not to judge your patient's needs by how you feel working in a warm environment.
- Provide a head covering whenever possible—in bed, out of bed, and particularly out-of-doors.
- Cover patients well when in bed or bathing. The standard—a light bath blanket over a naked body—is not enough protection for frail elders.
- Cover patients with heavy blankets for transfer to and from showers; dry quickly and thoroughly before leaving shower room; cover head with a dry towel or hood while wet. Shower rooms and bathrooms should have warming lights.
- Dry wet hair quickly with warm air from an electric dryer. Never allow the hair of frail elders to air-dry.
- Use absorbent pads for incontinent patients rather than allowing urine to wet large areas of clothing, sheets, and bedcovers.
- Provide as much exercise as possible to generate heat from muscle activity.
- Provide hot, high-protein meals and bedtime snacks to add heat and sustain heat production throughout the day and as far into the night as possible.

❖ IMPLICATIONS FOR GERONTOLOGICAL NURSING AND HEALTHY AGING

Recognition of clinical signs and severity of hypothermia and hyperthermia is an important nursing responsibility. Nurses are responsible for keeping frail elders in environments with appropriate temperatures for comfort and prevention of problems. It is important to closely monitor body temperature and pay particular attention to lower or higher than normal readings compared with the person's baseline reading. The potential risk of hypothermia and its associated cardiorespiratory and metabolic exertion make prevention important and early recognition vital. Nurses must advocate for resources in the community to ensure appropriate temperatures in the homes of older people and surveillance when temperature changes occur.

VULNERABILITY TO NATURAL DISASTERS

Natural disasters such as hurricanes, tornadoes, floods, and earthquakes claim the lives of many people worldwide each year (Green et al., 2013; Wolfe & McGregor, 2013). In addition, human-made or human-generated disasters include chemical, biological, radiological, and nuclear terrorism and food and water contamination. Older people are at great risk during and after disasters and have the highest casualty rate during disaster events when compared with all other age groups (Burnett et al., 2008). The older and poorer the individual, the more likely he or she is to be isolated and vulnerable (Feather, 2013).

Older adults at most risk include, but are not limited to, those who depend on others for daily functioning; those with limited mobility; and those who are socially isolated, cognitively impaired, or institutionalized. Older people may be less likely to seek formal or informal help during disasters and may not get as much assistance as younger individuals. Nursing home residents compose a particularly vulnerable group because of their frailty, and nursing homes need to be prepared for disasters. The U.S. Department of Health and Human Services provides resources for emergency and disaster preparedness for special populations, including older adults (Box 16.1).

TRANSPORTATION SAFETY

Available transportation is a critical link in the ability of older adults to remain independent and functional. The lack of accessible transportation may contribute to other problems, such as social withdrawal, poor nutrition, depressive symptoms, and health decline (Dugan & Lee, 2013). Urban buses and subways can be physically hazardous and often dangerous. Rural and suburban areas may not have accessible transportation systems, making transportation by car essential. Even walking can be dangerous, and older people have more pedestrian crashes than anyone except children and are more likely to be injured or killed as pedestrians than as car drivers (Rosenbloom, 2009). Suggested pedestrian improvements include raised pavement markings, median islands, larger street signs with bigger lettering, increased time for pedestrian crossings, and lowered speed limits (Dugan & Lee, 2013).

A "crisis in mobility" exists for many older people because of the lack of an automobile, an inability to drive, limited access to public transportation, health factors, geographical location, and economic considerations. Neither public transit services nor special demand services will come anywhere near meeting the mobility needs of the country's aging population (Rosenbloom, 2009).

County, state, or federally subsidized transportation is being provided in certain areas to assist individuals in reaching social services, nutrition sites, health services, emergency care facilities, recreational centers, day care programs, physical and vocational rehabilitation centers, grocery stores, and library services. Some senior centers also offer transportation services. Although transportation can often be found for special needs, it is virtually impossible to locate transportation for pleasure or recreation, and many of these services are restricted to individuals with serious physical or mental impairments. A very small percentage of older individuals use these services.

Driving

Driving is one of the instrumental activities of daily living (IADLs) for most elders because it is essential to obtaining necessary resources. Driving is the preferred means of travel for most Americans, especially older adults. Almost 90% of people 65 years of age and older continue to drive, and these numbers are expected to grow as "baby boomers" age and more people live into their eighties and nineties. For many older people, alternate transportation is not available and, consequently, they may continue driving beyond the time when it is safe. Rosenbloom (2009) suggests that the most promising mobility option would be to modify the auto-based infrastructure so that older people can drive safely longer. This would include vehicle adaptations, sensory aids, elder driving training, and driving assessment programs (Box 16.5). The CarFit program (Box 16.1) is an educational program to improve driver-car fit.

Driving is a highly complex activity that requires a variety of visual, motor, and cognitive skills. As individuals age, the risk for impairments that affect driving skills increases because of changes related to normal aging, as well as disease-related changes (e.g., arthritis, Parkinson's disease, stroke, dementia). Sensory impairments affect driving ability, and older drivers with dual sensory impairment are at greater accident risk than those with a visual acuity or hearing deficit alone (Dugan & Lee, 2013).

Driving Safety

Older drivers typically drive fewer miles than younger drivers and tend to drive less at night, during adverse weather conditions, or in congested areas. Generally, they choose familiar routes, and fewer older drivers speed or drive after drinking alcohol than drivers of other ages. However, when compared with younger age

BOX 16.5 Adaptations for Safer Driving

- Wider rear-view mirrors
- Pedal extensions
- Less complicated, larger, and legible instrument panels
- Electronic detectors in front and back that signal when the car is getting too close to other cars, drifting into another lane, or likely to hit center dividers or other highway infrastructure
- Technology that facilitates left turns by warning drivers when it is safe to make the turn
- Better protection on doors
- Booster cushions for shorter-stature drivers
- "Smart" driving assistants (under development) that automatically plan a safe driving route based on the person's driving habits
- GPS devices

Modified from Dugan E, Lee C: Biopsychosocial risk factors for driving cessation: Findings from the Health and Retirement study, *J Aging Health* 25:1313–1328, 2013; Hooyman N, Kiyak H: *Social gerontology: A multidisciplinary perspective,* Boston, 2011, Allyn & Bacon.

groups, older people have more accidents per mile driven and have a ninefold increased risk of traffic fatality (Servat et al., 2011). The leading cause of injury-related deaths among drivers 65 to 74 years of age is a motor vehicle accident; for those older than 75 years of age, motor vehicle accidents are the second leading cause of death, after falls (Hooyman & Kiyak, 2011).

The legal regulations regarding driver's license renewal in older drivers and the responsibility of medical practitioners to identify unsafe drivers vary among states and countries (Mathias & Lucas, 2009). Driver's license renewal procedures may include accelerated renewal cycles, renewal in person rather than electronically or by mail, and vision and road tests. The issues of driving in the older adult population are the subject of a great deal of public discussion. Many older drivers and their families struggle with issues related to continued safety in driving and when and how to tell older people they are no longer safe drivers.

Driving and Dementia

Driving has been identified as one in ten tough ethical issues associated with dementia (Dobbs et al., 2009). Dementia, even in the early stages, can impair cognitive and functional skills required for safe driving. Evidence from some studies of motor vehicle crashes suggests that drivers with dementia have at least a twofold risk of crashes compared with those without cognitive impairment (Carr & Ott, 2010; Gray-Vickrey, 2010a,b). Many individuals early in the course of dementia are still able to pass a driving performance test, so a diagnosis of dementia should not be the sole justification for revocation of a driver's license (Carr & Ott, 2010). However, discussions should begin about the inevitability of driving cessation. Additionally, driving evaluations should be conducted every 6 months or as needed as the disease progresses.

Silver Alert systems. Many states have implemented the Silver Alert system. Similar to Amber Alerts for missing children, the Silver Alert is designed to create a widespread lookout for older adults who have wandered from their surroundings while driving a car. Silver Alert features a public notification system to broadcast information about missing persons, especially older adults with Alzheimer's disease or other mental disabilities, in order to aid in their return. Silver Alert uses a wide array of media outlets, such as commercial radio stations, television stations, and cable TV, to broadcast information about missing persons. Silver Alert also uses message signs on roadways to alert motorists to be on the lookout for missing elders and provides the car's make, model, and license information.

Driving Cessation

Relinquishing the mobility and independence afforded by driving one's own car has many psychological ramifications and inconveniences. Giving up driving is a major loss for an older person both in terms of independence and pleasure as well as in feelings of competence and self-worth. Driving cessation has been associated with decreased social integration, decreased out-of-home activities, increased depressive and anxiety symptoms, decreased quality of life, and increased risk of nursing home placement (Carr & Ott, 2010; Dugan & Lee, 2013).

Women are more likely than men to stop driving for less pressing reasons than health, and at a younger age (Dugan & Lee, 2013; Oxley & Charlton, 2009). Older men seem to place more value on the ability to drive, as well as owning a car, than older women. Therefore, one can expect more stress involved with the decision not to drive for older men. Other factors associated with driving cessation include IADL difficulties, poorer cognitive function, poor vision, being a member of a minority race or ethnicity, and having lower income and education (Dugan & Lee, 2013).

Planning for driving cessation should occur for all older adults before their mobility situations become urgent (Carr & Ott, 2010; Counsell, 2016). Health care providers should encourage open discussion of issues related to driving with the older person and his or her family and should identify impairments that affect safe driving, correct them when possible, and offer alternatives for transportation. Matching individuals to volunteer drivers and using car-sharing programs have been successful in some communities. It is generally agreed that voluntarily giving up a driver's license, rather than having it revoked, is associated with more positive outcomes (Oxley & Charlton, 2009). Specialized driving cessation support groups aimed at the transition from driver to nondriver may also be beneficial in decreasing the negative outcomes associated with this decision (Dobbs et al., 2009).

❖ IMPLICATIONS FOR GERONTOLOGICAL NURSING AND HEALTHY AGING

Assessment of functional capacities often neglects driving ability. Assessment should include evaluation of whether an individual can drive, feels safe driving, and has a driver's license. The mnemonic SAFE DRIVE (McGregor, 2002) addresses key components in screening older drivers (Box 16.6). Box 16.7 presents a self-assessment of driving that can be shared with individuals. The American Automobile Association also provides an interactive driving evaluation available on-line or in DVD format (Box 16.1). These kinds of tools can be effective in raising awareness of threats to driving fitness (Dugan & Lee, 2013). Box 16.8 presents other suggestions in assessment of driving safety.

There is no gold standard for determining driving competency, but driving evaluations are offered by driver rehabilitation specialists through local hospitals and rehabilitation centers and private or university-based driving assessment programs. State Departments of Motor Vehicles (DMVs) also conduct performance-based road tests.

EMERGING TECHNOLOGIES TO ENHANCE SAFETY OF OLDER ADULTS

Advancements in all types of technology hold promise for improving quality of life, decreasing the need for personal care, and enhancing independence and the ability to live safely at home and age in place. Emerging technologies will play a larger role in ensuring care for older people in the future. Assistive technology is any device or system that allows a person to perform a task independently or that makes the task easier and safer to perform. Assistive technology is decreasing the number of older people who depend on others for personal care in ADLs and presents cost-effective alternatives to human services and institutionalization (Daniel et al., 2009). Gerotechnology is the term used to describe assistive technologies for older people, and these technologies are expected to significantly influence how we live in the future. Health care technologies, robotics,

BOX 16.6 Safe Driving

S Safety record
A Attention skills
F Family report
E Ethanol use
D Drugs
R Reaction time
I Intellectual impairment
V Vision and visuospatial function
E Executive functions

BOX 16.7 Driving Skills and Safety Factors

Directions

If you answer "yes" to one or more of the following questions, you may want to limit your driving or take steps to improve a problem.

If you answer "yes" to most of the questions, it may be time to consider letting someone else do your driving.

- Does driving make you feel nervous or physically exhausted?
- Do you have difficulty seeing pedestrians, signs, and vehicles?
- Do cars frequently seem to appear from nowhere?
- At night, does the glare from oncoming headlights temporarily "blind" you?
- Do you find intersections confusing?
- Are you finding it harder to judge the distance between cars?
- Do you have difficulty coordinating your hand and foot movements?
- Do you have difficulty staying in a lane?
- Are you slower than you used to be in reacting to dangerous situations?
- Do you sometimes get lost in familiar neighborhoods?
- Do other drivers often honk at you?
- Have you had any tickets?
- Have you been pulled over by the police?
- Have you had an increased number of traffic violations, accidents, or near-accidents in the past year?
- Do you have any vision problems?
- Do you have any hearing problems?
- Do you take any of the following medications: antihistamines, antipsychotics, tricyclic antidepressants, benzodiazepines, barbiturates, sleeping medications, muscle relaxants?
- Do you have any memory impairment?
- Do you have any muscle stiffness or weakness?

Adapted from Carr D, Ott B: The older adult driver with cognitive impairment: "It's a very frustrating life," *JAMA* 303:1632–1641, 2010.

BOX 16.8 Tips for Best Practice

Driving Safety

- Include the person in all discussions about driving safety.
- Encourage the individual to conduct a self-assessment of driving abilities.
- Assess vision and hearing and ensure appropriate use of corrective lenses and hearing devices.
- Evaluate medical conditions that may interfere with driving ability (arthritis, Parkinson's disease, dementia, stroke) and ensure appropriate treatment, as well as adaptations that may be necessary to enhance driving safety.
- Discuss the impact of medical conditions and sensory impairments on driving safety.
- Suggest vehicle adaptations and elder driving assessment programs if indicated.
- Encourage the individual to modify driving habits, such as not driving on unfamiliar roads, during rush hour, at dusk or at night, in inclement weather, or in heavy traffic.
- Discuss strategies to decrease the need to drive, including arranging for home-delivered groceries, prescriptions, and meals; having personal services provided in the home; asking a caregiver to obtain needed supplies or act as a copilot; and exploring community resources for transportation.
- If the individual has driving safety risk factors and should not be driving, ask the individual's health care provider to "prescribe" driving cessation. This may be better received than reporting the individual to the DMV.
- Ask the family to have the family lawyer discuss with the individual the financial and legal implications of a crash or injury.

From Carr D, Ott B: The older adult driver with cognitive impairment: "It's a very frustrating life," *JAMA* 303:1632–1641, 2010; Gray-Vickrey P: Enhancing driver safety in dementia, *Alzheimers Care Today* 11:147–148, 2010.

telemedicine, mobility and activities of daily living (ADL) aids, and environmental control systems (smart houses/intelligent homes) are some examples of assistive technology.

Telehealth

Telehealth (telemedicine) is defined as "the use of electronic information and telecommunication technologies to support long-distance clinical health care, patient and professional health-related education, public health, and health administration" (Grady, 2014, p. 39). Telehealth offers exciting possibilities for managing medical problems in the home or other setting, reducing health care costs, and promoting self-management of illness, particularly in rural and underserved areas. The number of telehealth programs is increasing worldwide, and these programs offer exciting possibilities for nurses, particularly advanced practice nurses (Mars, 2010; Rutledge et al., 2014; Wamala & Augustine, 2013).

Telehealth nurses may practice in any setting in which on-site access to health care providers is limited. Remote-monitoring devices allow patients to connect with telehealth nurses from their homes or from a community setting such as a senior center. Remote physical assessment (pulse oximeters, weight scales, blood glucose monitors, and intelligent toilets that collect data on weight, blood pressure, and urine glucose level) allow nurses and primary care providers to track trends in patient data. The nurse may use a digital stethoscope to auscultate lung sounds or a digital camera to assess and document wound healing. A home care telehealth nurse can "see" many more patients through virtual visits (Grady, 2014; Rutledge et al., 2014).

A number of studies have reported that telehealth technology improves patient outcomes and decreases hospital readmissions and health care costs (Grady, 2014; Rutledge et al., 2014). Factors driving the adoption of telehealth include rising health care costs, the desire to age in place, increasing comfort with technology, the new generation of nurses who expect to incorporate technology into their practice, and the profit motive of device manufacturers. Factors slowing widespread development include concerns about privacy, fear of diminishing human contact and caring, and limited reimbursement (Fuji et al., 2014; Grady, 2014).

Smart Homes

Smart medical homes are being studied as a way to aid in the prevention and early detection of disease through the use of sensors and monitors. These devices keep data on vital signs and other measures such as gait, behavior, and sleep and provide an interactive medical-advising system. Devices to monitor gait and detect balance problems, such as the iShoe and the "smart carpet" (a sensor system embedded in the carpet that detects gait abnormalities that may predispose the person to falls, and also detects falls and summons assistance), are being developed (Aud et al., 2010; Rantz et al., 2008). SmartSoles, shoe insoles with an embedded GPS device, are being developed and may be an aid to locate individuals with dementia who wander from their home.

Remote-controlled houses are becoming more popular and allow the individual to control the house from anywhere (e.g., devices that turn lights on and off, automatically water plants, or feed pets; motion detectors; and leak detectors). The first of a series of smart houses to enable older people to live safely in their own homes is already on the market. An example is the

QuietCare 24-hour monitoring service. This system uses an ordinary home security infrastructure to monitor the house and transfers information about the occupant's daily living activities, triggering when a normal routine is broken. Caregivers and family can perform virtual check-ins with their older relative over the Internet (Bezaitis, 2009).

Motion and pressure sensors may be useful in the homes of older adults with cognitive impairment. These sensors can detect movement and the absence of movement. If there has been no movement for a period of time, a monitoring system is activated and a plan of action initiated depending on the person's response or lack of response. Pressure sensors can be used under the mattress and can turn on bedside lights when the individual gets out of bed or activate an alarm if he or she does not return to bed in a specified period of time. Sensors placed in entry doors can detect if a person leaves the home and can send messages to caregivers that the individual has left the house (Daniel et al., 2009). Medical alert devices are now available that automatically call for help in the event of a fall, without requiring the user to push a button (American Association of Retired Persons Bulletin, 2015).

In hospitals and long-term care facilities, devices such as wireless pendants that track people's movements, load cells built into beds that create an alert when individuals get out of bed, and monitor weight and sleep patterns, and bed lifts that allow individuals to go from lying down to standing up with the push of a button are being used. Wheelchair technology that enables the user to go down stairs, move to an upright position, be reminded to change positions to alleviate pressure, or use mechanical arms to change a light bulb or get things out of the refrigerator are other developing technologies.

Robots

Robotic technology for health care is more advanced in Europe and Japan than in the United States at this time, but we can expect to see increased development and use of robotics in nursing. On the horizon are technology developments such as robots that can help lift both individuals and objects, remind patients to take their medicine or administer the medication, check a person's vital signs, provide help in the event of a fall, and assist with baths and meals. A child-size therapist robot on wheels with a humanlike torso is being developed for use in homes and long-term care facilities to assist with the high level of attention individuals with dementia require for safety and function. Many ethical issues have been raised about the use of robots, and nurses will play an important role in ensuring that technological competence is balanced with caring to enhance the well-being of the individual (Campling et al., 2007; Fuji et al., 2014).

As the baby boomers and future generations age, comfort with technology will be increased, and people will seek options for better, safer, and more independent ways not yet imagined. At this time, many of the assistive technologies can be cost-prohibitive for older people, but with advances in development they may be more accessible and affordable for more people. Research is needed on assistive technologies and their acceptance among older people. It is important for nurses to be aware of available technology to improve safety.

ELDER-FRIENDLY COMMUNITIES

Developing elder-friendly communities and providing increasing opportunities to age in place can lead to enhanced health and well-being. Aging in place is the ability to live in one's own home and community safely, independently, and comfortably, regardless of age, income, or ability level (CDC, 2013). Many state and local governments are assessing the community and designing interventions to enhance the ability of older people to remain in their homes and familiar environments. These interventions range from adequate transportation systems to home modifications and universal design standards for barrier-free housing.

Components of an elder-friendly community include the following: (1) addresses basic needs; (2) optimizes physical health and well-being; (3) maximizes independence for the frail and disabled; and (4) provides social and civic engagement. Fig. 16.1 presents elements of an elder-friendly community. An outgrowth of age-friendly communities is the Dementia Friendly America Initiative to foster dementia-friendly communities across the United States, which will support those living with dementia and their caregivers and families (Weiss, 2016) (see Chapter 25) (Box 16.1).

KEY CONCEPTS

- Thermoregulatory changes, chronic illness, and medications may predispose the older adult to hypothermia and hyperthermia. Careful attention must be paid to temperature monitoring and provision of adequate heat and cooling in weather extremes.
- Transportation for older adults is critical to their physical, psychological, and social health.
- Driving safety for older people is an important issue and health care professionals must be knowledgeable about assessment, safety interventions, and transportation resources.

Addresses Basic Needs

- Provides appropriate and affordable housing
- Promotes safety at home and in the neighborhood
- Ensures no one goes hungry
- Provides useful information about available services

Promotes Social and Civic Engagement

- Fosters meaningful connections with family, neighbors, and friends
- Promotes active engagement in community life
- Provides opportunities for meaningful paid and voluntary work
- Makes aging issues a community-wide priority

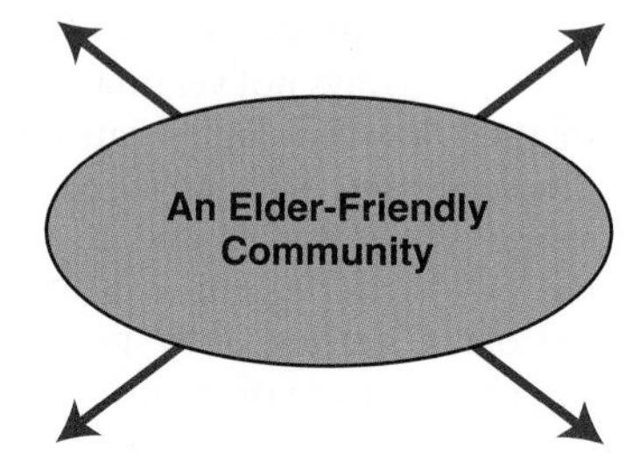

Optimizes Physical and Mental Health and Well-Being

- Promotes healthy behaviors
- Supports community activities that enhance well-being
- Provides ready access to preventive health services
- Provides access to medical, social, and palliative services

Maximizes Independence for Frail and Disabled

- Mobilizes resources to facilitate "living at home"
- Provides accessible transportation
- Supports family and other caregivers

FIGURE 16.1 Essential elements of an elder-friendly community. (From AdvantAge Initiative, Center for Home Care Policy and Research, Visiting Nurse Service of New York.)

- Technology advances hold promise for improving quality of life, decreasing need for personal care assistance, and enhancing independence and ability to live safely.
- Efforts to make communities more elder friendly are underway across the globe. New and innovative ideas for aging in community will continue to change living options for older adults.

ACTIVITIES AND DISCUSSION QUESTIONS

1. What interventions are important to prevent hypothermia in an elder undergoing surgery? In a frail elder residing in a long-term care facility?
2. Locate low-cost housing in your area and assess for convenience and safety.
3. Evaluate the safety of your living quarters or the living quarters of your parents/grandparents.
4. What types of support does your community provide to assist elders safely age in place?

REFERENCES

American Association of Retired Persons Bulletin: *Help from tech breakthroughs,* November 2015.

American College of Surgeons: American Geriatrics Society: *Optimal perioperative management of the geriatric patient: Best practices guidelines from ACS NSQIP/American Geriatrics Society,* 2016. Available at https://www.facs.org/quality-programs/acs-nsqip/geriatric-periop-guideline. Accessed January 2016.

Aud M, Abbott C, Tyrer H, et al: Smart carpet: Developing a sensor system to detect falls and summon assistance, *J Gerontol Nurs* 36:8–12, 2010.

Bezaitis A: Robot technologies: Exciting new frontier, *Aging Well* 2:10, 2009.

Burnett J, Dyer CB, Pickins S: Rapid needs assessment for older adults in disasters, *Generations* 31:10–15, 2008.

Campling A, Tanoika T, Locsin R: Robots and nursing: Concepts, relationships and practice. In Barnard A, Locsin R, editors: *Technology and nursing,* New York, 2007, Palgrave Macmillan, pp 73–99.

Carr D, Ott B: The older adult driver with cognitive impairment: "It's a very frustrating life," *JAMA* 303:1632–1641, 2010.

Centers for Disease Control and Prevention: *Health places terminology,* 2013. Available at http://www.cdc.gov/healthyplaces/terminology.htm. Accessed January 2016.

Counsell S: Driving expert eldercare forward—on and off the road, *J Gerontol Nurs* 42(5):47–48, 2016.

Daniel K, Cason CL, Ferrell S: Emerging technologies to enhance the safety of older people in their homes, *Geriatr Nurs* 30:384–389, 2009.

Dobbs B, Harper L, Wood A: Transitioning from driving to driving cessation: The role of specialized driving cessation support groups for individuals with dementia, *Top Geriatr Rehabil* 25:73–86, 2009.

Dugan E, Lee C: Biopsychosocial factors for driving cessation: Findings from the Health and Retirement Study, *J Aging Health* 25:1313–1328, 2013.

Feather J: Why older adults face more danger in natural disasters, *The Blog,* Dec 18, 2013. Available at http://www.huffingtonpost.com/john-feather-phd/why-older-adults-face-mor_b_4461648.html. Accessed January 2016.

Fuji S, Ito H, Yasuhara Y, et al: Discussion of nursing robot's capability and ethical issues, *Information* 17(1):349–353, 2014.

Grady J: Telehealth: A case study in disruptive innovation, *Am J Nurs* 114(4):38–45, 2014.

Gray-Vickrey P: Enhancing driver safety in dementia, *Alzheimer's Care Today* 11:147–148, 2010a.

Gray-Vickrey P: Research updates: Driving and dementia, *Alzheimer's Care Today* 11:149–150, 2010b.

Green M, Prior N, Capeluto G, et al: Climate change and health in Israel: Adaptation policies for extreme weather events, *Isr J Health Policy Res* 2:23, 2013.

Hogan T, Rios-Alba T: Emergency care. In Ham R, Sloane PD, Warshaw GA, et al, editors: *Primary care geriatrics*, ed 6, Philadelphia, 2014, Elsevier, pp 177–192, 2014.

Hooyman N, Kiyak H: *Social gerontology: A multidisciplinary perspective*, Boston, 2011, Allyn & Bacon.

Mars M: Health capacity development through telemedicine in Africa, *Yearb Med Inform* 2010:87–93, 2010.

Mathias J, Lucas L: Cognitive predictors of unsafe driving in older drivers: A meta-analysis, *Int Psychogeriatr* 21:637–653, 2009.

McGregor D: Driving over 65: Proceed with caution, *J Gerontol Nurs* 28:221–226, 2002.

Outzen M: Management of fever in older adults, *J Gerontol Nurs* 35:17–23, 2009.

Oxley J, Charlton J: Attitudes to and mobility impacts of driving cessation, *Top Geriatr Rehabil* 25:43–54, 2009.

Rantz M, Aud M, Alexander G, et al: Falls, technology, and stunt actors: New approaches to fall detection and risk fall assessment, *J Nurs Care Qual* 23:195–201, 2008.

Rosenbloom S: Meeting transportation needs in an aging-friendly community, *Generations* 33(2):33–41, 2009.

Rutledge C, Haney T, Bordelon M, et al: Telehealth: Preparing advanced practice nurses to address healthcare needs in rural and underserved populations, *Int J Nurs Educ Scholarsh* 11(1):1–9, 2014.

Servat J, Risco M, Nakasato Y, et al: Visual impairment in the elderly: Impact on functional ability and quality of life, *Clin Geriatr* 19(7):2011.

University of Maryland Medical Center: *Hypothermia*, 2013. Available at https://umm.edu/health/medical/altmed/condition/hypothermia. Accessed January 2016.

Wamala D, Augustine K: A meta-analysis of telemedicine success in Africa, *J Pathol Inform* 4:6, 2013.

Weiss J: Response to the commentary: Aging in community, *Res Gerontol Nurs* 9(1):14–15, 2016.

Wolf T, McGregor G: The development of a heat wave vulnerability index for London, United Kingdom, *Weather Climate Extremes* 1:59–68, 2013.

17

Living With Chronic Illness

Kathleen Jett

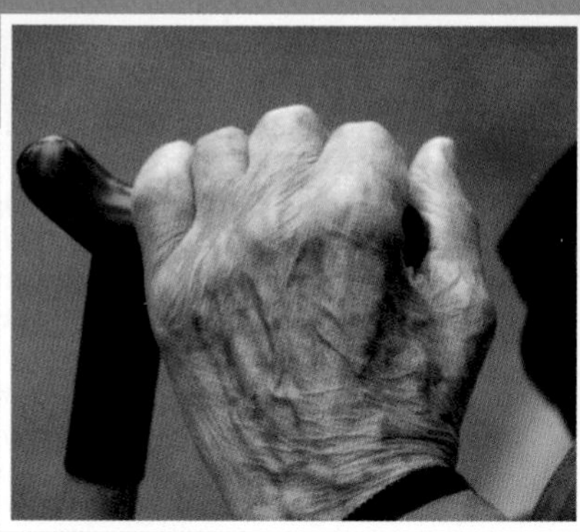

 evolve.elsevier.com/Touhy/gerontological

LEARNING OBJECTIVES

Upon completion of this chapter, the reader will be able to:

- Differentiate between chronic and acute illness.
- Discuss the factors that influence the experience of chronic illness.
- Identify competencies to improve care for those with chronic conditions.
- Discuss models to enhance self-care management of chronic illness.
- Discuss nursing interventions to maximize wellness in the presence of chronic illness.

THE LIVED EXPERIENCE

Just because you think you understand my disease doesn't mean you understand me. You do not know how I experience my illness. I am unique. I think and feel and behave in a combination that is unique to me.

Judith, age 87

During the past century, a major shift has occurred in the leading causes of death for all age groups—from infectious diseases and acute illnesses to chronic diseases and degenerative illnesses (Centers for Disease Control and Prevention [CDC], 2015a). The number of individuals with chronic illnesses is increasing rapidly and is influenced by many factors—from advances in medical sciences in treating illness and prolonging life to the "globalization" of lower income countries as diets change to those with more sugars, fats, and salt (World Health Organization [WHO], 2015).

A dramatic escalation in the numbers of persons with chronic illnesses is a global health concern. It accounts for more than half of the global health burden. Each year 17 million persons younger than age 70 and 22 million older than age 70 die of a noncommunicable disease, especially one of the cardiovascular diseases. Many of these deaths are preventable, especially for persons living in low- and middle-income countries (WHO, 2015).

Seven out of 10 deaths among Americans each year are from chronic diseases (CDC, 2015b). In 2008 41% of older Americans had three or more chronic conditions, 51% had one or two, and only 8% had perfect health (National Institutes of Health [NIH], 2014). Vulnerable and socially disadvantaged people of any age get sicker and die sooner as a result of chronic illness. A host of social determinants, especially education, age, income, gender, and ethnicity, influences levels of chronic illness.

Sixty-six percent of the country's overall health care budget is spent treating those with chronic conditions (CDC, 2015a). Among health care costs for older Americans, 95% are for chronic diseases. The cost of providing health care for one person age 65 or older is three to five times higher than the cost for someone younger than 65 (CDC, 2015a). One-fourth of Medicare (see Chapter 7) dollars are spent annually in the last year of the life of a ≥65-year-old person (Kaiser Family Foundation [KFF], 2015). Forty-three percent of Medicaid (see Chapter 7) dollars are spent in providing personal and nursing care in a nursing facility. The potential estimated loss in economic output as a whole between 2006 and 2015 for 23 nations totaled $84 billion (National Institute of Aging [NIA], 2015). Diminished quality of life is a major personal cost of living with chronic conditions for both the individual and his or her family and significant others. Disability is common, especially for those with advanced heart disease or arthritis. In turn, this disability results in social costs in terms of reduced financial productivity and in any number of other roles (see Chapter 26).

This chapter addresses chronic illness as a life experience and discusses how gerontological nurses can work with the person in secondary and tertiary prevention strategies (that is, detecting any new problems or exacerbations promptly and maximizing function and quality of life and promoting healthy aging).

ACUTE ILLNESS

Before chronic disorders can be discussed, their relationship to acute illness must be addressed. They cannot really be separated in the health of older adults because so many conditions are intricately intertwined. A previously stable chronic condition can and often does worsen when an acute illness occurs. An episode of pneumonia may trigger acute congestive heart failure even though before the episode the failure had been present but controlled through diet and medications.

Sudden changes in the functional, physiological, cognitive, psychological, or spiritual status of an older adult call for immediate and prompt nursing and medical assessment to determine the possibility of a reversible condition. A person with cognitive impairments attributable to dementia suddenly becomes more confused or less alert than usual and is found to have a urinary tract infection or constipation. Once the underlying condition is treated the person may return to his or her prior state. Unfortunately, as a result of age-related diminished physiological reserves (see Chapter 3), it takes longer to "bounce back," or the person never does fully return to the prior state of health and/or dies (Box 17.1). Further complicating a return to full functioning is the common situation that the person has several chronic disorders simultaneously (comorbidities).

BOX 17.1 Walking on Air

I have been walking about 4 miles a day for most of my life, but over the last year it is becoming more difficult. The bottoms of my feet tingle and sometimes it just doesn't feel like I can feel the ground as well and I am afraid I will miss a bump in the sidewalk and fall. My doctor says it is because my diabetes is getting worse. I don't quite understand that; I have had it for 20 years.

Helena at age 86

BOX 17.2 ADLs and IADLs

Activities of Daily Living (ADLs)
Bathing, dressing, eating, and getting around the house

Instrumental Activities of Daily Living (IADLs)
Preparing meals, shopping, managing money, using the telephone, doing housework, and taking medication

CHRONIC ILLNESS

"Chronic health problems are not fixable with shiny new technology, and do not promise the suspense, exhilarating hope, and dramatic ending that acute medical crises often do. They simply continue day after day, [they are] often invisible or misunderstood" (Hodges et al., 2001, p. 390). Chronic illnesses are those that occur slowly and progress slowly (WHO, 2015). They have an irreversible presence and may be hidden to outsiders. The presence of a chronic illness may be as little as an inconvenience or as great as an impairment of one's ability to perform even the most basic self-care activities (see Chapter 8). In 2013, 30% of community-resident Medicare beneficiaries ages 65 and older reported difficulty in performing one or more activities of daily living (ADLs), and an additional 12% reported difficulty with one or more instrumental activities of daily living (IADLs) (Box 17.2). By contrast, 95% of Medicare beneficiaries living in nursing facilities had difficulties with one or more ADLs, and 81% of them had difficulty with three or more ADLs (Fig. 17.1). According to the U.S. Census Bureau's American Community Survey, some type of disability was reported by 36% of people age 65 and older in 2014 (AOA, 2015).

For those with multiple chronic illnesses who are also frail (Box 17.3), the nurse is called upon to minimize the effect of any of the complications of the geriatric syndromes that may also be present (Box 17.4). The person with dementia and osteoporosis develops a urinary tract infection, and although he or she may have

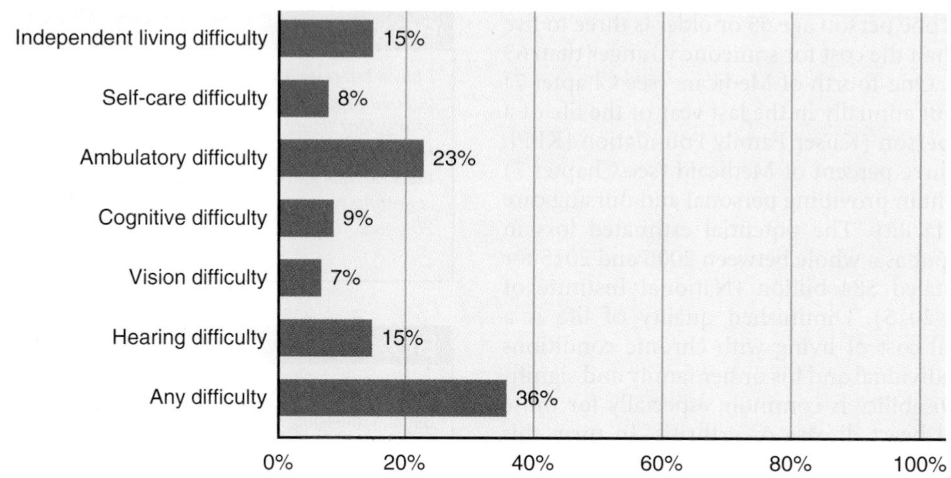

FIGURE 17.1 Percentage of persons 65+ with a disability, 2014. (Redrawn from Administration on Aging: *Profile of older Americans: 2015: Disability and activity limitations.* Available at http://www.aoa.acl.gov/Aging_Statistics/Profile/2015/16.aspx. Accessed June 2016.)

BOX 17.3 Tips for Best Practice

Assessing Frailty

Frailty is loosely defined as evidence of three of the following: unexplained weight loss, self-reported exhaustion, weak grip strength, slow walking speed, and low activity. It is better to ask specifically about each one of these symptoms. Many people consider the signs as "just a normal part of aging." To provide a method of quantifying frailty to the extent possible, a number of scales have been developed and some of them tested. Most are available free of charge for educational and professional practice use.

BOX 17.4 Most Common Conditions Referred to as "Geriatric Syndromes"*

- Falls and gait abnormalities
- Frailty
- Delirium
- Urinary incontinence
- Sleep disorders
- Pressure ulcers

*Note that there is considerable discussion about the exact "conditions" that are considered a "geriatric syndrome." There is agreement that a syndrome is something that does not neatly fit into another disease category.

From Brown-O'Hara T: Geriatric syndromes and their implications for nursing, *Nursing* 43(1):1–3, 2013.

been ambulatory, he or she falls and breaks a bone before treatment for the first acute condition is effective. The subsequent hospitalization for the fall leads to acute delirium in an unfamiliar environment and possibly death (see Chapter 15).

If not triggered by an acute event such as a seizure or a stroke, the onset of a chronic disease or a disability may be insidious and identified only during a wellness health screening. The person may have long periods of remission, times when symptoms are under control and function is at the highest level possible. Many persons continue to work and perform their usual activities and roles. The illness may only be identified when symptoms reach a level noticeable to the person (e.g., diminishing sensation to the feet, indicating years of hyperglycemia) (see Chapter 20) or to others (e.g., memory loss); or when the damage caused by the condition results in an acute event, such as an acute myocardial infarction (heart attack) indicative of many years of untreated, undertreated, or unknown hypertension (see Chapter 22).

Between 2012 and 2014, the most frequently occurring chronic conditions among older persons were high blood pressure (71% between 2009 and 2012), arthritis (49%), all types of heart disease (31%), and diabetes (21% between 2009 and 2012). Of those older than age 65, 25% had cancer (AOA, 2015). Worldwide, the most common conditions are cardiovascular disease of any kind, cancer, respiratory illnesses, and diabetes (WHO, 2015).

More than two out of every three older Americans have multiple chronic conditions. At all ages, the health status of Hispanics, Asian Americans, African Americans, and other minority population groups, such as American Indians/Alaska Natives and Native Hawaiians/Other Pacific Islanders, lags behind that of non-Hispanic whites. For a variety of reasons, older adults in these groups may experience the effects of health disparities more than younger people. Language barriers, reduced access to health care, historically low economic status, and different cultural norms can be major challenges to promoting health in an increasingly diverse older population (CDC, 2015a).

Symptoms of chronic illness interfere with many normal activities and routines, make medical regimens necessary, disrupt patterns of living, and frequently make it necessary for the individual to incorporate significant lifestyle changes. Physical suffering, loss, worry, grief, depression, functional impairment, and increased dependence on family or friends for support are among the potential negative consequences of chronic illnesses.

The current generation of persons 65 and older is living longer with more chronic diseases. A dramatic example of this phenomenon is the changing trajectory for persons with human immunodeficiency virus (HIV). Only a short time ago, those infected with HIV died of acquired immunodeficiency syndrome (AIDS) quickly, due to delayed diagnoses and absence of treatment. Since the advent of HIV-specific antiviral medications more persons will be living into later life with HIV. It is one more chronic disease that will be superimposed on hypertension, diabetes, dementia, and other disorders that commonly develop with aging.

Prevention

It is perhaps most accurate to say that many of the chronic diseases in late life are the result of our lifestyle choices at an earlier age. Most people in their sixties and seventies today can remember eating (or "smoking") candy in the shape of tiny cigarettes in imitation packaging when they were children. In doing so, they were emulating their parents and celebrities. Smoking tobacco early in life was often condoned rather than criticized. This explains the high levels of heart and lung disease after many years of tobacco exposure as children and younger adults.

Preventive practices were not emphasized until the very youngest of the baby boomers (born between approximately 1947 and 1964) became older (see Chapter 1). The document *Healthy People 2000* (CDC, 2009) was published in 1997 and proposed a national agenda for the achievement of improving the health of the nation. This was updated with *Healthy People 2010* (CDC, 2011) and with *Healthy People 2020* (Office of Disease Prevention and Health Promotion [ODPHP], 2015). The current edition is the first one that adds a section specific to improving the health of older adults.

BOX 17.5 Major Risk Factors for the Development of Chronic Diseases

- Smoking or exposure to second-hand smoke
- Lack of exercise
- High sugar and fat diet
- Obesity

In a document that builds on the *Healthy People* work, the *State of Aging and Health in America* provides intermittent status updates of 15 different indicators. The report of 2013 indicates that some areas have exceeded goals: (1) leisure time in the past month, (2) reduced obesity, (3) reduced smoking, (4) taking medications for diagnosed high blood pressure, (5) had mammogram within past 2 years, and (6) had timely colorectal cancer screenings. However, many other goals remain unmet, including no state having met the 2020 goal for flu or pneumonia vaccinations (CDC, 2013).

Both many chronic illnesses and their associated acute events are not inevitable consequences of aging. They may be prevented through healthy lifestyle choices at any age, the reduction of factors that increase one's risk for illness (Box 17.5), early detection, and careful attention to minimize a disease from advancing or causing other associated conditions. The use of preventive strategies has the potential to reduce morbidity (associated disability) and premature mortality (death sooner than would have occurred without the condition). As the emphasis continues to shift toward healthy lifestyle choices, it is anticipated that future cohorts of older adults, including the younger baby boomers, will be healthier and more functional longer than their predecessors.

THEORETICAL FRAMEWORKS FOR CHRONIC ILLNESS

Several theoretical frameworks have been used to understand the effect of chronic illness and organize the nurse's response: the Chronic Illness Trajectory (Corbin & Strauss, 1992; Strauss & Glaser, 1975) and the Shifting Perspectives Model (Paterson, 2001).

Chronic Illness Trajectory

The trajectory model, originally conceptualized by Anselm Strauss and Barney Glaser (1975) and later expanded by Corbin and Strauss (1992), has long aided health care providers to better understand the realities of chronic illness and its effect on individuals. According to this theoretical approach, chronic illness can be viewed from a life course perspective or along a trajectory. In this way, the course of a person's illness can be viewed as an integral part of the person's life rather than as an isolated event. The nurse's response is then holistic rather than isolated. The time between the diagnosis of an illness and death is divided into eight phases for the purpose of identifying goals and developing interventions (Table 17.1). The shape and stability of the trajectory are influenced by the combined efforts, attitudes, and beliefs held by the older person, family members, and significant others, and the involved health care providers (Box 17.6). Although it appears linear, it is instead fluid as crises reappear and are addressed and as instability becomes stable again until this is no longer possible.

TABLE 17.1 The Chronic Illness Trajectory and Nursing Reponses

Phase	Definition
1. Pretrajectory	Before the illness course begins, the preventive phase, no signs or symptoms present
2. Trajectory onset	Signs and symptoms are present, includes diagnostic period
3. Crisis	Life-threatening situation
4. Acute	Active illness or complications that require hospitalization for management
5. Stable	Controlled illness course/symptoms
6. Unstable	Illness course/symptoms not controlled by regimen but not requiring or desiring hospitalization
7. Downward	Progressive decline in physical/mental status characterized by increasing disability/symptoms
8. Dying	Progressive decline in physical/mental status characterized by increasing disability/symptoms Immediate weeks, days, hours preceding death

Examples of goals that nurses might establish include the following:

1. To assist a client in overcoming a plateau by increasing adherence to a regimen so that he or she might reach the highest level of functional ability possible within limits of the disability
2. To assist a client in making the attitudinal and lifestyle changes that are needed to promote health and prevent disease
3. To assist a client who is in a downward trajectory to be able to maintain sense of self and receive expert palliative care
4. To assist with advance care planning to ensure wishes are met
5. To assist the client who is in an unstable phase to gain greater control over symptoms that are interfering with his or her ability to carry out everyday activities

The Shifting Perspectives Model of Chronic Illness

The Shifting Perspectives Model (Paterson, 2001) is derived from a synthesis of qualitative research findings of living with chronic illness as an ongoing, continually shifting process in which the person moves between the perspectives of wellness in the foreground or illness in the foreground. This model is more reflective of an "insider" perspective on chronic illness as opposed to the more traditional "outsider" view. At any point in time, one may take precedence over the other, but the goal is to move toward the highest level of well-being even in the presence of illness through appropriate interventions.

The focus is on health within illness rather than illness first (Larsen et al., 2006; Paterson, 2001). People's perspective of the chronic illness is neither right nor wrong but is a reflection of their needs and situation. How people perceive the chronic illness at any given time influences how they interpret and respond to the disease, themselves, caregivers, and situations affected by the illness (Lindqvist et al., 2006; Paterson, 2001).

Chronic illness contains elements of both illness and wellness, and people with chronic illness live in the "dual kingdoms of the well and the sick" (Donnelly, 2003, p. 6). The illness in the foreground perspective is triggered when threats to control are perceived (signs of disease progression, lack of skills to manage the symptoms, and fear of suffering, loss, and the burden the illness may cause). This perspective has a protective function, may assist in conserving energy, and may help a person learn

BOX 17.6 Key Points in the Chronic Illness Trajectory Framework

- The majority of health problems in late life are chronic.
- Chronic illness and its management often profoundly affect the lives and identities of both the individual and the family members or significant others.
- The acute phase of illness management is designed to stabilize physiological processes and return to a state of stability.
- Maintaining stable phases is central in the work of managing chronic illness.
- A primary care nurse often has the role of coordinator of the multiple resources that may be needed to promote quality of life at any point along the trajectory.

more about the illness and try to adjust and come to terms with it (Paterson, 2001).

Those who are able to bring wellness to the foreground in the face of chronic illness exhibit courage and resilience and are able to develop strategies and draw on resources to adjust to the changes that are occurring and those that are anticipated. The shift from illness to wellness is an active process triggered by the need to return to the wellness perspective.

In the wellness in the foreground perspective, the focus is centered more on the self than the disease and its consequences. The illness becomes part of who a person is but it does not define the person. The illness is seen as an opportunity for growth and meaningful changes in relationships with the environment and others. This perspective is fostered by learning as much as possible about the illness, creating supportive environments, paying attention to one's own patterns of response to the illness, and sharing one's knowledge of the disease with others. With this perspective, one is able to focus on the emotional, spiritual, and social aspects of life while still attending to disease management and the effects of the illness on one's life. Paterson (2001) suggests that the shifting perspectives model calls for understanding the person's perspective and the reasons the person varies in his or her attention to symptoms; the nurse supports persons with, or at, either perspective.

IMPLICATIONS FOR GERONTOLOGICAL NURSING AND HEALTHY AGING

The goals of caring for persons with chronic disease are to minimize worsening, provide comfort when this is not possible, and be alert at all times for an added, reversible condition requiring prompt treatment. A multimodal approach is always necessary, including expert medical and nursing care and social, psychological, and spiritual support. Regardless of the setting, from acute care to home care, the nurse is usually the person who ensures that the best care of all types is provided, including functional rehabilitation (see Chapter 6).

Assessment

Assessment of the elder with a chronic illness is a holistic and interactive process. In no other situation is it necessary to consider all aspects of a person: physiological, psychological, social, spiritual, and functional. Each aspect is affected by the presence of the disease and in the context of the person's culture (see Chapter 2). Tools can be found throughout the text that can be used for assessment purposes, both comprehensive (see Chapter 8) and specific related to the chronic condition and development of an acute process (e.g., risk for fall in Chapter 15).

Since a chronic disease is an evolving one, so is the need for, and type of, assessment. There is the need for nursing skills to conduct ongoing evaluation of responses and outcomes, careful observation, periodic monitoring, alert watchfulness, and (most importantly) discussion and collaboration with elders about their perceptions, the meaning of their illness, and their plans for the future. The assessment helps identify the gap between the existing patient self-care abilities and needed self-care resources.

Interventions

Caring for patients with chronic illness is a combination of addressing acute events that are superimposed on underlying conditions. It is curing what can be cured, providing comfort, and assuring that the person receives optimal, evidence-based care for that which is chronic. Individuals with chronic conditions need care that is coordinated across time and centered on their needs, values, and preferences. They need self-management skills to minimize long-term complications and that help them know when to seek help. They need health care providers (including nurses) who understand the fundamental differences between episodic illness to be cured and chronic conditions to be managed over many years and over periods of stability and instability (WHO, 2015). Interventions must take into consideration all of the information learned in the assessment to work with the individual and significant others to help the person develop personal goals and achieve these whenever possible (see Chapter 4, Box 4.10).

The traditional medical care model and models of public health have not been effective in dealing with the complexity of chronic illness. The training, education, and skill of today's health care personnel have been inadequate in providing evidence-based care to older adults with chronic illnesses (WHO, 2015). The updated version of *Healthy People 2020* notes this need for improved training with a new objective aimed toward improving the health of older adults by increasing the proportion of the health care work force with geriatric certification.

Nursing roles may include direct caregiver, resource person, advisor, teacher, facilitator, and student (of the person who usually has years of experience dealing with the ups and downs of the illness) (Box 17.7). Gerontological nurses are care coordinators regardless of setting; they help people navigate through the maze of disparate financing and delivery systems that are complex and confusing and where care is often fragmented, less effective, and more costly than it could be (Box 17.8).

BOX 17.7 Nursing Roles in Caring for Persons With Chronic Illness

Counselor: Listen to the story, and come to know the person and what gives him or her meaning in life. Help person set realistic goals and expectations. Focus on potential rather than limitations.

Educator: Regarding the illness, its management and skills required for effective self-care.

Nursing practice: Ongoing with a focus on prevention of complications. Ensure delivery of the highest, evidence-based medical and nursing care at all times.

Coordinator: Assist with obtaining access to resources. Refer appropriately and when needed. Refer and coordinate palliative care as needed.

BOX 17.8 Challenges for the Person With a Chronic Illness

- Long-term and uncertain nature of the illness
- Costs associated with care including preventive and long-term personal care
- Little coordination of care across the continuum
- Lack of health care professionals with expertise in geriatrics and chronic care
- Focus of health care system on acute and episodic care
- Continued disparities in health care outcomes for vulnerable groups

Gerontological nurses develop and work with self-management programs to help persons with chronic illnesses function as independently as possible and prevent unnecessary hospitalizations. Several of the newest models are a result of changes to Medicare options under the Affordable Care Act (http://www.innovations.cms.gov/initiatives/index.html). Other current models include the Geriatric Resources for Assessment and Care of Elders model (GRACE) (Counsell et al., 2006; Indiana University, 2015), the Guided Care Results (http://www.guidedcare.org), and the Program of All-Inclusive Care for the Elderly (PACE) (CMS, n.d.) (Box 17.9).

Nurses work toward the achievement of the goals of *Healthy People 2020* to prepare individuals for a healthier later life and to enhance health and wellness for those already in later life. Progress is not measured in attempts to achieve cure, but rather in prompt responses to new acute events and maintenance of a steady state or regression of the chronic condition while remembering that the condition does not define the person.

Nursing's response of caring instead of curing brings the highest level of expertise to assist people in adapting, continuing to grow, and attaining a level of wellness and wholeness despite their illness and, ultimately, their functional limitations. Gerontological nurses know that understanding and caring for those with chronic illnesses and long-term disabilities require close caring relationships in order to accompany the person on his or her journey with hope, courage, and joy, day after day and year after year.

BOX 17.9 Characteristics of Successful Chronic Illness Management Models

- Interdisciplinary team of health care professionals, often led by a nurse
- Ability to conduct initial and intermittent comprehensive assessments
- Skill in the development of a comprehensive care plan that is individualized, incorporates evidence-based protocols, and is culturally appropriate
- Adequate funding to implement the plan over time
- Actively engages the patient and family caregivers in care
- Proactive monitoring of the patient's clinical status and ability and willingness to modify the care plan as needed
- Success in facilitating transitions across settings
- Facilitation of the patient's access to community resources

Healthy aging does not mean the absence of disease; rather, it means moving toward wellness in spite of disease. Someone once said that a chronic illness is like a grain of sand in an oyster; it irritates and creates a pearl, or the oyster just dies. Part of nursing intervention is aimed at helping create that pearl.

KEY CONCEPTS

- Declines in mortality, a growing older adult population, increasing medical expertise, and sophisticated technological developments have resulted in a great increase in the survival of the very old with multiple chronic disorders.
- The effects of chronic illness range from mild to life-limiting, with each person responding to unique circumstances in a highly individualized manner.
- The Chronic Illness Trajectory and the Shifting Perspectives Model of Chronic Illness offer useful frameworks to understand chronic illness and design nursing interventions.
- People with chronic illnesses can achieve wellness, and the role of the nurse is critical in the promotion of wellness.
- The goals of healthy aging include rapidly responding to acute and curable illnesses, minimizing risk for

disease, encouraging health promotion, and, in the presence of disease, alleviating symptoms, delaying or avoiding the development of complications, and maximizing function and quality of life.
- New models of cost-effective care are needed that increase access and improve outcomes and quality of life for persons with chronic illness. Nurses are particularly well prepared to assume major roles in chronic illness care.

ACTIVITIES AND DISCUSSION QUESTIONS

1. What type of education and counseling might the nurse provide to a 30-year-old person in anticipation of a healthier late life?
2. What would be the most devastating loss to you should you develop a chronic condition that affects day-to-day life?
3. What are some nursing interventions to assist a person with chronic illness to deal with loss? Practice or role-play various ways that these issues can be addressed.
4. How would you encourage an individual toward maximal participation in self-care?
5. What would be the measures of wellness during chronic illness?

REFERENCES

Administration on Aging (AOA): *Profile of older Americans*, 2015. Available at http://www.aoa.acl.gov/Aging_Statistics/Profile/index.aspx. Accessed August 2016.

Centers for Disease Control and Prevention (CDC): *Healthy People 2000*, 2009. Available at http://www.cdc.gov/nchs/healthy_people/hp2000.htm. Accessed December 2015.

Centers for Disease Control and Prevention (CDC): *Healthy People 2010*, 2011. Available at http://www.cdc.gov/nchs/healthy_people/hp2010.htm. Accessed December 2015.

Centers for Disease Control and Prevention (CDC): *The state of aging and health in America*, 2013. PDF and interactive version available at http://www.cdc.gov/aging. Accessed December 2015.

Centers for Disease Control and Prevention (CDC): *Chronic disease prevention and health promotion*, 2015a. Available at http://www.cdc.gov/chronicdisease/index.htm.

Centers for Disease Control and Prevention (CDC): *Chronic diseases: The leading causes of death and disability in the United States*, 2015b. Available at http://www.cdc.gov/chronicdisease/overview/. Accessed 2015.

Centers for Medicare and Medicaid Services (CMS): *The program of all-inclusive care for the elderly(PACE)*, n.d. Available at https://www.medicaid.gov/medicaid-chip-program-information/by-topics/long-term-services-and-supports/integrating-care/program-of-all-inclusive-care-for-the-elderly-pace/program-of-all-inclusive-care-for-the-elderly-pace.html. Accessed December 2015.

Corbin JM, Strauss A: A nursing model for chronic illness management based upon the trajectory framework. In Woog P, editor: *The chronic illness framework: The Corbin and Strauss nursing model*, New York, 1992, Springer.

Counsell SR, Clark DO, Frank KI: Geriatric Resources for Assessment and Care of Elders (GRACE): A new model of primary care for low-income seniors, *J Am Geriatr Soc* 54(7):1136–1141, 2006.

Donnelly G: Chronicity: Concepts and reality, *Holist Nurs Pract* 8(1):1–7, 2003.

Hodges HF, Keeley AC, Grier EC: Masterworks of art and chronic illness experiences in the elderly, *J Adv Nurs* 36(3):389–398, 2001.

Indiana University: *GRACE Team care*, 2015. Available at http://graceteamcare.indiana.edu/publications/publications.html. Accessed December 2015.

Keiser Family Foundation (KFF): *10 FAQs: Medicare's role in end-of-life care*, 2015. Available at http://kff.org/medicare/fact-sheet/10-faqs-medicares-role-in-end-of-life-care/. Accessed December 2015.

Larsen P, Lewis P, Lubkin I: Illness behavior and roles. In Lubkin I, Larsen P, editors: *Chronic illness: Impact and interventions*, Sudbury, MA, 2006, Jones & Bartlett.

Lindqvist O, Widmark A, Rasmussen B: Reclaiming wellness—Living with bodily problems, as narrated by men with advanced prostate cancer, *Cancer Nurs* 29(4):327–337, 2006.

National Institute of Aging (NIA): *Assessing the cost of aging and health*, 2015. Available at https://www.nia.nih.gov/research/publication/global-health-and-aging/assessing-costs-aging-and-health-care. Accessed December 2015.

National Institutes of Health (NIH): *NIH-commissioned Census Bureau report highlights effect of aging on boomers*, 2014. Available at http://www.nih.gov/news-events/news-releases/nih-commissioned-census-bureau-report-highlights-effect-aging-boomers. Accessed December 2015.

Office of Disease Prevention and Health Promotion (ODPHP): *Healthy People 2020*, 2015. Available at http://www.healthypeople.gov/. Accessed December 2015.

Paterson BL: The shifting perspectives model of chronic illness, *J Nurs Scholarsh* 33(1):21–26, 2001.

Strauss A, Glaser B: *Chronic illness and the quality of life*, St Louis, 1975, Mosby.

World Health Organization (WHO): *Noncommunicable diseases, fact sheet*, 2015. Available at http://www.who.int/mediacentre/factsheets/fs355/en/. Accessed December 2015.

18

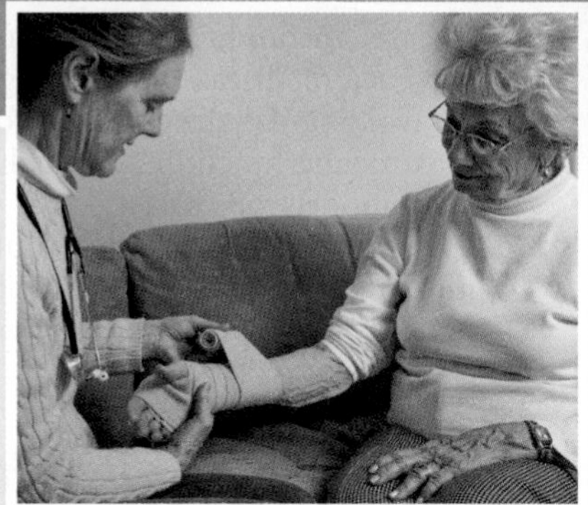

Pain and Comfort

Kathleen Jett

 evolve.elsevier.com/Touhy/gerontological

LEARNING OBJECTIVES

Upon completion of this chapter, the reader will be able to:

- Define the concept of pain and explain how this may be interpreted by the older adult.
- Compare the pain assessment in an older adult with that of a younger adult.
- Describe pharmacological and nonpharmacological measures to promote comfort for the person in pain.
- Discuss the special circumstances of pain in those with cognitive or communication limitations.
- Discuss the potential influence of culture on the expressions of pain.

THE LIVED EXPERIENCE

Ms. S. had cancer and was in severe pain most of the time. When she was referred to the local hospice, the nurse assessed the level of pain, the type of pain, and the level of relief that was acceptable. After a careful titration of her medications, it was found that only a long-acting morphine provided her comfort and an improved quality of life. However, at the dose needed she also hallucinated, seeing several puppies in the room with her. When asked if she wanted to reduce the dosage to eliminate this side effect, she responded, "No—I'll keep the puppies, I know they are not real and they don't hurt anything. I'd rather have them with me than the pain."

Helen, age 93

Pain is a subjective sensation of physical, psychological, or spiritual distress. It is a multidimensional phenomenon, and usually one type of pain is intertwined with another. Pain has many consequences, including questioning the meaning of one's life (Box 18.1). Physical pain is intensified when accompanied by any of the other types of pain (Molton & Terrill, 2014).

More than 50%, or about 18.7 million, older adults in the United States report that they live with "bothersome" pain to the extent that it reduces their function (Patel et al., 2013). In a study of primarily white elders with dementia, more than 60% were assessed to have pain and only about 30% were prescribed pain medications (Hunt et al., 2015).

How pain is expressed is highly influenced by the unique history of the individual and the meaning he or she ascribes to the pain. Some are only able to express pain in terms of "not feeling well"; others are highly articulate but controlled; still others are highly vocal and expressive. It is important for the nurse to realize that an individual responds to pain in a way that reflects his or her own cultural expectations and understanding of acceptable behavior (Box 18.2). How we respond to pain is part of who we are—part of our very core. Even the words we use to describe it are personal. Pain may be referred to as an ache, a hurt, "pester," nuisance, a bother, and so forth, with the language and the willingness to express it a manifestation of the person's relationship to

BOX 18.1 Tips for Best Practice

Potential Impact of Persistent Pain in the Older Adult

Depression
Sleep disturbances
Loss or worsening of physical function and fitness
Loneliness attributable to loss of social support/withdrawal from social activities
Loss of ability to perform usual role activities
Loss of ability to perform prior leisure activities
Potential for drug/alcohol abuse or misuse

Adapted from Epplin JJ, Higuchi M, Gajendra N, et al: Persistent pain. In Ham RJ, Sloane PD, Warshaw GA, et al, editors: *Primary care geriatrics: a case-based approach,* ed 6, pp 306–314, Philadelphia, 2014, Elsevier.

BOX 18.2 Examples of Possible Effect of Culture on Expressions of Pain

Stoic and unemotive
"Grin and bear it" approach—withdrawn, prefers to be alone
When asked about pain, it is minimized
Generalized to Northern European and Asian heritage

Emotive
Wants others around to validate feelings
Readily cries out in pain
Generalized to Hispanic, Middle Eastern, Mediterranean

Data from Carteret M: *Cultural aspects of pain management,* 2011. Available at http://www.dimensionsofculture.com/2010/11/cultural-aspects-of-pain-management/. Accessed January 2015.

whom he or she is speaking. The communication of pain is not always straightforward. Some do not, cannot, or will not verbalize their pain in ways that the nurse understands (see Chapter 2). Instead, the nurse must be alert to the cues that suggest that pain or discomfort is present.

Expert pain management is now part of evidence-based practice (The Joint Commission, 2015). Health care providers, especially nurses, are expected to adequately address patients' pain. In this chapter the types of pain are briefly reviewed and considered in the context of aging. The barriers to comfort are discussed, especially for those with cognitive impairments. Finally, interventions that the nurse can use to promote comfort are proposed.

BOX 18.3 Types of Physical Pain Sensations

- **Nociceptive pain** is associated with injury to the skin, mucosa, muscle, or bone and is usually the result of stimulation of pain receptors. This type of pain arises from tissue inflammation, trauma, burns, infection, ischemia, arthropathies (rheumatoid arthritis, osteoarthritis, gout), nonarticular inflammatory disorders, skin and mucosal ulcerations, and internal organ and visceral pain from distention, obstruction, inflammation, compression, or ischemia of organs. Nociceptive mechanisms usually respond well to common analgesic medications and nonpharmacological interventions.
- **Neuropathic pain** involves a pathophysiological process of the peripheral or central nervous system and presents as altered sensation and discomfort. This type of pain may be described as stabbing, tingling, burning, or shooting.
- **Mixed or unspecified pain** usually has mixed or unknown causes. A compression fracture causing nerve root irritation, common in older people with osteoporosis, is an example of a mix of nociceptive and neuropathic pain.

ACUTE AND CHRONIC PAIN

For many years there was a commonly held belief that older adults experienced pain less often than younger persons and that those with dementia had the least amount of pain of all. There now is a significant amount of research that refutes this, although the nuances of understanding are difficult. A normal change with aging is decreased tactile sensation, especially at the periphery such as the finger tips. Another age-related change is delayed reaction time. When these are combined the slight delay in the recognition of pain can lead to very serious consequences. There appears to be an increase in sensitivity to pain that is caused by pressure and must be considered in the protection of skin and muscle (e.g., pressure ulcer formation), especially in those who are frail (Kaye et al., 2010).

The most common type of pain in later life is chronic, also referred to in the literature as "persistent." Consistent with the most common cause of disability, pain in later life is often musculoskeletal in nature, from arthritis and degenerative spinal conditions such as degenerative joint disease (see Chapter 21) (Molton & Terrill, 2014). Overall pain may be differentiated as nociceptive, neuropathic, idiopathic, or mixed types (Box 18.3).

Acute Pain

Acute pain in late life is essentially the same as it is in earlier life: temporary, postoperative, procedural, or posttraumatic (e.g., fractures). A major difference is that acute pain at some point is a universal experience for the older adult attributable to increasing risk for traumatic injury (e.g., falls) and the development of pain-producing illnesses that defy comfort measures (e.g., arthritis). Further, as one ages if is much more likely that acute pain is superimposed on preexisting chronic pain.

Chronic Pain

Late-life pain is most often chronic and described as moderate to severe (Molton & Terrill, 2014). It may develop insidiously as a disease progresses or may be a sequela to an episode of acute pain. For example, after the acute pain of an outbreak of shingles, a specific kind of neuropathic pain (i.e., postherpetic neuralgia) may last a lifetime. The pain of more than 75% of those persons living in the community is thought to be chronic in nature (Molton & Terrill, 2014; Schofield, 2010). The number of those living in long-term care facilities with chronic pain is much higher, somewhere between 75% and 85%, the majority of which are untreated or undertreated (Horgas et al., 2012; Robinson, 2010).

Chronic pain is not time-limited and may vary in intensity throughout the day or with changes in activity. For example, persons with the emotional pain of depression usually feel worse in the morning with a lifting of mood as the day progresses (see Chapter 24). For those with the nociceptive pain of rheumatoid arthritis, pain is the most intense in the morning with slow but limited improvement with movement (see Chapter 21). Neuralgias occur frequently from long-standing diabetes, peripheral vascular disease, and other syndromes such as stroke, and iatrogenic side effects of treatment such as following chemotherapy. For those with persistent pain the only realistic goals may be reducing the sensation to a level that is possible and minimizing its effect on the person's quality of life and independence.

BARRIERS TO PROVIDING COMFORT FOR THOSE IN PAIN

Providing expert care to those in pain is a considerable challenge for gerontological nurses. The barriers are many and include attitudes and practices of nurses and other health care providers and of those in pain (Burns & McIlfatrick, 2015). Although the current cohort is usually quite compliant taking other medications, they often report that this is not the case with their analgesic prescriptions. The oldest adults may underreport pain and undertreat themselves because of the cost of the medications, the belief in an associated stigma, the association of pain to normal burdens of "old age," or the fear of addiction (AGS, 2009; Molton & Terrill, 2014). The nurse and patient may have incongruent personal beliefs and expectations of how pain is expressed. Both patients and nurses are influenced by their beliefs regarding the expression of pain. The influences come from the nurses' personal experiences, professional experiences, culture-associated values, and beliefs.

As a result of these and other barriers (Box 18.4) there remains a significant inadequacy of assessment and ultimately the undertreatment of pain, especially when the patient is from a social/racial/cultural/ethnic group other than those who comprise the majority in the setting (Inelman et al., 2012). The Centers for Medicare and Medicaid Services (CMS) have tried to address this issue in long-term care facilities by requiring periodic pain assessment of residents using standardized instruments. The results must be used to revise the plan of care (Ahn et al., 2015; CMS, 2015).

Special Circumstances: Pain in Elders With Cognitive and Communication Limitations

Study after study has shown that older adults who are cognitively impaired receive less pain medication, even

BOX 18.4 Barriers to Pain Management in Older Adults

Health Care Professional Barriers

- Lack of education regarding pain assessment and management
- Concern regarding regulatory scrutiny
- Fears of opioid-related side effects/addiction
- Belief that pain is a normal part of aging
- Belief that cognitively impaired elders have less pain
- Personal beliefs and experiences with pain
- Inability to accept the person's report of pain without "objective" signs

Patient and Family Barriers

- Fear of medication side effects
- Concerns related to addiction
- Belief that pain is a normal part of the aging process
- Belief that nothing can be done to adequately relieve pain
- Fear of being a "bad patient" if complaining or fear of what pain may signal

Health Care System Barriers

- Cost
- Time
- Cultural bias regarding opioid use

Modified from Hanks-Bell M, Halvey K, Paice JA: Pain assessment and management in aging, *Online J Issues Nurs* 9(3), 2004; Barber JB, Gibson SJ: Treatment of chronic non-malignant pain in the elderly: Safety considerations, *Drug Saf* 32(6):457–474, 2009.

though there is no convincing evidence that peripheral transmission of the sensation of pain to the brain is altered when affected by dementia (Ahn & Horgas, 2013; Epplin et al., 2014; Herr & Decker, 2004, pp. 47–48; Herr et al., 2006a, 2006b; Kovach et al., 2006a, 2006b; Ware et al., 2006). However, they may not understand why or where they are hurting and their expressions of pain are most likely different than those who can express themselves. It is a best practice to assume "that any condition that is painful to cognitively intact persons would also be painful to those with advanced dementia who cannot express themselves" (Herr, 2010, p. S1). Research has suggested that older people with mild to moderate cognitive impairment can provide valid reports of pain using self-report scales, but people with more severe impairment and loss of language skills may be unable to communicate the presence of pain in a manner that is easily understood.

For persons who are no longer able to express themselves verbally either because of dementia or as a result of other neurological conditions such as aphasia, communication of pain usually occurs through changes in behavior, such as changes in ambulation, agitation, aggression, increased confusion, or passivity (Ahn & Horgas, 2013). Caregivers should be educated to be particularly alert for the latter because the person is less disruptive and this may not be recognized as a change that may indicate pain. Providing comfort to those who cannot express themselves requires careful observation of behavior and attention to caregiver reports, knowledge of when subtle changes have occurred, and a willingness to help (Box 18.5). In nursing homes, the certified nursing assistants (CNAs) play an important role in pain assessment.

BOX 18.5 Pain Cues in the Person With Communication or Cognitive Limitations

Changes in Behavior

Restlessness and/or agitation or reduction in movement
Repetitive movements
Unusually cautious movements, guarding

Activities of Daily Living

Sudden resistance to help from others
Decreased appetite
Decreased sleep

Vocalizations

Person groans, moans, or cries for unknown reasons
Person increases or decreases usual vocalizations

Physical Changes

Pleading expression
Grimacing
Pallor or flushing
Physical tension such as clenching teeth or hands
Diaphoresis (sweating)
Increased pulse, respirations, or blood pressure

BOX 18.6 Fact and Fiction About Pain in Older Adults

MYTH: Pain is a normal part of aging.
FACT: Pain is not part of the normal changes with aging; however, its occurrence increases with age.
MYTH: If patients do not complain of pain, they do not have pain.
FACT: There are multiple barriers to the report and interpretation of expressions of pain in all persons.
MYTH: Narcotic medications are inappropriate for use in the older population.
FACT: Opioid analgesics are often the best treatment for moderate to severe persistent pain in order to help restore the person's ability to function and have some quality of life.

IMPLICATIONS FOR GERONTOLOGICAL NURSING AND HEALTHY AGING

Nurses and CNAs are usually the most attuned to the needs of patients and can become skilled at the recognition of pain in their patients. The nurse is responsible for assuring that the patient is comfortable and has the highest possible health-related quality of life regardless of cognitive or functional status or disease state. The nurse counters myths, stereotypes, and generalizations about aging and pain (Box 18.6). Care of the person in pain begins with assessment and continues through to the evaluation of the effectiveness of the interventions.

Assessment

Pain management begins with a complete assessment specific to pain with expert communication between the patient and the nurse to detail the pain: **o**nset, **l**ocation, **d**uration, **c**haracteristics, **a**ggravating and **r**elieving factors, and **t**reatment (OLD CART) such as the following questions: "When did it start?" "Do you have pain (discomfort based on descriptors acceptable to the individual) now?" "Where is your pain?" "Do you have pain every day?" "How would you describe it?" "What makes it worse?" "What makes it better (including a medication history, prescribed medication, herbs and supplements, over-the-counter drugs, and street drugs)?" (Box 18.7). Essential to the assessment is to determine how the pain is affecting function, sleep, appetite, activity, mood, relationships with others, and other factors particularly pertinent to older adults. A significant number of persons with pain are chronically sleep deprived and depressed (Box 18.8) (Molton & Terrill, 2014). Verbal descriptors should be obtained, that is, asking how the pain feels, such as burning or stabbing or aching. This information contributes to the diagnosis of the type of pain (e.g., neuropathic pain almost always is described as "burning," "tingling," or "shooting").

BOX 18.7 Basic Pain Assessment

1. **Self-report of pain intensity (rating):** ________
2. **OLD CART**
   Onset: ________
   Location: ________
   Duration: ________
   Characteristics: ________
   Aggravating factors: ________
   Relieving factors: ________
   Treatment previously tried: ________
3. **Comfort level goal:** ________

BOX 18.8 Additional Factors to Consider When Assessing Pain in Older Adults

Function: How is the pain affecting the ability to participate in usual activities and perform activities of daily living and instrumental activities of daily living?

Alternative expression of pain: Have there been recent changes in cognitive ability or behavior, such as increased pacing, grimacing, or irritability? Is there an increase in the number of complaints? Are the complaints vague and difficult to address? Has there been a change in sleep-wake patterns? Is the person resisting certain activities, movements, or positions?

Social support: What are the resources available to help the person cope and tolerate treatment? How is pain affecting the person's usual role? How is pain affecting relationships with others?

Pain history: How have previous experiences with pain been managed? What is the perceived meaning of the past and the present pain? What are the cultural factors that affect the belief in the meaning of the pain and the ability to express pain and receive relief?

For those who are able to express themselves, spoken analog scales are used most often; the person is asked to rate her or his pain on a scale of 1 (or "0") to 10, with 1 being no pain and 10 the worst imaginable, what is the worst it has ever been, and what it is today, now, and this week, for example. It should be noted that the use of numbers differs by culture and individuals. There may be specific numbers with specific meanings (e.g., "lucky number") that may skew this assessment (Booker, 2015).

For chronic pain, it is recommended to go a step further to ask, "If your pain could not be relieved completely, what would be an acceptable level?" The nurse may be very surprised at the high levels of pain that people have become accustomed to living with. For example, a person who is not outwardly expressive and does not "appear" to be in pain may describe it as 8 out of 10.

Written or visual analog scales have been developed; most can be used cross-culturally or with a person with limited English proficiency. Although they have been clinically tested, not all agree that they are best to use in the older population (Taylor et al., 2005) (Fig. 18.1). Scales using a series of facial expressions have been used as well (Fig. 18.2). Although some have been tested more broadly than others, the uniqueness of emotional expression associated with culture cannot be understated (Booker, 2015).

The use of scales may help those who would otherwise not report pain directly. Regular, repeated assessments, use of standardized tools with consistent documentation, and communication are the most important components of pain assessment. This leads to the ability to adjust the plan of care promptly, consistently, and expertly in the promotion of comfort. For more information on pain assessment, see the *Try This:* materials available at the website for the Hartford Institute for Geriatric Nursing (http://www.hartfordign.org).

Assessment of Pain in Those With Cognitive or Communication Limitations

When the person has cognitive impairments or difficulties with communication, assessment is particularly challenging and an alternate approach is needed (Box 18.9). In 2008 and 2010, Dr. Herr and colleagues conducted reviews of pain assessment tools for use with nonverbal patients in the nursing home setting. The *Pain Assessment in Advanced Dementia Scale* (PAINAD) and the *Pain Assessment Checklist for Seniors with Limited Ability to Communicate* (PACSLAC) were recommended for use. They are complementary to the Minimum Data Set 3.0 (MDS 3.0), which is already required for use in skilled nursing facilities (see Chapter 8). If the person cannot rate his or her pain (including by pointing), it is recommended that both tools be used to determine the presence or absence of pain based on behavior at initial assessment and following treatment.

The PAINAD is a simple, short, focused tool that has been found to demonstrate sensitivity to change in response to an intervention or over time (Warden et al., 2003) (Table 18.1). Four behaviors are rated by an observer on a scale of 0 to 2: breathing when not speaking, negative vocalizations, facial expression and body language, and if the person can be comforted. The tool is described in detail at a number of sites easily available on-line. It is in use in its original form internationally.

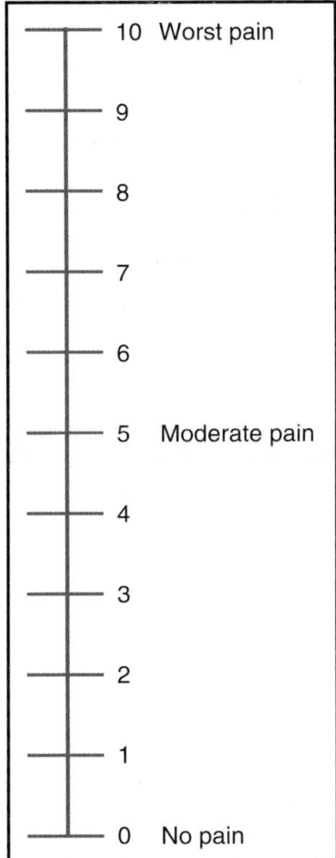

FIGURE 18.1 Example of a numeric rating/visual analog scale (can also be verbally administered). (From Pasero C, McCaffery M: *Pain assessment and pharmacologic management,* St Louis, 2011, Elsevier.)

The PACSLAC includes four domains of observation: facial expression, activity/body movement, social/personality/mood, and physiological/sleeping/eating/vocal. The CNA in any care setting can use the PACSLAC to assess pain (Fuchs-Lachelle & Hadjistavropoulos, 2004; Herr, 2010). Detailed instructions and downloads of the PACSLAC are available on-line in various formats. Understanding what the person is trying to communicate through his or her behavior is an essential skill for all staff caring for older people with limitations in ability to communicate.

Interventions

The goals of pain management in the older adult are to promote comfort, maintain the highest level of functioning and self-care possible, and balance the risks and benefits of the various treatment options. Careful use of pharmacological and nonpharmacological approaches helps to achieve these goals. A holistic approach is necessary because of the complex and pervasive nature of pain in later life.

Reducing suffering calls for first determining if there is a reversible cause, such as a urinary tract infection or a fracture, and then addressing these accordingly. If pain persists, the nurse and certified nursing assistant (CNA) intervene with expert assessment, careful listening, unconditional positive regard, ongoing support, and mobilization of resources. Use of pillows for support or body positioning, appropriate and comfortable seating and mattresses, frequent rest periods, and pacing of

BOX 18.9 Hierarchy of Pain Assessment in the Cognitively Impaired

Patient report, even if "yes" or "no"
Evaluate and treat all potential causes of pain
Observe for behaviors that may indicate pain
Surrogate report of behavior change
Observe response to analgesic trial

Data from Hadjistavropoulos T, Herr K, Turk DC, et al: Interdisciplinary expert consensus statement of pain in older persons, *Clin J Pain* 23(1 Suppl):S1–S43, 2007.

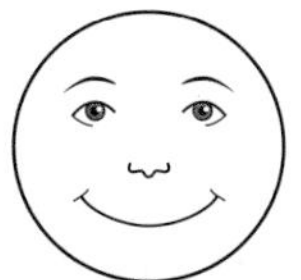 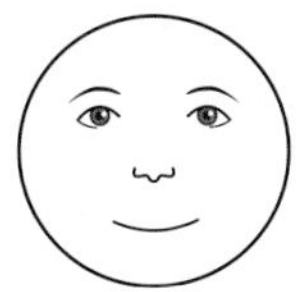 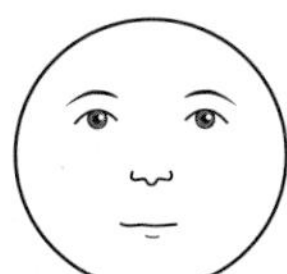 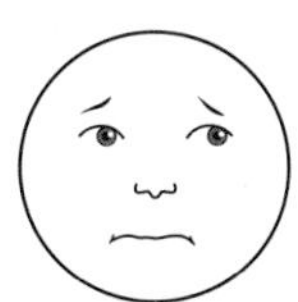 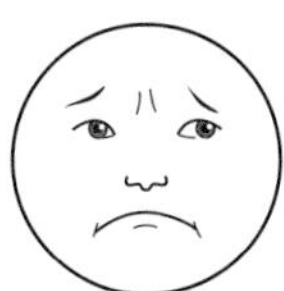

FIGURE 18.2 Example of a face pain-rating scale. (From Swartz MH: *Textbook of physical diagnosis,* ed 7, St Louis, 2014, Elsevier.)

TABLE 18.1 Pain Assessment in Advanced Dementia (PAINAD)

Items	0	1	2	Score
Breathing independent of vocalization	Normal	Occasional labored breathing Short period of hyperventilation	Noisy labored breathing Long period of hyperventilation Cheyne-Stokes respirations	
Negative vocalization	None	Occasional moan or groan Low level of speech with a negative or disapproving quality	Repeated trouble calling out Loud moaning or groaning Crying	
Facial expression	Smiling or inexpressive	Sad Frightened Frowning	Facial grimacing	
Body language	Relaxed	Tense Distressed pacing Fidgeting	Rigid Fists clenched Knees pulled up Pulling or pushing away Striking out	
Consolability	No need to console	Distracted or reassured by voice or touch	Unable to console, distract, or reassure	
			TOTAL*	

*Total scores range from 0 to 10 (based on a scale of 0 to 2 for five items), with a higher score indicating more severe pain (0 = no pain, 10 = severe pain).
From Warden V, Hurley AC, Volicer V: Development and psychometric evaluation of the Pain Assessment in Advanced Dementia (PAINAD) Scale, *J Am Med Dir Assoc* 4:9–15, 2003.

activities to balance activity and rest are important aspects of providing comfort.

The nurse encourages elders and their significant others to have an active role in pain management. The patient can keep a diary of levels of pain; this includes the times, types, and doses of medication taken; its effect and the duration of its benefit; and which activities increase or decrease the pain regardless of the type. This information helps establish patterns that may be useful in improving comfort by adjusting activity, providing medications at the right times, and helping the patient feel in control of some aspect of his or her life. A pain graph provides a visual picture of the highs and lows of the pain. The diary should be reviewed with the care provider and used to adjust dosages or timing of activities for optimal relief. The website http://www.optimismonline.com provides an excellent tool for chronicling and recording the highs and lows of psychological pain.

The nurse also encourages patients to stay as active as possible within their comfort range. The nurse learns the patient's ability to cope with pain and works within those parameters. When a person has pain with a needed specific activity (e.g., as in rehabilitation or psychotherapy), anticipation anxiety may decrease both the motivation and the ability to participate fully. In this case, the plan of care may include both pharmacological and nonpharmacological interventions such as relaxation before the scheduled activity. Administering an effective short-acting medication 30 to 40 minutes before the specific activity, such as physical therapy, may eventually lessen or eliminate the fear of discomfort and can greatly enhance the individual's capacity for that activity for those at all levels of cognitive functioning (Box 18.10) (see Chapter 13).

BOX 18.10 "Did My Back Hurt?"

Ms. R. had moderate dementia; she mistook her son for her husband, and did not know that she was in a nursing home. She began moaning from time to time, grimacing and pacing, and spending less time "visiting" with the other residents she believed were her guests. While she did not complain of pain, she began holding her back and refusing to get out of bed, and when up, she paced with more intensity of motion. An x-ray study of her back showed severe osteoporosis. She was started on a multidisciplinary approach to pain management. Ms. R. began resuming her usual activities and was much more cheerful than she had been in a long time. When asked if her back still hurt she responded, "Did my back hurt?"

Pharmacological Interventions

A pharmacological approach to pain relief is aimed at altering sensory transmission to the brain, specifically the cerebral cortex. This approach is most effective when the treatment plan involves teamwork between the patient and the health care providers (especially nurses), caregivers, and significant others. In some cultures the patient is not the decision-maker regarding treatment. With permission of the patient, the tribal elder, oldest son, or others may need to be consulted first (see Chapter 2).

The American Geriatrics Society published their last update of the management of persistent physical pain in 2009. There is a significant amount of evidence of the risks and benefits of the use of pharmacological agents in treating pain in older adults (AGS, 2009; Flaherty & Resnick, 2014). Analgesics (nonopioid and opioid agents) and adjuvant medications (antidepressants, anticonvulsants, and herbal preparations, including cannabinoids) have all been found to have a role in addressing both acute and chronic pain; however, several age-related changes and common conditions need to be considered, especially reduced kidney function, increased fat to muscle ratio, and decreased gastric motility (see Chapter 3) (Flaherty & Resnick, 2014). Nonopioid nonsteroidal anti-inflammatory drugs (NSAIDs) must be used with more caution than was previously thought (see Chapter 9).

To achieve the highest level of pain control, the goal is to erase the "memory of pain." This means that it is necessary to consistently both relieve and prevent the pain. The most effective way to do this is to provide around-the-clock (ATC) dosing at the appropriate dosage and at the right time (Portenoy et al., 2006).

In gerontological nursing it is essential that medications are started at the lowest dose possible. However, it is equally as important for the dosages to be titrated up as needed to the level that pain is relieved to a point that is acceptable to the patient and the relief is *continuous* (Drew et al., 2014).Too often, while a low dose is started, increases are delayed and suffering is unnecessarily prolonged. The adage "Start low, go slow, but go!" is important to remember.

Nonopioid analgesics. Acetaminophen (Tylenol) and NSAIDs are the non-narcotic analgesics most often used for relief of physical pain in older adults. Acetaminophen has been found to be effective for the most common causes of physical pain, such as osteoarthritis and back pain, and should always be considered a first-line approach unless contraindicated (AGS, 2015). If acetaminophen is used for persistent pain, ATC dosing may provide adequate relief. When used appropriately, it is not associated with gastrointestinal (GI) bleeding or adverse renal or cardiac effects.

SAFETY ALERT

The maximum dose of acetaminophen is 4 g (4000 mg) in 24 hours from **all sources** and is reduced for people with renal or hepatic dysfunction or who drink alcohol; the dose is easily reached when "extra-strength" formulations are taken at 1000 mg per tablet.

When chronic pain is from inflammation or from a short arthritic flare, one of the NSAIDs is sometimes used. However, older adults have been found to be at a higher risk for adverse drug effects from NSAIDs than younger adults, especially in persons with heart or renal disease, in persons with preexisting gastric irritation, or in those with low albumin levels (AGS, 2012). In the summer of 2015 the U.S. Food and Drug Administration (FDA) reiterated the findings that NSAIDs alone may increase blood pressure, reduce renal function, worsen heart failure, or contribute to a stroke (see Chapter 9) (U.S. FDA, 2015). A significant number of NSAID-related hospitalizations for adverse drug reactions have occurred, especially when co-administered with aspirin (AGS, 2009; Papaleontiou et al., 2010). The recent Beers Criteria lists the NSAIDs as inappropriate for use in the older adult because of these reasons (AGS, 2015).

SAFETY ALERT

In 2006, the Food and Drug Administration in the United States issued a warning regarding the use of aspirin (81 mg) and ibuprofen (Advil) at the same time. When taken together, the aspirin is less cardioprotective (i.e., there is less antiplatelet effect), and the person's risk for a cardiac event increases. For persons who take immediate-release aspirin with even a single dose of ibuprofen (400 mg), the ibuprofen should be taken at least 30 minutes after or 8 hours before the aspirin.

Data from Food and Drug Administration: *Information for healthcare professionals: Concomitant use of ibuprofen and aspirin,* 2006. Updated 2013. Available at http://www.fda.gov/Drugs/DrugSafety/PostmarketDrugSafetyInformationforPatientsandProviders/ucm125222.htm.

An approach that has been used to address the potential adverse drug reactions to NSAIDs is to alternatively use cyclooxygenase-2 (COX-2) inhibitors. COX-2 selective inhibitors appear to be as effective and have fewer GI side effects. However, other potential side effects do not differ from the other NSAIDs; cautions from the American Geriatrics Society remain, and renal function in particular must be monitored. Two of the three originally in this group have been taken off the market for their risk of adverse cardiac effects; only celecoxib (Celebrex) remains. Co-administration of any of the gastric agents available (histamine-2 [H_2] antagonists or proton pump inhibitors) may be helpful and reasonable, especially for persons at a higher risk for GI bleeding. NSAIDs cannot be used by persons taking anticoagulants such as warfarin and only for a short time in persons with hypertension.

Opioid analgesics. Acute traumatic physical pain is usually easily controlled by common analgesic medications, especially opioids. In the hospital setting an analgesic pump controlled by the patient is used for a restricted period. At the same time, the older a person is, the more likely it is that the person will have an adverse reaction to a medication (see Chapter 9). For example, most analgesics cause sedation, which increases the risk for falls, delirium, and any of the geriatric syndromes (see Chapter 17).

Opioid analgesics effectively treat both acute and persistent physical pain and have a very important role in the management of the latter yet require utmost caution in their use with older adults (Makris et al., 2015). They may produce a greater analgesic effect, a higher peak effect, and a longer duration of effect in older adults when compared to younger adults attributable in part to prolonged half-lives (see Chapter 9). However, responses to opioids are highly individualized, especially in aging. Depending on their metabolism, a standard dose in one person may prove toxic and have no effect in another (see Chapter 9). The recommendation is to start with the lowest anticipated effective dose, monitor the response frequently, and titrate slowly to the desired effect, especially applicable with the use of opioid pain relievers. They are available in oral, parenteral, and transdermal delivery methods.

Relief of chronic pain should be planned for the "around the clock" approach with a combination of long-acting sustained-release analgesics and generous use of as-needed (PRN) medications for "breakthrough" pain. The doses of the PRN medications are monitored so that the long-acting doses can be adjusted to the point that breakthrough pain is at a minimum. If breakthrough medication is needed on a regular basis, this is an indication that the long-acting medication dosage needs adjustment. Breakthrough pain may occur occasionally during a stable regimen of long-acting medication, and additional medication should always be available. Opioids used long term for chronic pain control should be convenient and easy to administer or take. As with all other medications, the simplest regimen is the one most likely to be effective and to be followed more consistently, and least likely to be misused (see Chapter 9).

Side effects should be expected and transient or treatable; all are particularly dangerous to older adults, especially the frail adults. These include gait disturbance, dizziness, sedation, falls, nausea, pruritus, and constipation. Side effects may be lessened or prevented when the prescribing provider works closely with the patient and nurse to slowly increase the dosage of the drug to a point where the best relief can be obtained with the fewest side effects. Sedation and impaired cognition do occur when opioid analgesics are started or when dosages are increased. This often causes great concern from patients, families, and nurses but is usually temporary. Patients and caregivers should be cautioned about the potential for falls, and appropriate safety precautions should be instituted.

The nurse provides close observation of the person's response and works to prevent and promptly treat side effects or adverse drug reactions. Since constipation is almost universal when opioids are used in older patients, the nurse can ensure that an appropriate bowel regimen is begun at the same time as the opioids. A daily dose of a combination stool softener and mild laxative may be very helpful, along with ensuring adequate fluid intake and exercise.

Although many of the opioid pain relievers can be used in later life, albeit with caution, *the use of meperidine (Demerol) is absolutely contraindicated* (AGS, 2015). The metabolites of meperidine can quickly produce confusion, psychotic behavior, and seizures. The same can be said for pentazocine (Talwin) and the nonopioid methadone. The nurse can refer to the Agency for Healthcare Research and Quality guidelines for acute and chronic pain management as well as the latest equianalgesic charts if they are needed (http://www.ahrq.gov).

Adjuvant drugs. There are a number of drugs developed for other purposes that have been found to be useful in the management of physical pain, sometimes alone, but more often in combination with an analgesic; these are referred to as *adjuvant drugs*.

Adjuvant drugs are thought to be most effective for neuropathic pain syndromes such as postherpetic neuralgia and diabetic nephropathy (pain described as sharp, shooting, piercing, or burning). Cannabinoids are being used with increased frequency as they become legal for use in states across the United States. They have been found to be especially useful for this type of pain as well (Vargas-Schaffer, 2010).

The tricyclic antidepressants such as amitriptyline had been used widely; however, because of their potential for adverse effects, they are now used less often. Although the mechanism is unknown, anticonvulsants (e.g., gabapentin [Neurontin]) and the mixed serotonin and norepinephrine reuptake inhibitors (SNRIs) (e.g., duloxetine [Cymbalta]) seem to be helpful with fewer problems (AGS, 2009).

Other agents. Topical agents (e.g., capsaicin, lidocaine patch) may have mild to moderate local effects; skin must be intact and the area watched for signs of irritation.

Nonpharmacological Measures of Pain Relief

Nurses have a long history of comforting patients through nonpharmacological measures. This may be either in the form of a caring and supportive relationship or through the use of specific techniques performed by the nurse or at the recommendation of the nurse. Several methods that elders use are briefly reviewed here, but it must be acknowledged that this represents only a small sample of what is available (http://www.nccih.nih.gov).

Cutaneous stimulation. Nurses have long provided massage, vibration, heat, cold, and ointments. Heat and cold temporarily interrupt the transmission of pain impulses to the cerebral pain center; however, caution must be used in consideration of the cause of the pain. Heat provides comfort but will also increase the circulation to the area and therefore is contraindicated in occlusive vascular disease and in nonexpansive tissue such as bursae (some joints), where it may increase pain (Cherian et al., 2016). Intermittent application of cold packs is especially recommended for pain related to muscle strain, a common complaint in older patients. Care must be taken when applying heat and cold to older skin to prevent skin damage because of normal age-related thinning (see Chapter 3).

Several forms of cutaneous nerve stimulation involve the application of small amounts of electricity to the skin to achieve the same purpose. The best known of these is TENS (transcutaneous electrical nerve stimulation) and has been used in a variety of settings to treat a range of conditions. Patients often reported anecdotally that at least they were doing "something" for their pain. The effectiveness of TENS and similar devices has been study and thus far shown to be inconclusive (Beaulieu & Schneider, 2013; Moreno-Duarte et al., 2014). Subcutaneous stimulation may be more helpful and is being used with increasing frequency for musculoskeletal pain that does not respond to anything else.

Acupuncture and acupressure. Pain is registered as impulses pass through the theoretical pain gate in the spine and register the sensation in the brain, which in turn signals the central mechanism of the brain to return counter-impulses, which close the gate. Acupuncture uses tiny needles inserted along specific meridians or pathways in the body (National Center for Complementary and Integrative Health [NCCIH], 2016). Acupressure is pressure applied with the thumbs or tip of the index finger at the same locations. It is thought that acupuncture and acupressure stimulate nerve clusters that cause the "pain gate" to close more quickly or that trigger the release of the body's own opiate substances, enkephalins (endorphins). Acupuncture and acupressure have been used for thousands of years, and scientific evidence of their effectiveness in the treatment of persistent pain is growing, but usefulness for other illness is still under investigation (NCCIH, 2016; Vickers et al., 2012). There has been some evidence that acupuncture is effective for specific conditions (i.e., pain associated with back, neck, and shoulder; osteoarthritis; and chronic headaches) (NCCIH, 2016).

Touch. Some say the use of touch therapies is a legacy in nursing. Over the years, different kinds of touch have been formalized to include those referred to as Healing Touch, Therapeutic Touch, Reiki, and others. When combined with purposeful relaxation, touch may decrease anxiety, reduce muscle tension, and help relieve pain. The acceptability of touch by individual and culture varies considerably. Some touch may never be acceptable, such as cross-gender touch in strict Muslim or Orthodox Jewish traditions (International Strategy and Policy Institute [ISPI], 1999). The culturally sensitive nurse always requests permission before touching a patient.

Biofeedback. Biofeedback is a cognitive-behavioral approach that has been applied to pain control. It is based on the theory that an individual can learn voluntary control over some body processes and alter them by changing the physiological correlates appropriate to them. Training and equipment of some type are needed to learn how to alter one's body response through biofeedback. It requires full cognitive functioning and manual dexterity for self-treatment.

Distraction. Distraction is a behavioral strategy that temporarily lessens the perception of pain by drawing the person's attention away from the pain. In some instances the individual is completely unaware of the pain; in other instances the intensity of pain is significantly diminished. Pain messages are more slowly transmitted to the pain center in the brain, and therefore less pain is felt. The most common forms of distraction include slow rhythmical breathing, slow rhythmical massage, rhythmical singing or tapping, active listening, guided imagery, and humor (Steele & Steele, 2009).

Relaxation, meditation, and imagery. As a behavioral strategy, relaxation enables the quieting of the mind and the muscles, providing the release of tension and anxiety. Relaxation should be adjunctive to all pharmacological interventions and for all types of pain. Meditation and imagery are two methods of promoting relaxation. Several studies using guided imagery have shown that there was a decrease in pain perception in foot pain and abdominal pain. It was suggested that a strong image of a pain-free state effectively alters the autonomic nervous system's responses to pain (NCCIH, 2016).

Pain Clinics

Pain clinics provide a specialized, often comprehensive, multidisciplinary approach to the management of pain that has not responded to the usual, more standard approaches as described earlier. The use of pain clinics by elders has been limited. However, their use should be encouraged when appropriate. The number and types of pain clinics and programs have increased as a response to continued poor pain management in general health care practice. Pain center programs may be inpatient, outpatient, or both. Pain clinics are generally one of three types: syndrome-oriented, modality-oriented, or comprehensive. Syndrome-oriented centers focus on a specific chronic pain problem, such as headache or arthritis pain. Modality-oriented centers focus on a specific treatment technique, such as relaxation or acupuncture/acupressure. The comprehensive centers tend to be larger and associated with medical centers. These centers include many services and provide a thorough initial assessment (physical, mental, psychosocial) of the person in pain. More and more centers are utilizing an integrated health approach including any or all of the strategies described previously.

The goals of the centers are to decrease pain intensity to a tolerable limit or eliminate it, if possible; improve functionality and activities of daily living (ADLs); increase involvement in family and social activities; decrease depression; and improve mood. This is accomplished by improving quality and frequency of assessment, improving optimal use of analgesics, assisting in minimizing analgesic adverse reactions, selecting nonpharmacological interventions, and evaluating outcomes associated with treatment (Fine, 2012). The nurse should be familiar with the types of pain management clinics available in their communities to provide the patient and family with necessary information to make a decision.

Evaluation

The nurse, the patient, and the significant others work together to find comfort for the patient with pharmacological and nonpharmacological interventions working in harmony (Box 18.11). Evaluation of pain relief strategies requires repeated reassessment of the patient's status and comfort level. Indicators of comfort include relaxation of skeletal muscles that were tense and rigid during pain, increased activity level and sense of self-worth, and the ability to better concentrate, focus, and increase attention span, regardless of cognitive status. The individual is better able to rest, relax, and sleep. Verbal indicators reflect the patient referring to the decrease in pain or the absence of pain during conversation.

BOX 18.11 General Principles of Pharmacological Management of Pain in Older Adults

1. When pain is assessed, negotiate a pain relief or comfort goal with the patient.
2. Be aware of other conditions that may affect assessment and management of pain.
3. Anticipate age-associated, but unpredictable, differences in sensitivities and toxicities related to medication use.
4. Always start at a low dose and slowly titrate to around-the-clock pain relief.
5. Use the least-invasive possible route of administration first.
6. Plan timing of medication administration to meet the needs of the patient.
7. Never use placebos.
8. Consider complementary, nonpharmacological, and pharmacological approaches.

The evaluation of pain management and relief is also measured with the same instruments used in the initial assessment for a means of comparison. Reevaluations of the frequency and intensity of pain and response to pharmacological and nonpharmacological interventions are done. Adjustments of treatment regimens and interventions are based on reassessment findings and continue until optimal comfort is produced and maintained and in doing so health is promoted at any stage of life and wellness. It has now been shown that a combination of pharmacological and nonpharmacological interventions appears to be most effective in the relief of both acute and chronic pain. In one study it was found that up to 50% of the older adults reported using at least three different strategies at the same time to control their pain (Barry et al., 2005). The basic approach to pain control is to encourage whatever strategies have been effective in the past without causing harm. This is particularly applicable for older adults with a lifetime of experience at managing their own pain and that of others. In some cases, what is now referred to as complementary and alternative or integrative medicine (CAM) is actually the formalization of approaches that people have used for years. More and more of what is considered CAM is gaining acceptance by insurers such as Medicare.

Regardless of the care setting or role played, nurses have a responsibility to let go of their own expectations and promote comfort to those who are suffering, regardless of the cause and manner of expression of this suffering. The best gerontological nursing care is that provided in a nonjudgmental manner with the goal of comfort always—not just to lessen pain but to relieve it and prevent its reoccurrence.

KEY CONCEPTS

- The absence of expressed pain does not necessarily imply comfort. Comfort is a state of ease and satisfaction of bodily needs and self-worth.
- The experience of pain is not limited to that which is of physical origin. Pain related to psychological or spiritual factors can have the same effect and is often combined with that arising from physical causes.
- Assessment of pain is influenced by many misconceptions, myths, and stereotypes about pain.
- Culture, ethnicity, family, and individual characteristics all influence one's tolerance and expression of pain as well as the acceptance of relief interventions.
- Older adults with cognitive or communication limitations may demonstrate pain by increased levels of confusion, restlessness, aggression, or withdrawal.
- The nursing goal is to assist in pain relief. Some pain medications are more appropriate than others for use with elders.
- Acute and persistent/chronic pain may necessitate different therapeutic approaches. Chronic pain predominates in the lives of most older adults.
- Various combinations of pharmacological and nonpharmacological pain control can be effective but must be individually designed with the elder and significant others involved in the decision-making process.

ACTIVITIES AND DISCUSSION QUESTIONS

1. Select a culture other than your own and research how pain is expressed by persons who hold traditional beliefs in that culture.
2. How does assessment of pain differ in cognitively impaired older people?
3. What pharmacological and nonpharmacological therapy is available, and how can each type work with the other to relieve pain?

REFERENCES

Ahn H, Garvan C, Lyon D: Pain and aggression in nursing home residents with dementia: Minimum Data Set 3.0 analysis, *Nurs Res* 64(4):256–263, 2015.

Ahn H, Horgas A: The relationship between pain and disruptive behaviors in nursing home residents with dementia, *BMC Geriatr* 13:14, 2013.

American Geriatrics Society (AGS): Pharmacological management of persistent pain in older persons: American Geriatrics Society panel on the pharmacological management of persistent pain in older persons, *J Am Geriatr Soc* 57:1331, 2009.

American Geriatrics Society (AGS): American Geriatrics updated Beers Criteria for potentially inappropriate medication use in older adults, *J Am Geriatr Soc* 60(4):616–631, 2012.

American Geriatrics Society (AGS): American Geriatrics updated Beers Criteria for potentially inappropriate medication use in older adults, *J Am Geriatr Soc* 63(3):2227–2246, 2015.

Barry L, Gill T, Kerns R, et al: Identification of pain reduction strategies used by community-dwelling older persons, *J Gerontol A Biol Sci Med Sci* 60(12):1569–1575, 2005.

Beaulieu L, Schneider C: Effects of repetitive peripheral magnetic stimulation on normal or impaired motor control: A review, *Neurophysiol Clin* 43(4):251–260, 2013.

Booker S: The state of "cultural validity" of self-report pain assessment tools in diverse older adults, *Pain Med* 16:232–239, 2015.

Burns M, McIlfatrick S: Nurses' knowledge and attitudes towards pain assessment for people with dementia in a nursing home setting, *Int J Palliat Nurs* 21(10):479–487, 2015.

Centers for Medicare and Medicaid Services (CMS): *Quality measures*, 2015. Available at https://www.cms.gov/Medicare/Quality-Initiatives-Patient-Assessment-instruments/NursingHomeQualityInits/NHQIQualityMeasures.html. Accessed January 2016.

Cherian JJ, Jauregui JJ, Leichliter AK, et al: The effects of various physical non-operative modalities on the pain in osteoarthritis of the knee, *Bone Joint J* 98-B(1 Suppl A):89–94, 2016.

Drew D, Gordon D, Renner L: The range of "as needed" range orders for opioid analgesics in the management of pain: A consensus statement of the American Society of Pain Management Nurses and the American Pain Society, *Pain Manag Nurs* 15(2):551–554, 2014.

Epplin JJ, Higuchi M, Gajendra N, et al: Persistent pain. In Ham RJ, Sloan PD, Warshaw GA, et al, editors: *Primary care: A case-based approach*, ed 6, Philadelphia, 2014, Elsevier, pp 306–314.

Fine PG: Treatment guidelines for the pharmacological management of pain in older persons, *Pain Med* 13(Suppl 2):S57–S66, 2012.

Flaherty E, Resnick B, editors: *Geriatric nursing review syllabus: A core curriculum in advanced practice geriatric nursing*, ed 4, 2014, American Geriatric Society.

Fuchs-Lachelle S, Hadjistavropoulos T: Development and preliminary validation of the Pain Assessment Checklist for Seniors with Limited Ability to Communicate (PACSLAC), *Pain Manag Nurs* 5:37, 2004. Available at http://e-pacslac.com.

Herr K: Pain in the older adult: An imperative across all health care settings, *Pain Manag Nurs* 11(2 Suppl):S1, 2010.

Herr K, Decker S: Assessment of pain in older adults with severe cognitive impairment, *Ann Longterm Care* 12:46, 2004.

Herr K, Coyne PJ, Key T, et al: Pain assessment in the nonverbal patient: Position statement with clinical practice recommendations, *Pain Manag Nurs* 7:44, 2006a.

Herr K, Bjoro K, Decker S: Tools for assessment of pain in nonverbal older adults with dementia: A state of the science review, *J Pain Symptom Manage* 31:170, 2006b.

Horgas A, Yoon SL, Grall M: *Pain: Nursing standards of practice protocol: Pain management in older adults*, 2012. Available at http://www.consultgerirn.org/topics/pain/want_to_know_more. Accessed January 2016.

Hunt LJ, Covinsky KE, Yaffe K, et al: Pain in community-dwelling adults with dementia: Results from the National Health and Aging Trends study, *J Am Geriatr Soc* 63(8):1503–1511, 2015.

Inelman EM, Mosele M, Sergi G, et al: Chronic pain in the elderly with advanced dementia. Are we doing our best for their suffering?, *Aging Clin Exp Res* 23(3):207–212, 2012.

International Strategy and Policy Institute (ISPI): *Guidelines for health care providers interacting with Muslim patients and their families,* 1999. Available at http://www.ispi-usa.org/guidelines.htm. Accessed January 2016.

Kaye AD, Baluch A, Scott JT: Pain management in the older population: A review, *Ochsner J* 10(3):179–187, 2010.

Kovach C, Logan BR, Noonan PE, et al: Effects of the Serial Trial Intervention on discomfort and behavior of nursing home residents with dementia, *Am J Alzheimers Dis Other Demen* 21:147, 2006a.

Kovach C, Noonan PE, Schlidt AM, et al: The Serial Trial Intervention: An innovative approach to meeting the needs of individuals with dementia, *J Gerontol Nurs* 32:18, 2006b.

Makris UE, Pugh MJ, Alvarez CA, et al: Exposure to high-risk medications is associated with worse outcomes in older veterans with chronic pain, *Am J Med Sci* 350(4):279–285, 2015.

Molton IR, Terrill AL: Overview of persistent pain in older adults, *Am Psychol* 69(2):197–207, 2014.

Moreno-Duarte I, Morse L, Alam M, et al: Targeted therapies using electrical and magnetic neural stimulation for the treatment of chronic pain in spinal cord injury, *Neuroimage* 85(Pt 3):1003–1013, 2014. doi: 10.1016/j.neuroimage.2013.05.097. [Epub 2013 May 30].

National Center for Complementary and Integrative Health (NCCIH): *Acupuncture in depth,* 2016. Available at https://nccih.nih.gov/health/acupuncture/introduction. Accessed January 2016.

Papaleontiou M, Henderson CR, Turner BJ, et al: Outcomes associated with opioid use in the treatment of chronic noncancer pain in older adults: A systematic review and meta-analysis, *J Am Geriatr Soc* 58:1353, 2010.

Patel KV, Guralnik JM, Dansie EJ, et al: Prevalence and impact of pain among older adults in the United States: Findings from the 2011 National Health and Aging Trends Study, *Pain* 154(12):2649–2657, 2013.

Portenoy RK, Bennett DS, Rauck R, et al: Prevalence and characteristics of breakthrough pain in opioid-treated patients with chronic cancer pain, *J Pain* 7:583, 2006.

Robinson P: Pharmacological management of pain in older persons, *Consult Pharm* 25(Suppl A):11, 2010.

Schofield P: "It's your age": The assessment and management of pain in older adults, *CEACCP* 10:93, 2010.

Steele LL, Steele JR: Chronic pain. In Larsen PD, Lubkin IM, editors: *Chronic illness: Impact and intervention*, ed 7, Boston, MA, 2009, Jones & Bartlett, pp 395–412.

Taylor L, Harris J, Epps C, et al: Psychometric evaluation of selected pain-intensity scales for use with cognitively impaired and cognitively intact older adults, *Rehabil Nurs* 30:55–61, 2005.

The Joint Commission: *Facts about pain management*, 2015. Available at http://www.jointcommission.org/pain_management. Accessed January 2016.

U.S. Food and Drug Administration (FDA): *Non-aspirin nonsteroidal anti-inflammatory drugs (NSAIDS): Drug safety communication—FDA strengthens warning of increased chance of heart attack or stroke,* 2015. Available at http://www.fda.gov/Safety/MedWatch/SafetyInformation/SafetyAlertsforHumanMedicalProducts/ucm454141.htm. Accessed June 2016.

Vargas-Schaffer G: Is the WHO analgesic ladder still valid?, *Can Fam Physician* 56(6):514–517, 2010.

Vickers AJ, Cronin AM, Maschino AC, et al: Acupuncture for chronic pain: Individual patient data meta-analysis, *Arch Intern Med* 172(19):1444–1453, 2012.

Warden V, Hurley AC, Volicer L: Development and psychometric evaluation of the Pain Assessment in Advanced Dementia (PAINAD) scale, *J Am Med Dir Assoc* 4:9, 2003. Available at http://www.amda.com/publications/caring/may2004/painad.cfm. Accessed January 2016.

Ware LJ, Epps CD, Herr K, et al: Evaluation of the revised Faces Pain Scale, verbal descriptor scale, numeric rating scale, and Iowa pain thermometer in older minority adults, *Pain Manag Nurs* 7:117, 2006.

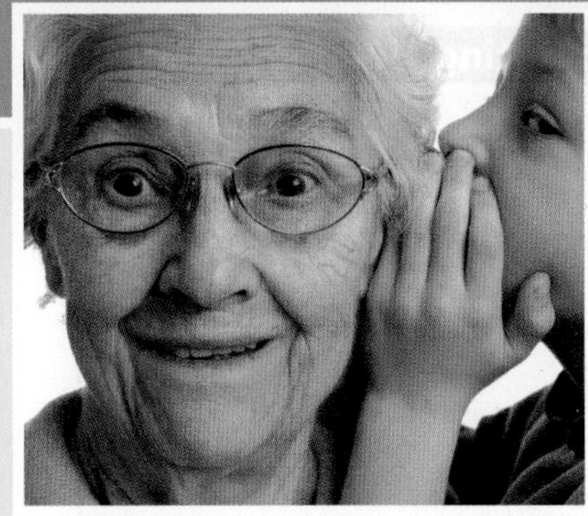

19

Diseases Affecting Vision and Hearing

Theris A. Touhy

evolve.elsevier.com/Touhy/gerontological

LEARNING OBJECTIVES

Upon completion of this chapter, the reader will be able to:

- Describe the impact of hearing and vision changes on quality of life and function and quality of life.
- Describe the importance of health education and screening for hearing and vision problems.
- Identify effective communication strategies for individuals with vision and hearing impairment.
- Discuss nursing interventions for older adults with diseases of the eye.

THE LIVED EXPERIENCE

One of the great frustrations is the matter of eyesight. One can get used to large print and hope for black letters on white paper, but why do modern publishers seem to prefer the shiny, slick off-white paper and pale ink in minuscule print? Thank goodness for restaurants with lighted menus and my new iPhone with a bright light. And my new prescription glasses have not restored my ability to cut my own toenails without danger of wounding myself.

Lyn, age 85

This chapter discusses changes in hearing and vision with age, diseases that affect vision, and adaptations to enhance communication for those with vision and hearing impairments. *Healthy People 2020* (U.S. Department of Health and Human Services [USDHHS], 2012) has set goals for vision and hearing (Box 19.1).

VISUAL IMPAIRMENT

Vision loss is not an inevitable part of the aging process, but age-related changes contribute to decreased vision (see Chapter 3). Even older adults with good visual acuity (20/40 or better) and no significant eye disease show deficits in visual function and need accommodations to enhance vision and safety (Johnson & Record, 2014). As we age there is a higher risk of developing age-related eye diseases and other conditions (hypertension, diabetes) that can result in vision losses if left untreated.

Vision loss is a leading cause of age-related disability. More than two-thirds of those with visual impairment are more than 65 years of age, and adults older than 80 years account for 70% of the cases of severe visual impairment Visual impairment among nursing home residents ranges from 3% to 15% higher than for adults of the same age living in the community (Johnson & Record, 2014). The World Health Organization (WHO, 2013) defines visual impairment as visual acuity worse than 20/70 but better than 20/400 (legal blindness) in the better eye, even with corrective lenses.

Visual impairment worldwide has decreased since the 1990s as a result of increased availability of eye care services (particularly cataract surgery), promotion of eye care education, and improved treatment

BOX 19.1 *Healthy People 2020*

Objectives Vision and Hearing—Older Adults

- Increase the proportion of adults who have had a comprehensive eye examination, including dilation, within the past 2 years.
- Reduce visual impairment due to diabetic retinopathy, glaucoma, cataract, and macular degeneration.
- Increase the use of vision rehabilitation services by persons with visual impairment.
- Increase the use of assistive and adaptive devices by persons with visual impairment.
- Increase the proportion of persons with hearing impairment who have ever used a hearing aid or assistive listening device or who have cochlear implants.
- Increase the proportion of adults 70 years of age who have had a hearing examination in the past 5 years.
- Increase the number of persons who are referred by their primary care physician or other health care provider for hearing evaluation and treatment.
- Increase the proportion of adults bothered by tinnitus who have seen a health care professional.

From U.S. Department of Health and Human Services, Office of Disease Prevention and Health Promotion: *Healthy People 2020,* 2012. Available at http://www.healthypeople.gov/2020.

of infectious diseases. However, vision impairment is a major public health problem across the globe that is expected to increase substantially with the aging of the population. Rates of blindness and visual impairment in disadvantaged, minority populations, particularly African American and Latino subpopulations who have an increased prevalence of diabetes and hypertension, are expected to increase even further (Servat et al., 2011). In the United States, the leading causes of visual impairment are cataracts, glaucoma, diabetic neuropathy, and age-related macular degeneration (AMD).

Consequences of Visual Impairment

Visual problems have a negative impact on quality of life, equivalent to that of life-threatening conditions such as heart disease and cancer. Loss of vision also impacts a person's ability to function in most daily activities such as driving, reading, maneuvering safely, dressing, cooking, and taking medications, as well as participating in social activities. Decreased vision has also been found to be a significant risk factor for falls and other accidents and is associated with cognitive decline and depression, as well as increased risk of institutionalization and death (Gopinath et al., 2013).

BOX 19.2 Promoting Healthy Eyes

- Do not smoke.
- Eat a diet rich in green, leafy vegetables and fish.
- Exercise.
- Maintain normal blood pressure and blood glucose measurements.
- Wear sunglasses and a brimmed hat anytime you are outside in bright sunshine.
- Wear safety eyewear when working around your house or playing sports.
- See an eye care professional routinely.

From the National Eye Institute, National Eye Health Education Program: *Make vision health a priority.* Available at http://www.nei.nih.gov/healthyeyestoolkit/pdf/VisionAndHealth_Tagged.pdf. Accessed October 31, 2014.

Prevention of Visual Impairment

Many age-related eye diseases have no symptoms in the early stages but can be detected early through a comprehensive dilated eye exam. However, knowledge about eye disease and treatments remains inadequate among both laypersons and medical professionals. Socioeconomic position and educational position are important social determinants that may influence access to and use of effective and appropriate eye care, thus influencing disease identification and treatment (MacLennan et al., 2014; Zhang et al., 2013).

At all ages, attention to eye health and protection of your vision are important (Box 19.2). Estimates are that 80% of all visual impairments can be avoided or cured. Prevention and treatment of eye disease are important priorities for nurses and other health professionals. The National Eye Health Education Program (NEHEP) of the National Eye Institute (NEI) provides a program for health professionals with evidence-based tools and resources that can be used in community settings to educate older adults about eye health and maintaining healthy vision (NEI, NEHEP, 2015a) (http://www.nei.nih.gov/SeeWellToolkit) (Box 19.3).

DISEASES AND DISORDERS OF THE EYE

Cataracts

A cataract is an opacification (cloudiness) in the eye's normally clear crystalline lens, causing the lens to lose transparency or scatter light. Cataracts can occur at any age (babies can be born with them), but they are most common later in life. In the United States, about 70% of people older than age 75 have cataracts. Cataracts are

BOX 19.3 Resources for Best Practice

Vision Impairment

Cacchione P: Sensory changes. In Boltz et al, editors: *Evidence-based geriatric nursing protocols for best practice,* New York, 2012, Springer

CDC: Educational materials, videos illustrating vision with AMD, glaucoma, diabetic retinopathy

Eye Care America: On-line referral center for eye care resources

Lighthouse International: Educational resources, professional development, public policy center

National Eye Health Education Program (NEHEP) and National Eye Institute (NEI): Educational and professional resources, vision and aging program: *See Well for a Lifetime Toolkit,* vodcasts on common visual problems, videos on eye disease

National Federation for the Blind: Educational information, resources

USDHHS/AHRQ: Evidence-based practice guideline: Care of the patient with open-angle glaucoma

Vision Aware (American Foundation for the Blind): Resources for independent living with vision loss, Getting started kit for people new to vision loss, How to walk with a guide

the leading cause of blindness in economically challenged countries, largely as a result of limited services and treatment (WHO, 2013).

Cataracts are categorized according to their location within the lens: nuclear, cortical, and posterior subcapsular (in the rear of the lens capsule). Nuclear cataracts are the most common type and their incidence increases with age and cigarette smoking. Cortical cataracts also are more common with age, and their development is related to a lifetime of exposure to ultraviolet light. Cataracts are also more likely to occur after glaucoma surgery or other types of eye surgery.

Cataracts form painlessly over time. The most common symptom is cloudy or blurred vision. Everything becomes dimmer, as if seen through glasses that need cleaning. Other symptoms include glare, halos around lights, poor night vision, a perception that colors are faded or that objects are yellowish, and the need for brighter light when reading. The red reflex may be absent or may appear as a black area. Fig. 19.1B illustrates the effects of a cataract on vision.

Treatment of Cataracts

The treatment of cataracts is surgical, and cataract surgery is the most common surgical procedure performed in the United States. The surgery involves removal of the lens and placement of a plastic intraocular lens (IOL). Most often, cataract surgery involves only local anesthesia and is done on an outpatient basis. If the eye is normal except for the cataract, surgery will improve vision in 95% of the cases. Significant postsurgical complications such as inflammation, infection, bleeding, retinal detachment, swelling, and glaucoma are rare. Individuals with medical problems such as diabetes and other eye diseases are most at risk for complications.

Presurgical and Postsurgical Interventions

Nursing interventions when caring for the person experiencing cataract surgery include preparing the individual for significant changes in vision and adaptation to light and ensuring that the individual has received adequate counseling regarding realistic postsurgical expectations. Most people experience a small amount of discomfort after surgery. Some redness, scratchiness, or discharge from the eye may occur during the first day after surgery. There may also be a few black spots or shapes (floaters) drifting through the field of vision. A protective patch may be used over the eye for 24 hours after surgery, and for several days to a few weeks glasses should be worn during the day and an eye shield at night to prevent trauma from rubbing the eye. Vision remains blurred for several days or weeks and then gradually improves as the eye heals.

Following surgery, the individual needs to avoid heavy lifting, straining, and bending at the waist. Eye drops may be prescribed to aid healing and prevent infection. Teaching fall prevention techniques and ensuring home safety modifications are also important because some research suggests that the risk of falls increases after surgery, particularly between first and second cataract surgeries (Meuleners et al., 2013). The vision imbalance that can occur if the person has one "good" eye and one "bad" eye contributes to the risk of falls. If the person has bilateral cataracts, surgery is performed first on one eye with the second surgery on the other eye a month or so later to ensure healing.

Glaucoma

Glaucoma is a group of diseases that can damage the optic nerve. Glaucoma is the second leading cause of blindness in the United States. Glaucoma affects as many as 2.3 million Americans age 40 years and older and 6% of those older than age 65. Because the most common form of the condition, primary open-angle glaucoma (POAG), affects side vision first, it may remain unnoticed for years. At least half of all persons with glaucoma are unaware they have the disease. The risk of glaucoma varies with age and race. The condition is four

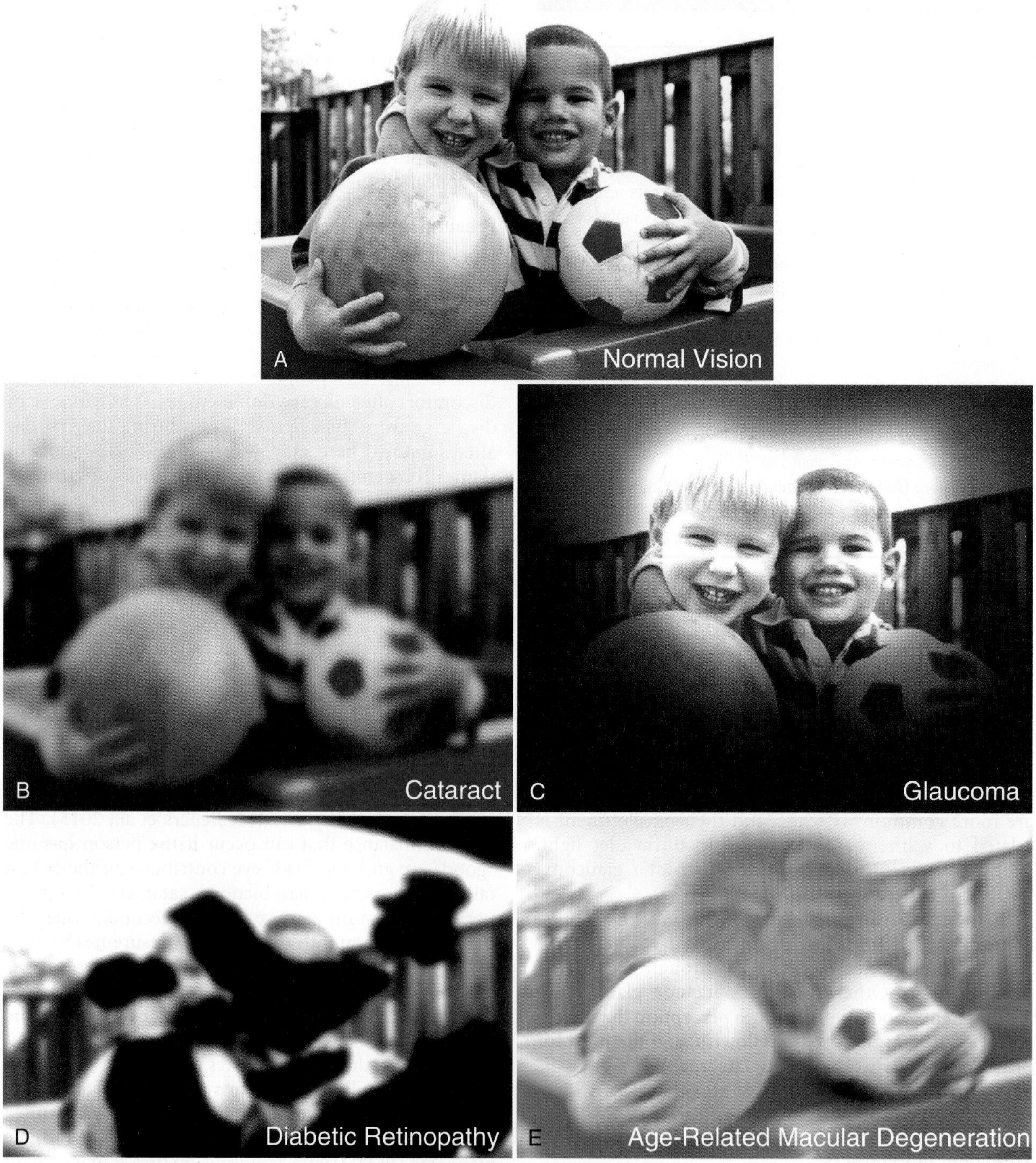

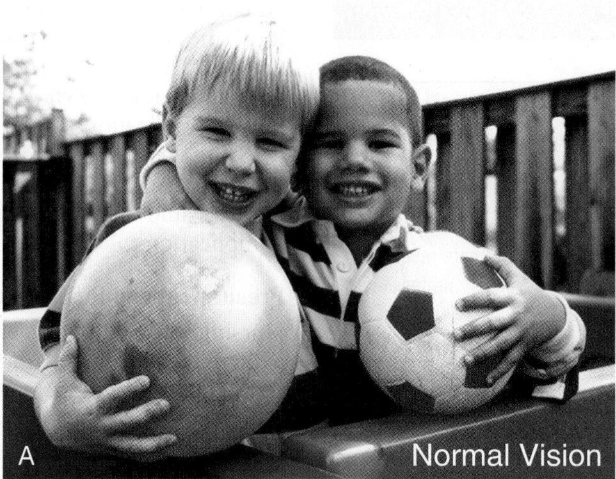

FIGURE 19.1 A, Normal vision. **B,** Simulated vision with cataracts. **C,** Simulated vision with glaucoma. **D,** Simulated vision with diabetic retinopathy. **E,** Simulated vision with age-related macular degeneration (AMD). (From National Eye Institute, National Institutes of Health, 2015.)

times more common in Hispanics and five times more common in blacks than whites, and it occurs more frequently with increasing age. African Americans are at risk of developing glaucoma at an earlier age than other racial and ethnic groups, with projections of a 66% increase in the number of cases by 2030 (Johnson & Record, 2014; NEI, 2016). Other high-risk groups are individuals with diabetes, hypertension, a history of corticosteroid use, and a family history of glaucoma (NEI, 2016).

If detected early, glaucoma can usually be controlled and serious vision loss prevented. Signs of glaucoma can include headaches, poor vision in dim lighting, increased sensitivity to glare, "tired eyes," impaired peripheral vision, a fixed and dilated pupil, and frequent changes in prescriptions for corrective lenses. Fig. 19.1C illustrates the effects of glaucoma on vision.

Angle-closure glaucoma is not as common as POAG and occurs when the angle of the iris causes obstruction of the aqueous humor through the trabecular network. Individuals with smaller eyes, Asians, and women are most susceptible. It may occur as a result of infection or trauma. Intraocular pressure (IOP) rises rapidly accompanied by redness and pain in and around the eye, severe headaches, nausea and vomiting, and blurring of vision. It is a medical emergency and blindness can occur in 2 days. Treatment is an iridectomy to ease pressure. Many drugs with anticholinergic properties, including antihistamines, stimulants, vasodilators, and sympathomimetics, are particularly dangerous for individuals predisposed to acute-closure glaucoma.

SAFETY ALERT

Redness and pain in and around the eye, severe headaches, nausea and vomiting, and blurring of vision occur with angle-closure glaucoma. It is a medical emergency and blindness can occur in 2 days.

Screening and Treatment of Glaucoma

A dilated eye examination and tonometry are necessary to diagnose glaucoma. Adults older than age 65 should have annual eye examinations with dilation, and those with medication-controlled glaucoma should be examined at least every 6 months. Annual screening is also recommended for African Americans and other individuals with a family history of glaucoma who are older than 40 years. Although standard Medicare does not cover routine eye care, it does cover 80% of the cost for dilated eye exams for individuals at higher risk for glaucoma and those with diabetes.

Management of glaucoma involves medications (oral or topical eye drops) to decrease IOP and/or laser trabeculoplasty and filtration surgery. Medications lower eye pressure either by decreasing the amount of aqueous fluid produced within the eye or by improving the flow through the drainage angle. Beta blockers are the first-line therapy for glaucoma followed by prostaglandin analogs. Second-line agents include topical carbonic anhydrase inhibitors and alpha$_2$-agonists (Johnson & Record, 2014). The patient may need combinations of several types of eye drops. There is ongoing research on the development of a contact lens to deliver glaucoma medication continuously for a month (Ciolino et al., 2014).

In the hospital or long-term care setting, it is important to obtain a medical history to determine if the person has glaucoma and to ensure that eye drops are given according to the person's treatment regimen. Without the eye drops, eye pressure can rise and cause an acute exacerbation of glaucoma. Usually medications can control glaucoma, but laser surgery (trabeculoplasty) and filtration surgery may be recommended for some types of glaucoma. Surgery is usually recommended only if necessary to prevent further damage to the optic nerve.

Diabetic Retinopathy

Diabetes has become an epidemic in the United States, and diabetic retinopathy occurs in both type 1 and type 2 diabetes mellitus (see Chapter 20). Diabetic retinopathy is a disease of the retinal microvasculature characterized by increased vessel permeability. Blood and lipid leakage leads to macular edema and hard exudates (composed of lipids). In advanced disease, new fragile blood vessels form and hemorrhage easily. Because of the vascular and cellular changes accompanying diabetes, there is often rapid worsening of other pathologic vision conditions as well (Fig. 19.1D).

Almost all people with type 1 diabetes will eventually develop retinopathy. People with type 2 diabetes are less likely to develop more advanced retinopathy than those with type 1. Estimates are that 40.8% of adults aged 40 and older with diabetes have diabetic retinopathy, and the incidence increases with age. It is more common in people with poorly controlled diabetes. Diabetic retinopathy is the leading cause of new blindness for Americans between the ages of 20 and 74.

Screening and Treatment of Diabetic Retinopathy

Early detection and treatment of diabetic retinopathy is essential. There are no symptoms in the early stages of diabetic retinopathy. Early signs are seen in the fundoscopic examination and include microaneurysms, flame-shaped hemorrhages, cotton wool spots, hard exudates, and dilated capillaries. Constant, strict control of blood glucose levels, cholesterol levels, and blood pressure measurements and laser photocoagulation treatments can halt progression of the disease.

Annual dilated fundoscopic examination of the eye is recommended beginning 5 years after diagnosis of diabetes type 1 and at the time of diagnosis of diabetes type 2. Nurses need to provide education to diabetic patients about the risk of diabetic retinopathy and the importance of early identification, as well as good control of diabetes. Some experts are encouraging mass screening efforts. There is good treatment that can reverse vision loss and improve vision, but individuals must have access to screenings and eye examinations.

Diabetic Macular Edema (DME)

Thickening of the center of the retina—diabetic macular edema—is the most common cause of visual loss attributable to diabetes. The disease affects 1 in 25 adults age 40 and older with diabetes and the incidence is higher in African Americans and Hispanics. It is the leading cause of legal blindness. Treatment includes medications (often cortisone-type drugs) and laser therapy to cauterize leaky blood vessels and reduce accumulated fluid within the macula. Laser treatment is very effective, reducing the risk of substantial worsening of vision.

Anti–vascular endothelial growth factor (anti-VEGF) therapy (Lucentis) is used alone or in conjunction with laser treatment to treat diabetic retinopathy in individuals with diabetic macular edema. The treatment appears to be well tolerated but requires about 12 to 15 injections into the eye over 36 months (NEI, 2015a).

Strict control of blood glucose, cholesterol, and blood pressure values; completion of annual dilated retinal examinations; and education about eye disease and diabetes are essential. However, in a recent study, only 44.7% of adults 40 years and older with DME reported that they were told by a physician that diabetes had affected their eyes and 59.7% had received a dilated eye examination in the last year (Bressler et al., 2014).

Age-Related Macular Degeneration

Age-related macular degeneration (AMD) is the most common cause of new visual impairment among people age 50 years and older, although it is most likely to occur after age 60 (Johnson & Record, 2014; NEI, 2015b). The prevalence of AMD increases drastically with age, with more than 15% of white women older than age 80 years having the disease. Whites and Asian Americans are more likely to lose vision from AMD than African Americans or Hispanics/Latinos. With the number of affected older adults projected to increase over the next 20 years, AMD has been called a growing epidemic.

AMD is a degenerative eye disease that affects the macula, the central part of the eye responsible for clear central vision. The disease causes the progressive loss of central vision, leaving only peripheral vision intact. The early and intermediate stages usually start without symptoms and only a comprehensive dilated eye exam can detect AMD. Objects may not appear to be as bright as they used to be and individuals may attribute their vision problems to normal aging or cataracts.

As AMD progresses, a blurred area near the center of vision is a common symptom. Over time, the blurred areas may grow larger and blank spots can develop in the central vision. AMD does not lead to complete blindness, but the loss of central vision interferes with everyday activities such as the ability to see faces, read, drive, or do close work, and can lead to impaired mobility, increased risk of falls, depression, and decreased quality of life (Johnson & Record, 2014; NEI, 2015b). Fig. 19.1E illustrates the effects of AMD on vision.

AMD results from systemic changes in circulation, accumulation of cellular waste products, atrophy of tissue, and growth of abnormal blood vessels in the choroid layer beneath the retina. Fibrous scarring disrupts nourishment of photoreceptor cells, causing their death and loss of central vision. Risk factors for AMD are similar to those for coronary artery disease (hypertension, atherosclerosis). Smoking doubles the risk of AMD. Other risk factors are thought to include genetic predisposition, inflammation, and diet. A genetic link for AMD is suspected in 50% of new cases (Johnson & Record, 2014; Wang et al., 2015).

There are three stages of AMD defined in part by the size and number of drusen under the retina. An individual can have AMD in one eye only or have one eye with a later stage than the other. Not everyone with early AMD will develop the later stage of the disease. In individuals with early AMD in one eye and no signs of AMD in the other eye, about 5% will develop advanced AMD after 10 years. For people who have early AMD in both eyes, about 14% will develop late AMD in at least one eye after 10 years. Having late AMD in one eye puts an individual at increased risk for late AMD in the other eye.

In late AMD, there is vision loss attributable to damage to the macula. There are two types of late AMD: geographic atrophy (dry AMD) and neovascular AMD (wet AMD). Neovascular AMD occurs when abnormal blood vessels behind the retina start to grow under the macula. These new blood vessels are fragile and often leak blood and fluid, which raise the macula from its normal place at the back of the eye. With wet AMD, the severe loss of central vision can be rapid and many people will be legally blind within 2 years of diagnosis.

Screening and Treatment of AMD

Early diagnosis is the key. An Amsler grid (Fig. 19.2) is used to determine clarity of vision. A perception of wavy lines is diagnostic of beginning macular degeneration. In the advanced forms, the person may see dark or empty spaces that block the center of vision. People with AMD are usually taught to test their eyes daily using an Amsler grid so that they will be aware of any changes. AMD occurs less in individuals who exercise, avoid smoking, and consume a diet high in green, leafy vegetables and fruits. In early AMD, adopting some of these habits may help keep vision longer (NEI, 2015b).

The National Eye Institute Age-Related Eye Disease Studies (AREDS/AREDS2) found that daily intake of certain high-dose vitamins and minerals can slow progression of the disease in individuals with intermediate AMD and those with late AMD in one eye. Supplementation with these formulations will not help people with early AMD and will not restore vision already lost. Individuals should discuss the supplementation with AREDS formulations with their eye physician.

Treatment of wet AMD includes photodynamic therapy (PDT), laser photocoagulation (LPC), and anti-VEGF therapy. In 2010 the FDA approved an implantable telescope (IMT) to help individuals 65 years of age and older with vision loss attributable to AMD. The IMT helps individuals with advanced AMD by enlarging objects in the center of the visual field.

Lucentis and Avastin (anti-VEGF therapy) are biological drugs that are the most common form of treatment in neovascular AMD. Abnormally high levels of a specific growth factor occur in eyes with wet AMD, which promote the growth of abnormal blood vessels. Anti-VEGF therapy blocks the effect of the growth factor. These drugs are injected into the eye as often as once a month and can help slow vision loss from AMD and, in some cases, improve sight. Photodynamic therapy with laser treatment is also used to manage AMD (NEI, 2015b).

Detached Retina

A retinal detachment can occur at any age but is more common after the age of 40 years. Emergency medical treatment is required or permanent visual loss can result. There may be small areas of the retina that are torn (retinal tears or breaks) and can lead to retinal detachment. This condition can develop in persons with cataracts or recent cataract surgery or trauma, or it can occur spontaneously. Symptoms include a gradual increase in the number of floaters and/or light flashes in the eye. It also manifests as a curtain coming down over the person's field of vision. Small holes or tears are treated with laser surgery or a freeze treatment called *cryopexy*.

Retinal detachments are treated with surgery. More than 90% of individuals with a retinal detachment can be successfully treated, although sometimes a second treatment is needed. However, the visual outcome is not always predictable and may not be known for several months following surgery. Visual results are best if the detachment is repaired before the macula detaches, so immediate treatment of symptoms is essential (NEI/NEHEP, 2016).

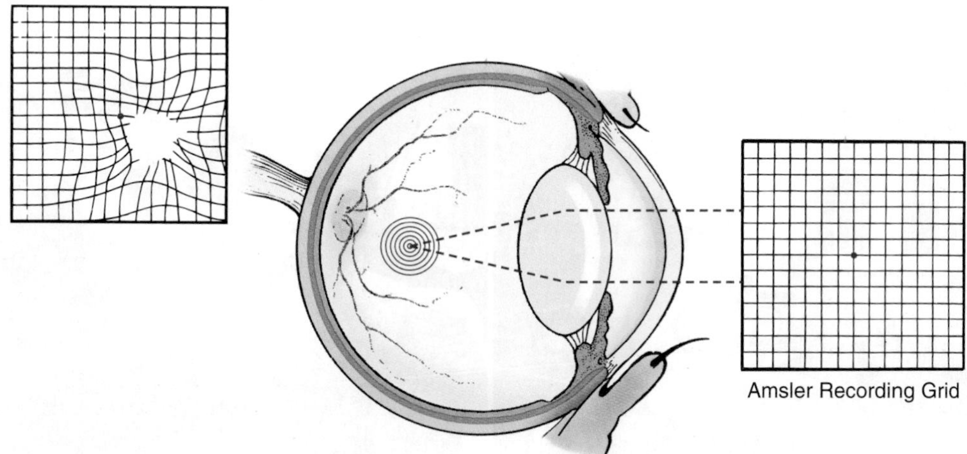

FIGURE 19.2 Macular degeneration: distortion of center vision, normal peripheral vision. (Illustration by Harriet R. Greenfied, Newton, MA.)

Dry Eye

Dry eye is not a disease of the eye but is a frequent complaint among older people. Tear production normally diminishes as we age. The condition is termed *keratoconjunctivitis sicca*. It occurs most commonly in women after menopause. There may be age-related changes in the mucin-secreting cells necessary for surface wetting, in the lacrimal glands, or in the meibomian glands that secrete surface oil, and all of these may occur at the same time. The older person will describe a dry, scratchy feeling in mild cases (xerophthalmia). There may be marked discomfort and decreased mucus production in severe situations.

Medications can cause dry eye, especially anticholinergics, antihistamines, diuretics, beta blockers, and some hypnotics. A common treatment is artificial tears or a saline gel, but dry eyes may be sensitive to them because of preservatives, which can be irritating. The ophthalmologist may close the tear duct channel either temporarily or permanently. Other management methods include keeping the house air moist with humidifiers, avoiding wind and hair dryers, and using artificial tear ointments at bedtime. Vitamin A deficiency can be a cause of dry eye, and vitamin A ointments are available for treatment.

❖ IMPLICATIONS FOR GERONTOLOGICAL NURSING AND HEALTHY AGING

◆ Assessment

Vision impairment is common among older adults in connection with aging changes and eye diseases and can significantly affect communication, functional ability, safety, and quality of life. To promote healthy aging and quality of life, nurses who care for elders in all settings can improve outcomes for visually impaired elders by assessing for vision changes, adapting the environment to enhance vision and safety, communicating appropriately, and providing health teaching and referrals for prevention, treatment, and assistive devices.

◆ Interventions

General principles in caring for persons with visual impairment include the following: use warm incandescent lighting; increase intensity of lighting; control glare by using shades and blinds; suggest yellow or amber lenses to decrease glare; suggest sunglasses that block all ultraviolet light; recommend reading materials that have large, dark, evenly spaced printing; and select colors with good contrast and intensity. Color contrasts are used to facilitate location of items. Sharply contrasting colors assist the partially sighted. For instance, a bright towel is much easier to locate than a white towel hanging on a beige wall. When choosing color, it is best to use primary colors at the top end of the spectrum rather than those at the bottom. If you think of the colors of the rainbow, it is more likely that people will see reds and oranges better than blues and greens. Fig. 19.3 beautifully illustrates the use of color in a nursing home in Copenhagen, Denmark. Box 19.4 presents tips for communicating with elders with visual impairment.

◆ Special Considerations in Long-Term Care Settings

Nursing homes and assisted living facilities (ALFs) care for a large number of individuals who are visually impaired and many also experience hearing and

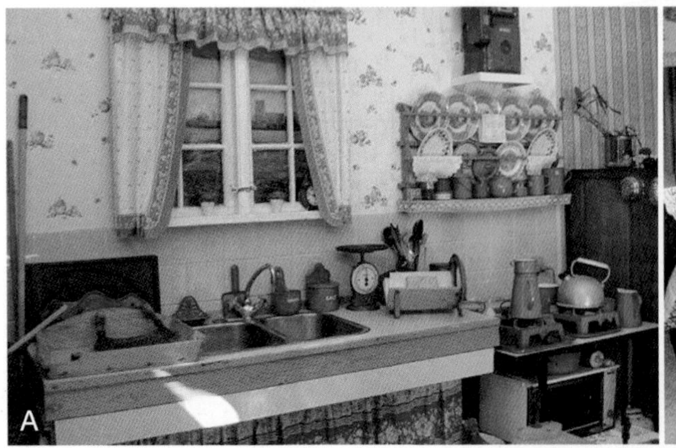

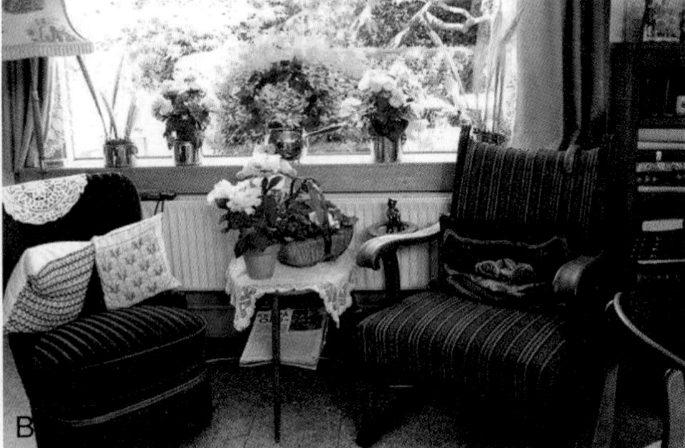

FIGURE 19.3 A, Reminiscence kitchen. **B,** Sitting room. (Højdevang Sogns Plejejem, Copenhagen, Denmark. Photos courtesy Christine Williams, PhD, RN.)

BOX 19.4 Tips for Best Practice

Communicating With Elders Who Have Visual Impairment

- Assess for vision loss.
- Make sure you have the person's attention before speaking.
- Clearly identify yourself and others with you.
- Position yourself at the person's level when speaking.
- When others are present, address the visually impaired person by prefacing remarks with his or her name or a light touch on the arm.
- Ensure adequate lighting and eliminate glare.
- Select colors for paint, furniture, pictures with rich intensity (e.g., red, orange).
- Use large, dark, evenly spaced printing.
- Use contrast in printed material (e.g., black marker on white paper).
- Use a night light in bathroom and hallways and use illuminated switches.
- Do not change room arrangement or the arrangement of personal items without explanations.
- If in a hospital or nursing home, use some means to identify patients who are visually impaired and include visual impairment in the plan of care.
- Use the analogy of a clock face to help locate objects (e.g., describe positions of food on a plate in relation to clock positions, such as meat at 3 o'clock, dessert at 6 o'clock).
- Label eyeglasses and have a spare pair if possible; make sure glasses are worn and are clean.
- Be aware of low-vision assistive devices such as talking watches, talking books, and magnifiers, and facilitate access to these resources.
- If the person is blind, ask the person how you can help. If walking, do not try to push or pull. Let the person take your arm just above the elbow, and give directions with details (e.g., the bench is on your immediate right); when seating the person, place his or her hand on the back of the chair.

cognitive impairment (Elliott et al., 2013). Routine eye care is sorely lacking in nursing homes and is related to functional decline, decreased quality of life, and depression. Estimates are that approximately one-third of vision impairment in this setting is reversible with currently available treatments such as correction of refractive errors and performance of cataract surgery (Elliott et al., 2013). Even in individuals with dementia who have clinically significant cataracts, surgery was found to improve visual acuity, slow the rate of cognitive decline, decrease neuropsychiatric symptoms, and reduce caregiver stress (Cassels, 2014). Although it may sound like common sense, it is especially important that individuals who wear glasses are wearing them and that the glasses are cleaned regularly. Also important is asking the person or the person's family/significant other if the person routinely wears glasses and if the person is able to see well enough to function.

◆ Low-Vision Optical Devices

Technology advances in the past decade have produced some low-vision devices that may be used successfully in the care of the visually impaired individual. These devices are grouped into devices for "near" activities (such as reading, sewing, writing) and devices for "distance" activities (such as attending movies, reading street signs, and identifying numbers on buses and trains). Nurses can refer individuals with low vision or blindness to vision rehabilitation services, which may include assistance with communication skills, counseling, independent living and personal management skills; independent movement and travel skills; training with low-vision devices; and vocational rehabilitation. It is important to be familiar with agencies in your community that offer these services. Persons with severe visual impairment may qualify for disability and financial and social services assistance through government and private programs including vision rehabilitation programs.

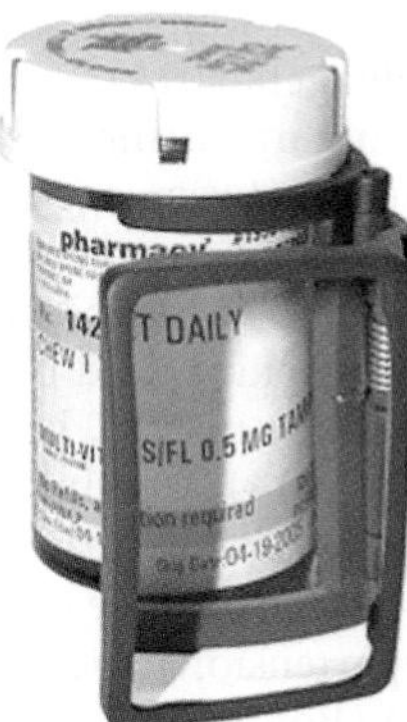

Prescription bottle magnifier. (Reprinted with permission from Carson Optical.)

An array of low-vision assistive devices is now available, including insulin delivery systems, talking clocks and watches, large-print books, magnifiers, telescopes (handheld or mounted on eyeglasses), electronic magnification through closed circuit television or computer software, and software that converts text into artificial voice output. iPods have a setting for audio menus; Microsoft and Apple computer programs allow a person to change color schemes, select a high-contrast display, and magnify and enlarge print. Many websites also have an option for audio text. The e-Reader product from Kindle allows the user to increase font sizes up to 40 points in e-books and offers a Text-to-Speech feature. The iPad from Apple can enlarge text up to 56 points and includes VoiceOver, a feature that reads everything displayed on the screen for you, making it fully usable for people with low to no vision. More and more mobile phones have speech-enabled features, and the Jitterbug phone comes with a live operator whose actions can be directed. As individual needs are unique, it is recommended that before investing in vision aids, the individual consult with a low-vision center or low-vision specialist. Other vision resources are presented in Box 19.3.

HEARING IMPAIRMENT

Hearing loss is the third most prevalent chronic condition and the foremost communicative disorder of older adults in the United States. Hearing loss is an under-recognized public health issue. Among adults between the ages of 60 and 69 years of age, 31% have bilateral hearing loss of at least mild severity. In those older than 70 years of age, the prevalence is 63%, and in those older than age 85, the prevalence is 80%. In all age groups, men are more likely than women to be hearing impaired, and black Americans have a lower prevalence of hearing impairment than either white or Hispanic Americans (Bainbridge & Wallhagen, 2014).

Age-related hearing impairment is a complex disease caused by interactions between age-related changes (see Chapter 3), genetics, lifestyle, and environmental factors. Factors associated with hearing loss include noise exposure, ear infections, smoking, and chronic disease (e.g., diabetes, chronic kidney disease, heart disease) (Bainbridge & Wallhagen, 2014). Hearing loss may not be an inevitable part of aging, and increased attention is being given to the links between lifestyle factors (e.g., smoking, poor nutrition, hypertension) and hearing impairment (Heine et al., 2013) (Box 19.5).

BOX 19.5 Promoting Healthy Hearing

- Avoid exposure to excessively loud noises.
- Avoid cigarette smoking.
- Maintain blood pressure/cholesterol levels within normal limits.
- Eat a healthy diet.
- Have hearing evaluated if any changes are noticed.
- Avoid injury with cotton-tipped applicators and other cleaning materials.

Consequences of Hearing Impairment

The broad consequences of hearing loss have functional and clinical significance and should not be viewed as something a person accepts as part of aging. Hearing loss diminishes quality of life and is associated with multiple negative outcomes, including decreased function, increased likelihood of hospitalizations, miscommunication, depression, falls, loss of self-esteem, safety risks, and cognitive decline (Bainbridge & Wallhagen, 2014; Lin et al., 2013). Growing evidence supports an association between age-related hearing loss and cognitive decline and dementia (Bainbridge & Wallhagen, 2014; Lin, 2012; Lin et al., 2013).

Hearing impairment increases feelings of isolation and may cause older adults to become suspicious or distrustful or to display feelings of paranoia. Because older persons with hearing loss may not understand or respond appropriately to conversation, they may be inappropriately diagnosed with dementia. All of these consequences of hearing impairment further increase social isolation and decrease opportunities for meaningful interaction and stimulation.

Types of Hearing Loss

The two major forms of hearing loss are conductive and sensorineural. *Sensorineural hearing loss* results from damage to any part of the inner ear or the neural pathways to the brain. *Presbycusis* (also called age-related hearing impairment or ARHI) is a form of sensorineural hearing loss that is related to aging and is the most common form of hearing loss. Presbycusis progressively worsens with age and is usually permanent. The cochlea appears to be the site of pathogenesis, but the precise cause of presbycusis is uncertain (Lewis, 2014).

Noise-induced hearing loss (NIHL) is the second most common cause of sensorineural hearing loss among older adults. Direct mechanical injury to the sensory hair cells of the cochlea causes NIHL, and continuous noise exposure contributes to damage more than intermittent exposure (Lewis, 2014). NIHL is permanent but considered largely preventable.

The rate of hearing impairment is expected to rise because of the growing number of older adults and also because of the increased number of military personnel who have been exposed to blast exposure in combat situations. Noise-induced hearing loss may be reduced through the development of better ear-protection devices, education about exposure to loud noise, and emerging research into interventions that may protect or repair hair cells in the ear, which are essential to the

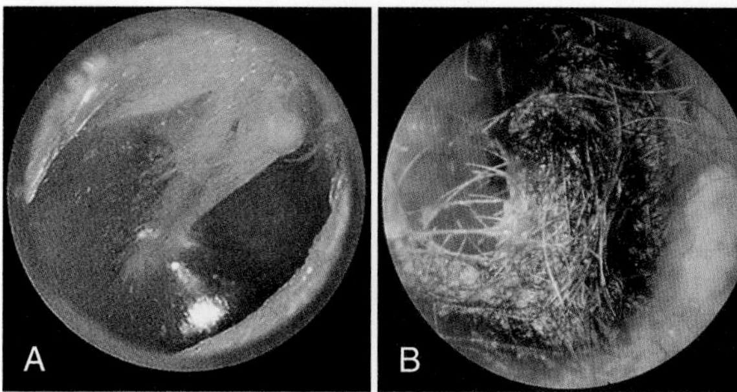

FIGURE 19.4 **A,** Normal eardrum. **B,** Eardrum impacted with cerumen. (**A,** From Ball JW, Dains JE, Flynn FA, et al: *Seidel's guide to physical examination,* ed 8, St Louis, 2015, Mosby. **B,** From Swartz MH: *Textbook of physical diagnosis,* ed 7, Philadelphia, 2014, Saunders.)

body's ability to hear (National Institute on Deafness and Other Communication Disorders [NIDCD], 2014).

Conductive hearing loss usually involves abnormalities of the external and middle ear that reduce the ability of sound to be transmitted to the middle ear. Otosclerosis, infection, perforated eardrum, fluid in the middle ear, tumors, or cerumen accumulations cause conductive hearing loss. Cerumen impaction is the most common and easily corrected of all interferences in the hearing of older people (Fig. 19.4). Individuals at particular risk of impaction are African Americans, individuals who wear hearing aids, and older men with large amounts of ear canal tragi (hairs in the ear) that tend to become entangled with the cerumen. When hearing loss is suspected, or a person with existing hearing loss experiences increasing difficulty, it is important first to check for cerumen impaction as a possible cause. After accurate assessment, if cerumen removal is indicated, it may be removed through irrigation, cerumenolytic products, or manual extraction.

INTERVENTIONS TO ENHANCE HEARING

Hearing Aids

A hearing aid is a personal amplifying system that includes a microphone, an amplifier, and a loudspeaker. There are numerous types of hearing aids with either analog or digital circuitry. The size, appearance, and effectiveness of hearing aids have greatly improved (decreasing stigma), and many can be programmed to meet specific needs. Digital hearing aids are smaller and have better sound quality and noise reduction, as well as less acoustic feedback; however, they are expensive. The behind-the-ear hearing aid looks like a shrimp and fits around and behind the ear; a small tube sits in the canal to direct the amplified sound. It is less commonly used now than the small, in-the-ear aid, which fits in the concha of the ear. Completely-in-the-canal (CIC) hearing aids fit entirely in the ear canal. These types of devices are among the most expensive and require good dexterity. Some models are invisible and placed deep in the ear canal and replaced every 4 months. New hearing aids can be adjusted precisely for noisy environments and telephone usage through software built into smartphones.

Most individuals can obtain some hearing enhancement with a hearing aid. The kind of device chosen depends on the type of hearing impairment and the cost, but most users will experience hearing improvement with a basic to midlevel hearing aid. The investment in a good hearing aid is considerable, and a good fit is critical. Hearing aids can range in price from about $500 to several thousand dollars per aid, depending on the technology. The cost of hearing aids is usually not covered by health insurance or Medicare, which can be a barrier to purchase.

Adjustment to Hearing Aids

Nearly 50% of people who purchased hearing aids either never wore them or stopped wearing them after a short period. Factors contributing to low hearing aid use after purchase include difficulty manipulating the device, annoying loud noises, being exposed to sensory overload, developing headaches, and perceiving stigma. Hearing aids amplify all sounds, making things sound different. People often delay acquiring hearing aids because the loss occurs gradually and they often ignore or deny the loss. Individuals wait on average 7 to 10 years between signs of hearing loss and audiological consultation (Lewis, 2014). This delay makes adjustment to the device even more challenging (Lane & Conn, 2013).

Age-related hearing loss (ARHL) is like any other physical impairment and requires counseling, rehabilitative training, environmental accommodations, and patience. Audiology centers, often attached to hospitals, medical centers, and universities, are excellent places for aural rehabilitation programs but costs are usually not covered by Medicare. The Internet may be a valuable tool for aural rehabilitation, as well as for improving adjustment to hearing aids and communication (Lewis, 2014).

It is important for nurses who work with individuals wearing hearing aids to be knowledgeable about the care and maintenance. They can teach the individual, family, or formal caregiver proper use and care of hearing aids (Box 19.6). Many older people experience unnecessary

BOX 19.6 Tips for Best Practice

Hearing Aid Care and Use

- When a hearing aid is first purchased: Initially it is advisable to wear for 15 to 20 minutes per day until the person is adjusted to the new sounds.
- Gradually increase the wearing time to 10 to 12 hours.
- Be patient and realize that the process of adaptation is difficult but ultimately will be rewarding.
- Make sure your fingers are dry and clean before handling hearing aids. Use a soft dry cloth to wipe your hearing aids.
- Each day, remove any earwax that has accumulated on the hearing aids. Use the brush that is included with the aid to clean difficult-to-reach areas.
- You will be instructed how to best insert the model you purchase.
- If it is not pre-programmed, adjust the volume to a level that is comfortable for you. You may be able to adjust the volume for different environments, depending on the model.
- Use great caution to avoid getting the aid wet; do not wear when swimming or taking a shower or bath.
- Also avoid use when around fine particles that can clog the microphone such as hair spray, make-up, or blowing sand and dirt.
- Many aids will slowly decrease in volume and may make a "peep" when it is time to change the battery. Check the battery by turning the hearing aid on, turning up the volume, cupping your hand over the ear mold, and listening. A constant whistling sound indicates that the battery is functioning. A weak sound indicates that the battery is losing power and needs replacement.
- Be sure to remove the battery and return the aid to its case when not in use. This will extend the life of the battery and protect the aid.

Data from Johns Hopkins Medicine: *Caring for your hearing aid,* 2007. Available at http://www.hopkinsmedicine.org/hearing/hearing_aids/caring_for_hearing_aids.htm. Accessed March 2014.

communication problems when in the hospital or nursing home because their hearing aids are not inserted and working properly, or they are lost.

Cochlear Implants

Cochlear implants are increasingly being used for older adults with sensorineural loss who are not able to gain effective speech recognition with hearing aids. Cochlear implants are safe and well tolerated and improve communication. The surgery is now commonly done bilaterally (Lewis, 2014). A cochlear implant is a small, complex electronic device that consists of an external portion that sits behind the ear and a second portion that is surgically placed under the skin (Fig. 19.5).

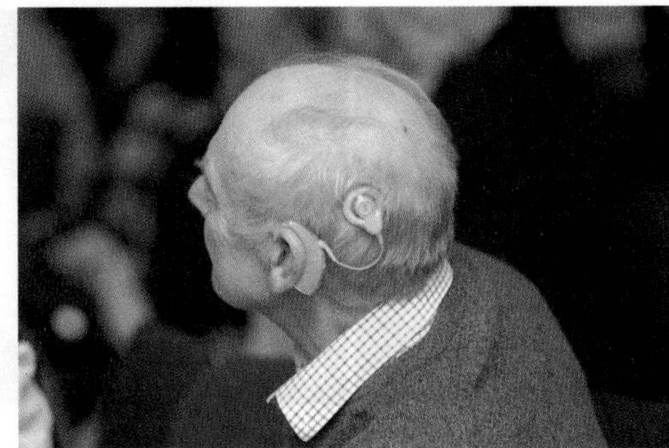

FIGURE 19.5 Cochlear implant. (Photo courtesy of the patient. Available at http://ais.southampton.ac.uk/new-programme-launched-help-cochlear-implant-users-enjoy-music/.)

Unlike hearing aids that magnify sounds, the cochlear implant bypasses damaged portions of the ear and directly stimulates the auditory nerve. Hearing through a cochlear implant is different from normal hearing and takes time to learn or relearn. Most insurance plans cover the cochlear implant procedure. The transplant carries some risk because the surgery destroys any residual hearing. Therefore, cochlear implant users can never revert to using a hearing aid. Individuals with cochlear implants need to be advised to never have a magnetic resonance imaging (MRI) scan because it may dislodge the implant or demagnetize its internal magnet.

Assistive Listening and Adaptive Devices

Assistive listening devices (also called personal listening systems) should be considered as an adjunct to hearing aids or used in place of hearing aids for people with hearing impairment. These devices are available commercially and can be used to enhance face-to-face communication and to better understand speech in large rooms such as theaters, to use the telephone, and to listen to television. Many movie theaters have both sound amplifiers and personal subtitle devices available.

Other examples of assistive listening and adaptive devices include text messaging devices for telephones and closed-caption television. Alerting devices, such as vibrating alarm clocks that shake the bed or activate a flashing light, and sound lamps that respond with lights to sounds, such as doorbells and telephones, are also available. Special service dogs ("hearing dogs") are trained to alert people with a hearing impairment about sounds and intruders. Dogs are trained to respond to different sounds, such as the telephone, smoke alarms, alarm clock, doorbell/door knock, and name call, and lead the individual to the sound.

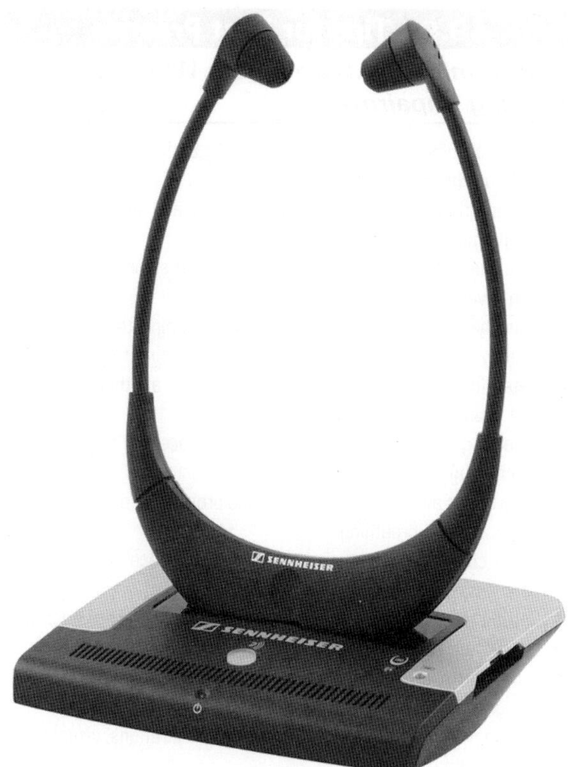

Voice-clarifying headset system for TV listening. (© Sennheiser electronic GmbH & Co. KG.)

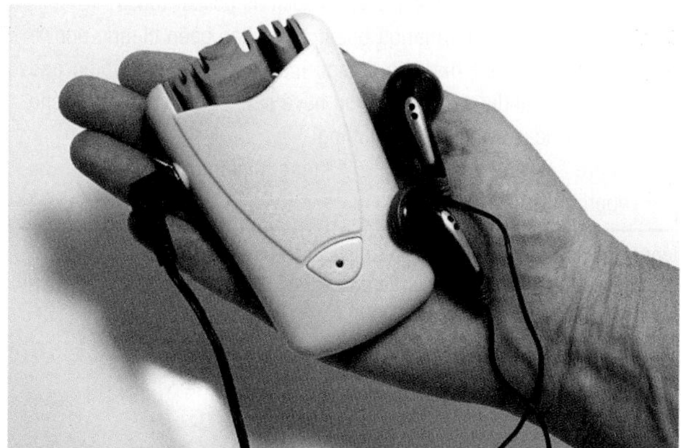

Pocket-sized amplifier. (With permission from Sonic Technology Products.)

The use of computers and email also assists individuals with hearing impairment to communicate more easily. Programs such as Skype and FaceTime are also beneficial because they may allow the person to lip read and to adjust volume. Pocket-sized amplifiers (available at retail stores) are especially helpful in improving communication in health care settings, and nurses should be able to obtain appropriate devices for use with hearing-impaired individuals.

BOX 19.7 Do I Have a Hearing Problem?

- Do I have a problem hearing on the telephone?
- Do I have trouble hearing when there is noise in the background?
- Is it hard for me to follow a conversation when two or more people talk at once?
- Do I have to strain to understand a conversation?
- Do many people I talk to seem to mumble (or not speak clearly)?
- Do I misunderstand what others are saying and respond inappropriately?
- Do I have trouble understanding the speech of women and children?
- Do people complain that I turn the TV volume up too high?
- Do I hear a ringing, roaring, or hissing sound a lot?
- Do some sounds seem too loud?

From National Institute on Deafness and Other Communication Disorders: *Hearing loss and older adults,* 2014. Available at http://www.nidcd.nih.gov/health/hearing/pages/older.aspx#2. Accessed October 31, 2014.

❖ IMPLICATIONS FOR GERONTOLOGICAL NURSING AND HEALTHY AGING

◆ Assessment

Hearing impairment is underdiagnosed and undertreated in older people (Bainbridge & Wallhagen, 2014). Older people may be initially unaware of hearing loss because of the gradual manner in which it develops and, therefore, not report any problems. Screening for hearing impairment and appropriate treatment are considered an essential part of primary care for older adults. Assessment of hearing includes a focused history and physical examination and also screening assessment for hearing impairment. Ask the person if he or she has any difficulty understanding speech in noisy situations, during telephone use, or in daily conversation. Obtaining information from the significant other about hearing problems can also be useful. Self-assessment instruments (Box 19.7) and the Hearing Handicap Inventory for the Elderly (HHIE-S) can also be included (Box 19.8). Question the patient about prolonged noise exposure, past ear injuries, and use of potentially ototoxic medications as well.

Physical examination includes assessing the external ear to determine any evidence of infection and using an

BOX 19.8 Resources for Best Practice

Hearing Impairment

American Tinnitus Association: Sounds of tinnitus

Hartford Institute for Geriatric Nursing (*Try This:* General Assessment Series): Hearing handicap for the elderly: Screening version (HHIT-S)

NIDCD (National Institute on Deafness and Other Communication Disorders): Hearing loss and older adults; Interactive sound ruler: how loud is too loud (experience noise levels)

NIH Senior Health: Hearing loss (patient information)

Sight and Hearing Association: Unfair hearing test/filtered speech (experience presbycusis)

otoscope to visualize the inner ear, looking for any possible causes of conductive hearing loss such as cerumen impaction or the presence of foreign objects. Inspect the tympanic membrane (TM) for integrity. Depending on findings, the patient may need to be referred for follow-up by a specialist. If no problems are identified, perform a few basic screening tests. These may include the Rinne and Weber tests to differentiate between conductive and sensorineural hearing loss. Other tests include the whisper and finger rub test.

◆ Interventions

Nursing actions are based on assessment findings and may include referral to an audiologist, education on hearing loss (including prevention and consequences), and provision of information about hearing aids, assistive listening devices, and communication techniques. If cerumen impaction is found, cerumen removal may be indicated. There are many evidence-based resources available that can be used to educate the patient and family and assist the nurse in designing educational materials (Box 19.8). Using the information presented in this chapter, nurses can play an important role in providing older adults the information they need to improve their hearing and avoid the negative consequences of untreated hearing loss. Effective communication strategies when working with individuals who are hearing-impaired are presented in Box 19.9.

BOX 19.9 Tips for Best Practice

Communicating With Elders Who Have Hearing Impairment

- Never assume hearing loss is from age until other causes are ruled out (infection, cerumen buildup).
- Inappropriate responses, inattentiveness, and apathy may be symptoms of a hearing loss.
- Face the individual, and stand or sit on the same level; do not turn away while speaking.
- Gain the individual's attention before beginning to speak. Look directly at the person at eye level before starting to speak.
- Determine if hearing is better in one ear than another, and position yourself appropriately.
- If hearing aid is used, make sure it is in place and batteries are functioning.
- Keep hands away from your mouth and project voice by controlled diaphragmatic breathing.
- Avoid conversations in which the speaker's face is in glare or darkness; orient the light on the speaker's face.
- Careful articulation and moderate speed of speech are helpful.
- Lower your tone of voice and articulate clearly.
- Label the chart, note on the intercom button, and inform all caregivers that the patient has a hearing impairment.
- Use nonverbal approaches: gestures, demonstrations, visual aids, and written materials.
- Pause between sentences or phrases to confirm understanding.
- When changing topics, preface the change by stating the topic.
- Reduce background noise (e.g., turn off television, close door).
- Utilize assistive listening devices such as pocket talker.
- Verify that the information being given has been clearly understood. Be aware that the person may agree to everything and appear to understand what you have said even when he or she did not hear you (listener bluffing).
- Share resources for the hearing-impaired and refer as appropriate.

From Adams-Wendling L, Pimple C: Evidence-based guideline: Nursing management of hearing impairment in nursing facility residents, *J Gerontol Nurs* 34(11):9–16, 2008.

TINNITUS

Tinnitus is defined as the perception of sound in one or both ears or in the head when no external sound is present. It is often referred to as "ringing in the ears" but may also manifest as buzzing, hissing, whistling, cricket chirping, bells, roaring, clicking, pulsating, humming, or swishing sounds. The sounds may be constant or intermittent and are more acute at night or in quiet surroundings. The most common type is high-pitched tinnitus with sensorineural loss; less common is low-pitched tinnitus with conduction loss such as is seen in Meniere's disease.

Tinnitus generally increases over time. It is a condition that afflicts many older people and can interfere with hearing, as well as become extremely irritating. It is estimated to occur in nearly 11% of elders with presbycusis. Tinnitus is a growing problem for America's military personnel and is the leading cause of service-connected disability of veterans returning from Iraq or Afghanistan (American Tinnitus Association, 2016).

The exact physiological cause or causes of tinnitus are not known, but there are several likely factors that are known to trigger or worsen tinnitus. Exposure to loud noises is the leading cause of tinnitus, and the exposure can damage and destroy cilia in the inner ear. Once damaged, the cilia cannot be renewed or replaced. Other possible causes of tinnitus include head and neck trauma, certain types of tumors, cerumen accumulation, jaw misalignment, cardiovascular disease, and ototoxicity from medications. More than 200 prescription and nonprescription medications list tinnitus as a potential side effect, aspirin being the most common. There is some evidence that caffeine, alcohol, cigarettes, stress, and fatigue may exacerbate the problem.

Interventions

Some persons with tinnitus will never find the cause; for others the problem may arbitrarily disappear. Hearing aids can be prescribed to amplify environmental sounds to obscure tinnitus, and there is a device that combines the features of a masker and a hearing aid, which emits a competitive but pleasant sound that distracts from head noise. Therapeutic modes of treating tinnitus include transtympanal electrostimulation, iontophoresis, biofeedback, tinnitus masking with alternative sound production (white noise), cochlear implants, and hearing aids. Some have found hypnosis, cognitive behavioral therapy, acupuncture, and chiropractic, naturopathic, allergy, or drug treatment to be effective.

Nursing actions include discussing with the client about times when the noises are most irritating and having the person keep a diary to identify patterns. Assess medications for possibly contributing to the problem. Discuss lifestyle changes and alternative methods that some have found effective. Also, refer clients to the American Tinnitus Association for research updates, education, and support groups (Box 19.8).

KEY CONCEPTS

- Vision loss is a leading cause of age-related disability.
- The leading causes of visual impairment in the United States are diseases that are common in older adults: age-related macular degeneration (AMD), cataracts, glaucoma, and diabetic retinopathy.
- Many causes of visual impairment are preventable, so attention to keeping eyes healthy throughout life and early detection and treatment of eye disease are essential.
- Nurses who care for visually impaired elders in all settings can improve outcomes by assessing for vision changes, adapting the environment to enhance vision and safety, communicating appropriately, and providing appropriate health teaching and referrals for prevention, treatment, and assistive devices.
- Age-related hearing impairment is a complex disease caused by interactions among age-related changes, genetics, lifestyle, and environment.
- *Presbycusis* (also called age-related hearing impairment or ARHI) is a form of sensorineural hearing loss that is related to aging and is the most common form of hearing loss.
- Hearing loss diminishes quality of life and is associated with multiple negative outcomes including decreased function, increased likelihood of hospitalizations, miscommunication, depression, falls, reduced self-esteem, safety risks, and cognitive decline.
- Screening for hearing loss is an essential component of assessment in older adults.
- Nurses need to know how to operate hearing aids and assist individuals with hearing impairment to access assistive listening devices to enhance communication.

ACTIVITIES AND DISCUSSION QUESTIONS

1. How can nurses enhance awareness and education about vision and hearing disorders?
2. What is the role of a nurse in the acute care setting in screening and assessment for eye and ear diseases?
3. What type of resources could a nurse in any setting offer to an older adult who has vision and hearing loss?
4. Which of the various sensory/perceptual changes of aging would you find most difficult to handle?

REFERENCES

American Tinnitus Association: *Demographics,* 2016. Available at https://www.ata.org/understanding-facts/demographics. Accessed January 2016.

Bainbridge K, Wallhagen M: Hearing loss in an aging American population: Extent, impact, management, *Annu Rev Public Health* 35:139–152, 2014.

Bressler N, Varma R, Doan Q, et al: Underuse of the health care system by persons with diabetes mellitus and diabetic macular edema in the United States, *JAMA Ophthalmol* 132(2):168–173, 2014.

Cassels C: Cataract surgery may cut cognitive decline in dementia, *Medscape Medical News,* July 14, 2014. Available at http://www.medscape.com/viewarticle/828188. Accessed January 2016.

Ciolino J, Stefanescu C, Ross A, et al: In vivo performance of a drug-eluting contact lens to treat glaucoma for a month, *Biomaterials* 35(1):432–439, 2014.

Elliott A, McGwin G, Owsley C: Vision impairment among older adults residing in assisted living, *J Aging Health* 25(2):364–378, 2013.

Gopinath B, Schneider J, McMahon C, et al: Dual sensory impairment in older adults increases the risk of mortality: A population-based study, *PLoS ONE* 8(1):2013. doi: 10.1371/journal.pone.0055054. [Epub ahead of print]. Available at http://www.plosone.org/article/info%3Adoi%2F10.1371%2Fjournal.pone.0055054. Accessed January 2016.

Heine C, Browning C, Cowlishaw S, et al: Trajectories of older adults' hearing difficulties: Examining the influence of health behaviors and social activity over 10 years, *Geriatr Gerontol Int* 13(4):911–918, 2013.

Johnson K, Record S: Visual impairment and eye problems. In Ham R, Sloane R, Warshaw G, et al, editors: *Primary care geriatrics*, ed 6, Philadelphia, 2014, Elsevier Saunders, pp 301–305.

Lane K, Conn V: To hear or not to hear, *Res Gerontol Nurs* 6(2):79–80, 2013.

Lewis T: Hearing impairment. In Ham R, Sloane P, Warshaw G, et al, editors: *Primary care geriatrics*, ed 6, Philadelphia, 2014, Elsevier Saunders, pp 291–300.

Lin F: Hearing loss in older adults—Who's listening?, *JAMA* 307(11):1147–1148, 2012.

Lin F, Yaffe K, Xia Y, et al: Hearing loss and cognitive decline in older adults, *JAMA Intern Med* 173(4):293–299, 2013.

MacLennan P, McGivin G, Heckemeyer C, et al: Eye care use among a high-risk diabetic population seen in a public hospital's clinics, *JAMA Ophthalmol* 132(2):162–167, 2014.

Meuleners L, Fraser M, Ng J, et al: The impact of first- and second-eye cataract surgery on injurious falls that require hospitalization: A whole population study, *Age Ageing* 2013. doi: 10.1093/ageing/aft177. [Epub ahead of print]. Available at http://www.ncbi.nlm.nih.gov/pubmed/24192250. Accessed January 2016.

National Eye Institute (NEI): *Facts about diabetic eye disease,* 2015a. Available at https://nei.nih.gov/health/diabetic/retinopathy. Accessed January 2016.

National Eye Institute (NEI): *Facts about macular degeneration,* 2015b. Available at https://nei.nih.gov/health/maculardegen/armd_facts. Accessed September 2016.

National Eye Institute (NEI): *Facts about glaucoma,* 2016. Available at https://nei.nih.gov/health/glaucoma/glaucoma_facts. Accessed September 2016.

National Eye Institute, National Eye Health Education Program (NEI, NEHEP), 2015a. Available at https://nei.nih.gov/nehep. Accessed January 2016.

National Eye Institute, National Eye Health Education Program (NEI, NEHEP): *Facts about retinal detachment,* 2015b. Available at https://nei.nih.gov/health/retinaldetach/retinaldetach. Accessed January 2016.

National Institute on Deafness and Other Communication Disorders (NIDCD): Noise-induced hearing loss *(NIH publication no. 14-4233)*, 2014. Available at http://www.nidcd.nih.gov/health/hearing/pages/noise.aspx. Accessed January 2016.

Servat J, Risco M, Nakasato Y, et al: Visual impairment and the elderly: Impact on functional ability and quality of life, *Clin Geriatr* 19(7):1–12, 2011.

U.S. Department of Health and Human Services, Office of Disease Prevention and Health Promotion: *Healthy People 2020* (2012). Available at http://www.healthypeople.gov/2020.

Wang S, Mitchell P, Chiha J, et al: Severity of coronary artery disease is independently associated with the frequency of early age-related macular degeneration, *Br J Ophthalmol* 99(3):365–370, 2015.

World Health Organization: Visual impairment and blindness *(fact sheet no. 282)*, 2013. Available at http://www.who.int/mediacentre/factsheets/fs282/en/. Accessed March 2014.

Zhang X, Beckles G, Chou C-F, et al: Socioeconomic disparity among US adults with age-related eye diseases: National Health Interview Survey 2002 and 2008, *JAMA Ophthalmol* 131(9):1198–1206, 2013.

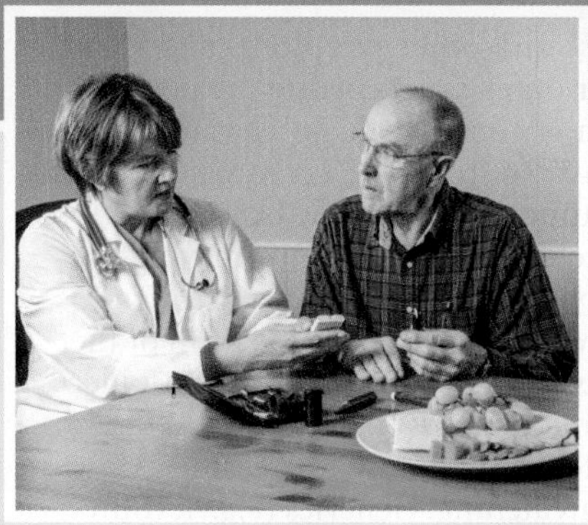

20 Metabolic Disorders

Kathleen Jett

evolve.elsevier.com/Touhy/gerontological

LEARNING OBJECTIVES

Upon completion of this chapter, the reader will be able to:

- Explain the risks for and complications of endocrine disorders in older adults.
- Describe the assessment necessary in the screening and monitoring of persons with diabetes.
- Identify the unique aspects of diabetes management in older adults.
- Develop a nursing care plan for elders with endocrine disorders.
- Discuss the nurse's role in care for persons with endocrine disorders.
- Propose a reason for the significantly higher rate of diabetes among those more than 75 years of age when compared to those between 50 and 74.

THE LIVED EXPERIENCE

I can see that Anna is going to need a lot of help learning to manage her diabetes. I know now that I have already overwhelmed her with brochures and information. She just looked frightened to death, and she just has a mild elevation in blood sugar; it could probably be controlled with diet and exercise. I will call her tomorrow and see if she is less anxious.

Anna's gerontological clinical nurse specialist

The endocrine system works with multiple body organs to regulate and integrate body activities through the release of hormones. Among other things, the hormones provide for cell metabolism and energy balance. Although the exact relationship between normal changes with aging and changes in endocrine function is unknown, they are most likely attributable to normal age-related reduced immune function (see Chapter 5). Because of the large number of elders who are affected, the gerontological nurse should have a working knowledge of these conditions to provide the care needed to promote healthy aging. In this chapter thyroid disease and diabetes mellitus are reviewed.

THYROID DISEASE

The thyroid is a small gland in the neck that stores and secretes thyroid hormones, which regulate metabolism and affect nearly every organ in the body. Although only a small percentage of persons in the United States have thyroid disease, the prevalence increases significantly with age. About 2.7% of those older than age 65 have hyperthyroidism but up to 20% have hypothyroidism (Shegal et al., 2014). Thyroid disorders are fairly easy to diagnose in younger adults, but many of the signs and symptoms mirror those of other health problems commonly found with aging, especially in those who are frail

BOX 20.1 Symptoms of Hypothyroidism: Differences in Older Adults Compared to Younger Adults

Probably Less Common in Older Adults

Fatigue
Weakness
Depression
Dry skin

Significantly Less Common in Older Adults

Weight gain
Cold intolerance
Muscle cramps

From Campbell JW: Thyroid disorders. In Ham RJ, Sloane PD, Warshaw GA, et al, editors: *Ham's primary care geriatrics: A case-based approach*, ed 6, p 442, St Louis, 2014, Elsevier.

(Box 20.1). These may be nonspecific, atypical, or absent. Such changes may be incorrectly attributed to normal aging, to another disorder, or to side effects of medications when the problem is actually a life-threatening thyroid disturbance. They may be found only when the person is screened for depression, anxiety, functional or cognitive changes, or cardiac disease.

Blood tests are used to make a diagnosis of a thyroid disturbance with the measurement of thyroid-stimulating hormone (TSH) the major indicator. The free T_3 (triiodothyronine) and the free T_4 (thyroxine) levels may also be used in making a diagnosis.

Hypothyroidism

The most common thyroid disturbance in older adults is hypothyroidism, that is, the failure of the thyroid gland to produce an adequate amount of the hormone thyroxine. The onset is often subtle, is slow in development, and is thought to be caused most frequently by chronic autoimmune thyroiditis. It may be iatrogenic, resulting from radioiodine treatment, a subtotal thyroidectomy, or medications. It can also be caused by a pituitary or hypothalamic abnormality (Campbell, 2014).

SAFETY ALERT

Amiodarone is an antidysrhythmic agent that is still in use. It is associated with multiple toxicities including thyroid disease. All persons taking amiodarone must be monitored regularly for hypothyroidism (AGS, 2015).

An older adult may complain of heart palpitations, slowed thinking, gait disturbances, fatigue, weakness, or cold intolerance. These and other symptoms and signs are often evaluated for other causes before the possibility of hypothyroidism is considered. An elevated TSH level combined with a low free T_4 (FT_4) measurement indicates that the pituitary is working extra hard to make the thyroid secrete thyroxine when it may not be able to do so (Campbell, 2014). The treatment is to replace the missing thyroxine, usually in the form of the medication levothyroxine. The usual dose in an older adult is 0.025 mg (25 micrograms [mcg]) and it is rarely necessary to advance to a higher dose. Increasing a dose rapidly could be life threatening. Generics (e.g., levothyroxine) are not equivalent to trade formulations (e.g., Synthroid) (Hamilton, 2015).

Hyperthyroidism

Hyperthyroidism is an excessive presence of thyroxine in the body. While it does not occur often, women are 2 to 10 times more likely to develop it than men (National Institute of Diabetes and Digestive and Kidney Diseases [NIDDK], 2012). Graves' disease is the most common cause in later life. It can also result from ingestion of iodine or iodine-containing substances, such as those found in some seafood, radiocontrast agents, the medication amiodarone, or too high a dose of prescribed levothyroxine. The same blood tests are done: this time the TSH level would be very low and the FT_4 level would be high. However, FT_4 levels are closely associated with protein levels in the blood. If the protein level is too low, the FT_4 level will be artificially low, making diagnosis difficult, especially in the large number of medically frail elders with hypoproteinemia (Pagana & Pagana, 2010).

Compared to hypothyroidism, the onset of hyperthyroidism may be quite sudden. The signs and symptoms in the older adult include unexplained atrial fibrillation, heart failure, constipation, anorexia, muscle weakness, and other vague complaints. Symptoms of heart failure or angina may cloud the clinical presentation and prevent the correct diagnosis. The person may be misdiagnosed as being depressed or having dementia. On examination, the person is likely to have tachycardia, tremors, and weight loss. In elders a condition known as apathetic thyrotoxicosis, rarely seen in younger persons, may occur in which usual hyperactivity is replaced with slowed movement and depressed affect. If left untreated it will increase the speed of bone loss and is as life threatening as hypothyroidism.

Complications

Complications occur both as the result of treatment and as the result of failure to diagnose or treat in a timely manner. Myxedema coma is a serious complication of untreated hypothyroidism in the older patient. If the disease is not detected until quite advanced, even with the best treatment, death may ensue.

Rapid replacement of the missing thyroxine is not possible because of the risk of drug toxicity. Thyroxine increases myocardial oxygen consumption; therefore, the elevations found in hyperthyroidism produce a significant risk for atrial fibrillation and exacerbation of angina in persons with preexisting heart failure or may precipitate acute congestive heart failure (see Chapter 21).

❖ IMPLICATIONS FOR GERONTOLOGICAL NURSING AND HEALTHY AGING

The management of thyroid disturbances is largely one of careful pharmacological intervention and, in the case of hyperthyroidism, one of surgical or chemical ablation. As advocates, nurses can ensure that a thyroid screening test be done anytime there is a possibility of concern, including when addressing any symptoms that are "vague." Nurses caring for frail elders can be attentive to the possibility that the person who is diagnosed with atrial fibrillation, anxiety, dementia, or depression may instead have a thyroid disturbance. Although little can be done to prevent thyroid disturbances, organizations such as the Monterey Bay Aquarium have launched campaigns to inform consumers of the iodine and mercury found in seafood (http://www.seafoodwatch.org).

The nurse may be instrumental in working with the person and family to understand both the seriousness of the problem and the need for very careful adherence to the prescribed regimen. If the elder is hospitalized for acute management, the life-threatening nature of both the disorder and the treatment can be made clear so that advanced planning can be done that will account for all possible outcomes.

The nurse works with the person and significant others in the correct self-administration of medications (Box 20.2). The nurse who is responsible for the administration of thyroxine must take care to follow these same instructions especially for those who are fed artificially.

BOX 20.2 Appropriate Administration of Levothyroxine

Levothyroxine should always be taken early in the morning, on an empty stomach and at least 30 minutes before a meal. It should be taken with a full glass of water to ensure it does not begin to dissolve in the esophagus. It cannot be taken within 4 hours of anything containing a mineral, such as calcium (including fortified orange juice), antacids, or iron supplements. It is always dosed in micrograms and care must be taken that it is not confused with milligrams. Twenty-five mcg/day (0.25 mg) is the most common dose used in adults older than age 50. The same brand of levothyroxine should be used with each refill.

From PharMerica: Specialized long-term care nursing drug handbook, Hudson, Ohio, 2016, Lexicomp.

DIABETES

Diabetes mellitus (DM) is a syndrome of disorders of glucose metabolism resulting in hyperglycemia. The two main types of diabetes are type 1 and type 2. Either the body is unable to produce the insulin needed to move glucose into the cells (type 1), or it does not make enough insulin to keep up with the needs of the body (type 2), as in the case of obesity. In other words, insulin is available, but the cells, especially in the muscles, liver, and fat, are not able to use it. This is referred to as insulin-resistant diabetes and comprises 90% to 95% of all cases (Centers for Disease Control and Prevention [CDC], 2015a). It is now viewed on a continuum from asymptomatic prediabetic insulin resistance, to mild postprandial hyperglycemia and/or mild fasting hyperglycemia, to diagnosable diabetes. Because glucose is necessary for life, DM is a life-threatening condition.

In most cases diagnosis requires the results of two of three possible tests on two different days. Prediabetes is indicated when the fasting plasma glucose (FPG) (not finger stick) level is 100 to 125 mg/dL or the hemoglobin A_{1c} (HgbA1c) value is 5.7% to 6.4%. Diabetes is diagnosed with a FPG of ≥126 mg/dL or an HgbA1c ≥6.5%, or a random blood glucose measurement of ≥200 mg/dL. When a person has a random blood glucose measurement of ≥200 mg/dL and is also symptomatic, no further testing is necessary (NIDDK, 2014a). The glucose tolerance test (GTT) is rarely used in this population.

The HgbA1c test is used to monitor the effects of treatment since it is an indicator of the average plasma glucose level over the previous 90 days (Table 20.1). However, there is newer information suggesting that because of genetic differences the HgbA1c value may not be a true measurement of glucose level in some subpopulations (National Glycohemoglobin Standardization Program [NGSP], 2015; NIDDK, n.d.). Because of the high prevalence and incidence of DM in older adults, when risk factors are present, diagnostic testing should be done (Box 20.3). This is especially important for the high number of older adults with any type of cardiovascular disease including hypertension (even if controlled).

In 2014 21 million people had been diagnosed with DM, the majority between the ages of 50 and 79

TABLE 20.1 Hemoglobin A_{1c} Readings Compared to the Calculated Estimated Average Glucose (eAG)

A_{1c} (%)	eAG (mg/dL)
6	126
7	154
8	183
9	212
10	240
11	269
12	298

From National Institute of Diabetes and Digestive and Kidney Diseases: Health information: Health communication programs: National Diabetes Educational Program: Health care professionals: Guiding Principles: *Principle 6: Control blood glucose to prevent or delay diabetes.* Available at http://www.niddk.nih.gov/health-information/health-communication-programs/ndep/health-care-professionals/guiding-principles/principle-06-control-blood-glucose/Pages/principle-06-control-blood-glucose.aspx. Accessed June 2016.

TABLE 20.2 Diabetes by Race/Ethnicity

Race/Ethnicity	Percentage of Diagnosed Diabetes
Non-Hispanic whites	7.6
Asian Americans	9.0
Chinese	4.4
Fillipinos	11.3
Asian Indians	13.0
Other Asian Americans	8.8
Hispanics	12.8
Central and South Americans	8.5
Cubans	9.3
Mexican Americans	13.9
Puerto Ricans	14.8
Non-Hispanic blacks	13.2
American Indians/Alaskan Natives	15.9

Data from American Diabetes Association: *Statistics about diabetes,* April 2016. Available at http://www.diabetes.org/diabetes-basics/statistics/. Accessed June 2016.

BOX 20.3 Risk Factors for Diabetes Mellitus

- High-risk population (evolving knowledge)
- More than 45 years of age
- Blood pressure ≥140/90 mm Hg
- First-degree relative (parent, sibling, child) with DM
- Prediabetes
- Overweight or obese: body mass index (BMI) >25 kg/m^2
- Previous gestational DM or having had a child with a birth weight >9 pounds
- History of cardiovascular disease of any kind
- Undesirable lipid levels: high-density lipoproteins (HDLs) ≤35 mg/dL or triglycerides ≥250 mg/dL
- Inactivity
- Taking atypical antipsychotics or glucocorticoids

(Fig. 20.1). Another 8 million people had the disease but had not yet been diagnosed. For those ages 65 to 74 years, the rates changed little from 1980 to 1993 and then increased by 113% (from 10.1 to 21.5 per 100) from 1993 to 2014. Similarly, for those ages 75 years or older, the rates changed little from 1980 to 1990 and then increased by 140% (from 8.0 to 19.2 per 100) from 1990 to 2014 (CDC, 2015b). Another 86 million people in the United States (37% of the population) have prediabetes, and only 11% know they have it (CDC, 2015a). The person still has a chance to prevent the disease from fully developing. Nonetheless, until the blood glucose measurement is consistently within a normal range, the older adult is still at a higher risk of developing the same complications of someone who already has the disease. There is an online quiz for those who wish to know their risk of developing diabetes at http://www.doihaveprediabetes.org.

There is a wide variation of the prevalence of diabetes among ethnic/racial groups and subgroups (Table 20.2). American Indian/Alaskan Native, non-Hispanic black, Hispanic, Asian American, and non-Hispanic white rank in order of prevalence from highest to lowest. However, an important caveat is the diversity within any one group. For example, persons of Chinese descent have a rate of about 4% compared to 13% among Asian Indians. Those from Central and South America have a prevalence of only about 9%, but this value increases to almost 15% among persons from Puerto Rico (American Diabetes Association [ADA], 2015a). As more is learned about Native Hawaiians and Pacific Islanders special concern is raised about the very high percentages that are being found (Kirkland et al., 2015).

Signs and Symptoms

The onset of type 2 diabetes mellitus (T2DM) in late life is usually insidious with few if any symptoms until end-organ damage (e.g., blindness) or an acute event (e.g., stroke) has occurred (Box 20.4). Older adults with T2DM often have other health issues, including problems with the metabolism of lipids and proteins. Other

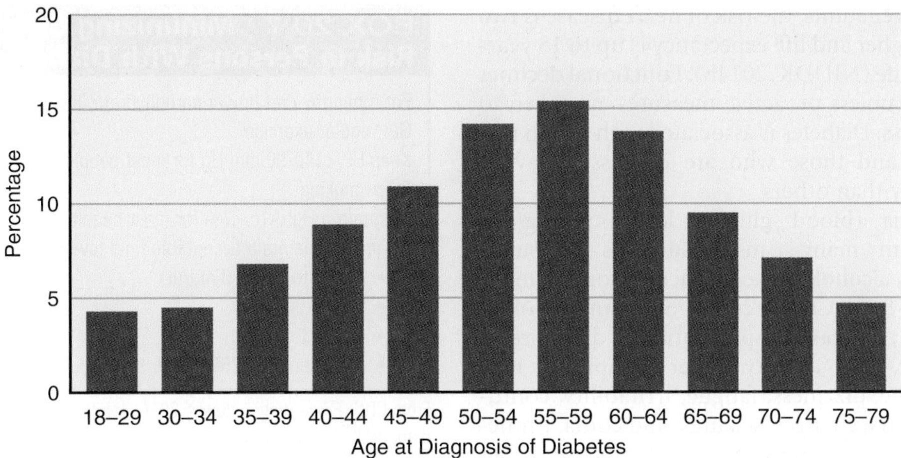

FIGURE 20.1 Distribution of age at diagnosis of diabetes among adult incident cases ages 18 to 79 years, United States, 2011. (From Centers for Disease Control and Prevention: *Diabetes public health resource,* 2015. Available at http://www.cdc.gov/diabetes/statistics/age/fig1.htm. Accessed June 2016.)

BOX 20.4 Signs of End-Organ Damage in DM

Decreased visual acuity	Heart disease
Paresthesia	Stroke
Neuropathy	Periodontal disease

From Razzaque I, Morley JE, Nau KC, et al: Diabetes mellitus. In Ham RJ, Sloane PD, Warshaw GA, et al, editors: *Ham's primary care geriatrics: A case-based approach,* ed 6, pp 431–439, St Louis, 2014, Elsevier.

BOX 20.5 Diabetes-Related Functional Disabilities in Later Life

Mobility impairment	Muscle weakness
Falls	Fatigue
Incontinence	Weight loss
Cognitive impairments	

From Razzaque I, Morley JE, Nau KC, et al: Diabetes mellitus. In Ham RJ, Sloane PD, Warshaw GA, et al, editors: *Ham's primary care geriatrics: A case-based approach,* ed 6, pp 431–439, St Louis, 2014, Elsevier.

signs more specific in the older population are changes in functional abilities (Box 20.5). Both the diagnosis and the care provided to those with diabetes in later life are considerably complex.

The classic signs and symptoms of diabetes include thirst and excessive urinating as the body tries to reduce the relative concentration of glucose in the blood. Yet hyperglycemia appears to be well tolerated in later life and there may be no early warning symptoms until the person is found to be in a life-threatening (hyperosmolar nonketotic) coma. For unknown reasons diabetic coma is more common among African American elders. It is not unusual to find asymptomatic older persons with fasting glucose levels of ≥300 mg/dL or as low as 50 mg/dL. In the older adult the early signs may be dehydration, confusion, or delirium instead; death may result when these signs are mistaken as worsening dementia (Razzaque et al., 2014). Instead of urinary frequency, the high amount of glucose in the urine may cause incontinence.

BOX 20.6 Complications of DM More Common in Older Adults

Dry eyes	Anorexia
Dry mouth	Dehydration
Confusion	Delirium
Incontinence	Nausea
Weight loss	Delayed wound healing

From Razzaque I, Morley JE, Nau KC, et al: Diabetes mellitus. In Ham RJ, Sloane PD, Warshaw GA, et al, editors: *Ham's primary care geriatrics: A case-based approach,* ed 6, pp 431–439, St Louis, 2014, Elsevier.

Complications

The development of complications in older adults with DM is compounded by aging itself and the presence of multiple comorbid diseases and disorders (Box 20.6). Although the same types of complications occur in both older and younger adults, the risk of heart disease is two to four times higher and life expectancy is up to 15 years shorter in later life (NIDDK, 2014b). Functional declines are more likely unless proactive measures are taken to promote wellness. Diabetes is associated with a high rate of depression, and those who are depressed have a higher mortality than others.

Hypoglycemia (blood glucose level <60 mg/dL) can occur from many causes, such as unusually intense exercise, alcohol intake, or medication mismanagement (Rote & McCance, 2014). Signs in the older adult include tachycardia, palpitations, diaphoresis, tremors, pallor, and anxiety. Later symptoms may include headache, dizziness, fatigue, irritability, confusion, hunger, visual changes, seizures, and coma. Immediate care involves giving the patient glucose either orally or intravenously.

With aging there is a higher tolerance for elevated levels of circulating glucose, making hyperglycemia harder to detect. It is not unusual to find persons with fasting glucose levels of 200 to 600 mg/dL or higher. This level of unrecognized hyperglycemia increases the risk for hyperosmolar hyperglycemic nonketotic coma. This is especially important in persons who are otherwise medically frail and should be considered in any older adult with diabetes who is difficult to arouse (ADA, 2015b). This is always a medical emergency.

❖ IMPLICATIONS FOR GERONTOLOGICAL NURSING AND HEALTHY AGING

Diabetes is a chronic disease that even in the best of circumstances will ultimately damage the body's organs. When it is untreated or undertreated, complications develop more quickly and more severely in the older adult. Therefore, the goals are twofold: control the blood glucose level as appropriate and reduce the risk for complications, especially those associated with cardiovascular disease (Box 20.7).

It is now recommended that the degree of glycemic control be based on the condition of the person rather than a universal number (NIDDK, n.d.). For healthy elders with a reasonably long life expectancy, the same evidence-based practice as younger adults should be followed. However, for those who are very medically fragile and whose life expectancy is limited, such as those in nursing homes, some flexibility may be more appropriate, with an emphasis on quality of life rather than length of life. Tight control of glucose levels in these circumstances may lead to life-threatening hypoglycemia. There is now some discussion that a hemoglobin A_{1c} goal of >8% for the very frail may be adequate (Zarowitz, 2011). Unfortunately, this leads to an increase in urinary tract infections (UTIs) in the presence of glucosuria, especially *Klebsiella* and *Escherichia coli.*

BOX 20.7 Minimizing Cardiovascular Risk in Persons With Diabetes

Eat a healthy diet (lower carbohydrate, lower sodium)
Get regular exercise
Keep BP <140/90 mm Hg for most people
Stop smoking
Maintain a HgbA1c <7% for most people
Attain and maintain acceptable lipid levels:

- Cholesterol <200 mg/dL
- LDL <100 mg/dL
- HDL >35 mg/dL
- Triglycerides <250 mg/dL

From CDC: *Preventing diabetes,* 2015. Available at http://www.cdc.gov/diabetes/basics/prevention.html. Accessed January 2016.

The goals of promoting healthy aging in persons with diabetes are to maintain the best health that is realistically possible and to ensure that evidence-based care is received (Box 20.8). Care of elders in any setting relative to diabetes begins with early detection—both of disease and of prediabetes. The nurse can participate in early detection through public screenings or pay attention to the need for screening of persons residing in communal settings such as nursing homes and assisted living centers. All persons with an elevated blood pressure (treated or untreated) should be screened for DM at least every 3 years. More frequent screening is individually determined and includes the presence of other risk factors and consideration of life expectancy (Veterans Administration/Department of Defense [VA/DOD], 2010). The nurse can promote healthy aging by helping people address all of the modifiable risk factors that are appropriate (Box 20.9).

◆ Assessment

The nurse begins with the assessment for risk factors for conditions leading to worsening of the DM and the development of complications. A full functional assessment is necessary for documentation of a baseline. Smoking status, nutritional status, weight history, and exercise history are important to identify lifestyle choices, all of which can provide clues for realistic education. Assessing economic resources helps establish the person's ability to purchase the equipment, materials, and foods that are needed to maintain diabetes control. This is especially important for older adults who have very limited incomes. Assessment of access to transportation provides information about the ability to obtain the foods necessary for a diabetic diet and health

BOX 20.8 Evidence-Based Practice

Minimal Standards of Medical/Nursing Care for the Person With Diabetes

At Each Visit
- Monitor weight and BP.
- Inspect feet.
- Review self-monitoring glucose record.
- Review/adjust medications as needed.
- Review self-management skills/goals.
- Assess mood.

Quarterly Visits
- Obtain hemoglobin A_{1c} measurement (biannually if stable).

Annual Visits
- Obtain fasting lipid profile and serum creatinine values.
- Obtain albumin-to-creatinine ratio.
- Refer for dilated eye exam.
- Perform foot exam for evidence of neuropathy.
- Refer to dentist for comprehensive exam and cleaning.

Immunizations
- Check for pneumococcal vaccination (once, repeat in 5–10 years as appropriate).
- Assess for streptococcal vaccine (once, per Medicare cannot be within 12 months of above).
- Obtain high-dose influenza vaccine annually.

Extracted from NIDDK: *What's new in diabetes*, 2016. Available at http://www.cdc.gov/diabetes/new/index.html. Accessed January 2016.

BOX 20.9 *Healthy People 2020*

Goals for Persons With Diabetes or Pre-Diabetes

- Reduce annual number of new cases.
- Reduce death rate.
- Reduce number of lower extremity amputations.
- Improve glycemic control.
- Improve lipid control.
- Increase the proportion of persons with controlled hypertension.
- Increase the number of persons with at least annual dental, foot, and dilated eye exams.
- Increase the proportion of persons with at least biannual glycosylated hemoglobin measurement.
- Increase the proportion of persons who obtain an annual microalbumin measurement.
- Increase the number of persons who perform self-monitoring of blood glucose levels at least twice a day.
- Increase the number of persons who receive formal diabetes education.
- Increase the number of persons who have been diagnosed with diabetes mellitus.
- Increase preventive measures in persons at high risk or with prediabetes.

Data from U.S. Department of Health and Human Services, Office of Disease Prevention and Health Promotion: *Healthy People 2020: Diabetes: Objectives*, 2014. Available at http://www.healthypeople.gov/2020/topics-objectives/topic/diabetes/objectives. Accessed June 2016.

care. History of alcohol and tobacco use provides information related to the risk for complications, especially cardiovascular.

The nursing assessment also includes paying attention for the earliest signs and symptoms of complications. This includes careful measurement of blood pressure, visual acuity, gross neurological function, and depression. Distant vision can be checked with a Snellen chart and near vision with a newspaper. The skin and feet should be thoroughly inspected for any injury, such as corns, calluses, blisters, cracks, or fungal infections.

◆ Management

The goals of health promotion for older adults with DM are often different than those for younger adults. Multiple factors confound decision-making about almost every aspect, including comorbid conditions, life expectancy, and ability to comply with a treatment plan. If the person is frail, management is difficult; and if there is not a consistent caregiver or one who has not obtained the necessary diabetes education on behalf of, or with, the older adult, diabetes control will be impossible.

Promoting healthy aging in older adults with diabetes requires an array of interventions and an effective interdisciplinary team working together with the patient and significant others. Management of such a disease requires expertise in medication use, diet, exercise, counseling, and finding ways to support while empowering (Bowen et al., 2015). The care team includes the person, his or her care partner, and the bedside and office nurses as well as nutritionists, pharmacists, podiatrists, ophthalmologists, physicians or nurse practitioners, and counselors. If the person's disease is hard to control, endocrinologists are involved, and as complications develop, more specialists, such as nephrologists, cardiologists, and wound care specialists, are required. Nurses with a special interest in diabetes can become certified diabetic educators.

The focus of management is now geared more toward life expectancy and the recognition of the importance of cardiovascular health–promoting strategies. The benefits of better control of blood pressure and lipids can be seen in 2 to 3 years. In comparison, research has indicated that it may take 8 years of glycemic control before benefits are seen.

Diabetes Self-Management (DSM)

The skills needed for self-management are many, and the nurse and dietitian are often the cornerstones of related education (Box 20.10). The nurse encourages patient empowerment and supports the elder and significant others while they struggle with a complicated and very serious disease (Bowen et al., 2015).

Experiential teaching and mastery are important to successful self-management. However, there are multiple factors related to aging that can affect this goal (Box 20.11). Standards have now been established for diabetes self-management education (DSME), and the cost is covered by many insurance companies including Medicare. Medicare pays 100% of the costs of an initial 10 hours of education and 2 hours each year after that. Limited diabetic supplies are now covered by Medicare as well (see Chapter 5).

DSM includes self-monitoring blood glucose (SMBG). Older adults with arthritis, low vision, or peripheral neuropathy (regardless of cause) will have difficulties with the mechanics of SMBG and will require creative teaching, perhaps enlisting friends or neighbors in the tasks that are necessary; however, new technologies and drug delivery systems are being designed to make these tasks easier. Daily foot care and foot examination should be discussed and demonstrated. Persons who are not particularly flexible will have difficulty reaching and inspecting their feet, and a family member

BOX 20.10 Evidence-Based Practice

Minimal Self-Care Skills Needed for the Person With Diabetes

Glucose Self-Monitoring

- Obtaining a blood sample correctly
- Using the glucose monitoring equipment correctly
- Troubleshooting when results indicate an error
- Recording the values from the machine
- Understanding the timing and frequency of the self-monitoring
- Understanding what to do with the results
- Knowing signs and symptoms of high and low blood glucose level and what to do about either one

Medication Self-Administration

Where Appropriate, Insulin Use

- Selecting appropriate injection site
- Using correct technique for injections
- Disposing of used needles and syringes correctly
- Storing and transporting insulin correctly

Oral Medication Use

- Knowing drug, dose, timing, and side effects
- Knowing drug-drug and drug-food interactions
- Recognizing side effects and knowing when to report

Foot Care and Examination

- Selecting and using appropriate and safe footwear

Handling Sick Days

- Understanding the effects illness and new medications may have on glycemic control

Note: See also http://www.niddk.nih.gov/health-information/health-communication-programs/ndep/health-care-professionals/guiding-principles/principle-03-provide-self-management-education-support/Pages/default.aspx.

BOX 20.11 Interaction Between Diabetes and the Aging Process

1. A decline in visual acuity can affect the individual's ability to read printed educational material, medication labels, markings on a syringe, and blood glucose monitoring devices.
2. Auditory impairments can lead to difficulty in hearing instructions.
3. Altered taste can affect food choices and nutritional status.
4. Poor dentition or changes in the gastrointestinal system can lead to difficulties with food ingestion and digestion needed to maintain a stable diet.
5. Altered ability to recognize hunger and thirst may lead to weight loss, dehydration, and increased risk for hyperosmolar nonketotic syndrome.
6. Unrecognized changes in hepatic or renal function occur more frequently in later life and affect anti-hyperglycemic drug dosing.
7. Arthritis or tremors can affect ability to self-administer medications and to use monitoring devices.
8. Polypharmacy complicates medication choices.
9. Diabetes and chronic disease–related depression reduce the motivation for self-management.
10. Cognitive impairment and dementia decrease self-care ability and necessitate a care-partner who has complete diabetes education and can act on behalf of the person as needed.
11. Low levels of education and low health literacy call for modifications in the method of teaching about diabetes care.
12. Reduced access to care because of financial limitations or geographic isolation can occur.

or friend can be asked to do this. As long as vision is adequate, checking can also be done by placing a **non-breakable mirror** on the floor to examine the sole. Attention to foot care can reduce the risk of amputation. Awareness of the need for good shoes that fit well is essential. Those with Medicare are eligible for one pair of specially made shoes annually.

Knowledge about the disease and its effects includes knowing what affects blood glucose levels, such as eating high-carbohydrate foods and skipping meals. The elder should have a list of warning signs for high and low blood glucose levels, especially one that reflects the signs and symptoms he or she typically experiences, and know that extra SMBG should be done any time the person feels clammy or cold, sweaty, shaky, or confused, all signs of low blood glucose level. An identification bracelet is highly recommended, especially because of the quick misdiagnosis that can occur if the person is found to be confused and mistakenly believed to have dementia.

◆ Nutrition

Adequate and appropriate nutrition is a key aspect in diabetes management. An initial nutrition assessment with a 24-hour recall will provide some clues to the person's dietary habits and style of eating. This may not be possible for persons who are independent but have some memory limitations. It is always necessary to know who shops for and prepares the food, and this person is included in, at the very least, all aspects of nutrition-related education. If the person is from an ethnic group different from that of the nurse, the nurse will need to learn more about the usual ingredients and methods of food preparation to be able to give reasonable instructions. Ideally, all persons with diabetes should have medical nutrition therapy by a registered dietitian who is a certified diabetic educator on an annual basis. This service is covered by Medicare (see Diabetes Self-Management [DSM]).

All guidelines focus on a healthful diet with attention to an adequate variety of foods with portion control. Recommended daily caloric intake ranges from 1600 to 2000 calories for women and from 2000 to 2600 calories for men more than 60 years of age, depending on activity level. The goal is to keep the glucose level under control by balancing exercise with eating, by losing weight (if overweight), and by limiting saturated fats in the diet (CDC, 2015a). Carbohydrates are included, but these are restricted to those that are full-grain. There is detailed and consumer-friendly dietary information on many websites, including that of the National Institutes of Health (http://diabetes.niddk.nih.gov/index.htm). Working with elders, whose dietary habits have been formed over a lifetime, can be difficult but is not impossible.

◆ Exercise

Daily exercise is an important aspect of therapy for T2DM because it decreases blood glucose level by increasing insulin production and decreasing insulin resistance. Walking is an inexpensive and beneficial way to exercise. Unfortunately, in some communities, environmental conditions prevent walking in one's neighborhood. This is most applicable to elders who live in areas of extremes of climates or in communities with high crime rates. Walking in a local mall, where it is climate controlled and environmentally safe, has proved to be a good alternative. Those who have limited mobility can still do chair exercises or, if possible, use exercise machines that permit sitting and holding on for support.

Exercise in conjunction with an appropriate diet may be sufficient to maintain blood glucose levels within normal limits. A more intensive exercise program should not be started until the person has had a physical examination, including a stress test and electrocardiogram (ECG). A physician or nurse practitioner and a diabetic educator will then have the information necessary to develop a safe and individualized exercise plan. If the person is using insulin, exercise must be done on a regular rather than an erratic basis, and blood glucose level should be tested before and after exercise to avoid hypoglycemia.

◆ Medications

Oral medications are the mainstay of pharmacological treatment of T2DM in later life. The sulfonylureas have been used the longest but also present the greatest risk for hypoglycemia, especially glyburide. They must be used with utmost caution in older adults who may appear to tolerate the lower range of blood glucose level, but it is nonetheless as life-threatening at any age (American Geriatrics Society [AGS], 2015; see Chapter 9). The biguanide metformin is frequently prescribed for both diabetes and prediabetes. It has been found to be very safe and effective but can only be used by people with good renal functioning. It is not recommended for use in persons more than 80 years of age (VA/DoD, 2010). Renal function must be monitored periodically and whenever there is a dose change. Several other classes of anti-hyperglycemics are used, all with their own risks and levels of effectiveness.

If oral medications do not achieve the necessary effect (usually lowering the post-prandial blood glucose level to <200 mg/dL), then insulin may be added. It is important to note that the use of insulin by someone with T2DM does not "convert" them to a type 1 diabetic, because the diagnosis is made on the type of disorder rather than on the treatment. The current practice is to use long-acting formulations, and the use of sliding-scale dosing is considered inappropriate in this population (AGS, 2015). The same DSM skills used by all persons with diabetes are required with additional skills specific to the use of insulin (Box 20.10). For those who can afford them, insulin pens require less manual dexterity and visual acuity.

If any other medications are prescribed, they must be carefully reviewed. The effect of drugs on blood glucose level must be given serious consideration because a number of medications commonly used for elders adversely affect blood glucose levels, especially psychotropics, antibiotics, and steroids. Therefore older adults should be advised to ask if a particular drug prescribed affects their therapy and should check with their primary care provider or pharmacist before taking any over-the-counter medications.

◆ Long-Term Care and the Elder With Diabetes

Many of the persons cared for by gerontological nurses in long-term care facilities have diabetes. In this setting the nurse may be responsible for many of the activities that would otherwise be the responsibility of the patient or a home caregiver. Nutritional status, intake and output, and exercise and activity are monitored. The nurse regularly assesses the person for signs of hypoglycemia and hyperglycemia as well as evidence of complications. The nurse ensures that evidence-based practice is followed. The nurse monitors the effect and side effects of diet, exercise, and medication use and encourages self-care whenever possible.

KEY CONCEPTS

- Signs and symptoms of endocrine disorders in the older adult may be vague or suggestive of other medical conditions or considered as part of "old age" rather than the usual and expected symptoms.
- Although thyroid disorders only affect a small number of persons, the incidence increases with age and is life threatening when not treated appropriately.
- Any time a person is being evaluated for depression, atrial fibrillation, dementia, or confusion, the assessment should include consideration of a thyroid disturbance.
- Very low doses of thyroid replacement are usually adequate in older adults. When dose changes are necessary, they must be made very slowly.
- Consideration of the person's life expectancy and the risks and benefits of treatment are taken into account when determining the appropriate level of glycemic control in the older adult with DM.
- Management of diabetes is a comprehensive team effort and should include the elder as much as he or she can realistically participate. If this is not possible, the caregiver, if not the nurse, will need to ensure that the medical regimen is followed and is effective.
- Caring for persons with DM includes working with them to reduce their risk for complications, especially cardiovascular diseases.
- Preventive foot care is essential for prevention of the possibility of future problems.

ACTIVITIES AND DISCUSSION QUESTIONS

1. What are the risks and complications of DM for the older adult?
2. What are the risks of treatment of the older adult with DM?
3. State the components of diabetes management, and explain what each component entails.
4. Describe the nurse's role in the management of endocrine disorders in older adults.

REFERENCES

American Diabetes Association (ADA): *Statistics about diabetes,* 2015a. Available at http://www.diabetes.org/diabetes-basics/statistics/. Accessed February 2016.

American Diabetes Association (ADA): *DKA (ketoacidosis) & ketones,* 2015b. Available at http://www.diabetes.org/living-with-diabetes/complications/ketoacidosis-dka.html. Accessed February 2016.

American Geriatrics Society (AGS): American Geriatrics 2015 update Beers criteria for potentially inappropriate medication use in older adults, *J Am Geriatr Soc* 63:2227–2246, 2015.

Bowen PG, Clay OJ, Lee LT, et al: Associations of social support and self-efficacy with quality of life in older adults with diabetes, *JGN* 41(12):21–29, 2015.

Campbell JW: Thyroid disorders. In Ham RJ, Sloane PD, Warshaw GA, et al, editors: *Primary care geriatrics: A case-based approach,* ed 6, Philadelphia, 2014, Elsevier, pp 440–444.

Centers for Disease Control and Prevention (CDC): *Rates of diagnosed diabetes per 100 civilian, non-institutionalized population, by age, United States, 1980–2014,* 2015a. Available at http://www.cdc.gov/diabetes/statistics/prev/national/figbyage.htm. Accessed January 2016.

Centers for Disease Control and Prevention (CDC): *National diabetes report card 2014,* 2015b. Available at http://www.cdc.gov/diabetes/pdfs/library/diabetesreportcard2014.pdf. Accessed January 2016.

Hamilton RJ, editor: *Tarascon pocket pharmacopoeia,* ed 16, Burlington, MA, 2015, Jones & Barlett.

Kirkland KA, Cho P, Geiss LS: Diabetes among Asians, Native Hawaiians and other Pacific Islanders, United States 2011–2014, *MMWR* 64(45):1261–1266, 2015.

National Glycohemoglobin Standardization Program (NGSP): *Harmonizing hemoglobin A1c testing,* 2015. Available at http://www.ngsp.org/interf.asp. Accessed January 2015.

National Institute of Diabetes and Digestive and Kidney Diseases (NIDDK): *Hyperthyroidism,* 2012. Available at http://www.niddk.nih.gov/health-information/health-topics/endocrine/hyperthyroidism/Pages/fact-sheet.aspx. Accessed January 2016.

National Institute of Diabetes and Digestive and Kidney Diseases (NIDDK): *Diabetes A-Z,* 2014a. Available at http://www.niddk.nih.gov/health-information/health-topics/diabetes/Pages/default.aspx. Accessed January 2016.

National Institute of Diabetes and Digestive and Kidney Diseases (NIDDK): *Complications of diabetes,* 2014b. Available at http://www.cdc.gov/diabetes/statistics/complications_national.htm. Accessed February 2016.

National Institute of Diabetes and Digestive and Kidney Diseases (NIDDK): *Consider needs of special populations,* n.d. Available at http://www.niddk.nih.gov/health-information/health-communication-programs/ndep/health-care-professionals/guiding-principles/principle-09-consider-special-populations/Pages/principle-09-consider-special-populations.aspx. Accessed February 2016.

Pagana KD, Pagana TJ: *Mosby's manual of diagnostic and laboratory tests*, ed 4, St Louis, 2010, Mosby.

Razzaque I, Morley JE, Nau KC, et al: Diabetes mellitus. In Ham RJ, Sloane PD, Warshaw GA, editors: *Primary care geriatrics: A case-based approach*, ed 6, Philadelphia, 2014, Elsevier.

Rote NS, McCance KL: Alterations in immunity and inflammation. In McCance KL, Huether SE, editors: *Pathophysiology: The biologic basis for disease in adults and children*, ed 7, St Louis, MO, 2014, Elsevier, pp 262–297.

Shegal V, Sukhminder JSB, Shegal R, et al: Clinical conundrums in management of hypothyroidism in critically ill older adults, *Int J Endocrinol Metab* 12(1):e13759, 2014.

Veterans Administration/Department of Defense: *Clinical practice guideline for the management of diabetes mellitus,* 2010. Available at http://www.healthquality.va.gov/guidelines/CD/diabetes/DM2010_FUL-v4e.pdf. Accessed January 2016.

Zarowitz B: The ADA focus on diabetes, *Geriatr Nurs* 32(2):119–122, 2011.

21

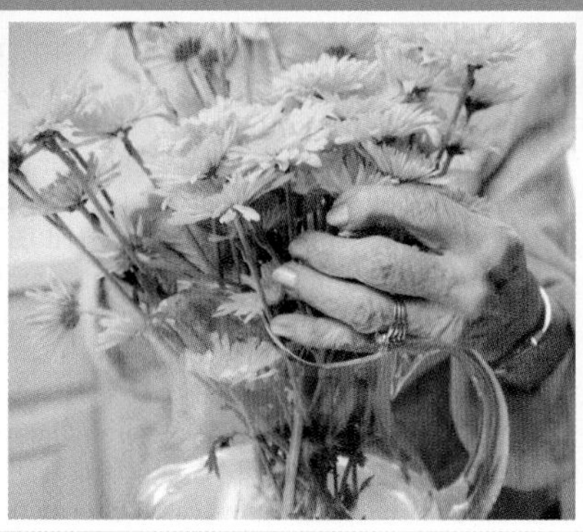

Bone and Joint Problems

Kathleen Jett

 evolve.elsevier.com/Touhy/gerontological

LEARNING OBJECTIVES

Upon completion of this chapter, the reader will be able to:

- Describe the most common bone and joint problems affecting older adults.
- Discuss the potential dangers of osteoporosis.
- Recognize postural changes that suggest the presence of osteoporosis.
- Explain some effective ways of preventing or slowing the progression of osteoporosis.
- Compare the differences in common arthritic conditions.
- Describe the nurse's responsibility in caring for the person with arthritic conditions.
- Name several methods of promoting healthy aging in the person with pain and disability from joint and bone disorders.

THE LIVED EXPERIENCE

I was always so athletic; I can't understand how I have become so crippled up. Now I understand what my grandmother used to say about the weather affecting her rheumatism. I can feel it when a storm is coming.

Mabel, age 80

I don't know how folks with arthritis can stand being uncomfortable so much of the time. I know Mabel takes medications, but she still seems to be in a lot of pain and has so much trouble moving about. I try to be as gentle as possible when I help her.

Elva, student nurse

MUSCULOSKELETAL SYSTEM

A healthy musculoskeletal system not only allows the body to be upright but also is necessary for carrying out the most basic activities of daily living (ADLs). For some, later life is an opportunity to explore the limits of their ability and become master athletes. For others, later life is a time of significant restriction in movement. However, both athletes and nonathletes have to deal with the challenges of one or more of the musculoskeletal problems commonly encountered in later life.

The gerontological nurse attends to the needs of older adults with musculoskeletal problems and works to promote healthy bones and joints. In this chapter we discuss osteoporosis, several forms of arthritis, and their implications for nursing interventions to promote healthy aging.

OSTEOPOROSIS

In the normal process of growth, the bones increase in structural density and strength through the accumulation of calcium and other minerals. At the same time, the bones are weakened as calcium and minerals return to the bloodstream. Peak bone mass is reached at about 30 years of age. After that, the loss of bone mineral density (BMD) is quite minimal at first but accelerates with age. For women, the period of fastest loss of BMD is in the 5 to 7 years immediately following menopause.

Osteoporosis means *porous bone.* Primary osteoporosis is so common in women that it is sometimes thought to be part of the normal aging process. Secondary osteoporosis is caused by another disease, such as Paget's disease, or by medications, such as long-term steroid use. In *osteopenia,* BMD has been lost but not to the extent it is in osteoporosis. Both are characterized by deterioration of the bone structure and changes in posture (Fig. 21.1). More than 53 million Americans either have osteoporosis or are at risk for it because of low BMD, the majority of whom are women (NIH, 2015). African American women have the highest BMD but are still at risk.

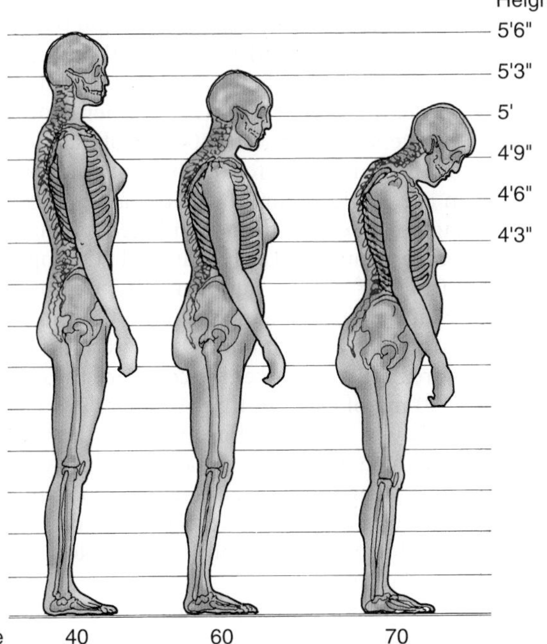

FIGURE 21.1 Age-related changes in the spine as a result of bone loss. (From Ignatavicius DD, Workman ML: *Medical-surgical nursing: Patient-centered collaborative care*, ed 8, St Louis, 2016, Elsevier. Data from Sattin RW, Easley KA, Wolf SL, et al: Reduction in fear of falling through intense tai chi exercise training in older, transitionally frail adults, *J Am Geriatr Soc* 53:1168–1178, 2005.)

Osteoporosis is a silent disorder; the person may never know he or she has a fracture. It is diagnosed through a dual-energy x-ray absorptiometry (DEXA) scan but is presumed in older adults with nontraumatic fractures, a loss of 3 inches or more in height, and/or kyphosis (see Fig. 21.1). Often referred to as a "fragility fracture," a non or low traumatic fracture is one resulting from an activity that would not normally cause one, such as falling from a standing height or from coughing, sneezing, or laughing (National Osteoporosis Guideline Group [NOGG], 2014). The nurse may be the person to identify the changes that indicate osteoporosis. The most serious complication of osteoporosis is the increased risk for a fracture and subsequent death or disability, usually the result of a fall (see Chapter 15).

A number of factors increase or decrease a person's risk for both osteopenia and osteoporosis. Some of these cannot be changed but others are amenable to change (Box 21.1). The U.S. Preventive Services Task Force (USPSTF) recommends that all women 65 years of age or older and younger women with significant risk factors (e.g., family history) be screened for osteoporosis. For those at risk, Medicare will pay for a DEXA scan every 2 years (Centers for Medicare and Medicaid Services [CMS], 2014).

There is currently insufficient evidence to make a recommendation about screening in men (USPSTF, 2011). If the screening is positive, the nurse can advocate for the elder to receive appropriate treatment. The nurse should always recommend preventive measures, such as

BOX 21.1 Risk Factors for Osteoporosis

Nonmodifiable Factors

Gender (female)
Race
Age
Family history of osteoporosis

Modifiable Factors

Weight (underweight)
Diet (low calcium, excessive caffeine, ethyl alcohol)
Hormonal deficiencies
Activity level (low)
Medications (steroids, anticonvulsants, thyroid preparations)
Cigarette smoking

increased intake of adequate amounts of calcium and vitamin D and cessation of smoking.

❖ IMPLICATIONS FOR GERONTOLOGICAL NURSING AND HEALTHY AGING

With the treatments and interventions now available, some osteoporosis can be prevented or treated and stabilized to some extent. It is always possible to promote healthy aging for the person with osteoporosis. However, for those already with osteoporosis it becomes paramount to reduce osteoporosis-related injury.

Reducing Osteoporosis-Related Risk and Injury

Measures to prevent osteoporosis-related injury or progression of the disease include exercise, nutrition, and lifestyle changes to reduce known risk factors. As with many other diseases, smoking is one risk factor that can be changed. Home safety inspection and education regarding injury prevention strategies are essential (see Chapter 16). An assortment of print and interactive educational materials for both the lay and professional audience can be found at http://www.niams.nih.gov/Health_Info/Bone/Osteoporosis/default.asp.

Patient teaching includes key aspects of the prevention and treatment of osteoporosis. Weight-bearing physical activity, such as brisk walking carrying light weights, helps to maintain bone mass by applying mechanical force to the spine and long bones. Muscle-building exercises help to maintain skeletal architecture by improving muscle strength and flexibility.

Information about the sites most vulnerable to injury should be provided. Explanation should be given about changes in the upper spine that occur when vertebrae are weakened, and about the pain that results from strain on the lower spine that is caused by the effort to compensate for balance and height changes attributable to alteration of the upper spine. Education also includes the appropriate way to take medications and their side effects.

Fall prevention is especially important to decrease the morbidity and mortality associated with osteoporosis. Environmental safety and fall prevention are addressed in detail in Chapters 15 and 16.

Pharmacological Interventions

Considerable progress has been made in the last decade in the development of pharmacological treatments for both the prevention and the treatment of osteoporosis. Adequate intake of calcium and vitamin D is recommended for persons of all ages and must be taken with all of the prescribed treatments currently available.

For optimal bone mass in later life, a healthy diet, especially one with adequate calcium and vitamin D intake earlier in life, is necessary (see Chapter 10). The diet during adolescence and young adulthood is a key to healthy bones later. A balanced diet that includes food sources of calcium is best (Box 21.2). Women more than 50 years of age should ingest 1200 mg of calcium per day (men 1000 mg/day); for both men and women older than age 70, 1200 mg of calcium a day is recommended and can come from combined dietary and supplementary sources (NIH/National Osteoporosis Center, 2014). If using supplements, combination calcium–vitamin D supplements (e.g., Caltrate D or calcium carbonate with vitamin D) are recommended. The doses are best spread over the course of the day (for example, 400 mg of calcium three times a day). Constipation, already a problem for many as they age, is worsened by calcium supplementation and may reduce the person's willingness to take calcium. Good nursing care includes working with the person to develop an effective bowel regimen. It usually includes stool softeners and plenty of water.

BOX 21.2 Sources of Calcium

- Dairy products (e.g., yogurt, milk, cheese)
- Chinese cabbage or bok choy
- Tofu (calcium fortified)
- Soy milk (calcium fortified)
- Orange juice (calcium fortified)
- Dried figs
- Cheese pizza
- Green, leafy vegetables (e.g., broccoli, brussels sprouts, mustard greens)
- Beans/legumes
- Tortillas
- Cooked soybeans
- Sardines or salmon with edible bones
- Nuts (especially almonds)
- Bread

From National Institutes of Health: *Sources of calcium,* 2014. Available at http://www.niams.nih.gov/Health_Info/Bone/Bone_Health/bone_health_for_life.asp. Accessed February 2016.

It is recommended that persons younger than 70 years of age ingest 600 supplemental units of vitamin D a day and those older than age 70, 800 international units The goal is to achieve blood levels of vitamin D greater than or equal to 50 nmol/L and less than 125 nmol/L (NIH/National Osteoporosis Center, 2014). Older adults are at particularly high risk for vitamin D deficiencies because of changes in the skin that reduce the ability to synthesize vitamin D efficiently. For those living in institutional settings or northern climates where the skin is covered, the reduced opportunities for sunlight exposure only increase the risk for deficiencies.

Patient teaching includes discussion of the factors that inhibit calcium absorption (e.g., excess alcohol, protein, or salt) or enhance excretion (e.g., caffeine; excess fiber; phosphorus in meats, sodas, and preserved foods); and the influence of the body's response to stress (decreased calcium absorption, increased excretion of calcium in the urine).

SAFETY ALERT

Neither calcium nor any other product containing a metal may be taken at the same time as thyroid preparations. They will chemically bind together and the thyroxine with be inactivated.

There are a number of medications currently available for both preventing the development of osteoporosis and slowing its progression. All increase bone mass, reduce bone turnover, or both (Kennel, 2014). They are available in oral and injectable forms and are taken daily, monthly (oral, subcutaneous), to yearly (intravenous). Calcitonin is available in a spray formulation. Only the medications Prolia and Forteo have been found to actually reverse BMD loss but can only be used in unique circumstances and are very expensive. The effectiveness of the class of drugs called bisphosphonates longer than 5 years is unknown. The nurse is often the one to notice that this time period has been reached.

SAFETY ALERT

Because of the seriousness of the risk for esophageal erosion, bisphosphonates must be taken on an empty stomach, with a full glass of water, and with the person completely upright for a half hour after ingestion. They are not appropriate for the person with memory loss or for anyone else who cannot be depended upon to comply with these directions.

The medication Evista is used as a substitute for estrogen as a bone protector and decreases the risk for breast cancer. It is approved for both the prevention and the treatment of bone loss, but it can cause hot flashes and coagulation disorders and is contraindicated for use by anyone with a history of a deep venous thrombosis (DVT) or who is taking blood thinners.

THE ARTHRITIDES

Arthritis is the term used to apply to more than 100 musculoskeletal conditions. It is significantly more common in women in all age groups and increases dramatically after about 45 years of age. Arthritis of some kind affects at least 52.5 million Americans older than age 18; two-thirds of these are younger than 65 years of age. This number is expected to rise to 67 million by 2030, and 37% of these have an arthritis-associated disability (Centers for Disease Control and Prevention [CDC], 2015a). The most common forms of arthritis that the gerontological nurse will encounter are osteoarthritis (OA), polymyalgia rheumatica (PMR), rheumatoid arthritis (RA), and gout (Table 21.1).

Osteoarthritis

OA, the most common type of arthritis, is a degenerative joint disorder. Risk factors include genetic predisposition (family history), local inflammation, joint integrity, mechanical forces, and cellular and biochemical processes. After the age of 65 more women than men are affected and will have radiographic evidence of OA even if they are asymptomatic. There is considerable racial and ethnic variability in prevalence (Table 21.2). For example, within the Hispanic subpopulation, the range of those with diagnosed arthritis ranges from 21.1% in Cuban Americans to 41.6% in Mexican Americans (Murphy et al., 2011).

TABLE 21.1 Comparison of Osteoarthritis, Rheumatoid Arthritis, and Gout

	Osteoarthritis	Rheumatoid Arthritis	Gout
Onset	Insidious	More acute in older adults than in younger adults	Sudden/acute
Classic symptoms	Stiffness of joint resolved in less than 20 minutes after rest	Stiffening lasting more than 20–30 minutes after rest	Acute pain
Classic signs	Affects distal interphalangeal joints, knees, hips, and vertebrae	Affects proximal joints; may be systemic	Inflammation, especially at the base of the great toe
Key management	Initial treatment may be nonpharmacological such as heat and exercise; later acetaminophen and NSAIDs	Use of DMARDs as soon as diagnosis is made	NSAIDs

TABLE 21.2 Prevalence of Arthritis by Race/Ethnicity

Race/Ethnicity	Prevalence
Non-Hispanic white	22.9%
Non-Hispanic black	22.4%
Hispanic	15.9%
Asian/Pacific Islander	12.1%
Other races	27.9%

From Barbour KE, Helmick CG, Theis KA, et al: Prevalence of doctor-diagnosed arthritis and arthritis-attributable activity limitation—United States, 2010–2012, *MMRW* 62(440):869–873, 2013.

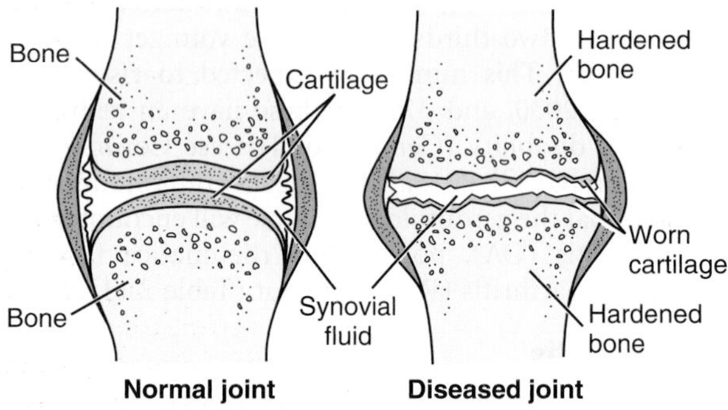

FIGURE 21.2 Normal joint and diseased joint.

The osteoarthritic joint is one in which the normal soft and resilient cartilaginous lining becomes thin and damaged. This causes the joint space to narrow and, ultimately, the bones of the joint rub together, causing destruction, pain, swelling, and loss of motion. Bone spurs (osteophytes) may develop in the spaces, causing deformation and deterioration (Fig. 21.2).

In classic OA there is stiffness with inactivity that is relieved by activity. At the same time, the activity may lead to pain relieved by rest. The stiffness is greatest in the morning after the disuse during sleep, but should resolve within 30 minutes of use. Pain at rest develops as the disease advances and more joints become involved. Crepitus (that is, a crunching or popping sound or sensation) may be detected during an exam, indicating joint instability. This is an indication of the deterioration of the joint. The joint will enlarge as osteophytes develop and range of motion will be reduced. The most common location for OA is the knee, followed by the hands, hip, and feet (CDC, 2015b). OA of the cervical spine affects its curvature in a classic fashion (see Fig. 21.1). The neck (cervical spine), the lower back (lumbar spine), the fingers, and the thumbs may also be affected

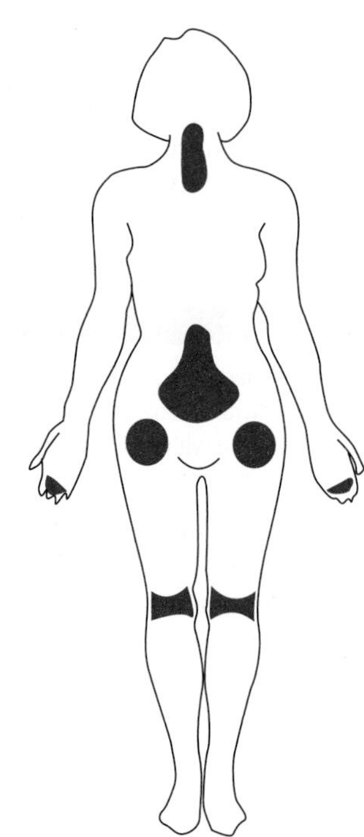

FIGURE 21.3 Common locations for osteoarthritis. (From National Institutes of Health: *Handout on health: Osteoarthritis,* 2015. Available at http://www.niams.nih.gov/hi/topics/arthritis/oahandout.htm. Accessed February 2016.)

(Fig. 21.3). OA is found in the shoulders less often. Depression, anxiety, joint stiffening, pain, and decreased functional status are all associated with OA.

Early treatment is palliative (that is, geared toward promoting comfort and slowing the decline in function). When the associated pain cannot be controlled or one's function is impaired to the point that quality of life is unacceptable, a joint replacement procedure (arthroplasty) may be done for osteoarthritis in the knee, shoulder, or hip. These are often highly successful and restore the person to his or her previous or higher level of functioning. In select cases joint replacement surgery is recommended for even the very old when pain cannot be controlled. The nurse is involved in the preoperative and perioperative periods and rehabilitation while the person is learning to use the new joint.

Polymyalgia Rheumatica and Giant Cell Arteritis

Polymyalgia rheumatica (PMR) is one of the more common inflammatory diseases seen in older adults, especially Caucasian women. For unknown reasons

PMR may occur at the same time as giant cell arteritis (GCA). Their causes are unknown, but they are associated with immune disorders and have genetic factors (National Institute of Arthritis and Musculoskeletal and Skin Diseases [NIAMS], 2015a).

While PMR may develop as suddenly as overnight, it often develops slowly. Classic symptoms are stiffening and pain beginning in the neck and upper arms and possibly evolving to the pelvic and pectoral girdles, fatigue, and low-grade fever. Pain is usually greatest at night and in the early morning, but usually without joint inflammation. It usually resolves on its own in 1 to 2 years. The exact cause of polymyalgia rheumatica is not known. However, it is associated with immune system problems and genetic factors and may be triggered by a sudden event such as an infection. It is rare in people younger than age 50 and becomes more common as age increases, suggesting that it may be linked to the aging process (NIAMS, 2015a).

Giant cell arteritis (GCA) (also known as *temporal arteritis*) may occur at the same time as PMR. It is primarily an acute inflammation of the arteries of the scalp in the temporal area but medium to large vessels may be involved as well. The inflammation causes restricted blood flow and may cause very serious and permanent damage such as stroke or blindness.

Early symptoms of GCA are flu-like, such as fatigue, loss of appetite, and fever. Other symptoms that are specifically related to inflamed arteries in the head include headaches, pain and tenderness over the temples, double vision or vision loss, dizziness, or problems with coordination. Pain may also affect the jaw and tongue, especially when eating and opening the mouth to chew (NIAMS, 2015a). Initial treatment is high-dose steroids and later low-dose steroids continuing for years or indefinitely. *Sudden changes in vision are always a medical emergency.*

Rheumatoid Arthritis

Rheumatoid arthritis (RA) is a chronic, systemic, inflammatory joint disorder. It is considered an autoimmune disease in which products from the inflamed lining of the joint invade and destroy the cartilage and bone within the joint. The cause is unknown and it affects about 1.5 million people, or 0.6% of the U.S. adult population and predominantly most often starts in midlife between 40 and 60 years of age (NIAMS, 2014).

RA is characterized by pain and swelling in symmetrical joints (for example, both hands, both sides of the hip). It generally affects the small joints of the wrist, the ankle, or the hand, although it can affect large joints as well. Whereas morning stiffness in OA lasts less than 30 minutes, in RA it lasts longer than 30 minutes. RA is a systemic disease; therefore the person may feel generalized fatigue and malaise and have occasional unexplained fevers. The joints are warm and tender. Weight loss is common. The natural course of RA is highly variable, with good and bad days. The disease may last a few months or years or may become a chronic condition with progressive damage to the joints. Risk factors include environmental and genetic factors.

In the past, nonsteroidal anti-inflammatory drugs (NSAIDs) were used for treatment early in the disease and RA-specific drugs were "saved" for later. However, it has been found that prompt efforts may halt or slow the damage (NIAMS, 2014). Persons diagnosed with RA usually are under a rheumatologist's care, which involves aggressive therapy primarily using a class of drugs called disease-modifying antirheumatic drugs (DMARDs) and the newer biological response modifiers and *jak* kinase inhibitors. All the DMARDs are potentially toxic and are administered with care by a registered nurse, such as the charge nurse in a nursing home, or by a physician.

As with OA, care is palliative. It includes providing comfort and support and monitoring the progression of the disease and the effectiveness, side effects, and potential toxicity of treatment (Box 21.3). Support groups specific for persons with RA may help to empower, which in turn may improve their quality of life.

Gout

Gout is a common form of inflammatory arthritis in older adults. It appears to result from the accumulation of uric acid crystals in a joint. Uric acid is produced when purines found in food break down.

Gout typically starts with an acute attack. The person complains of sudden and *exquisite* or *severe* pain in the

BOX 21.3 Partial List of Potential Side Effects of Medications Used to Treat Rheumatoid Arthritis

- Nausea, stomatitis (common), bone marrow suppression, liver disease, intestinal pneumonitis (rare)
- Nausea, rash, Stevens-Johnson syndrome (life-threatening), neutropenia, aplastic anemia
- Nausea, rash, bone marrow suppression, agranulocytosis, plastic anemia, corneal and retinal damage at higher doses
- Frequent infections, rash, pain, headache, cough, heart failure

From National Institute of Arthritis and Musculoskeletal and Skin Diseases: *Handout on health: Rheumatoid arthritis,* 2014. Available at http://www.niams.nih.gov/health_info/Rheumatic_Disease/default.asp. Accessed February 2016.

BOX 21.4 Examples of Foods High in Purines

Asparagus	Herring, mackerel, and sardines
Game meat	Sweetbread
Beef kidneys	Mushrooms
Gravy	Dried beans and seeds
Brain	Scallops

 **BOX 21.5 *Healthy People 2020***

Goals for Musculoskeletal Wellness

- Reduce the mean level of joint pain among adults with doctor-diagnosed arthritis.
- Reduce the number of adults with doctor-diagnosed arthritis who find it "very difficult" to perform joint-related activities.
- Reduce the number of adults with doctor-diagnosed arthritis who have difficulty in performing two or more personal care activities, thereby preserving independence.
- Increase the proportion of adults with doctor-diagnosed arthritis who receive health care provider counseling.
- Reduce hip fractures among older adults.

Data from U.S. Department of Health and Human Services, Office of Disease Prevention and Health Promotion: *Healthy People 2020.* Available at http://www.healthypeople.gov/2020/topics-objectives/topic/Arthritis-Osteoporosis-and-Chronic-Back-Conditions/objectives. Accessed February 2016.

affected joint, often starting in the middle of the night during sleep. The joint is bright purple-red, hot, and too painful to touch. The most common treatments for an acute attack are NSAIDs; however, these are associated with a high risk for adverse drug events (see Chapter 9). For some, corticosteroids are necessary. If there is still no relief, colchicine is used as a last resort and with much caution (NIAMS, 2015b).

After an acute attack, gout may become chronic with periodic acute "attacks." Risk factors include alcohol abuse, high blood pressure, a diet high in purines (Box 21.4), and certain medications, especially thiazide diuretics, salicylates (e.g., aspirin), niacin, cyclosporines, and levodopa (Sinemet) (NIAMS, 2015b). The medical goals are to prevent another attack, systemic spread of the disease, and the development of chronic gout. This may be done with the avoidance of risk-elevating drugs or of foods that are high in purine and alcohol, both of which increase uric acid levels; also, medications can be used to either decrease uric acid production (e.g., allopurinol) or increase its excretion (e.g., probenecid) (American Society of Health-System Pharmacists [ASHSP], 2010). The nurse ensures that the person ingests enough fluids to help flush the uric acid through the kidneys (2 L/day if not contraindicated).

The proximal joint of the great toe is the most typical site, although sometimes the ankle, the knee, the wrist, or the elbow is involved. The development of gout and the body's response to uric acid accumulation are highly individual. It is important to note that some people have elevated levels of uric acid and do not get gout, a clinical picture described as asymptomatic hyperuricemia, and others have gout and low levels of uric acid. The uric acid level itself does not result in a diagnosis of gout.

❖ IMPLICATIONS FOR GERONTOLOGICAL NURSING AND HEALTHY AGING

Gerontological nurses have a direct impact on promoting musculoskeletal health in a number of ways. They are active at all levels of health promotion and disease prevention (Box 21.5).

◆ Assessment

When assessing the musculoskeletal system, the nurse examines the joints and muscles for tenderness, swelling, warmth, and redness. The hands are examined for the presence or absence of osteophytes. If they appear in the distal joints as deformities of the fingers, they are called Heberden's nodes, and they are called Bouchard's nodes in the proximal joints (Fig. 21.4). The nurse questions their effect on function. In GCA, the temporal arteries enlarge and become tender to touch. The osteoporosis risk assessment instrument (ORAI) can be used to help determine an individual's risk for osteoporosis (OsteoEd, 2016).

Both passive and active range of motion is evaluated. How far can the person reach and bend all joints without assistance? The degrees of flexion, extension, rotation, abduction, and adduction are measured and documented. The testing of passive range of motion must go only to the point of discomfort and never to that of inducing pain. Ask if there are any activities of daily living (ADLs) or instrumental activities of daily living (IADLs) that are limited or not possible because of musculoskeletal issues. For example, can the person comb the hair or tie a shoe; can a woman fasten her bra; can food and other needed materials be taken from cabinets; is the person able to get up and down from the toilet, open medicine bottles, and hold and use eating utensils?

◆ Interventions

The goals of intervention and management of the different forms of musculoskeletal problems are to obtain

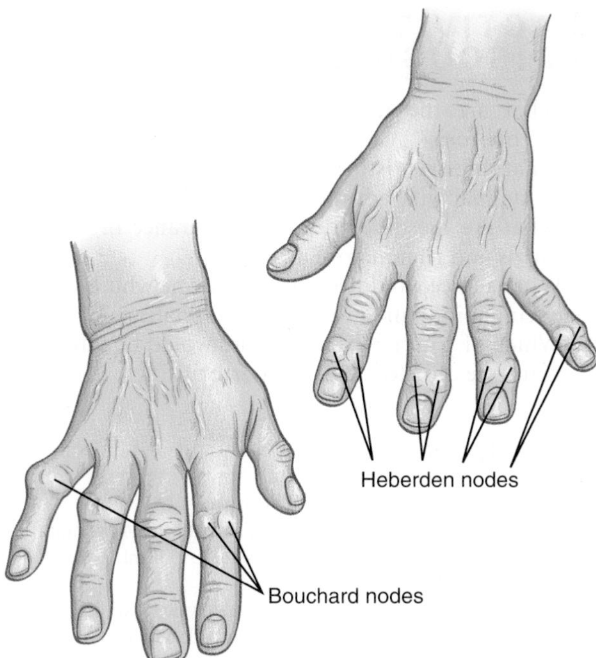

FIGURE 21.4 Hand deformities in arthritis. (From McCance KL, Huether SE, editors: *Pathophysiology: The biologic basis for disease in adults and children,* ed 7, St Louis, 2014, Elsevier.)

TABLE 21.3 Prevalence of Arthritis-Related Activity Limitation Among Adults by Race/Ethnicity

Race/Ethnicity	Prevalence
Non-Hispanic white	41.7%
Non-Hispanic black	49.3%
Hispanic	48.8%
Asian/Pacific Islander	41.1%
Other races	60.1%

From Barbour KE, Helmick CG, Theis KA, et al: Prevalence of doctor-diagnosed arthritis and arthritis-attributable activity limitation—United States, 2010–2012, *MMRW* 62(440):869–873, 2013.

treatment as soon as possible for inflammatory conditions, control pain, and minimize functional limitations (Table 21.3). The nurse is very involved in advocacy for adequate and prompt treatment, pain control (see Chapter 18), medication administration, evaluation, and patient teaching. Pain management and the minimization of disability are interconnected. In administering gout-related medications the nurse pays close attention to renal function and notifies the physician or nurse practitioner of any change so that the dosages can be adjusted.

It cannot be overstated that ongoing treatment from accredited physical therapists is necessary for persons with arthritic problems to retain joint use. Weight loss, if necessary, and muscle building are highly recommended. In joint replacement, outcomes depend on the timing of surgery, the number of procedures that the surgeon has performed, the nursing care received, and the patient's medical status before and after the surgery and the ability to participate in rehabilitation.

Exercise has been found to be the cornerstone to maintaining function with OA and RA. Regular exercise can improve flexibility and muscle strength, which in turn help support the affected joints, reduce pain, and reduce falls. Walking, swimming, and water aerobics are preferred by many, and the latter is often available in senior centers, public pools, and YMCAs in many communities.

Attention should also be given to diet (see Chapter 10). With the decreases in activity associated with pain in all forms of arthritis, it is easy for the person to gain weight. Excess weight significantly increases the pressure and wear and tear on the joints, leading to less activity and more weight gain. The nurse and the registered dietitian can work with the person to identify realistic weight and caloric goals and develop meal plans that are personally and culturally acceptable but still balanced and healthy.

The use of heat and cold is well known in the management of pain in OA and RA. It should not be used in GCA. Patient preference is important, but cold usually works best for an acute process, for example, the application of cold packs that decrease muscle spasm, decrease swelling, and relieve inflammatory pain. Heat may be applied superficially or deeply. Ultrasound provides deep heat and is usually administered by physical therapists. Hot packs, hydrotherapy, and radiant heat provide superficial heat. Liquid paraffin baths can be purchased in most drug stores for submerging the hands to provide deep heat and temporary relief.

To minimize disability with OA and RA, the joint must be used carefully, strengthened, and protected. Devices and techniques are available that relieve some of the pressure to the joints and protect the joints and muscles from further stress and, in doing so, possibly decrease pain and improve balance and function. Canes, crutches, walkers, collars, shoe orthotics, and corsets can relieve joint pressure and help support the person with the muscle weakness or resultant orthopedic abnormalities. A shoe lift can improve lumbar pain. A knee brace is useful if there is lateral instability (the knee "gives out"). The person can avoid carrying packages by the fingers or can use utensils and household equipment with larger rather than smaller grips if the hands are affected. The nurse works with the elder and the occupational therapist to maintain or improve the ability to independently perform activities of daily living to the extent possible. Preventing the exposure of the affected joints to cold temperatures may also help. The person is encouraged to wear leggings, gloves, or scarves as necessary while outside.

◆ Complementary and Alternative Interventions

A number of complementary and alternative medicine (CAM) interventions are used by persons around the globe to attempt to treat the pain associated with musculoskeletal problems, especially osteoarthritis. Among the most popular is the use of the dietary supplements glucosamine and chondroitin sulfate. There is now a large body of evidence that finds there is improvement in pain or function of joints when these products are used. There are promising (small) studies in Europe examining the use of avocado/soybean unsaponifiables (ASUs), that is, supplements made from avocado oil and soybean oil extracts. They have been found to reduce pain, increase function, and reduce the amount of NSAIDs taken (National Center for Complementary and Integrative Health [NCCIH], 2015). Research continues in finding useful and safe approaches to this significant problem for many older adults.

KEY CONCEPTS

- Most people more than 40 years of age will have osteoarthritis at some point in their lives.
- Osteoporosis can become a crippling problem for many elders, especially women. Although it cannot be completely prevented, it can be minimized by early interventions: weight-bearing exercise and calcium and vitamin D intake.
- The most serious outcomes of osteoporosis are fractures, and are associated with high mortality.
- Rheumatoid arthritis produces swelling, inflammation, intense pain, and distortion of the joints.
- Gout is both an acute and a chronic condition. One of the goals of treatment with gout is to minimize a future attack.
- Individuals have found certain types of complementary and alternative interventions very helpful for joint disorders and chronic discomfort.

ACTIVITIES AND DISCUSSION QUESTIONS

1. What are the most effective ways of preventing osteoporosis?
2. What lifestyle issues would you discuss with an individual with advanced osteoporosis?
3. What are the differences in appearance of osteoarthritis and rheumatoid arthritis?
4. What advice would you give someone who is experiencing joint pain and mobility limitations?
5. Which of your favorite activities would be difficult if you were afflicted with osteoarthritis?

REFERENCES

American Society of Health-System Pharmacists (ASHP): *MedLine plus: Probenecid*, 2010. Available at https://www.nlm.nih.gov/medlineplus/druginfo/meds/a682395.html. Accessed February 2016.

Barbour KE, Helmick CG, Theis KA, et al: Prevalence of doctor-diagnosed arthritis and arthritis-attributable activity limitation — United States, 2010–2012, *MMRW* 62(440):869–873, 2013.

Centers for Disease Control and Prevention (CDC): *Arthritis data and statistics*, 2015a. Available at http://www.cdc.gov/arthritis/data_statistics/index.htm. Accessed February 2016.

Centers for Disease Control and Prevention (CDC): *Osteoarthritis*, 2015b. Available at http://www.cdc.gov/arthritis/basics/osteoarthritis.htm. Accessed September 2015.

Centers for Medicare and Medicaid Services (CMS): *Preventive services chart*, 2014. Available at https://www.cms.gov/Medicare/Prevention/PrevntionGenInfo/Downloads/MPS-QuickReferenceChart-1TextOnly.pdf. Accessed February 2016.

Kennel KA: *Osteoporosis treatment: Medications can help*, 2014. Available at http://www.mayoclinic.org/diseases-conditions/osteoporosis/in-depth/osteoporosis-treatment/art-20046869?pg=1. Accessed September 2016.

Murphy LB, Hootman JM, Langmaid GA, et al: Prevalence of doctor-diagnosed arthritis and arthritis-attributable effects among Hispanic adults, by Hispanic subgroup—United States, 2002, 2003, 2006, and 2009, *MMWR* 60(06):167–171, 2011.

National Center for Complementary and Integrative Health: *Dietary supplements for osteoarthritis: What the science says*, 2015. Available at https://nccih.nih.gov/health/providers/digest/osteoarthritis-supplements-science. Accessed February 2016.

National Institute of Arthritis and Musculoskeletal and Skin Diseases (NIAMS): *Handout on health: Rheumatoid arthritis*, 2014. Available at http://www.niams.nih.gov/Health_Info/Rheumatic_Disease/default.asp. Accessed February 2016.

National Institute of Arthritis and Musculoskeletal and Skin Diseases (NIAMS): *Questions and answers about polymyalgia rheumatica and giant cell arteritis*, 2015a. Available at http://www.niams.nih.gov/Health_Info/Polymyalgia/default.asp#poly6. Accessed February 2016.

National Institute of Arthritis and Musculoskeletal and Skin Diseases (NIAMS): *Questions and answers about gout*, 2015b. Available at http://www.niams.nih.gov/Health_Info/Gout/default.asp. Accessed February 2016.

National Institutes of Health (NIH): *NIH senior health: Osteoporosis*, 2015. Available at http://nihseniorhealth.gov/osteoporosis/faq/faq3.html. Accessed February 2016.

National Institutes of Health/National Osteoporosis and Related Bone Disorders Resource Center: *Bone health for life: Health information basics for you and your family*, 2014. Available at http://www.niams.nih.gov/Health_Info/Bone/Bone_Health/bone_health_for_life.asp#c. Accessed February 2016.

National Osteoporosis Guideline Group [NOGG]: *Guideline for the diagnosis and management of osteoporosis in postmenopausal women and men from the age of 50 in the UK*, 2014. Available at http://www.shef.ac.uk/NOGG/NOGG_Pocket_Guide_for_Healthcare_Professionals.pdf. Accessed September 2016.

OsteoEd: *The osteoporosis risk assessment instrument (ORAI)*, 2016. Available at http://depts.washington.edu/osteoed/tools.php?type=orai. Accessed February 2016.

U.S. Preventive Services Task Force (USPSTF): *Osteoporosis: Screening*, 2011/2015. Available at http://www.uspreventiveservicestaskforce.org/uspstf10/osteoporosis/osteors.htm. Accessed September 2016.

22

Cardiovascular and Respiratory Disorders

Kathleen Jett

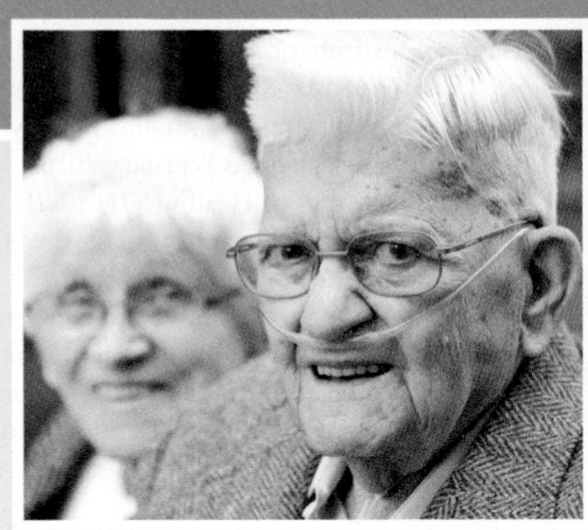

evolve.elsevier.com/Touhy/gerontological

LEARNING OBJECTIVES

Upon completion of this chapter, the reader will be able to:

- Identify the most common types of cardiovascular and respiratory diseases occurring in late life.
- Discuss how assessment and interventions for cardiovascular and respiratory diseases in older adults may differ from those for younger adults.
- Suggest ways to prevent cardiovascular and respiratory disease to the extent possible.
- Discuss the signs and symptoms of pneumonia and explain how they may differ in a frail elder.
- Propose how the nurse works with elders in the consideration of treatment plans in the presence of pneumonia.

THE LIVED EXPERIENCE

I came down to the clinic and told them that I felt kind of strange all night, but just a little pressure in the middle of my chest but otherwise the same as always. It was amazing how fast the nurse practitioner sent me to the emergency room. I had been having something they called "angina" and didn't even know it! They said I could have died and I am not quite ready for that.

Milly, age 93

We keep trying to tell dad he needs to stop smoking or it is going to kill him! He coughs all of the time and gets one infection after another. All he says is "I've been smoking all of my life, why should I stop now?"

Maria, daughter of José, age 69

Caring for older adults often means caring for persons with cardiovascular disease (CVD), respiratory problems, or both. These two systems are interconnected: a problem in one is likely to cause or complicate a problem in the other. When the nurse is addressing a cardiac problem, the respiratory system is addressed as well, and vice versa. For example, pneumonia may trigger heart failure. Nursing interventions frequently overlap. One carefully planned action must address several systems at the same time and achieve goals to meet basic physiological, psychological, and spiritual needs while promoting healthy aging in the face of very serious illnesses.

CARDIOVASCULAR DISEASE

The American Heart Association identifies the major cardiovascular diseases as hypertension (HTN); coronary heart disease (CHD), including myocardial infarction

(MI) and angina; and heart failure (HF). Although the numbers of deaths from heart disease have decreased, they remain the number one cause of death for Caucasians and African Americans in the United States (Centers for Disease Control and Prevention [CDC], 2015a; CDC, 2015b). The rate of deaths increases dramatically with age partly because of normal changes with aging (see Chapter 3) and the high prevalence of hypertension and diabetes. Older adults also undergo the majority of CVD-related procedures, but treatment approaches are highly variable by ethnicity and sex (Mehta et al., 2016).

Hypertension

Hypertension (HTN) is the most common chronic cardiovascular disease encountered by the gerontological nurse. Both the definition of and the guidelines for treatment of HTN are provided by the Joint National Committee on the Detection, Evaluation, and Treatment of High Blood Pressure (JNC 8). In the general population HTN is diagnosed any time the diastolic blood pressure reading is 90 mm Hg or higher or the systolic reading is 140 mm Hg or higher on two separate occasions. However, it has recently been suggested that a systolic reading up to 150 mm Hg is acceptable for those at least 65 years of age, except for those with diabetes (James et al., 2014).

Blood pressure increases slightly with age, with a leveling off or decrease in the diastolic pressure for persons about 60 years of age and older. Older adults most often have isolated systolic hypertension, that is, an elevation in only the systolic reading. This is quite different from the younger person, who is more likely to have an elevation in just the diastolic, or in both.

Although often treatable, and in some cases preventable, the rate of HTN has increased in approximately the last 15 years, especially for women; but significant disparities between groups persist. Although race, ethnicity, and a family history of hypertension cannot be changed, a number of other factors are within control of the individual to reduce this disparity and his or her risk for hypertension-associated heart disease (Box 22.1). A consistent research finding is that about 90% of those persons who are normotensive at the age of 50 develop HTN at some later time in life (Goroll & Mulley, 2014).

Most HTN is discovered during health screening or examination for another problem, when related complications may have already developed, referred to as "end-organ damage," especially to the heart (James et al., 2014). Older persons with HTN have an absolute higher risk for cardiac disease such as CHD, atrial fibrillation (irregular heartbeat), and heart failure, as well as increased likelihood for acute cardiovascular and cerebrovascular events such as myocardial infarction, stroke, and sudden death. Poorly controlled HTN can also lead to chronic renal insufficiency, end-stage renal disease, and peripheral vascular disease (Goroll & Mulley, 2014) (Box 22.2).

It is recommended that at least three separate readings be used in the diagnosis of hypertension in older adults because of the variability inherent with the less compliant vasculature associated with normal aging. It is preferable that a reading outside of the clinical setting, such as an accurate home measurement, be included before a diagnosis is made (U.S. Preventive Services Task Force [USPSTF], 2015) (Box 22.3). All adults at least 40 years of age should be screened at least once a year.

BOX 22.1 Modifiable Factors to Minimize Risk for Heart Disease

- Control blood pressure.
- Maintain healthy triglyceride and cholesterol levels.
- Prevent or control diabetes.
- Cease or never use tobacco products/reduce exposure to pollutants including tobacco smoke.
- Eat a healthy diet and maintain or attain acceptable weight.
- Engage in regular exercise.
- Control alcohol intake (1 drink daily for women and 2 for men).
- Reduce stress and treat depression.

BOX 22.2 Evidence-Based Practice

Benefits of Reducing Blood Pressure by 5%

- 34% fewer strokes
- 21% less ischemic heart disease

Data from Law M, Wald N, Morris J: Lowering blood pressure to prevent myocardial infarction and stroke: A new preventive strategy, *Executive Report: Health Technology Assessment* 7(31), 2003.

BOX 22.3 Tips for Best Practice

Home Measurement of Blood Pressure

- Observe the technique that the person uses in the measurement of blood pressure, in both arms, using his or her personal home device.
- Duplicate the measurement using the same device, but with the nurse conducting the measurement.
- Measure the BP using either a reliable and tested BP cuff or a cuff and a stethoscope.
- If there is a discrepancy even with a person using good technique, counsel the person regarding the replacement of the home device.

BOX 22.4 Evidence-Based Practice

Screening for Hypertension

Office measurement of blood pressure is done with a manual or automated sphygmomanometer. Proper protocol is to use the mean of two measurements taken while the patient is seated. Allow for ≥5 min between entry into the office and blood pressure measurement. Use an appropriately sized arm cuff and place the patient's arm at the level of the right atrium, with the patient's legs uncrossed and the patient not speaking. The measurements must be in contralateral arms. Multiple measurements over time have better positive predictive value than a single measurement.

BOX 22.5 Signs of Potential Exacerbation of Illness in an Older Adult With Coronary Heart Disease

- Light-headedness or dizziness
- Disturbances in gait and balance
- Loss of appetite or unexplained loss of weight
- Inability to concentrate or shortened attention span
- Changes in personality or mood
- Changes in grooming habits
- Unusual patterns in urination or defecation
- Vague discomfort, frequent bouts of anxiety
- Excessive fatigue, vague pain
- Withdrawal from usual sources of pleasure

Consideration of more frequent screenings should be made for those at high risk (i.e., smokers, those who are obese, and those of African American descent) (USPSTF, 2015) (Box 22.4).

Heart Disease

The beating heart, like other muscles, needs oxygen and other nutrients to survive. And like all other muscles, the heart receives its oxygen from adjacent arteries rather than from the blood passing through it.

Heart disease (HD) is also referred to as coronary heart disease (CHD) and coronary artery disease (CAD). It develops from a number of causes including *atherosclerosis* or "hardening of the arteries," or when cholesterol and other fats stick to the arterial walls (i.e., the lumen of an arterial wall). Both CHD and CAD reduce the blood flow through the heart vessels, limiting the amount of oxygen reaching the tissue. HD is also a direct consequence of chronic, untreated, or inadequately treated hypertension (Goroll & Mulley, 2014). The extent to which one suffers from HD is significantly affected by a personal history of exposure to smoke and pollutants, control of blood pressure, and the coexistence of diabetes or a family history of diabetes.

Heart disease can result in ischemia, that is, either partial or complete blockage of the delivery of oxygen to the heart muscle. When the blockage is sudden but shortly resolves on its own, it is called angina. A more serious and often permanent blockage is referred to as an acute myocardial infarction or acute MI (AMI). In younger adults, especially men, an AMI is described as gripping chest pain and radiation to the shoulder, left arm, or jaw. In women and in older adults the signs and symptoms are more likely to be mild and may be localized to the back or the abdomen, or manifest as a sensation of nausea or heartburn, but are nonetheless just as serious as "typical" AMI symptoms. These vague symptoms too often are not brought to the attention of a medical provider but may be "mentioned" to the nurse (Box 22.5). In the older adult, especially one who is medically frail, the AMI may be *silent*. There may be no noticeable signs or symptoms at all and the event is only noticed at the time of death or when an electrocardiogram (ECG) is performed for some other purpose, such as during an annual wellness visit.

BOX 22.6 Treatment of Chest Pain Differs by Sex and Ethnicity

The signs of an acute myocardial infarction in women, especially older women, have been found to be noticeably different from those of men. Women are more likely to report shortness of breath, weakness, fatigue, indigestion, and a sense of dread. Risk factors that influence women more than men are major life stressors and events, sense of loss of control, and the illness or death of significant others.

Data from Mehta LS, Becker TM, DeVon HA, et al: Acute myocardial infarction in women: A scientific statement from the American Heart Association, *Circulation,* published 2/25/16 ahead of print. Available at http://circ.ahajournals.org/content/early/2016/01/25/CIR.0000000000000351.

Death from CVD, specifically from an AMI, has been more common in women for many years. However, for the first time in 10 years the survival rate among older women is improving. This is attributed in large part to increased awareness and the use of evidence-based guidelines (Mehta et al., 2016) (Box 22.6).

Atrial Fibrillation

Atrial fibrillation (AF or afib) is a rapid and irregular heartbeat affecting about 30 million Americans (Unger,

2015). It may have some type of pattern or be completely random; it may occur once, intermittently, or persistently. Although it may occur in younger adults, it occurs much more often in (white) older adults and increases with each decade. The average age of onset is 67 for men and 75 for women (Davis, 2013). There are many causes including indications of advanced heart failure, diabetes, alcohol abuse, CHD, hypertension, and thyroid disease (Goroll & Mulley, 2014).

It is associated with a heightened risk for dementia and stroke-related mortality (Davis, 2013). If a younger adult has AF he or she is more likely to have it in the absence of other diseases; in an older adult it is most often a complication of another disease such as CAD. In many cases AF itself is completely asymptomatic and only identified by the nurse or other practitioner as part of a thorough auscultation of the heart. If symptoms occur, they are vague, such as fatigue, and because the person already has other underlying heart disease, this may be difficult to attribute specifically to the AF. The fatigue may be incorrectly attributed to "old age" or the onset of frailty. Occasionally people report the sensation of "palpations," intermittent shortness of breath, or nonspecific chest pain, especially if the fibrillation is intermittent.

Because the pulsations of the heart in AF are irregular, there is always a risk for pooling of blood in the atria when the time between the beats is prolonged. This pooling increases the risk for the development of tiny emboli. If an embolus leaves the heart, the risk for stroke is very high. Anticoagulation therapy remains the gold standard for treatment with a reduction in fibrillation-associated strokes by 50% (Unger, 2015).

Medications range from aspirin and clopidogrel (Plavix) for those at low risk for a stroke, to the long-used warfarin (e.g. Coumadin), to newer medications such as Pradaxa and Eliquis. Warfarin is highly effective but must be monitored closely and regularly to ensure that the level of anticoagulation is within a range that is effective at the same time the risk of bleeding is minimized (see Chapter 9). It interacts with many foods and medications. Vitamin K is the antidote and can quickly inactivate the effects of warfarin. Several of the newer anticoagulants have been found to be slightly more effective than warfarin but at the time of this writing only Pradaxa has an approved antidote (Unger, 2015). A person who is taking one of these anticoagulants should be directed to promptly seek emergency support with any obvious bleeding or the potential of bleeding (e.g., trauma to the head following a fall).

Nurses have important roles in helping patients understand the dangers and benefits of anticoagulation therapy, the impact of medication/food/herb/nutritional supplement interactions (see Chapter 9), and the need for strict adherence to the prescribed dosing regimen and prompt emergency care if even the potential for need is considered.

Heart Failure

Heart failure (HF) is a disease of the heart muscle in which it is damaged and malfunctions, and can no longer pump enough blood to meet the needs of the body. Causes of HF may include long-term hypertension, fever, hypoxia, anemia, metabolic disease, and infection. If the underlying problem (e.g., hypertension) is poorly controlled, further damage leads to increasingly severe HF, known as congestive heart failure (CHF). Lifestyle choices such as an unhealthy diet, smoking, and lack of exercise aggravate the development of heart disease and the extent of damage, especially for those who have a family (genetic) history of heart disease. There is no cure for HF, only the management of symptoms and the attempt to prevent worsening.

Although the signs and symptoms of heart failure are based on which side is damaged (right or left), both sides of the heart are often affected by the time one reaches late life. The gerontological nurse observes for fatigue, shortness of breath (dyspnea) with exertion, the person's inability to lie flat without getting short of breath (orthopnea), waking up at night gasping for air, weight gain, and swelling in the lower extremities. Dyspnea may occur at rest or on exertion (DOE), or it may appear intermittently at night (paroxysmal nocturnal dyspnea). The dyspnea may be relieved by sitting up or sleeping on multiple pillows, or with the head of the bed elevated. If a cough is present, it is worse at night. The New York Heart Association provides a clear way to classify the symptomatic experience of HF, from symptom-free to severely disabled (Box 22.7).

The nurse should be particularly alert for the atypical clinical presentation of exacerbations of HF in the elderly. The person may appear confused, or delirious; begin falling; or complain of insomnia or urinary frequency at night (nocturia). He or she may complain of dizziness or may have syncope (fainting). Or more often, the nurse will notice that the person has the "droops," or malaise and a subtle decline in activity tolerance or functional or cognitive abilities. The need for hospitalization is frequent. While the overall numbers are decreasing, in 2011 heart failure remained the number one cause for hospitalization for persons 85 and older and second for those between 65 and 85 after osteoarthritis (Pfunter et al., 2013). Affecting more than 5 million Americans, approximately 50% die within 5 years of diagnosis (CDC, 2015c) (Box 22.8).

BOX 22.7 Classification of Heart Failure

Class I: Asymptomatic
Cardiac disease without associated limitations of physical activity

Class II: Mild Heart Failure
Slight limitation of physical activity
Comfortable at rest
An increase in activity may cause fatigue, palpitations, dyspnea, or anginal pain

Class III: Moderate Heart Failure
Marked limitation in physical activity
Comfortable at rest
Ordinary walking or climbing of stairs can quickly trigger symptoms of fatigue, palpitations, dyspnea, or anginal pain
Substantial periods of bedrest required

Class IV: Severe Heart Failure
Almost permanently confined to bed
Inability to carry out any physical activity without discomfort or severe symptoms
Some symptoms occur at rest
Chronic shortness of breath is common

Data from the New York Heart Association in 1928. Disseminated broadly. Available at http://www.heart.org/HEARTORG/Conditions/HeartFailure/AboutHeartFailure/Classes-of-Heart-Failure_UCM_306328_Article.jsp#.VtSWUUko5Ms.

BOX 22.8 *Healthy People 2020*

Emerging issues in cardiovascular health include:

- Defining and measuring overall cardiovascular health.
- Assessing and communicating lifetime risk for cardiovascular disease.
- Addressing depression as a risk factor for and associated condition of heart disease and stroke.
- Examining cognitive impairment due to vascular disease.

From U.S. Department of Health and Human Services, Office of Disease Prevention and Health Promotion: *Healthy People 2020. Heart disease and stroke,* 2016. Available at http://www.healthypeople.gov/2020/topics-objectives/topic/heart-disease-and-stroke. Accessed February 2016.

SAFETY ALERT

One of the major ways that cardiac conditions differ from other chronic problems in older adults is that when they become acute, they can do so very rapidly, and often necessitate acute hospitalization and intensive treatment followed by rehabilitation. Many other chronic disorders are managed at home.

❖ IMPLICATIONS FOR GERONTOLOGICAL NURSING AND HEALTHY AGING

◆ Assessment

As with any assessment, obtaining a pertinent history of the events leading up to and including the presentation of cardiovascular problems is essential, whether the history is from the patient or a friend or family member. For the older adult in the acute or long-term care setting, monitoring of vital signs and kidney function has special meaning because of the high potential of long-standing comorbid conditions, especially diabetes. An auscultatory gap, or time when the second heart sound ceases, begins again, and then finally is not heard, is common in the older adult compared to a younger adult and may lead to underestimation of blood pressure (Hall, 2000). For elders with heart disease it is always recommended that they regularly monitor their blood pressure at home (with a reasonable frequency) and these results be reviewed with each office encounter. Instructions for assessment and care of the resident of a long-term care facility with heart disease can be purchased from the University of Iowa College of Nursing Evidence-Based Practice Guidelines (http://www.iowanursingguidelines.com/).

◆ Interventions

For the person with CVD, the goals of therapy are to provide relief of symptoms, improve the quality of life, reduce mortality and morbidity, and slow or stop progressive loss of function to the extent possible. Aggressive pharmacological therapy may be needed to prevent sudden death.

A key intervention to reduce heart attack–related disability and death is to teach all persons the warning signs, the effective and accurate use of automatic defibrillators (AEDs), and the importance of responding quickly in an emergency. When aggressive treatment is no longer effective, a change of focus to palliative care is appropriate and may include a referral to a hospice agency or palliative care service (see Chapter 28).

Nursing interventions assist the person to accomplish his or her goals and have been found to be highly effective (Sisk et al., 2006) (Box 22.9). Education includes information about healthy eating, an exercise plan consistent with one's cardiovascular ability, and other measures as needed such as how to balance rest and activity and the correct and safe use of supplemental oxygen. The specific interventions used depend on the severity of the disease and the desire for either palliative or aggressive care.

Fortunately, the American Heart Association and the American College of Cardiology Foundation provide

BOX 22.9 Skills Required for Promoting Healthy Aging in the Person With Cardiovascular Disease

- Knowing appropriate technique for obtaining a blood pressure measurement
- Monitoring response to prescribed exercise
- Administering medications and evaluating their effects correctly
- Monitoring for signs and symptoms of changes in cardiovascular condition
- Monitoring diet and also fluid intake and output
- Monitoring weight (either daily, biweekly, or weekly)
- Auscultating heart and lung sounds
- Monitoring laboratory values
- Educating patient and caregivers related to all of the above
- Providing palliative care (see Chapter 28)

detailed evidence-based treatment guidelines for older adults (Aronow et al., 2011). Unfortunately, less is known about the appropriate treatment of fragile older adults with CVD who are residing in long-term care facilities. A more careful risk-benefit analysis must be done related to treatment and outcomes in this setting. For someone with a limited life expectancy, the significant side effects of many medications and limited food choices may result in an unnecessary decrease in quality of life.

The potential for disability can progress rapidly after an acute event or episode of illness, especially if the person believes that any exertion overtaxes the heart and will cause acute CHF, another heart attack, or death. To prevent this, cardiac exercise rehabilitation programs are designed to address the physical, mental, and spiritual needs and overall health of the person and his or her family. Typical programs begin with self-management education and light activity progressing to moderate activity under the supervision of a rehabilitation nurse and physical therapist. For those who are more physically compromised, it is necessary to identify energy-conserving measures applicable to their daily tasks with the goal of maximizing independence.

The nurse and the person with CVD must be cautious about exercise. For those who have had an acute myocardial infarction of any kind, exercise-related orthostatic hypotension is more likely to occur as a result of age-related decreases in baroreceptor responsiveness, which controls the body's ability to respond to the need for changes in blood pressure (see Chapter 3). Because thermoregulation is also impaired, exercise intensity must be reduced in hot, humid climates (see Chapter 13). A healthy alternative is to encourage "mall walking" in local covered and climate-controlled shopping centers. In some locations this has become a social event as well as a safe way to exercise.

Risk reduction programs should be instituted with a clear understanding of the difficulties involved in attempts to alter harmful lifestyle practices such as smoking, overeating, habitual anger or irritation, and a sedentary lifestyle. These practices may have existed for a lifetime and are not easily changed by "education." The nurse's role in these instances is to discuss these practices in a nonjudgmental manner, providing acceptance, encouragement, resources, knowledge, and affirmation of both the difficulty of making lifestyle changes and the person's right to choose. The LEARN Model of communication (see Chapter 2) may be particularly useful for persons from any culture or background.

RESPIRATORY DISORDERS

The normal physical changes with aging (see Chapter 3) result in a greater risk for respiratory problems and when they occur, there is a higher risk for death in older persons than in younger persons (see Fig. 3.4). Diseases of the respiratory system are identified as infectious, as acute or chronic, and as involving the upper or lower respiratory tract. They are further defined as either *obstructive*—preventing airflow out as a result of obstruction or narrowing of the respiratory structures; or *restrictive*—causing a decrease in total lung capacity as a result of limited expansion.

Other than asthma, almost all chronic obstructive pulmonary diseases in late life arise from tobacco use or exposure to tobacco and other pollutants earlier in life. Although asthma may be triggered by environmental factors, there are strong genetic and allergic factors that contribute to its occurrence. The nurse's focus is on helping the person maintain function and quality of life, while being vigilant for early signs of infection, which become more and more atypical in later life.

Chronic Obstructive Pulmonary Disease

Chronic obstructive pulmonary disease (COPD) is a catch-all term used to encompass those conditions that affect airflow. It includes asthma, bronchitis, and emphysema, and as a group remains the third leading cause of death for both older men and women (CDC, 2015a).

The signs and symptoms vary with the type of COPD. For example, persons with emphysema have little sputum production and appear pink because they are actually able to get enough oxygen into the lungs. On the other hand, persons with chronic bronchitis have chronic sputum production and frequent cough and are pale and somewhat cyanotic, indicating low oxygen levels associated with difficulty getting oxygen into the lungs. In asthma, constrictions of the bronchial tubes keep air from exiting the lungs. Thorough discussions of these symptoms can be found in medical-surgical nursing and pathophysiology texts. What is crucial to gerontological nursing is the need to watch the person with COPD very closely for signs of worsening infection, of aggravation of any underlying heart disease, or changes in cognition or functional status.

An acute episode of emphysema or bronchitis is characterized by significantly worsened dyspnea and increased volume and change in the color of sputum. An acute episode of asthma is characterized by shortness of breath and wheezing. A number of factors, including viral or bacterial infections, air pollution or other environmental exposures, or changes in the weather, may trigger a change in the person's respiratory health.

Older adults with advanced COPD can expect to have periods of worsening of symptoms and functioning between periods of control. During periods of illness, medication changes are usually needed. Persons who have well-developed skills in self-management often will begin to deal with the changes before consulting a health care provider. Hospitalization is always a possibility with COPD exacerbations, especially when one has or is suspected of having an infection.

Pneumonia

Pneumonia is a bacterial or viral lower respiratory tract infection that causes inflammation of the lung tissue. Pneumonia and influenza are anywhere from the fourth to the seventh leading causes of death for persons older than age 65, depending on race and ethnicity (CDC, 2015a). Factors that increase risk for pneumonia are many including the normal changes of aging (Box 22.10; see Fig. 3.4). Elders with comorbid conditions such as alcoholism, asthma, COPD, or heart disease or those who live in communal settings or are homeless are particularly susceptible. Dental caries and periodontal disease are common in late life and both predispose one to develop pneumonia as a secondary infection. However, many cases of pneumonia can be either prevented or the lethality lessened by receipt of the two pneumonia immunizations available and the annual influenza immunization. Mortality is further reduced by effective, appropriate, and prompt interventions.

Pneumonia is classified either as a *community-acquired disease* (CAD), or as a *hospital-acquired condition* (HAC) (nosocomial), beginning while a patient is in a hospital or other institutional setting such as a nursing home. In the nursing home the most frequent causes of pneumonia are from aspirations of colonized oral secretions or from reflux of stomach contents from a feeding tube or other oral intake.

BOX 22.10 Evidence-Based Practice

Several Factors Increasing the Risk for Pneumonia

Worsening of another health condition at the same time
Respiratory rate >30 breaths/min
Systolic BP <70 mm Hg
Pulse rate >125 beats/min
Temperature <95°F
Current heart disease
Altered mental status
Age >50 years
Male gender
Living in a nursing home

From Patient Outcomes Research Trial; see Kormos WA: Approach to the patient with acute bronchitis or pneumonia in the ambulatory setting. In Goroll AH, Mulley AG, editors: *Primary care medicine: Office evaluation and management of the adult patient,* ed 7, pp 433–444, Philadelphia, 2014, Wolters Kluwer.

The usual signs and symptoms of pneumonia such as cough, fatigue, and dyspnea may easily be initially attributed to something else, such as the underlying COPD or medications. In older adults, the signs may include falling, mental status changes or signs of confusion, general deterioration, weakness, or anorexia and be incorrectly attributed to the appearance of a geriatric syndrome (see Chapter 17). When one appears to have pneumonia, an abnormal chest x-ray, fever, and elevated white blood count would be expected. However, these signs may be delayed in an older adult, and if treatment is not started until they are present, it may be too late and the result may be death attributable to sepsis. For the best possibility of survival of a frail elder with pneumonia, very prompt interventions are necessary as soon as an infection is determined to be a reasonable explanation for a sudden change (Gulick & Jett, 2006; Jett, 2006). Detailed risk algorithms are now available (Kormos, 2014).

❖ IMPLICATIONS FOR GERONTOLOGICAL NURSING AND HEALTHY AGING

◆ Assessment

Nursing assessment of the person with respiratory problems focuses on the objective observations of oxygen saturation, sputum production, and respiratory rate, and the subjective reports of dyspnea or shortness of breath, its effect on functional status, and quality of life. When respirations exceed about 20 per minute, the person with COPD is having a worsening of his or her baseline illness and prompt response by the nurse is necessary. It is not unusual for older adults with a history of COPD to have oxygen saturation rates between 90% and 95%; when it drops below this, there is always cause for concern. Rates below 88% are almost always respiratory emergencies and the person may be advancing to a state of respiratory failure. In an older adult, especially one who is frail or with multiple comorbid conditions, this advance may be quite rapid.

Only persons experiencing a problem can really tell us what it is like for them. Visual analog scales and numeric rating scales, similar to those used to assess pain, may be helpful (see Chapter 18). Persons can be asked how they would rate their breathing, from 1 (no dyspnea) to 10 (the worst dyspnea they can imagine), and so on.

When a bacterial infection is suspected and treatment is desired, it is never appropriate to use a "wait and see" approach; elevations in temperature or in white blood cell count may not occur until the person is septic and chest x-ray exams in debilitated persons are often falsely negative at the beginning of respiratory tract infections or if the person is dehydrated. Patients and their families should be told the seriousness of this or any infection in older adults. More timely diagnosis calls for sensitive clinical assessments by both the nurse and the other health care providers.

Assessment includes detailed information about cough. When did it start? How long are the episodes of coughing? Is there any associated pain? What seems to make it better, and what makes it worse? Is the person using anything to treat the cough? Is the person smoking (and how much) or exposed to smoke or other respiratory irritants? If the cough is productive, what is the color, texture, and odor of the mucus? Does the color change according to the time of the day? Pulmonary function testing is most definitive in terms of lung capacity but not always available and cannot be done in persons with cognitive impairments if the ability to follow instructions is compromised. Box 22.11 presents the key aspects of a respiratory assessment.

One of the most important questions a nurse asks in the assessment is if hospitalization is desired. If so, preparation for what will happen (e.g., possible need for IV therapy and intubation) is helpful. If hospitalization is declined by the patient and/or surrogate, then the consequences of this must also be discussed. The ultimate decision regarding the extent of treatment elected is always an emotionally charged one.

BOX 22.11 Respiratory Assessment

History

Family
Past medical
Symptoms

Physical Assessment Includes

Overall body configuration (e.g., posture, chest symmetry, shape)
Respirations, including ease of ventilation, use of accessory muscles
Detailed description of level of dyspnea per activity
Oxygenation (pulse oximetry, skin color, capillary refill, pallor)
Sputum (color, amount, consistency)
Palpation, percussion, and auscultation
Functional status
Cognitive status
Mood
Discussion of wishes for treatment and advance planning
Presence or absence of a living will and designated health care surrogate

Interventions

As with CVD, many chronic respiratory diseases in late life cannot be cured. Nursing interventions are based on palliative goals, namely, stabilizing the disease, reducing the risk of exacerbations and hospitalizations, promoting maximal functional capacity, and preventing premature disability. Education always includes smoking cessation, secretion clearance techniques, identification and management of exacerbations, breathing retraining, management of depression and anxiety, nutritional support, the proper use and administration of medications, and dealing with supplemental oxygen therapy if and when it is necessary. Except in severe cases, treatment can occur at home with home health or in a skilled nursing facility, as long as oxygen therapy, parenteral fluids, and antibiotics can be administered.

If the elder fails to improve or deteriorates in either setting, then hospitalization is often necessary if curative care is desired. If the person is hospitalized, a prolonged rehabilitation may be necessary, most often in a skilled nursing facility. Pharmacological and mechanical interventions for the treatment of infection are individually tailored based on the health status of the person before the infection, other health problems, expected outcomes of treatment, where treatment will be provided, and the wishes of the patient.

◆ Multidisciplinary Care

A multidisciplinary team of health professionals works collectively to help the older adult achieve the following goals:

- Increase the level of independence.
- Improve function in his or her environment.
- Decrease the number of hospitalizations and need for hospitalization.
- Increase exercise tolerance.
- Increase self-esteem and self-care skills.
- Improve quality of life and comfort.

The number of goals achieved depends on many factors, including extent of illness and coexisting conditions. For those recovering from pneumonia, the rehabilitative period is often prolonged in older adults.

Education is a part of every aspect of pulmonary care (Box 22.12). The person is taught how to recognize the signs and symptoms of a respiratory tract infection; how to maintain adequate nutrition; how to use an inhaler, nebulizer, and a peak flow meter; how to clean their equipment; and the importance of good oral care afterward. Patients and caregivers are taught the safe use of oxygen; the type of exercise that is beneficial; how to pace activities; coping strategies; and about other issues, such as sexual function. Each of these areas calls for sensitive teaching and indicates specific interventions that will help older adults engage in self-care management.

BOX 22.12 Instructions for Persons With Chronic Obstructive Pulmonary Disease

Nutrition

Eat small, frequent meals with high protein and caloric content.*

Select foods that do not require a lot of chewing or cut food in bite-size pieces to conserve energy.

Drink 2 to 3 L of fluid daily.*

Weigh self at least twice each week and report change as directed.

Activity Pacing to Conserve Energy

Plan exertion during the best periods of the day.

Arrange regular rest periods.

Allow plenty of time to complete activities.

Schedule sexual activity around best breathing time of day.

- Use prescribed bronchodilators 20 to 30 minutes before sexual activity.
- Use a sexual position that does not require pressure on the chest or support of the arms.

General Instructions

Participate in regular exercise.*

Select and wear clothing and shoes that are easy to put on and remove.

Avoid indoor and outdoor pollutants.

Avoid exposure to others with illness.

Obtain an annual flu shot if not allergic.

Obtain pneumococcal and streptococcal immunizations as appropriate.

Notify health care provider of changes:

- Temperature elevation
- Sputum color or amount produced
- Increased shortness of breath

*As prescribed.

Dietary education addresses the reason for monitoring weight and the signs of malnutrition. Weight loss can occur rapidly because of the energy expenditure needed to breathe while eating. A sense of being full early in the meal (early satiation) is caused by congestion in the abdomen attributable to a flattened diaphragm. Anorexia occurs as a result of sputum production and gastric irritation from the use of bronchodilators and steroids. Monitoring nutrition and helping the person obtain nutritional consultation is the responsibility of the nurse in all settings. The nurse ensures that the person recovering from pneumonia is adequately nourished and hydrated while monitoring fluid volume. Overload is a risk for persons with coexisting heart disease.

Activity and exercise tolerance are assessed by the occupational and respiratory therapists, and activities are prescribed to increase endurance and improve respiratory status. Exercise may be done with or without oxygen as a supplement to control symptoms so that the older adult can spend enough time in exercise to benefit from it. Mobilizing the older person and referring him or her for physical and occupational therapy to prevent or stop functional decline should occur as soon as the person's condition allows. The person should be informed that sexual activity is still possible, and education and counseling information should be provided, either by the rehabilitation nurse or by a professional medical counselor.

Medications are used to treat infection and control dyspnea, cough, and sputum production. As with any medication teaching, the nurse makes sure that the person knows the purpose and the correct dosage and regimen of any medication he or she is taking, its side effects, and what to do if complications occur (see Chapter 9). Inhalers are difficult for those with limited manual dexterity and/or strength, as with arthritis in the hands. However, special adaptive devices and nebulizers are available.

Economic issues are always a concern for persons with chronic disease (see Chapter 7). A number of medications are used and can be very expensive, especially when needed for an indefinite period of time as they are for COPD. The gerontological nurse should know the options available to the older adult who is no longer driving or on a very limited income.

Medicare coverage for oxygen and equipment such as nebulizers is determined by their oxygen saturation rates (<88%, which improves with oxygen); supplemental oxygen is never covered by insurance for comfort only. The expense of therapy for persons with a limited income or no insurance (see Chapter 7) will interfere with the adequacy of therapy and result in feelings of anxiety and a focus on the lowest level biological needs.

Rehabilitation is an important aspect of maximizing quality of life for the person with respiratory problems, as it is for those with cardiovascular problems. An older adult with COPD would be considered a candidate for pulmonary rehabilitation as long as he or she has pulmonary reserve and stable heart disease. Rehabilitation programs for the older adult with COPD consist of drug therapy, reconditioning exercises, and counseling.

Mouth care is very important, especially for the person receiving supplemental oxygen or inhaled steroids, and for all persons who are medically or physically debilitated. Inadequate mouth care leads to the propagation of bacteria and fungi, which compounds an already serious situation. Inadequate oral care may lead to aspiration pneumonia or an oral thrush infection. Colored sputum is considered potentially infectious and must be handled appropriately.

Prevention is an important aspect of care of the person with respiratory problems, and the nurse also has an important role in the prevention of complications and infections. Adults older than 65 years of age and those with chronic conditions should be encouraged to receive the pneumococcal vaccine (Pneumovax) unless it is contraindicated. While it is most often a one-time dose, their health care providers may recommend a second dose at a later time. A second type of vaccine specific to streptococcal strains of pneumonia (Prevnar) was approved in 2014 for use in persons at least 65 years of age. Streptococcal pneumonia is the most lethal form and is rarely effectively treated in the outpatient setting. At the time of this writing, Prevnar is approved for one-time administration only and can only be given at least 1 year before or after Pneumovax in order for it to be covered by Medicare.

Annual influenza immunizations are especially important for those with COPD. Normally one is received each fall. In years when there is a particularly intense infection outbreak in the fall, an additional immunization may be recommended by public health officials. Finally, the nurse can be aware of the pertinent goals of *Healthy People 2020* and play a part in helping the nation to achieve them (Box 22.13).

 BOX 22.13 ***Healthy People 2020***

Goals for Those With Chronic Obstructive Pulmonary Disease (COPD)

Reduce COPD-related activity limitations in persons ≥45 years of age:
From 23.2% in 2008 to 18.7% in 2020
Reduce the number of COPD-related deaths in persons ≥45 years of age:
From 113.9 per 100,000 in 2007 to 102.6 by 2020
Reduce COPD-related hospitalizations in persons ≥45 years of age:
From 56 per 100,000 in 2007 to 50.1 by 2020

From U.S. Department of Health and Human Services, Office of Disease Prevention and Health Promotion: *Healthy People 2020,* 2016. Available at http://www.healthypeople.gov/2020.

KEY CONCEPTS

- Heart disease is the most common cause of death for most persons in the United States.
- The underlying cause for the majority of cardiovascular and pulmonary disease is smoking.
- Pneumonia and influenza are particularly important health problems for those more than 65 years of age and significantly more so for those who are frail, immunocompromised, have human immunodeficiency virus (HIV), or are otherwise decompensated.
- The mortality associated with pneumonia can be minimized through the use of pneumonia and influenza vaccinations and excellent oral hygiene.
- The goal of therapy for older adults with cardiac and respiratory disorders is not curative. It is to relieve symptoms, improve the quality of life, reduce mortality, stabilize and slow the progression of the disease, reduce the risk of exacerbation, and maximize functional capacity.
- There is a high correlation between heart disease and diabetes.

ACTIVITIES AND DISCUSSION QUESTIONS

1. How are heart failure and congestive heart failure different in older adults compared to younger adults?
2. How is the assessment of elders with cardiovascular and respiratory problems different from that of younger adults?
3. What is the range of complications of pneumonia in older adults and how would you address these with the patient and significant others?
4. What preventive measures can be instituted to prevent or lessen the severity of pneumonia?

REFERENCES

Aronow WS, Fleg JL, Pepine CJ, et al: American College of Cardiology Foundation/American Heart Association (ACCF/AHA): 2011 Expert consensus document on hypertension in the elderly, *J Am Coll Cardiol* 57(20):2037–2114, 2011.

Centers for Disease Control and Prevention (CDC): *Mortality tables*, 2015a. Available at http://www.cdc.gov/nchs/nvss/mortality_tables.htm. Accessed February 2016.

Centers for Disease Control and Prevention (CDC): *Heart disease facts*, 2015b. Available at http://www.cdc.gov/heartdisease/facts.htm. Accessed February 2016.

Centers for Disease Control and Prevention (CDC): *Heart failure fact sheet*, 2015c. Available at http://www.cdc.gov/dhdsp/data_statistics/fact_sheets/fs_heart_failure.htm. Accessed February 2016.

Davis LL: Contemporary management of atrial fibrillation, *J Nurse Pract* 9(110):623–652, 2013.

Goroll AH, Mulley AG: *Primary care medicine*, ed 7, Philadelphia, 2014, Wolters Kluwer, pp 93–95.

Gulick G, Jett KF: Applying evidence-based findings to practice: Caring for older adults in subacute units, *Geriatr Nurs* 27(5):280–283, 2006.

Hall WD: Pitfalls in the diagnosis and management of systolic hypertension, *South Med J* 93(1):1–3, 2000.

James PA, Oparil S, Carter BL, et al: Evidence-based guideline for the management of high blood pressure in adults: Report from the panel members appointed to the eighth Joint National Committee (JNC 8), *JAMA* 311(5):507–522, 2014.

Jett KF: Examining the evidence: Knowing if and when to transfer a resident with pneumonia from the nursing home to the hospital or subacute unit, *Geriatr Nurs* 27(5):280, 2006.

Kormos WA: Approach to the patient with acute bronchitis or pneumonia in the ambulatory setting. In Goroll AH, Mulley AG, editors: *Primary care medicine: Office evaluation and management of the adult patient*, ed 7, Philadelphia, 2014, Wolters Kluwer, pp 433–444.

Law M, Wald N, Morris J: Lowering blood pressure to prevent myocardial infarction and stroke: A new preventive strategy, *Health Technol Assess* 7(31):1–94, 2003.

Mehta LS, Becker TM, DeVon HA, et al: Acute myocardial infarction in women: A scientific statement from the American Heart Association, *Circulation*, published 2/25/16 ahead of print. Available at http://circ.ahajournals.org/content/early/2016/01/25/CIR.0000000000000351. Accessed February 2016.

Pfunter A, Wier LM, Stocks C: *Most frequent conditions in U.S. hospitals, 2011,* AHRQ Statistical Brief *no. 162*, 2013.

Sisk J, Herbert P, Horowitz C, et al: Effects of nurse management on the quality of heart failure care in minority communities: A randomized clinical trial, *Ann Intern Med* 145(4):273–283, 2006.

Unger EF: *Atrial fibrillation, oral anticoagulant drugs, and their reversal agents*, 2015. Available at http://www.fda.gov/drugs/newsevents/ucm467203.htm.

U.S. Preventive Services Task Force [USPSTF]: *Hypertension screening in adults*, 2015. Available at http://www.uspreventiveservicestaskforce.org/Page/Document/UpdateSummaryFinal/high-blood-pressure-in-adults-screening. Accessed February 2016.

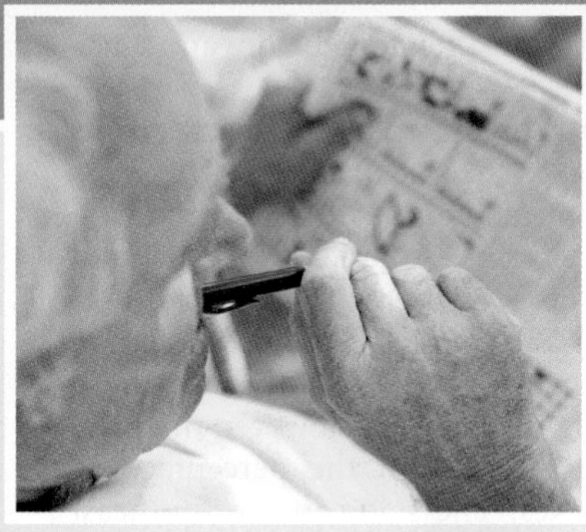

23

Neurological Disorders

Kathleen Jett

evolve.elsevier.com/Touhy/gerontological

LEARNING OBJECTIVES

Upon completion of this chapter, the reader will be able to:

- Differentiate a transient ischemic attack from a stroke.
- Differentiate a hemorrhagic stroke from an embolic stroke and understand the care implications of the differences.
- Identify strategies to decrease the likelihood of a stroke.
- Differentiate the early recognition of the neurodegenerative disorders Parkinson's disease and Alzheimer's disease.
- Develop a strategy to promote safety in persons with neurological disorders.
- Suggest ways to optimize communication with persons with communication difficulties attributable to a neurological impairment.

THE LIVED EXPERIENCE

People come up to me and talk to me like I should know them, and I know I should but it is just getting harder and harder to recognize them.

Henry, age 82

I just don't understand what she is trying to tell me. I know it must be very frustrating for her to feel kind of trapped inside and not being able to speak, but I am frustrated too, not knowing what she needs!

Angela, a new nurse

Neurological disorders are seen in older adults more than any other age group. In this chapter we discuss two of these: Parkinson's and Alzheimer's diseases. We have also chosen to include the cerebrovascular conditions of the transient ischemic attack (TIA) and stroke. Although these are cardiovascular in origin, their effects are universally neurological and the implications for nursing practice for all conditions covered herein are similar. All have the potential to significantly impair a person's function and affect every aspect of life at some point. Parkinson's and Alzheimer's diseases are neurodegenerative in nature in that they are terminal conditions and characterized by a progressive decline in function leading to death.

The nurse plays an active role in helping the patient and significant others navigate the health care system with care focused on rehabilitation whenever possible, and always on comfort. The goal is to minimize the loss of function for as long as possible. Care may occur in the acute care, long-term care, and rehabilitation settings and in the person's home. In the case of cerebrovascular disease, the nurse is active in health promotion and disease prevention by ensuring prompt diagnosis and treatment at the time of the acute event. Finally, the gerontological nurse helps elders and those who love them cope with the changes inherent in these disorders, including grief support (see Chapter 28).

CEREBROVASCULAR DISEASE

Cerebrovascular diseases are interruptions in blood supply to the brain resulting in neurological damage. They are either ischemic or hemorrhagic in nature and manifested as either strokes or TIAs. Because the initial signs and symptoms are similar but the outcomes are different, the rapid identification of the specific diagnosis takes precedence and must be done before any treatment can occur.

More than two-thirds of all strokes occur in persons older than 65 years of age. The rate of strokes is decreasing in all groups, yet they remain the fifth cause of death among Caucasian Americans, American Indians, and Alaskan Natives (Centers for Disease Control and Prevention [CDC], 2015). Each year 800,000 people in the United States have a stroke and 1 person dies from a stroke every 4 minutes (CDC, 2016); however, there are significant regional differences in the percentage of persons who have strokes. The states in the southeast portion of the United States are known as the "stroke belt" (Fig. 23.1).

Ischemic Events

The majority of all cerebrovascular events are ischemic in nature (CDC, 2013). The four main causes are arterial disease, cardioembolism events, hematological disorders, and systemic hypoperfusion. Cardioembolism

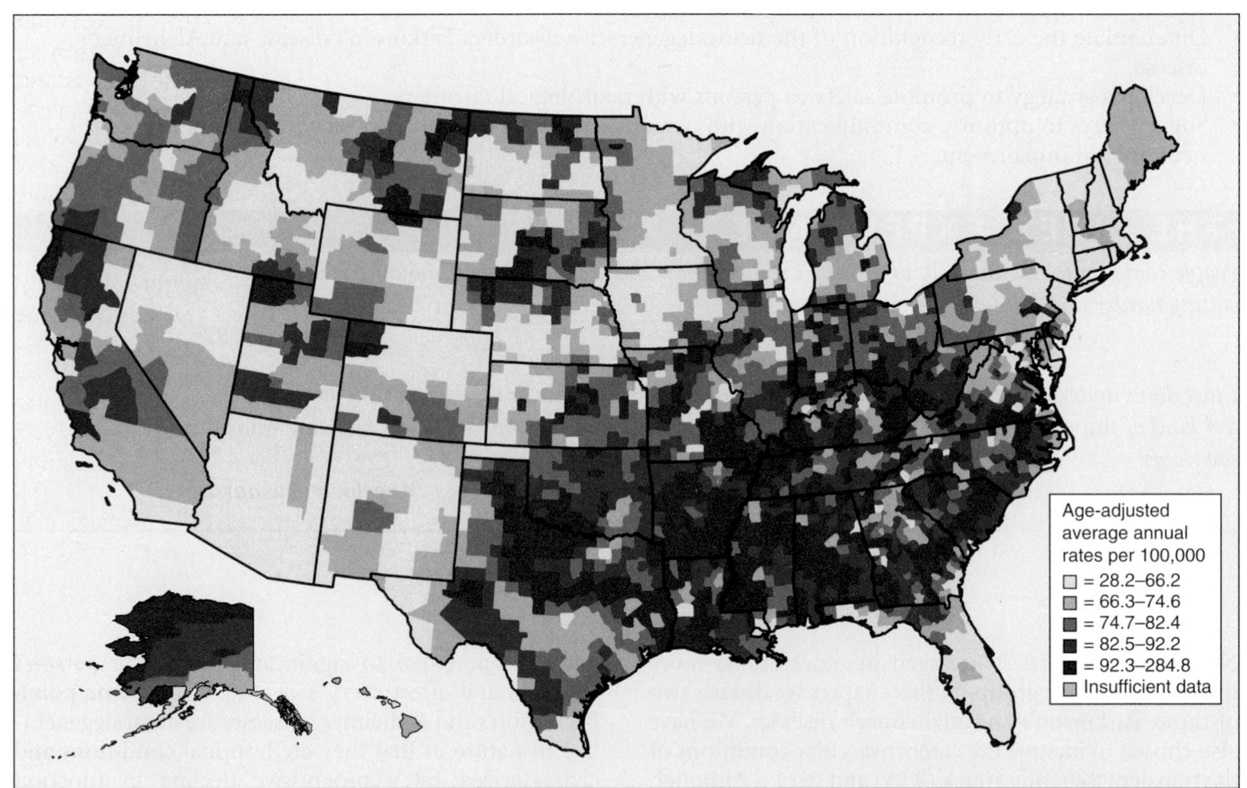

FIGURE 23.1 Stroke death rates of adults, ages 35+, 2011–2013. (Redrawn from Centers for Disease Control and Prevention, Division for Heart Disease and Stroke Prevention: *Stroke fact sheet,* 2016. Available at http://www.cdc.gov/dhdsp/data_statistics/fact_sheets/fs_stroke.htm.)

BOX 23.1 Relative Risk for a Major Stroke After a TIA

Age >60 years = 1 point
BP >140/90 mm Hg = 1 point
Resulting unilateral weakness = 2 points
Speech impairment, no weakness = 1 point
Duration of deficit 10–59 minutes = 1 point
Duration >1 hour = 2 points
Diabetes = 1 point

Risk
Score 6–7: High risk (8.1% chance of a major stroke in 2 days)
Score 4–5: Moderate risk (4.1% chance)
Score 0–3: Low risk (1% chance)

From Llinas R: Stroke. In Durso SC, editor: *Oxford American handbook of geriatric medicine,* New York, 2010, Oxford Press, p168.

events include those caused by a dysrhythmia such as atrial fibrillation (see Chapter 22). Hematological disorders include alterations in normal coagulation hyperviscosity. Hypoperfusion leading to a stroke can occur from dehydration, hypotension (including over-treatment of hypertension), cardiac arrest, or fainting (syncope) (Pruitt, 2014).

A TIA is ischemic but clinically different from a stroke in that all of the neurologically-associated symptoms begin to resolve within minutes. About one-third of persons who have a TIA and do not receive treatment are likely to have a major stroke within 1 year; 10% to 15% of these persons will have a major stroke within 3 months (CDC, 2013) (Box 23.1).

Hemorrhagic Events

Hemorrhagic strokes are less frequent than ischemic strokes but much more life threatening. They are primarily caused by uncontrolled hypertension and less often by malformations of the blood vessels (e.g., aneurysms). Although the exact mechanism is not fully understood, it appears that in some people chronic hypertension causes thickening of the vessel wall, microaneurysms, and necrosis. When enough damage to the vessel accumulates, a spontaneous rupture may occur. The rupture may be large and acute, or may be small with a slow leaking of blood into the adjacent brain tissue. Resolution of the event can occur only with the resorption of excess blood and damaged tissue.

Signs and Symptoms of Cerebrovascular Events

The first signs of both strokes and TIAs are acute neurological deficits consistent with the part of the brain affected and the type of event. Neurological changes may include alterations in motor, sensory, and visual function; coordination; cognition; and language. Persons with hemorrhage have more specific neurological changes, including seizures and more depressed level of consciousness, than those with an ischemic stroke. If a person is deeply unresponsive following a stroke he or she is unlikely to survive (Boss & Huether, 2014). Nausea and vomiting are suggestive of increased cerebral edema in response to an event of any type. Because TIAs are highly transient by nature they often resolve on their own and health care is not sought. Instead, the person reports (often to the nurse), "I think I had a small stroke last week/month, etc." Differentiation of type and damage is done through the use of a computed tomography (CT) scan or magnetic resonance imaging (MRI).

Complications

After a TIA resolves, there should be no residual effect other than an increased chance of recurrence and the increased risk for stroke as noted earlier. Early complications of a simple stroke include extension of the amount of damage and recurrence; brain edema could result in obstructive hydrocephalus (Pruitt, 2014).

The potential long-term effects of a stroke range from neurological changes noticed only by the person to paralysis or hemiparesis limiting or eliminating certain voluntary movements on the side of the body opposite to the brain injury. Speech may be limited by dysarthrias, dysphagias, and aphasias, as discussed later in this chapter. The development of spasticity or unusually tight muscles in the affected limb(s) is a risk if paralysis or hemiparesis occurs. Spasticity can lead to contractures if it is not managed well and even sometimes when it is. Pain in the affected side is not uncommon and may be treated with muscle medications specific for neuropathic pain (see Chapter 18). The medications, added to the potential limitations of the stroke, significantly increase the risk for falls. Other complications include blood clots (deep vein thrombosis [DVT]) in the affected limb, pressure ulcers, aspiration pneumonia (see Chapter 22), and urinary tract infections. Post-stroke depression is common and has been found to negatively affect both rehabilitation and mortality.

Management

All actual or potential cerebrovascular events are considered emergencies and should be treated as such (see Safety Alert). For ischemic strokes caused by an embolism, the compromised circulation to the brain must be restored rapidly. This is done in emergency departments through *reperfusion therapy* using recombinant tissue plasminogen activator (rt-PA) if the facility is equipped to do so.

SAFETY ALERT

Reperfusion therapy (using recombinant tissue plasminogen activator [rt-PA]) can only be used for ischemic occlusive (usually embolic) strokes and only if a CT scan or MRI confirms the absence of hemorrhage and is within 3 hours of the onset of the event (Llinas, 2010).

If the person has had a hemorrhagic stroke and it is misdiagnosed, the bleeding will be rapidly accelerated by the rt-PA, and the person will die. The initial response to the hemorrhagic stroke is to find a means to stop the bleeding if possible and rapidly replace the blood loss.

Rehabilitation following a stroke occurs in rehabilitation hospitals, in long-term care facilities, and at home depending on the location of the neurological damage, the extent of the damage, available support system, and the endurance of the person. Recovery to the extent possible may take as little as a few months or as long as years. The use of antithrombotics/anticoagulants (e.g., aspirin, warfarin) in persons with heart disease is an attempt to reduce the risk for stroke and has proven to prevent recurrent cardioembolic strokes and TIAs (see Chapter 22). Management is preventive and rehabilitative.

IMPLICATIONS FOR GERONTOLOGICAL NURSING AND HEALTHY AGING

The key aspect of the nurse's role related to persons at risk for stroke is to teach others how to minimize the risk for strokes, how to recognize the signs of a stroke, and when to seek immediate emergency care (Box 23.2). Nurses identify high-risk or stroke-prone elders at homes, in the community, or at the health facilities where they work; and nurses work with individuals and groups to reduce their stroke risk (Box 23.3).

Cessation of smoking, strict control of blood pressure and diabetes, and management of obesity are the most important factors that both the person and the nurse can influence to reduce the risk for any one person to suffer from a stroke. An individual's relative risk both before and after the age of 80 can be calculated using the information available through the National Institute for Neurological Diseases and Stroke (NINDS, 2016a).

In the acute period the nurse participates in patient assessment (Box 23.4). The assessment must be repeated routinely to carefully evaluate and document areas of progress, areas of need, and signs of depression, a common sequela.

The nurse works to prevent aspiration and the development of DVTs. Pneumatic stocking devices, compression stockings, and low-molecular-weight heparin may

BOX 23.2 Quick Assessment of the Person Who May Be Having a Stroke

If you think someone may be having a stroke, act F.A.S.T. and do the following simple test:

F—Face: Ask the person to smile. Does one side of the face droop?

A—Arms: Ask the person to raise both arms. Does one arm drift downward?

S—Speech: Ask the person to repeat a simple phrase. Is the person's speech slurred or strange?

T—Time: If you observe any of these signs, call 9-1-1 immediately.

BOX 23.3 *Healthy People 2020*

Goals

HDS-17.1 Increase the proportion of adults who are aware of the early warning symptoms and signs of a stroke and the importance of accessing rapid emergency care by calling 9-1-1 or another emergency number.

HDS-17.2 Increase the proportion of adults aged 20 years and older who are aware of the early warning symptoms and signs of a stroke.

HDS-17.3 Increase the proportion of adults aged 20 years and older who are aware of the importance of accessing rapid emergency care for a stroke by calling 9-1-1 or another emergency number.

From U.S. Department of Health and Human Services, Office of Disease Prevention and Health Promotion: *Healthy People 2020,* 2016. Available at http://www.healthypeople.gov/2020.

BOX 23.4 Assessment of the Person Following a Stroke or TIA

General

Vital signs
Cardiovascular
Respiratory
Abdominal

Neurological

Level of arousal, orientation, attention
Speech (dysarthria, dysphasia)
Cranial nerves
Motor strength
Coordination
Sensation
Gait (if possible)

be used (if ischemic). Early mobilization is also necessary and physical therapists are often involved even before the patient leaves the acute care setting. Eating may be a problem and a nasogastric (NG) tube may be required. If this is anticipated to be a persistent problem, the patient and family may elect to have a semi-permanent percutaneous endoscopic gastrostomy (PEG) tube inserted directly into the stomach, although this significantly increases the risk for aspiration pneumonia.

The nurse has an active role in the prevention and minimization of disability, that is, the promotion of healthy aging in persons with significant functional limitations following a stroke. A period of intense rehabilitation often takes place in a rehabilitation or skilled nursing facility setting and continues long after the person returns home or to an assisted living setting. Care of the person following a stroke is extremely complex; it is often coordinated by a rehabilitation nurse and includes a diverse multidisciplinary team. It may include a spiritual advisor or indigenous healer as the person copes with the associated losses (see Chapter 28). It always includes the person's significant other(s) who may be involved with meeting daily needs. Acute support services are now available in specialized stroke centers. These have been found to improve outcomes in persons with ischemic strokes (Llinas, 2010).

The nurse works to prevent iatrogenic complications such as skin breakdown, falls, and increased confusion or delirium from medications and infections. The nurse monitors the patient for changes in mental status and respiratory functioning and ensures and maximizes the capacity for self-care, especially related to mobility, activity, eating, maintaining adequate fluid intake, and promoting continence. The nurse is alert for problems with sleep, constipation, and depression. The nurse acts as an advocate, providing post-stroke recommendations regarding participation in support groups for both the person and the person's significant others or caregivers. The gerontological nurse is challenged to take an active role in improving the quality of life of elders with cerebrovascular disorders, especially those with functional limitations.

NEURODEGENERATIVE DISORDERS

The neurodegenerative disorders of Parkinson's and Alzheimer's diseases discussed here occur in older adults more than any other age group. Both are terminal conditions and characterized by a progressive decline in function. The declines may be barely noticeable in the beginning, with slight exacerbations and remissions, but the ultimate trajectory is always a downward slope. The impairments ultimately become so severe that the person cannot meet even his or her most basic self-care needs. However, there are interventions available to promote the healthiest aging possible for the elder, for the elder's significant others, and for those who will be providing care.

The evaluation leading to a diagnosis of a presumed neurodegenerative disorder is initiated by the person, significant other, or a health care provider, when changes are noted in comparison to a prior state of cognition, especially memory in the case of Alzheimer's disease and physical stability, such as balance or tremors, in the case of Parkinson's disease. The signs are slow to appear, which delays a diagnosis and therefore treatment.

The diagnostic process begins with the assessment of all potentially reversible causes for the changes such as delirium, infection, vitamin deficiencies, or endocrine disturbances. If a reversible cause is not found, or the signs remain after treatment, a more expanded, comprehensive exam is necessary to make a diagnosis and establish a baseline (see Chapter 8). The evaluation of people with signs or symptoms of any neurodegenerative disorder increases in complexity when the person has other confounding chronic diseases, is very frail, or has sensory limitations.

Parkinson's Disease

Approximately 1 million people have Parkinson's disease (PD) in the United States and 7 to 10 million people worldwide. Ninety-six percent of these persons are diagnosed after the age of 60 and more often in men than in women (Parkinson's Disease Foundation [PDF], 2016). PD is the second most common neurodegenerative disease after Alzheimer's disease. The median time between diagnosis and death is 9 years. In very late stages the person may also develop a form of dementia, especially those who develop the disease after the age of 70 (Boss & Huether, 2014).

PD is typically a slowly progressing movement disorder that is the result of destruction of the cells in the brain that produce the neurotransmitter dopamine. Dopamine plays a major part in controlling movement. By the time the first symptoms are seen, 80% of the specific brain cells have been lost and 70% to 80% of the dopamine needed for the control of involuntary movement and the initiation of voluntary, smooth movement has been lost (Boss & Huether, 2014). The exact cause of PD is unknown. It is thought to be a combination of factors including exposure to viruses and toxins such as pollutants (including smoking) and other external factors such as repeated head trauma (NINDS, 2016b) (Box 23.5). Specific proteins in the cells have been found to be directly linked to hereditary PD

BOX 23.5 An Eye Into the Brain: Genetics and Parkinson's Disease

Although the exact cause is not yet known for the body's destruction of the neurons in the brain that lead to PD, scientists have identified several genes that are linked to PD. One gene *(LRRK2)* is the most common cause of the disease, about 10% inherited and 4% without genetic influence. However, a mutation of this gene *(G2019S)* is thought to cause 30% to 40% of PD cases in persons of North African Arabic descent.

From National Institutes of Health: *Insights into mutations that cause Parkinson's disease,* 2014. Available at http://www.nih.gov/researchmatters/april2014/04282014parkinson.htm. Accessed June 2016.

BOX 23.6 Other Symptoms Experienced by People With Parkinson's Disease

Frequent changes in body temperature
Problems with blood pressure
Dizziness
Fainting
Frequent falls
Sensitivity to heat and cold
Sexual dysfunction
Urinary incontinence
Constipation
Poor sense of smell
Sialorrhea (drooling)

(Lazarou et al., 2015). Older adults are especially prone to the development of PD-like symptoms as a side effect of antipsychotic medications. Any older adult receiving these medications should be routinely screened for extrapyramidal symptoms (EPSs), which look like PD (see Chapter 9).

Signs and Symptoms

The four major signs of PD are *resting tremor, muscular rigidity, bradykinesia,* and *asymmetrical* onset (Stallworth-Kolinas, 2014). Diagnosis is one of exclusion; that is, all possible other potential causes are excluded first. The diagnosis is then tested by a "challenge test" in which a person with symptoms is given a dose of levodopa. If there is a significant and rapid improvement, the diagnosis of PD is thought to be confirmed. Early falls, poor response to levodopa, symmetry of motor symptoms, lack of tremor, and early autonomic dysfunction (e.g., incontinence) suggest other illnesses (Boss & Huether, 2014).

Resting tremor is the first sign in the majority of those with PD. The tremors are asymmetrical and disappear briefly during voluntary movement. The arm and hand are most commonly affected; the leg, foot, and head less often. They are not present during sleep but increase with stress and anxiety.

Muscular movement in an affected limb is "cogwheel." That means that smooth movement alternates with resistance when passive range of motion is performed. Severe muscle cramps may occur in the toes or hands because of the lack of free and regular movement. Bradykinesia, or slowed movement, affects the person's ability to perform fine motor tasks. This early sign may have the most dramatic effect on the person's ability to independently perform day-to-day self-care functions.

Muscles in the extremities, trunk, ocular area, and face may be affected, including the muscles used in chewing, swallowing, and speaking. Handwriting is small (micrographia). As muscular rigidity and bradykinesia worsen, all of the striated muscles will ultimately be affected. The person with PD will sit for long periods or lie motionless with few shifts in position and few changes in facial expression (Boss & Huether, 2014). This lack of movement makes the person at high risk for pressure ulcers.

Motor symptoms of special importance to independent functioning, safety, and the need for assistance with activities of daily living are related to gross movement and positioning. Downward gaze becomes more difficult, and there is an involuntary flexion of the head and neck, a stooped posture, and postural instability. The characteristic gait consists of very short steps and minimal arm movements (festination). Initiating and restarting movement is difficult (freezing) later in the disease, but once it starts the person moves forward with small steps and a forward lean, further increasing the person's risk for falling (see Chapter 15). Turning is difficult and may require many steps. If the person becomes unbalanced, correction is very slow. There are many other symptoms that are of particular importance to persons with PD, all of which decrease their quality of life (Box 23.6).

Symptoms, and the intensity of these, vary from person to person; some become severely disabled early in the disease and others experience only minor motor disturbances until much later. However, the number of symptoms and the degree to which they will affect a person's life and function will always increase over time.

Management

There is no cure for PD, only attempts to minimize the symptoms and the considerable nursing interventions that can promote safety. The most common medication given to treat the rigidity associated with PD is Sinemet, a levodopa-carbidopa combination drug. It is designed to increase the dopamine level in the brain and prevent the speed of its breakdown.

SAFETY ALERT

Levodopa-carbidopa must be taken on an empty stomach (i.e., 30–60 minutes before a meal or 45–60 minutes after a meal) in order for it to be effective. It is given on a set schedule to prevent fluctuations in symptoms.

Persons who are stable on Sinemet are often followed by their primary care providers. However, when it is no longer effective or additional treatment is necessary, they are cared for by neurologists specializing in PD whenever possible. Medication therapy is complicated and must be closely supervised. Hypotension, dyskinesia (involuntary movements), dystonia (lack of control of movement), hallucinations, sleep disorders, and depression are common side effects of both the disease and the medications used to treat it.

Deep brain stimulation (DBS) may be used in patients who have not responded to drug therapy or have intractable motor fluctuations, dyskinesias, or tremor (NINDS, 2015). Exercise therapy and speech therapy for patients with dysarthria should be considered.

Alzheimer's Disease

About 5 million people in the United States have a neurocognitive disorder (dementia), and between 60% and 80% of these have Alzheimer's disease (AD) (NIA, 2015). The incidence of AD increases dramatically with age: from 5% between 65 and 75 years to 50% after the age of 85 years. By 2050 the number of persons with AD is expected to grow to 16 million (NIA, 2016a). Although AD rarely occurs in persons younger than age 60, it is not a normal part of aging and should never be accepted as such. It is expected that the actual number of persons *diagnosed* will grow as they take advantage of the free annual wellness visit now available through the Affordable Care Act, where cognitive screening is part of the overall assessment (see Chapter 8). AD is the sixth leading cause of death overall in the United States; however, it is expected that it will soon be advancing to third place after heart disease and cancer. There are ethnic variations. In some cases the effects of genetics are strong (NIA, 2016b).

Persons with AD have an increased number of beta-amyloid proteins (plaques) outside the neurons and an accumulation of abnormal tau proteins inside the neurons (neurofibrillary tangles) that damage the cortical areas of the brain. As a result, the synapses, which normally connect the neurons, decline; and the neurons are deprived of nutrients, malfunction, and eventually die. As the number of beta-amyloid and tau proteins increases, more and more brain cells die. The initial damage is to the part of the brain where memories are stored; therefore, memory loss is seen in almost all persons with AD, specifically the ability to remember new information. Other signs are impaired thinking, the inability to find words (anomia), and changes in judgment and behavior.

A diagnosis of AD requires that there has been a decline in the person's cognitive functioning from a previous level, that it developed slowly, that the changes are "greater than expected for the person's age and educational background," and that these changes can be documented with standardized neuropsychological testing.

A person with a mild neurocognitive disease attributable to AD (sometimes referred to as mild cognitive impairment [MCI]) has only modest impairment in one or more of the cognitive areas. In amnestic AD the person has isolated memory loss but is at a higher risk to advancing to full AD than those with nonamnestic variation where the impairments are in areas other than memory (Box 23.7) (Stallworth-Kolinas, 2014).

Management

Like Parkinson's disease, Alzheimer's disease is neurodegenerative in nature and a cure is not possible. Pharmacological therapy is limited to two classes of drugs that have the potential to slow cognitive decline in some and therefore help persons continue to function to the best of their ability longer, maximizing their quality of life and that of their loved ones. Cholinesterase inhibitors, such as Aricept, are for those with early or middle AD and *N*-methyl-D-aspartate (NMDA) antagonists such as Namenda are for middle- to late-stage AD. The effectiveness of the medications and the side effects vary from person to person. They have not been found to extend the life of the person with AD.

Depression and other mental health issues are common in persons with AD. They may remain

BOX 23.7 "I Just Can't Seem to Remember ..."

Mr. Phillipe had been coming to see me regularly in the clinic. One day when we had a little extra time he looked at me and said, "You know a lot of people come up and talk to me like I should know them. I am polite and smile but more and more I don't know who they are. Sometimes I think I am losing my mind."

unrecognized and untreated, but the person should be monitored for these and treated appropriately and promptly should they be found (see Chapter 25).

❖ IMPLICATIONS FOR GERONTOLOGICAL NURSING AND HEALTHY AGING

Ongoing nursing care for persons with neurodegenerative disorders such as Alzheimer's and Parkinson's diseases focuses on making sure the person gets good care, preserving self-care abilities, preventing complications and injury, and providing support and guidance in dealing with progressive loss (see Chapter 28). A comprehensive evaluation should be done at least annually (Box 23.8).

Nurses caring for people with neurodegenerative disorders in the acute care setting must be knowledgeable about the person's baseline abilities and design interventions to prevent loss of function to the extent possible during episodes of acute illness. Because of the usually slow progression and disability that accompanies these disorders, individuals experience a change in activities and social participation. Persons with neurodegenerative disorders eventually experience changes in roles and may avoid social situations because of the accompanying signs and symptoms. For example, the tremors that accompany PD may produce embarrassing movements such as spilling food when eating in public. Drooling, a common problem with those with PD, is a socially unacceptable "behavior" in most societies. The expressionless face, slowed movement, and soft, monotone speech or aphasias of either PD or AD may give the impression of apathy, depression, and disinterest and therefore others are discouraged to continue long-time relationships. A sensitive nurse is aware that the visible symptoms produce an undesired façade that may hide an alert and responsive individual who wishes to interact but is trapped in a body or brain that no longer cooperates. It is important to see beyond the disease to the person within and provide nursing interventions that enhance hope and promote the highest quality of life despite disease. Whitney (2004) found that learning what gives persons purpose and meaning in life and helping them understand what is happening to their bodies can assist in coping with their losses.

Everyone, especially those with strong family histories of neurodegenerative disorders, would like to find ways to prevent them. Unfortunately, at this time this is not possible. Most of the potentially preventive strategies and nonpharmacological interventions to promote healthy aging in persons with neurodegenerative disorders involve the nurse working with the individual and those who are either already providing care or will be doing so. Early comprehensive health, fall risk, and gait assessments are important to help the caregivers and nursing staff provide the highest quality and most empowering care possible. The assessment is repeated periodically to monitor changes and make modifications to the plan of care as needed.

In the skilled nursing setting periodic reassessments are done through the RAI process (see Chapter 8); however, it is just as important in the outpatient setting. This information guides the discussions around end-of-life care, including legal preparation when the point of cognitive incapacity is reached (see Chapters 7 and 28).

To prepare those with PD for anticipated changes in muscular flexibility, early training in relaxation such as modified yoga or Zen techniques and exercises may be helpful. Tai chi has been found to increase balance skills (Gao et al., 2014; Li et al., 2014). Exercise, including walking, moving all of the joints, and improving balance, needs to be included early in the course of PD treatment; physical therapy evaluation and treatment are important. Rigidity of facial muscles and bradykinesia as well as advancing cognitive impairments effect eating ability, nutrition, swallowing, and communication. Occupational therapy can assist with adaptive equipment such as weighted utensils, nonslip dinnerware, and other self-care aids. Speech therapy is beneficial for dysarthria, dysphagia, and aphasia (see later in this chapter). Patients can be taught facial exercises and swallowing techniques. Regular pain assessments and appropriate management (see Chapter 18) are essential to address the often unnoticed problem of pain. This may be related to rigidity, contractures, dystonias, and central-pain syndromes in those with PD or pain that

BOX 23.8 Evidence-Based Practice

Components of an Annual Medical Exam for the Person With Parkinson's Disease

- Review of current medications
- Assessment of mental health (evidence of psychosis, depression, anxiety, impulse control disorders)
- Cognitive status
- Evidence of autonomic dysfunction: orthostatic hypotension, constipation, urinary or fecal incontinence or urinary retention, erectile dysfunction
- Sleep quality
- History of falls
- Outcome of rehabilitation if used
- Safety issues relative to the stage of the disease
- Safe use and effectiveness of current medications
- Psychosocial and support needs

the person with AD cannot understand or express but nonetheless experiences as anyone else would under the same circumstances. The nurse is aware of this and uses alternative means to observe for potential pain (see Chapter 18).

Nowhere in the care of elders is a skilled and caring multidisciplinary team more essential than in the care of persons with neurodegenerative disorders. It includes a nurse and neurologist; a physiatrist; speech, occupational, and physical therapists; an ophthalmologist; a rehabilitation specialist; a psychologist; a movement disorders specialist; and the hospice team. Ideally it includes a physician and a nurse practitioner working as a primary care team. It also may include a spiritual advisor or indigenous healer. It always includes the person's significant other(s), who will be involved in day-to-day life at some point in time.

Persons with neurodegenerative disorders watch their own decline over time, challenging self-esteem. The nurse can direct the person and care partners to formal programs in stress management or group support and urge them to attempt to maintain former relationships (see Chapter 26). The key factors in the care of those with neurodegenerative disorders are (1) appropriate use of available nonpharmacological and pharmacological interventions, (2) prompt treatment of all reversible conditions (e.g., infections) at any time, and (3) coordination between all care providers, including family members or partners.

COMMUNICATION AND PERSONS WITH NEUROLOGICAL DISORDERS

Three of the major categories of impaired verbal communication arise from neurological disturbances. These all deal with the person's ability to receive information as in a hearing deficit or altered level of consciousness, understand what is being said, or articulate (that is, speak in a way that is understood by others). Articulation is hampered by mechanical difficulties such as dysarthria, respiratory disease, destruction of the larynx, and strokes. Specific difficulties may include the following:

- *Anomia* is the difficulty to retrieve words. This may be in spontaneous speech, such as a conversation or when asked to name a particular object.
- *Aphasia* affects a person's ability to use and understand spoken or written words and is the results of damage to the side of the brain dominant for language.
- *Verbal apraxia* or *apraxia of speech* is a motor speech disorder that affects the ability to plan and sequence the voluntary muscle movements needed to produce speech. The muscles of speech are not paralyzed; instead there is a disruption in the brain's transmission of signals to the muscles. When thinking about what to say, the person may be unable to speak at all or may struggle to say words. In contrast, the person may be able to say many words or sentences correctly when not thinking about the words. Apraxia frequently occurs with aphasia.

The Aphasias

The most common language disorder associated with neurological impairments is one or more of the aphasias. Aphasia may occur suddenly such as following a stroke or slowly from advancing AD or PD. It may affect a person's ability to speak, to understand speech, and to read, write, or gesture in one or more ways and in varying degrees. Depending on the type and severity of the aphasia, there may be little or no speech, speech that is fragmented or broken, or speech that is fluent but empty in content. When the stroke affects the dominant half of the brain, some disruption will occur in the "word factories," which are specific to the Broca's and Wernicke's areas in the cerebral cortex. The National Aphasia Association categorizes the two major types of aphasia as fluent and nonfluent.

Fluent (Wernicke's) Aphasia

Fluent aphasia is caused by damage to a part of the brain adjacent to the primary auditory cortex (Wernicke's area). In some cases the person may not be able to speak. More often the person speaks easily with many long runs of words, but the content does not make sense. They have problems finding the correct word and often substitute an incorrect word without realizing it. The speech sounds like what is sometimes referred to as "jabberwocky," with unrelated words strung together or syllables repeated. The person may be unaware of his or her speech difficulties and cannot understand why others do not understand.

Nonfluent (Broca's) Aphasia

Nonfluent aphasia typically involves damage to the Broca's area. The person usually understands others but speaks very slowly and uses minimal numbers of words. The person often struggles to articulate a word and seems to have lost the ability to voluntarily control the movements of speech. Difficulties are experienced in communicating both orally and in writing.

Global Aphasia

Global aphasia is the result of large lesions in the left hemisphere of the brain and affects most or all aspects of language. Persons with global aphasia cannot understand words or speak intelligibly. They may use meaningless syllables repetitiously.

Anomic Aphasia

Anomic aphasia is associated with lesions of the dominant temporoparietal regions of the brain, although no single location has been identified. Persons with anomic aphasia understand and speak readily but may have severe word-finding difficulty. They may be unable to remember crucial content words. This is a frequent form of aphasia characterized by the inability to name objects. They struggle to provide the correct noun and often become frustrated at their inability to do so.

Dysarthria

Dysarthria, second in incidence only to aphasia, is most often seen in persons following a stroke or the neurological brain damage associated with another cause such as traumatic injury. It is an impairment in the ability to articulate words as the result of damage to the central or peripheral nervous system that affects the muscle control needed for speech. Muscle weakness or incoordination interferes with the clarity of speech and pronunciation. Speech may be slow, jerky, slurred, quiet, lacking in expression, and difficult to understand. It may involve a weakness in any one or more of the several mechanisms of speech, such as respiration, phonation, resonance, articulation, and prosody (the meter, or rhythm of speech). For example, if the respiratory system is weak, then speech may be too quiet or be produced one word at a time. If the laryngeal system is weak, speech may be breathy, quiet, and slow. If the articulatory system is affected, speech may sound slurred and be slow and labored.

Enhancing Communication

Treatment of communication disorders as a result of a neurological impairment depends on the cause, type, and severity of the symptoms with a goal of maximizing the effectiveness of the ability to express and understand language and meaning. A speech-language pathologist is the expert in this field and provides advice and instructions for the nurses, significant others, and affected persons.

Alternative or augmentative communication devices are frequently used and communication tools exist for every imaginable type of language disability (e.g., an alphabet or picture board that the individual can point to letters to spell out messages or point to pictures of common objects and situations). Speech-therapy software that displays a word or picture, speaks the word (using prerecorded human speech), records the user speaking it, and plays back the user's speech has been found to be especially helpful to those with some types of aphasia and with dysarthria.

For individuals with hemiplegic or paraplegic conditions, electronic devices and computers can be voice-activated or have specially designed switches that can be activated by just one finger or by slight contact with the ear, nose, or chin.

Communication with the older adult experiencing aphasia and dysarthria can be frustrating for affected persons and all others involved in their lives as they struggle to understand each other. It is important to remember that in most cases of aphasia, the person retains normal intellectual ability. Therefore, communication must always occur at an adult level but with special modifications. Sensitivity and patience are essential to promote effective communication (Box 23.9).

The nurse may encounter persons with communication difficulties across the continuum of care and illness but most often when working with persons with neurological disorders. It is most helpful if both formal and informal caregivers remain consistent so that they can come to know and understand the needs of the person and how these needs are communicated. It is exhausting for the person to have to continually try to communicate needs and desires to an array of different people.

In addition to being knowledgeable about appropriate communication techniques it is important for the nurse to be aware of equipment and resources available.

BOX 23.9 Tips for Best Practice

Communicating With Individuals Experiencing Dysarthria

- Pay attention to the speaker; watch the speaker as he or she talks.
- Allow more time for conversation, and conduct conversations in a quiet place.
- Be honest, and let the speaker know when you have difficulty understanding.
- If speech is very difficult to understand, repeat back what the person has said to make sure you understand.
- Repeat the part of the message you did not understand so that the speaker does not have to repeat the entire message.
- Remember that dysarthria does not affect a person's intelligence.
- Check with the person for ways in which you can help, such as guessing or finishing sentences or writing.

Adapted from information about coping with dysarthria from the American Speech-Language-Hearing Association and the Royal College of Speech and Language Therapists. Available at http://www.asha.org and www.rcslt.org.

Re-enforcing or teaching effective communication strategies is an important nursing role. Plans of care should include individualized communication strategies so that caregiving staff, health care providers, families, and significant others know the most effective way to enhance communication with persons with neurological disorders and maximize the quality of life for all persons who have experienced or will experience the consequences of these and other potentially debilitating circumstances.

KEY CONCEPTS

- There are a number of things that an individual can do to reduce his or her risk for cerebrovascular disease.
- Ischemic strokes are the result of temporary loss of oxygen to the brain, resulting in damage to the tissue.
- Hemorrhagic strokes are less common than ischemic strokes but much more deadly and result from a rupture in a blood vessel in the brain.
- For the best possible outcomes, immediate treatment is required for the person with a stroke; persons need to learn the signs and symptoms and how to activate the emergency response system.
- Correct diagnosis of the type of stroke is necessary before treatment can begin.
- Parkinson's disease and Alzheimer's disease are progressive and incurable at this time.
- Parkinson's disease is a disorder that affects voluntary control of movement.
- The signs and symptoms of Parkinson's disease initially may be mistaken for other common disorders seen in older adults.
- The first symptom of Alzheimer's disease is always loss of recent memory.
- Neurological disorders frequently affect one's ability to speak in a way that is understandable to others.
- Working with persons with neurological disorders requires a team approach that includes professionals, the patient, and significant others.

ACTIVITIES AND DISCUSSION QUESTIONS

1. What would you say to a person who tells you, "I thought I had a 'mini-stroke' the other day, but it did not last long and is not a problem today"?
2. You are teaching a class in the community on the signs of a stroke and what to do in response to them. What is the most important message you want to give?
3. Consider the things you can do in your life to reduce your risk for a stroke. Write them on a piece of paper and then share them with a friend or family member. When you do so, discuss which strategies you can commit to doing to reduce your risk (e.g., stop smoking, eat more vegetables, etc.).
4. Suggest strategies to optimize communication with persons who have communication difficulties as a result of a neurological problem.

REFERENCES

Boss B, Huether SE: Disorders of the central and peripheral nervous system and the neuromuscular junction. In McCance SE, Huether SE, editors: *Pathophysiology: The biological basis for disease in adults and children*, ed 7, St Louis, 2014, Elsevier.

Centers for Disease Control and Prevention (CDC): *Types of stroke*, 2013. Available at http://www.cdc.gov/stroke/types_of_stroke.htm.

Centers for Disease Control and Prevention (CDC): *American Indian and Alaska Native heart disease and stroke fact sheet*, 2015. Available at http://www.cdc.gov/dhdsp/data_statistics/fact_sheets/fs_aian.htm.

Centers for Disease Control and Prevention (CDC): *Stroke* 2016. Available at http://www.cdc.gov/Stroke/index.htm.

Gao Q, Leung A, Yanung A, et al: Effects of Tai Chi on balance and fall prevention in Parkinson's disease: A randomized clinical trial, *Clin Rehabil* 11(28):748–753, 2014.

Lazarou M, Sliter DA, Kane LA, et al: The ubiquitin kinase PINK1 recruits autophagy receptors to induce mitophagy, *Nature* 524(7565):309–314, 2015.

Li F, Harmer P, Liu Y, et al: A randomized controlled trial of patient-reported outcomes with tai chi exercise in Parkinson's disease, *Mov Disord* 29(4):539–545, 2014.

Llinas R: Stroke. In Durso SC, editor: *Oxford handbook of geriatric medicine*, New York, 2010, Oxford Press, pp 165–194.

National Institute of Aging (NIA): *2014–2015 Alzheimer's disease progress report: Advancing research toward a cure*, 2015. Available at https://www.nia.nih.gov/alzheimers/publication/2014-2015-alzheimers-disease-progress-report/introduction#dementias.

National Institute of Aging (NIA): *Alzheimer's disease fact sheet*, 2016a. Available at https://www.nia.nih.gov/alzheimers/publication/alzheimers-disease-fact-sheet.

National Institute of Aging (NIA): *Alzheimer's disease genetics fact sheet*, 2016b. Available at https://www.nia.nih.gov/alzheimers/publication/alzheimers-disease-genetics-fact-sheet.

National Institute of Neurological Disorders and Stroke (NINDS): *NINDS deep brain stimulation for Parkinson's disease information page*, 2015. Available at http://www.ninds.nih.gov/disorders/deep_brain_stimulation/deep_brain_stimulation.htm.

National Institute of Neurological Disorders and Stroke (NINDS): *Brain basics: Preventing stroke*, 2016a. Available at http://www.ninds.nih.gov/disorders/stroke/preventing_stroke.htm.

National Institute of Neurological Disorders and Stroke (NINDS): *NINDS Parkinson's disease information page*, 2016b. Available at http://www.ninds.nih.gov/disorders/parkinsons_disease/parkinsons_disease.htm.

Parkinson's Disease Foundation (PDF): *Statistics on Parkinson's*, 2016. Available at http://www.pdf.org/en/parkinson_statistics.

Pruitt AA: Management of transient ischemic attack and asymptomatic carotid bruit. In Goroll AH, Mulley AG, editors: *Primary care medicine: Office evaluation and management of the adult patient*, ed 7, New York, 2014, Walters Kluwer, pp 1233–1240.

Stallworth-Kolinas M: Parkinson's disease. In Ham RJ, Sloane D, Warshaw GA, et al, editors: *Primary care geriatrics: A case-based approach*, ed 6, Philadelphia, 2014, Elsevier, pp 554–562.

U.S. Department of Health and Human Services (USDHHS), Office of Disease Prevention and Health Promotion: *Healthy People 2020*, 2016. Available at http://www.healthypeople.gov/2020.

Whitney CM: Managing the square: How older adults with Parkinson's disease sustain quality in their lives, *J Gerontol Nurs* 30(1):28–35, 2004.

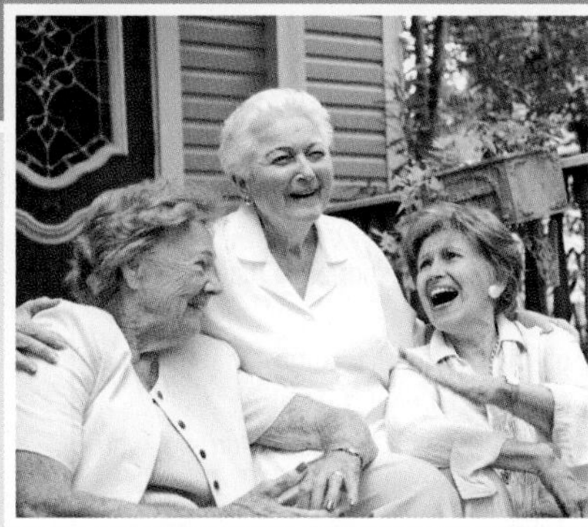

24

Mental Health

Theris A. Touhy

evolve.elsevier.com/Touhy/gerontological

LEARNING OBJECTIVES

Upon completion of this chapter, the reader will be able to:

- Discuss factors contributing to mental health and wellness in late life.
- Discuss the effect of chronic mental health problems on individuals as they age.
- List symptoms of anxiety and depression in older adults, and discuss assessment, treatment, and nursing interventions.
- Recognize elders who are at risk for suicide, and utilize appropriate techniques for suicide assessment and interventions.
- Specify several indications of substance abuse in elders, and discuss appropriate nursing interventions.

THE LIVED EXPERIENCE

I feel the older I get, the more I'm learning to handle life. Being on this quest for a long time, it's all about finding yourself.

Ringo Starr

MENTAL HEALTH

Mental health is not different in later life, but the level of challenge may be greater. Developmental transitions, life events, physical illness, cognitive impairment, and situations calling for psychic energy may interfere with mental health in older adults. These factors, though not unique to older adults, often influence adaptation. However, anyone who has survived 80 or so years has been exposed to many stressors and crises and has developed tremendous resistance. Most older people face life's challenges with equanimity, good humor, and courage. It is our task to discover the strengths and adaptive mechanisms that will assist them to cope with the challenges.

Some factors that influence one's ability to manage stress are presented in Box 24.1. Resilience is a factor that may explain the ability of some individuals to withstand stress. Resilience is defined as "flourishing despite adversity" (Hildon et al., 2009, p. 36). The process of resilience is characterized by successfully adapting to difficult and challenging life experiences, especially those that are highly stressful or traumatic. Resilient people "bend rather than break" during stressful conditions and are able to return to adequate (and sometimes better) functioning after stress ("bouncing back").

Characteristics associated with resilience include positive interpersonal relationships; a willingness to extend oneself to others; optimistic or positive affect; keeping things in perspective; setting goals and taking steps to achieve these goals; high self-esteem and self-efficacy; determination; a sense of purpose in life; creativity; humor; and a sense of curiosity. These are considered personality traits, as well as ways of

BOX 24.1 Factors Influencing Ability to Manage Stress

- Health and fitness
- A sense of control over events
- Awareness of self and others
- Patience and tolerance
- Resilience
- Hardiness
- Resourcefulness
- Social support
- A strong sense of self

BOX 24.2 *Healthy People 2020*

Mental Health and Mental Disorders (Older Adults)

- Reduce the suicide rate.
- Reduce the proportion of persons who experience major depressive episodes.
- Increase the proportion of primary care facilities that provide mental health treatment onsite or by paid referral.
- Increase the proportion of adults with mental disorders who receive treatment.
- Increase the proportion of persons with co-occurring substance abuse and mental disorders who receive treatment for both disorders.
- Increase depression screening by primary care providers.
- Increase the proportion of homeless adults with mental health problems who receive mental health services.

From U.S. Department of Health and Human Services, Office of Disease Prevention and Health Promotion: *Healthy People 2020*, 2012. Available at http://www.healthypeople.gov/2020.

responding to difficult events that have been learned and developed over time (Resnick & Inguito, 2011).

Individuals who have the ability to use personal resources and see the world beyond their own concerns are most likely to be resilient. Older people may demonstrate greater resilience and ability to maintain a positive emotional state under stress than younger individuals (Clapp, 2016). Social support from the community, family, and professionals; access to care; and availability of resources can facilitate resilience (van Kessel, 2012).

In the United States, including older adults with dementia, nearly 20% of people older than age 55 experience mental health disorders that are not part of normal aging (Baxter et al., 2013; World Health Organization, 2014). Many individuals in the baby boomer generation have experienced mental health consequences from military conflict, and the twentieth century drug culture will also add to the burden of psychiatric illnesses in the future. The baby boomer generation is also more aware of mental health concerns and more comfortable seeking treatment, which will add to the challenges facing the mental health care system.

The prevalence of mental health disorders may be even higher than reported statistics because these disorders are not always reported and not well researched, especially among non-white populations. Predictions are that the number of older people with mental illness will soon overwhelm the mental health system.

The most prevalent mental health problems in late life are anxiety, severe cognitive impairment, and mood disorders. Alcohol abuse and dependence are also growing concerns among older adults. Mental health disorders are associated with increased use of health care resources and overall costs of care. *Healthy People 2020* (U.S. Department of Health and Human Services [USDHHS], 2012) includes mental health and mental health disorders as a topic area (Box 24.2).

The focus of this chapter is on the differing presentation of mental health disturbances that may occur in older adults and the nursing interventions important in maintaining the mental health and self-esteem of older adults at the optimum of their capacity. Readers should refer to a comprehensive psychiatric–mental health text for more in-depth discussion of mental health disorders. A discussion of cognitive impairment and the behavioral symptoms that may accompany this disorder is found in Chapter 25.

FACTORS INFLUENCING MENTAL HEALTH CARE

Attitudes and Beliefs

Older individuals with evidence of mental health disorders, regardless of race or ethnicity, are less likely than younger people to receive needed mental health care (Institute of Medicine [IOM], 2012; Jiminez et al., 2012). Nearly half of people older than age 65 with a recognized mental or substance use disorder have unmet needs for services (Mental Health America, 2014a). Some of the reasons for this include reluctance on the part of older people to seek help because of pride of independence, stoic acceptance of difficulty, unawareness of resources, lack of geriatric mental health professionals and services, and lack of adequate insurance coverage for mental health problems. Stigma about having a mental health disorder ("being crazy"), particularly for older people, discourages many from seeking treatment. Ageism also affects identification and treatment of mental health disorders in older people.

Symptoms of mental health problems may be looked at as a normal consequence of aging or blamed on dementia by both older people and health care professionals. In older people, the presence of comorbid medical conditions complicates the recognition and diagnosis of mental health disorders. Also, the myth that older people do not respond well to treatment is still prevalent.

Other factors—including the lack of knowledge on the part of health care professionals about mental health in late life; inadequate numbers of geropsychiatrists, geropsychologists, and geropsychiatric nurses; and limited availability of geropsychiatric services—present barriers to appropriate diagnosis and treatment (IOM, 2012). Increased attention to the preparation of mental health professionals specializing in geriatric care is important to improve mental health care delivery to older adults.

Geropsychiatric nursing is the master's level subspecialty within the adult–psychiatric mental health nursing field. The *Geropsychiatric Nursing Collaborative,* a project of the American Academy of Nursing funded by the John A. Hartford Foundation, has developed geropsychiatric nursing competency enhancements for entry and advanced practice level education and will be developing a range of training materials and learning tools to improve the current knowledge and skills of nurses in mental health care for older adults.

Culture and Mental Health

Mental illness is found in all societies, but the frequencies of different types of mental illness vary as do the social connotations. The standards that define "normal" behavior for any culture are determined by that culture itself. What may be defined as mental illness in one culture may be viewed as normal behavior in another. Different cultures and communities also exhibit and explain symptoms of mental distress in various ways (Box 24.3). Cultural beliefs also influence who makes health care decisions, help-seeking behavior, preferences for type of treatment, and provider characteristics (Jimenez et al., 2012, 2013).

In the United States, disparities in mental health service use by racial and ethnic minority groups are well documented. Regardless of age, African American, Latino, and Asian American individuals have lower mental health treatment initiation, receive a lower quality of care, and experience a greater burden of unmet mental health needs than do non-Latino whites. African Americans and Latinos utilize mental health services at half the rate of non-Latino whites (Kim et al., 2012). These differences persist even when controlling for individual factors (language) and other considerations such as economic deprivation and education. Disparities may result from cultural variation in beliefs about the causes of mental illness and the effects of treatment, past discrimination, and the lack of mental health treatments that are congruent with preferences, values, and beliefs (Jimenez et al., 2012, 2013).

The newest version of the *Diagnostic and Statistical Manual of Mental Disorders (DSM-5)* (American Psychiatric Association, 2013) has an increased emphasis on culture and mental health, including the range of psychopathology across the globe, not just illnesses common in the United States, Western Europe, and Canada. In other words, it is less ethnocentric (Foundation for Psychocultural Research, 2013; Warren, 2013).

BOX 24.3 Cultural Variations in Expressing Mental Distress

- ***Ataque de nervios (attack of nerves):*** A syndrome among individuals of Latin descent, characterized by symptoms of intense emotional upset, including acute anxiety, anger, grief; screaming and shouting uncontrollably; attacks of crying, trembling, heat in the chest rising into the head; verbal and physical aggression. May include seizure-like or fainting episodes, suicidal gestures. Attacks frequently occur as a result of a stressful event relating to the family (such as death of a relative, conflict with spouse/children, witnessing an accident involving a family member). Symptoms are similar to acute anxiety, panic disorder. Related conditions are "blacking out" in southern United States and "falling out" in West Indies.
- ***Susto (fright):*** A cultural expression for distress and misfortune prevalent among some Latinos in the United States and among people in Mexico, Central America, and South America. Illness is attributed to a frightening event that causes the soul to leave the body and results in unhappiness, sickness, and difficulty functioning in social roles. Symptoms include appetite and sleep disturbances, feelings of sadness, low self-worth, lack of motivation. Symptoms are similar to PTSD, depression, and anxiety.
- ***Khyâl cap (wind attacks):*** A syndrome found among Cambodians in the United States and Cambodia. Symptoms include dizziness, palpitations, shortness of breath, and cold extremities. Concern that khyâl (a wind-like substance) may rise in the body, along with blood, and cause serious effects such as entering the lungs to cause shortness of breath/asphyxia or entering the brain to cause dizziness, tinnitus, and a fatal syncope. Attacks frequently brought about by worrisome thoughts. Symptoms include those of panic attacks, generalized anxiety disorder, and PTSD.

Another significant change in the *DSM-5* is the developmental approach and examination of disorders across the life span. This is particularly relevant for older individuals because symptoms of mental distress present differently from the presentation in younger individuals (Katz et al., 2013).

An increased understanding of the importance of cultural perspectives for individuals across the life span will facilitate more accurate assessment of mental health, wellness, and illness and lead to less misdiagnosis. Enhancing the cultural proficiency of health care professionals will assist in structuring more culturally appropriate services, thus improving treatment outcomes and decreasing disparities (Warren, 2013). Research on all aspects of culture and mental health is critical. Chapter 2 discusses culture in more depth.

Availability of Mental Health Care

Dedicated financing for older adult mental health is limited even though about 20% of all Medicare beneficiaries experience some mental disorder each year. Medicare spends five times more on beneficiaries with severe mental illness and substance abuse disorders than on similar beneficiaries without these diagnoses. More than half of dual-eligible persons (those with both Medicare and Medicaid) have mental or cognitive impairments. The 2008 mental health parity legislations ended Medicare's discriminatory practice of imposing a 50% coinsurance requirement for outpatient mental health services. In 2014, coinsurance was reduced to 20%, bringing payments for mental health care in line with those required for all other Medicare Part B services (Center for Medicare Advocacy, 2014).

The Affordable Care Act will improve access to important psychiatric medication by closing the "donut hole" coverage gap in Medicare Part D (in 2020) and will also offer incentives to enhance integration of physical and behavioral health services. Medicare also covers a yearly depression screening at no cost to beneficiaries. Concerns remain about the 190-day lifetime limit for care in inpatient psychiatric facilities and the high out-of-pocket costs of prescription drugs. More comprehensive and integrated mental health care is needed, especially in light of the aging of the "baby boomer" generation (Center for Medicare Advocacy, 2014). Nurses will need to assist older people to access appropriate mental health services and understand reimbursement issues.

Settings of Care

Older people receive psychiatric services across a wide range of settings, including acute and long-term inpatient psychiatric units, primary care, and community and institutional settings. More than 55% of older persons treated for mental health services receive care from primary care providers. Less than 3% receive treatment from mental health professionals. It is critical to integrate mental health and substance abuse with other health services including primary care, specialty care, home health care, and residential-community–based care. Successful models include mental health professionals in primary care offices; care managers; community-based, multidisciplinary geriatric mental health treatment teams; and use of advanced practice nurses (Mental Health America, 2014a; Reuben et al., 2013).

In acute care settings, nurses will encounter older adults with mental health disorders in emergency departments or in general medical-surgical units. Admissions for medical problems are often exacerbated by depression, anxiety, cognitive impairment, substance abuse, or chronic mental illness. Medical patients present with psychiatric disorders in 25% to 33% of cases, although they are often unrecognized by primary care providers. Nurses who can identify mental health problems early and seek consultation and treatment will enhance timely recovery. Advanced practice psychiatric nursing consultation is an important and effective service in acute care settings.

Long-term care facilities, and increasingly residential care/assisted living facilities (RC/ALFs), although not licensed as psychiatric facilities, are providing the majority of care given to older adults with psychiatric conditions. Estimates of the proportion of long-term care facility residents with a significant mental health disorder range from 65% to 91%, and only about 20% receive treatment from a mental health clinician (Grabowski et al., 2010). These facilities are also caring for younger individuals with mental illness, and the number of individuals admitted with mental illness other than dementia has surpassed the dementia admissions (Splete, 2009). It is often difficult to find placement for an older adult with a mental health problem in these types of facilities, and few are structured to provide best practice care to individuals with mental illness.

Along a range of different measures of quality, the treatment of mental illness in long-term care and residential care facilities is substandard (Grabowski et al., 2010). The following are some of the obstacles to mental health care: (1) shortage of trained personnel; (2) limited availability and access for psychiatric services; (3) lack of staff training related to mental health and mental illness; and (4) inadequate Medicaid and Medicare reimbursement for mental health services. Psychiatric services in nursing homes, when they are available, are commonly provided by psychiatric consultants who are not full-time staff members and are inadequate to meet the needs of residents and staff. Training and education of frontline staff in mental health care is essential. New models of mental health care and services are needed to address the growing needs of older adults in these settings.

MENTAL HEALTH DISORDERS

Anxiety Disorders

A general definition of anxiety is unpleasant and unwarranted feelings of apprehension, which may be accompanied by physical symptoms. Anxiety itself is a normal human reaction and part of a fear response; it is rational, within reason. Anxiety becomes problematic when it is prolonged, is exaggerated, and interferes with function.

Prevalence and Characteristics

Approximately 10% of adults aged 65 and older experience a diagnosable anxiety disorder. Epidemiological studies indicate that anxiety disorders are common in older adults; however, anxiety is not well studied in older adults and is often underrecognized and undertreated by health care professionals (Bryant et al., 2013). Anxiety symptoms that may not meet the *DSM-5* (American Psychiatric Association, 2013) criteria for anxiety disorders (subthreshold symptoms) are even more prevalent, with estimated rates from 15% to 20% in community samples, with even higher rates in medically ill populations (Byers et al., 2010; Friedman et al., 2013).

The prevalence of anxiety disorders is higher among individuals with physical illnesses, particularly those in need of home health care or who live in residential settings such as long-term care and assisted living facilities (Friedman et al., 2013). Anxiety symptoms are common in visually impaired older adults; approximately one-third of visually impaired older adults experience mild but clinically significant anxiety or depressive symptoms (van der Aa et al., 2013). Women have higher prevalence rates of symptoms of anxiety and coexisting depression-anxiety than men. Hispanic older adults are slightly more likely to report a lifetime diagnosis of an anxiety disorder compared with white non-Hispanics and African Americans.

Anxiety disorders are not considered part of the normal aging process, but the changes and challenges that older adults often face may contribute to the development of anxiety symptoms and disorders or reactivate prior anxiety disorders. Increasing frailty, medical illness, losses, pain, lack of social support, traumatic events, medications, poor self-rated health, the presence of another psychiatric illness, and an early-onset anxiety disorder are all risk factors for late-life anxiety disorders.

Late-life anxiety is often comorbid with major depressive disorder (MDD), cognitive decline and dementia, and substance abuse (Friedman et al., 2013). Current evidence suggests that anxiety is even more common than depression in community-dwelling older adults and may precede depressive disorders (Bryant et al., 2013). There is some evidence to suggest anxiety may be predictive of cognitive decline, but anxiety also develops in response to cognitive decline, and symptoms of anxiety may occur in 75% of individuals diagnosed with dementia (Clifford et al., 2015).

Geriatric anxiety is associated with more visits to primary care providers and increased average length of visit. Anxiety symptoms and disorders are associated with many negative consequences including increased hospitalizations, decreased physical activity and functional status, increased sleep disturbances, increased health service use, substance abuse, decreased life satisfaction, and increased mortality (Brenes et al., 2014; Bryant et al., 2013).

❖ IMPLICATIONS FOR GERONTOLOGICAL NURSING AND HEALTHY AGING

◆ Assessment

Data suggest that approximately 70% of all primary care visits are driven by psychological factors (e.g., panic, generalized anxiety, stress, somatization) (American Psychological Association, 2014). This means that nurses often encounter anxious older people and can identify anxiety-related symptoms and initiate assessments that will lead to appropriate treatment and management. Assessment of anxiety in older people focuses on physical, social, and environmental factors, as well as past life history, long-standing personality, coping skills, and recent events.

The general and pervasive nature of anxiety may make diagnosis difficult in older adults. In addition, older adults tend to deny the psychological symptoms, attribute anxiety-related symptoms to physical illness, and have coexistent medical conditions that mimic symptoms of anxiety. Because older people are more sensitive to the stigma associated with disclosing psychiatric symptoms, they are less likely than younger adults to report symptoms of anxiety unless prompted to do so by a well-informed clinician (Bryant et al., 2013). Avoiding previously enjoyed activities and increasing social isolation are major signs of both anxiety and depression. Often, health care providers may attribute

BOX 24.4 Medications That May Cause Anxiety Symptoms

- Anticholinergics
- Digitalis
- Theophylline
- Antihypertensives
- Beta-blockers
- Beta-adrenergic stimulators
- Corticosteroids
- Over-the-counter (OTC) medications such as appetite suppressants and cough and cold preparations
- Caffeine
- Nicotine
- Withdrawal from alcohol, sedatives, and hypnotics

these symptoms to "getting older" as a result of age-related stereotypes.

Some of the medical disorders that cause anxiety include cardiac arrhythmias, delirium, dementia, chronic obstructive pulmonary disease (COPD), heart failure, hyperthyroidism, hypoglycemia, postural hypotension, pulmonary edema, and pulmonary embolism. The presence of cognitive impairment also makes diagnosis complicated (Friedman et al., 2013). Anxiety is also a common side effect of many drugs (Box 24.4). A review of medications, including over-the-counter (OTC) and herbal or home remedies, is essential with elimination of those that cause anxiety if possible.

It is important to investigate all possible causes of anxiety, such as medical conditions and depression. Diagnostic and laboratory tests may be ordered as indicated to rule out medical problems. Cognitive assessment, brain imaging, and neuropsychological evaluation are included if cognitive impairment is suspected. When comorbid conditions are present, they must be treated.

Assessment of anxiety in older people focuses on physical, social, and environmental factors, as well as past life history, long-standing personality, coping mechanisms, and recent stress. Older people report more somatic complaints rather than cognitive symptoms such as excessive worrying.

When assessing anxiety reactions in individuals residing in long-term care, look for daily disturbances, such as with staff or caregiver changes, room changes, or events over which the individual feels a lack of control or influence. By themselves, these circumstances seldom provoke an anxiety reaction, but they may be "the straw that breaks the camel's back," particularly in frail elders. Nurses must be alert to the signs of anxiety in frail older people or those with dementia because they may be unable to tell us how they are feeling. Carefully observing behavior and searching for possible reasons for changes in behavior or patterns are important (see Chapter 25).

◆ Interventions

Although further research is needed to provide evidence to guide treatment, existing studies suggest that anxiety disorders in older people can be treated effectively. Treatment choices depend on the symptoms, the specific anxiety diagnosis, comorbid medical conditions, and any current medication regimen. Nonpharmacological interventions are preferred, but treatment may include a combination of psychotherapy, pharmacotherapy, and complementary and alternative therapies (Eells, 2014). If the individual has more than one anxiety disorder or suffers from comorbid depression, substance abuse, or medical problems, treatment may be complicated.

◆ Pharmacological Approaches

Pharmacotherapy is an important treatment option for many patients with anxiety disorders, either in combination with cognitive-behavioral therapy (CBT) or as stand-alone treatment. However, research on the effectiveness of medication in treating anxiety in older people is limited. Age-related changes in pharmacodynamics and issues of polypharmacy make prescribing and monitoring in older people a complex undertaking. Antidepressants in the form of selective serotonin reuptake inhibitors (SSRIs) are usually the first-line treatment. Within this class of drugs, those with sedating rather than stimulating properties are preferred. Careful monitoring of response and side effects is important.

Second-line treatment may include short-acting benzodiazepines (alprazolam, lorazepam, mirtazapine). Treatment with benzodiazepines should be used for short-term therapy only (less than 6 months) and relief of immediate symptoms, but it must be used carefully in older adults. Current guidelines recommend the use of benzodiazepine agents as a bridge to manage anxiety symptoms acutely until the long-term first-line medications (e.g., escitalopram) and treatments (e.g., CBT) reach therapeutic efficacy (Clifford et al., 2015).

Chronic use of benzodiazepines in older individuals can cause cognitive impairment, falls, and other serious side effects. Use of older drugs, such as diazepam or chlordiazepoxide, should be avoided because of their long half-lives and the increased risk of accumulation and toxicity in older people. Non-benzodiazepine anxiolytic agents (buspirone) may also be used. Buspirone has fewer side effects but requires a longer period of administration (up to 4 weeks) for effectiveness (see Chapter 9). Antianxiety medications must be monitored closely, and this class of drugs accounts for a significant portion of emergency department visits among adults that are attributable to adverse drug effects (Hampton et al., 2014).

◆ Nonpharmacological Approaches

Psychotherapeutic approaches include CBT, exposure therapy, mindfulness-based stress reduction (MBSR), and interpersonal therapy. Increasing evidence supports the effectiveness of psychotherapy in treating anxiety in older adults, often in combination with pharmacotherapy. CBT is designed to modify thought patterns, improve skills, and alter the environmental states that contribute to anxiety. CBT may involve relaxation training and cognitive restructuring (replacing anxiety-producing thoughts with more realistic, less catastrophic ones) in addition to education about signs and symptoms of anxiety (Katz et al., 2013).

MBSR is a new technique that introduces the concept of mindfulness through the practice of techniques such as yoga, mindful breathing, and other forms of meditation (Clifford et al., 2015). Exposure therapy, also used in treatment of posttraumatic stress disorder (PTSD) (discussed later in this chapter), involves controlled exposure to events/situations that cause anxiety until anxiety lessens and the body and mind are trained to view the situation with less distress than it is perceived to be.

Complementary and alternative therapies include biofeedback, progressive relaxation, acupuncture, yoga, massage therapy, art therapy, music therapy, dance therapy, meditation, prayer, and spiritual counseling. Music and singing have been found effective in reducing anxiety levels in older adults in a variety of settings and can be a valuable therapeutic nursing intervention (Eells, 2014). The therapeutic relationship between the patient and the health care provider is the foundation for any intervention. Support from family, referral to community resources and support groups, and provision of educational materials are other important interventions. Suggested interventions for anxiety in older adults are presented in Box 24.5.

BOX 24.5 Tips for Best Practice

Interventions for Anxiety in Older Adults

- Establish a therapeutic relationship and come to know the person.
- Listen attentively to what is said and unsaid; pay attention to nonverbal behavior; use a nonjudgmental approach.
- Support the person's strengths and have faith in his/her ability to cope, drawing on past successes.
- Encourage expression of needs, concerns, and questions.
- Screen for depression.
- Evaluate medications for anxiety side effects; adjust as needed.
- Manage physical conditions.
- Accept the person's defenses; do not confront, argue, or debate.
- Help the person identify precipitants of anxiety and their reactions.
- Teach the person about anxiety, symptoms, and their effects on the body.
- If irrational thoughts are present, offer accurate information while encouraging the expression of the meaning of events contributing to anxiety; reassure the person of his or her safety and your presence in supporting the person.
- Intervene when possible to remove the source of anxiety.
- Encourage positive self-talk, such as "I can do this one step at a time" and "Right now I need to breathe deeply."
- Teach distraction or diversion tactics; progressive relaxation exercises; deep breathing.
- Encourage participation in physical activity, adapted to the person's capabilities.
- Encourage the use of community resources such as friends, family, churches, socialization groups, self-help and support groups, and mental health counseling.

From Flood M, Buckwalter K: Recommendations for the mental health care of older adults: Part 1—An overview of depression and anxiety, *J Gerontol Nurs* 35(2):26–34, 2009.

Posttraumatic Stress Disorder

Although originally considered an anxiety disorder, the *DSM-5* removed PTSD from the classification of anxiety disorders and included it in a new chapter, Trauma- and Stressor-Related Disorders. PTSD was once considered a psychological condition of combat veterans who were "shell shocked" by and unable to face their experience on the battlefield. Individuals with PTSD were labeled as weak, faced rejection from their military peers and society in general, and were removed from combat zones or discharged from the military.

Today we know that PTSD is a psychobiological mental disorder associated with changes in brain function and structure and can affect survivors of combat experience but also survivors of terrorist attacks, natural disasters, serious accidents, assault or abuse, and even sudden and major emotional losses (National Institute of Mental Health, 2014a). Scientists are focusing on genes that play a role in creating fear memories as well as studying parts of the brain that deal with fear and stress (Clapp, 2016). The *DSM-5* criterion for PTSD has been expanded to include both direct and indirect exposure to potentially traumatic experiences (Uher et al., 2014).

Prevalence

Most of the research on PTSD has been conducted with male veterans of military combat. In the cohort of Vietnam veterans (now in the "baby boomer" cohort), 3 out of 10 experience PTSD. Among Afghanistan and

Iraq veterans, 11% to 20% experience PTSD (United States Department of Veterans Affairs, 2014). Only recently realized is the fact that many World War II veterans have lived most of their lives under the shadow of PTSD without realization of their disorder. PTSD occurs increasingly in women, although research is scarce. Rape, child abuse, and domestic violence are the most likely traumas that will result in PTSD in women. With more women serving in the military, combat-induced PTSD among women is expected to increase (Kaiser et al., 2014a).

Prevalence rates of PTSD among older adults have not been adequately studied, but estimates are that between 3% and 5% of individuals older than age 60 experience PTSD. Many older individuals may not meet the full criteria for a PTSD diagnosis but may still exhibit symptoms (partial or subsyndromal PTSD) (Chopra et al., 2014). The percentage of older individuals with subclinical levels of PTSD symptoms ranges from 7% to 15% (Kaiser et al., 2014a). Current estimates may underrepresent the prevalence of PTSD in older adults (Clapp, 2016).

In addition to military combat, seniors in our care now have also experienced the Great Depression, the Holocaust, and racism—events that also may precipitate PTSD. Although they may have managed to keep symptoms under control, a person who becomes cognitively impaired may no longer be able to control thoughts, flashbacks, or images. This can be the cause of great distress that may be exhibited by aggressive or hostile behavior. Older individuals who are Holocaust survivors may experience PTSD symptoms when they are placed in group settings in institutions. Bludau (2002) described this as the concept of second institutionalization. Older women with a history of rape or abuse as a child may also experience symptoms of PTSD when institutionalized, particularly during the provision of intimate bodily care activities, such as bathing. Box 24.6 provides some clinical examples of PTSD.

BOX 24.6 Clinical Examples of PTSD

Ernie's Story

Ernie may have had PTSD, although it was only speculative after his suicide. On his 18th birthday, Ernie joined the U.S. Army Air Corps (precedent to our present U.S. Air Force) in 1941. He was quickly trained and sent to Burma, China, and India. During his 3-year stint, Ernie survived two airplane crashes, saw several of his companions mutilated in crashes, watched the torture of captured Japanese soldiers, and witnessed the capture of some of his friends. When Ernie returned to the United States, his hair had turned from deep auburn to pure white. He retired from the service after 20 years but was never really able to work after his retirement.

Ernie's life was filled with episodes of alcoholic binges, outbursts of anger, and episodes of abusing others, all seemingly quite out of his control. One friend remained from his service days and visited him periodically until his death in 1996. Other relationships seemed to have been superficial and to have had little meaning for Ernie. On his 78th birthday, which he spent alone, Ernie shot himself. One must wonder how many of the elderly veterans of World War II (WWII), the most highly suicidal group in the United States, are suffering from PTSD.

Jack's Story

An 80-year-old WWII veteran resident with dementia was admitted to a large Veterans Administration (VA) nursing home. Jack's wife told the staff that he had been a high school principal who was very successful in his position. He had recurring frightening dreams throughout his life related to his war experiences and he would always turn off the radio or TV when there were programs about WWII. Now, because of his dementia, he was unable to control his thoughts and feelings. While in the nursing home, he would became very agitated and attempt to hit other residents around him when placed in the large day room. The staff recognized this as a PTSD reaction from his years as a prisoner of war. They always placed him in a smaller day room near the nursing station away from other residents, where he remained calm and pleasant. The aggression stopped without the need for medication.

PTSD, Posttraumatic stress disorder.

Symptoms

The *DSM-5* includes four major symptom clusters for diagnosis of PTSD: (1) reexperiencing; (2) avoidance; (3) persistent negative alterations in cognition and mood; and (4) alterations in arousal and receptivity (including irritable or aggressive behavior and reckless or self-destructive behavior) (American Psychiatric Association, 2013). Individuals often reexperience and relive the traumatic event in episodes of fear and experience symptoms such as helplessness, flashbacks, intrusive thoughts, dreams, images, avoidance of thoughts or situations that remind them of the traumatic event, poor concentration, irritability, increased startle reactions, and numbing of emotional responsiveness (detachment, flattened, or absent affect) (Clapp & Beck, 2012; Khouzam, 2013).

❖ IMPLICATIONS FOR GERONTOLOGICAL NURSING AND HEALTHY AGING

◆ Assessment

PTSD prevention and treatment are only now getting the research attention that other illnesses have received over the years. The care of the individual with PTSD involves awareness that certain events may trigger inappropriate reactions, and the pattern of these reactions should be identified when possible. Knowing the person's history and life experiences is essential in understanding behavior and implementing appropriate interventions. Research on resiliency may lead to ways to predict who is most likely to develop PTSD following highly stressful events (National Institute of Mental Health, 2014a).

Assessment of trauma and related symptoms should be routine in older patients because they may not report traumatic experiences or may minimize their importance. The Hartford Institute for Geriatric Nursing recommends the Impact of Event Scale–Revised (IES-R) (Christianson & Marren, 2013) (Box 24.7). Similar to other mental health concerns, elders may be more likely to report physical concerns, pain, sleep difficulties, or cognitive problems rather than emotional problems. Asking about issues or concerns may prompt a description of emotional reactions. Reports of physical issues should be followed with questions about changes in mood and activities. Cognitive screening for delirium/dementia is important, as well as assessment for depression and suicide (Kaiser et al., 2014b).

BOX 24.7 Resources for Best Practice

American Academy of Nursing: Geropsychiatric Nursing Collaborative

American Geriatrics Society: Geriatrics evaluation and management tools: Depression (GeriatricsCareOnline.org)

Hartford Institute for Geriatric Nursing: Geriatric nursing protocol: Depression in Older Adults; Impact of Event Scale-Revised (IES-R); Nursing standard of practice protocol: Substance misuse and alcohol use disorders

National Alliance on Mental Illness

National Center for PTSD

National Institute of Mental Health (NIMH): Older Adults and Mental Health

NIH Senior Health: Anxiety, Depression, PTSD, Alcohol Abuse (including educational videos for older adults: Problem drinking in older adults; Getting help for alcohol addiction; How can I cut back my drinking?)

Substance Abuse and Mental Health Services Administration: Promoting Mental Health and Preventing Suicide: A Toolkit for Senior Living Communities (SPARK Kit)

University of Iowa Hartford Center for Geriatric Nursing Excellence: Detection of depression in cognitively intact older adults

◆ Interventions

The understanding of how to treat PTSD among older adults is still developing (Clapp & Beck, 2012) but recommendations are that older patients can benefit from CBT and prolonged exposure (PE) therapy (Kaiser et al., 2014b). Other therapies shown to improve PTSD symptoms include cognitive processing therapy, eye movement desensitization and reprocessing, and narrative exposure therapy (Agency for Healthcare Research and Quality [AHRQ], 2013). Pharmacological therapy is also used, and sertraline and paroxetine have received approval by the U.S. Food and Drug Administration (FDA) to treat PTSD. Careful monitoring of these medications is necessary in older patients (see Chapter 9).

Cognitive therapy aims to isolate dysfunctional thoughts and assumptions about the trauma that seem to cause distress. Individuals are encouraged to challenge the truth of the beliefs and to substitute them with more balanced thoughts. Exposure therapy involves recalling distressing memories of the trauma/event via controlled exposure to reminders of the event. Exposure can be done by imagining the trauma, reading descriptions of the event, or visiting the site of the trauma until distress associated with the memory lessens and your body and mind are retrained to view the situation less dangerous than it was perceived to be. Therapies should be individualized to meet the specific concerns and needs of each unique patient and may include individual, group, and family therapy (Khouzam, 2013). Further research is necessary to understand the various presentations of PTSD in late life and validate and improve the effectiveness of available treatment approaches (Bottche et al., 2012; Thorp et al., 2009).

SCHIZOPHRENIA

Prevalence

Older adults are the fastest growing segment of the total schizophrenia population, and the numbers are expected to grow in the coming decades with the increased longevity of the population (Meesters, 2014). Although the onset of schizophrenia usually occurs between adolescence and the mid-30s, it can extend into and first appear in late life. The prevalence of schizophrenia in older people is estimated to be approximately 0.6%—about half of the prevalence in younger adults. There is limited research on schizophrenia in older adults, and until the middle of the twentieth century it was assumed that mental illness was a part of the aging process. In fact, schizophrenia was originally conceptualized as a dementing illness in younger people and labeled dementia praecox (Collier & Sorrell, 2011).

Types

Distinction is made between early-onset schizophrenia (EOS), occurring before age 40; midlife-onset schizophrenia (MOS), between ages 40 and 60; and late-onset schizophrenia (LOS), after age 60. There is some suggestion that there may be neurobiological differences between LOS and EOS and that LOS may be a subtype of schizophrenia (Wetherell & Jeste, 2011). LOS appears to have a better prognosis and requires lower daily doses of antipsychotics than EOS (Jeste & Maglione, 2013).

Patients with LOS are more likely to be women, and paranoia is the dominant feature of the illness. They tend to have a greater prevalence of visual hallucinations, less prevalence of a formal thought disorder, fewer negative symptoms, less cognitive impairment, and less family history of schizophrenia (Wetherell & Jeste, 2011). Individuals with EOS who have grown older may experience fewer hallucinations, delusions, and bizarre behavior, as well as inappropriate affect. Positive symptoms may wane, substance abuse becomes less common, and mental health functioning often improves (Osterweil, 2012).

Consequences

Individuals with severe persistent mental illnesses such as schizophrenia form a disenfranchised group whose access to medical care has been limited, leading to greater functional declines, morbidity, and mortality, as demonstrated by statistics that individuals with schizophrenia have a life expectancy 20 to 23 years shorter than that of an unaffected person. A concerning finding is that the incidence of dementia is twice as high in individuals with schizophrenia (Meesters, 2014). There have been few studies of the health status of older adults with schizophrenia and the effect of aging-related illnesses on their mental health–related disabilities (Hendrie et al., 2014).

Schizophrenia is a costly disease both in terms of personal suffering and with regard to medical care costs. An estimated 41% of older people with schizophrenia now reside in long-term care facilities (Leutwyler & Wallhagen, 2010). Interventions to improve independent functioning, irrespective of age, and implementation of community services to help individuals manage schizophrenia would decrease the expenses associated with institutionalization. The management of older adult patients with schizophrenia is expected to become a serious burden for our health care system, requiring the development of integrated models of care across the continuum.

❖ IMPLICATIONS FOR GERONTOLOGICAL NURSING AND HEALTHY AGING

◆ Interventions

Treatment for schizophrenia includes both medications and environmental interventions. Conventional neuroleptic medications (e.g., haloperidol) have been effective in managing the positive symptoms but are problematic in older people and carry a high risk of disabling and persistent extrapyramidal side effects. Extrapyramidal symptoms, also known as extrapyramidal side effects (EPSEs), are drug-induced movement disorders that include acute and tardive symptoms. These symptoms include dystonia (continuous spasms and muscle contractions), akathisia (motor restlessness), parkinsonism (characteristic symptoms such as rigidity, bradykinesia, tremor), and tardive dyskinesia (irregular, jerky movements).

The newer atypical antipsychotic medications (e.g., risperidone, olanzapine, quetiapine), given in low doses, are associated with a lower risk of EPSEs. As a result of the tendency for improvement in schizophrenia symptoms with age, reductions in dose or gradual tapering or discontinuation of antipsychotics may be possible in older patients (Jeste & Maglione, 2013).

Other important interventions include a combination of support, education, physical activity, and CBT. A positive approach on the part of health care professionals, patients, and their families—combined with interventions to enhance positive psychological traits such as resilience, optimism, social engagement, and wisdom—is important (Meesters, 2014; Osterweil, 2012). Families of older people with schizophrenia experience the burden of caring for a family member with a chronic disability, as well as dealing with their own personal aging. Community-based support services that include assistance with housing, medical care, recreation services, and services that help the family plan for the future of their relative are necessary. There are relatively few services in the community for older persons with schizophrenia. The National Alliance on Mental Illness (NAMI) (Box 24.7) is an important resource for clients and their families.

PSYCHOTIC SYMPTOMS IN OLDER ADULTS

The onset of true psychiatric disorders is low among older adults, but psychotic manifestations may occur as a secondary syndrome in a variety of disorders, the most common being Alzheimer's disease and other dementias, as well as Parkinson's disease (Catic, 2015). Psychotic symptoms (delusions, hallucinations) are seen in about 20% of individuals with Alzheimer's disease (Catic,

BOX 24.8 Clinical Examples of Delusions

Maggie's Story

Maggie persistently held onto the delusion that her son was a very important attorney and was coming to force the administration to discharge her from the nursing home. Her son, a factory worker, had been dead for 10 years. The events of her day, her hopes, and her status were all organized around this belief. It is clear that without her delusion she would have felt forlorn, lost, and abandoned.

Herman's Story

Herman was an 88-year-old man in a nursing home who insisted that he must go and visit his mother. His thoughts seemed clear in other respects (often the case with people who are delusional), and one of the authors (P. Ebersole) suspected that he had some unresolved conflicts about his dead mother or felt the need for comforting and caring. P.E. did not argue with Herman about his dead mother because arguing is never a useful approach to persons with delusions. Rather, she used the best techniques she could think of to assure Herman that she was interested in him as a person and recognized that he must feel very lonely sometimes. Herman continued to say that he must go and visit his mother. When P.E. could delay his leaving no longer, she walked with him to the nurses' station and found that his 104-year-old mother did indeed live in another wing of the institution and that he visited her every day.

2015) (see Chapter 25). Acute illness, delirium, medications, vision and hearing loss, social isolation, alcoholism, depression, the presence of negative life events, financial strain, and PTSD can also be precipitating factors of psychotic symptoms in older adults.

Delusions

Delusions are defined as a false perception or belief with little basis in reality. Delusions of older adults are often paranoid or persecutory. Common delusions of older adults are of being poisoned, of children taking their assets, of being held prisoner, or of being deceived by a spouse, partner, or lover. In older adults, delusions often incorporate significant persons rather than the global grandiose or persecutory delusions of younger persons. It is always important to determine if what "appears" to be delusional ideation is, in fact, based in reality. Box 24.8 presents some clinical examples.

Hallucinations

Hallucinations are best described as sensory perceptions of a nonexistent object and may be spurred by the internal stimulation of any of the five senses. When individuals have a hallucination, they see, hear, smell, taste, or even feel something that is not really there. The character and stages of hallucinatory experiences in late life have not been adequately defined. Many hallucinations are in response to physical disorders, such as dementia, Parkinson's disease, sensory disorders, and medications. Older people with hearing and vision deficits may also hear voices or see people and objects that are not actually present (illusions). Some have explained this as the brain's attempt to create stimulation in the absence of adequate sensory input. If illusions or hallucinations are not disturbing to the person, they do not necessitate treatment (Box 24.9).

BOX 24.9 Clinical Example: Is It Hallucinations?

One older woman in a nursing home who had Alzheimer's disease and was experiencing agnosia would look in the mirror and talk to "the nice lady I see in there." "Do you want to eat or go out for a walk with me?" she would ask. It was comforting to her, and therefore she did not need medication for her "hallucination," as some would have labeled her behavior. As is the case with many disease symptoms, frail elders do not typically manifest the cardinal signs we have been taught to associate with certain physical and mental disorders. Diagnostic criteria, and often evidence-based practice guidelines, have been developed as a result of observation and research with younger people and may not always fit the older person. Until knowledge and research on the unique aspects of aging increase, nurses and other health care professionals are urged to individualize their assessment and treatment of older people using available guidelines specific to older people.

IMPLICATIONS FOR GERONTOLOGICAL NURSING AND HEALTHY AGING

Assessment

The assessment dilemma is often one of determining if psychotic symptoms are the result of medical illnesses, medications, dementia, psychoses, or sensory deprivation or overload, because the treatment will vary accordingly. Treating the underlying cause of a secondary psychosis caused by medical illnesses, dementia, substance abuse, or delirium is a priority. Assessment of vision and hearing is also important because these impairments may predispose the older person to paranoia or suspiciousness.

Psychotic symptoms and/or paranoid ideation also present with depression, so depression screening should also be conducted. Assessment of suicide potential is also indicated because individuals experiencing paranoid symptoms are at significant risk for harm to self. It is never safe to conclude that someone is delusional or paranoid or experiencing hallucinations without thoroughly investigated his or her claims, evaluating physical and cognitive status, and assessing the environment for contributing factors to the behaviors.

◆ Interventions

Frightening hallucinations or delusions, such as feeling that one is being poisoned, usually arise in response to anxiety-provoking situations and are best managed by reducing situational stress; being available to the person; providing a safe, nonjudgmental environment; and attending to the fears more than the content of the delusion or hallucination. Direct confrontation is likely to increase anxiety and agitation and the sense of vulnerability; it also may disrupt the relationship. A more useful approach is to establish a trusting relationship that is nondemanding and not too intense.

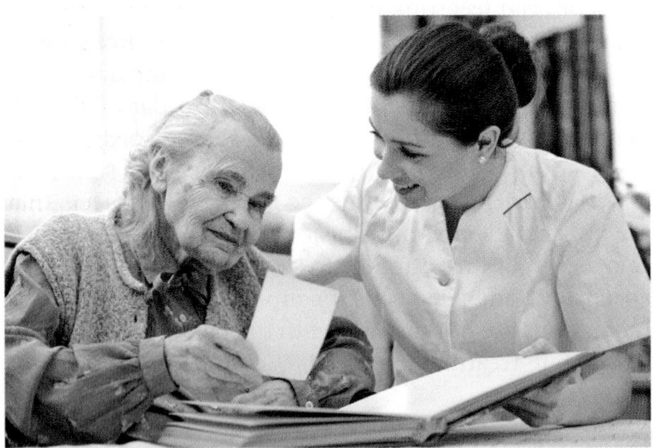

Demonstrating respect and a willingness to listen is the foundation for a caring nurse-patient relationship. (© iStock.com/AlexRaths.)

It is important to identify the client's strengths and build on them. Demonstrating respect and a willingness to listen to complaints and fears is important. It is important that the nurse be trustworthy, give clear information, and present clear choices. Do not pretend to agree with paranoid beliefs or delusions, but rather ask what is troubling to the person and provide reassurance of safety. It is important to try to understand the person's level of distress, as well as how he or she is experiencing what is troubling. Other suggestions are to avoid television, which can be confusing, especially if the person awakens and finds it on or has a hearing or vision impairment. In addition, reduce clutter in the person's room and eliminate shadows that can appear threatening. Provide glasses and hearing aids to maximize sensory input and decrease misinterpretations.

Nonpharmacological therapies are the preferred choice of treatment. In certain situations, medications may be considered in addition to nonpharmacological therapies. The newer atypical antipsychotics (risperidone, olanzapine) are preferred but must be used judiciously, with careful attention to side effects and monitoring of response. However, none of the antipsychotic medications are approved for use in treatment of behavioral responses in dementia. The benefits are uncertain, and adverse effects offset any advantages (Catic, 2015). In cognitively impaired individuals with paranoid ideation, there is some evidence suggesting that treatment with cognitive enhancer medications (cholinesterase inhibitors) may be of benefit. See Chapter 25 for further discussion of behavior and psychological symptoms in dementia and nonpharmacological interventions.

BIPOLAR DISORDER

The *DSM-5* defines bipolar disorder (BD) as a recurrent mood disorder that includes periods of mania or mixed episodes of mania and depression. The length of the phases of depression and mania varies, lasting from days to weeks (Dols et al., 2014; Murphy, 2013). BD is a lifelong disease that usually begins in adolescence, but 20% of older patients with BD experience their first episode after 50 years of age. With the aging of the population, predictions are that there will be a drastic increase of older individuals with BD in the coming decades. Bipolar disorders often stabilize in late life, and individuals tend to have longer periods of depression. Mania is a more frequent cause of hospitalization than depression, but depression may account for more disability. Similar to other psychiatric disorders in older adults, comorbidities often mask the presence of the disorder and it is frequently misdiagnosed, underdiagnosed, and undertreated.

❖ IMPLICATIONS FOR GERONTOLOGICAL NURSING AND HEALTHY AGING

◆ Assessment

Assessment includes a thorough physical examination and laboratory and radiological testing to exclude physical causes of the symptoms and identify comorbidities. A medication review should be conducted because symptoms can be a side effect of medications. Obtaining an accurate history from the individual, as well as the family, is important and should include

BOX 24.10 Focus on Genetics

Research on the genetic basis for mental health disorders such as depression, schizophrenia, and bipolar disorder is being conducted by the National Institute of Mental Health Center for Collaborative Genetic Studies on Mental Disorders (https://www.nimhgenetics.org/). The latest genome-wide study identified shared genetic risk factors between schizophrenia and bipolar disorder, bipolar disorder and depression, and schizophrenia and depression, the first evidence of overlap between these disorders. Continuous research on gene discovery for mental health disorders is ongoing.

assessment of symptoms associated with depression, mania, and hypomania and also a family history of bipolar disorder. Episodes of mania combined with depressed features and a family history of bipolar disorder are highly indicative of the diagnosis. There is a strong hereditary component to BD, and a person with a parent or sibling with BD is four to six times more likely to develop the illness (Murphy, 2013) (Box 24.10).

◆ Interventions

◆ Pharmacotherapy

Lithium, the most commonly used substance for individuals with bipolar disorders, has neurological effects that make it difficult for older people to tolerate. Lithium also has a long half-life (more than 36 hours), and dosing needs to be adjusted based on renal function. Medications that can affect urine production (diuretics) can alter lithium levels. Lithium levels, blood urea nitrogen (BUN) levels, and creatinine plasma levels need to be monitored closely (Murphy, 2013).

Anticonvulsant medications such as valproic acid, divalproex sodium, and lamotrigine are more commonly used in BD treatment. Medication levels must be monitored, as well as liver function. Many of the anticonvulsant medications have an FDA warning that their use may increase suicide risk, so careful monitoring for changes in mood and behavior and signs of suicidal ideation is important.

Antidepressants such as fluoxetine, paroxetine, and venlafaxine can be used to treat depression in BD disorder in combination with other medications. Because these medications can trigger mania, careful assessment is important. Atypical antipsychotic drugs are also sometimes used, but with the same safety warnings discussed earlier, and are not to be used if dementia is suspected. Olanzapine, aripiprazole, and quetiapine are all approved for the treatment of bipolar disorder and may relieve symptoms of severe mania and psychosis. Electroconvulsive therapy (ECT) may also be used when medication and/or psychotherapy is not effective (Murphy, 2013).

◆ Psychosocial Approaches

Patient and family education and support are essential, and the family must understand that the individual is not able to control mania and irritating behaviors because of a chemical imbalance in the brain. Treatment with medication and intensive psychotherapy; CBT; interpersonal and rhythm therapy (improving relationships with others and managing regular daily routines); and family-focused therapy have been reported to be effective in improving recovery rates (Crowe et al., 2010; Dols et al., 2014).

Psychoeducation is an important component of all psychosocial interventions, and nurses can assist patients in learning about BD and its treatment. Psychoeducation should include developing an acceptance of the disorder, becoming aware of factors influencing symptoms and signs of relapse, learning how to communicate with others, and establishing regular sleep and activity habits. Teaching patients to keep a log to monitor mood changes, activity levels, stressors, and amount of sleep is important. Medication regimens can be complicated, and many individuals struggle to remain adherent. An important nursing intervention is educating patients and families about the benefits and risks of prescribed medications, the importance of monitoring therapeutic effects and side effects, and the value of medication management systems (Carson & Yambor, 2012).

DEPRESSION

Depression is not a normal part of aging, and studies show that most older people are satisfied with their lives, despite physical problems (National Institute of Mental Health [NIMH], 2014b). To understand depression, the nurse must understand the influence of late-life stressors and changes and the beliefs older people, society, and health professionals may have about depression and its treatment.

Prevalence

Depression remains underdiagnosed and undertreated in the older population and is considered a significant public health issue (Abbasi & Burke, 2014). Depression is the fourth leading cause of disease burden globally and is projected to increase to the second leading cause by 2030 (World Health Organization, 2014). Approximately 1% to 2% of adults 65 years and older are diagnosed with major depressive disorder. An additional 25% have significant depressive symptoms that do not meet the criteria for major depressive disorder (Avari et al., 2014).

Symptoms that do not meet the criteria for major depressive disorder have been referred to as minor depression, subsyndromal depression, dysthymic depression, and mild depression. The *DSM-5* replaced the term *dysthymia* with the term *persistent* depressive disorder to describe symptoms that are long standing (lasting 2 years or longer) but do not meet the criteria for major depressive disorder. Recognition and treatment are important because persistent depressive disorder has a negative impact on physical and social functioning and quality of life for many older people and is associated with an increased risk of a subsequent major depression (Harvath & McKenzie, 2012; Uher et al., 2014).

Rates of depression are higher in older adults who experience physical illness, who have cognitive impairment, or who reside in institutional settings. Fourteen percent of patients receiving home care meet the criteria for depression, and nearly half of all nursing home residents receive antidepressants for depression (Abbasi & Burke, 2014; Smith et al., 2015). Depression is a major reason why older people are admitted to nursing homes.

Prevalence rates of depression in older adults likely underestimate the extent of the problem. The stigma associated with depression may be more prevalent in older people, and they may not acknowledge depressive symptoms or seek treatment. Many elders, particularly those who have survived the Great Depression, both world wars, the Holocaust, and other tragedies, may see depression as shameful, evidence of flawed character, self-centered, a spiritual weakness, and sin or retribution. Perceived stigma may be less of a concern for the future older population who are more aware of mental health concerns and more likely to seek treatment.

Health professionals often expect older people to be depressed and may not take appropriate action to assess for and treat depression. The differing presentation of depression in older people, as well as the increased prevalence of medical problems that may cause depressive symptoms, also contributes to inadequate recognition and treatment. Primary care providers accurately recognize depression in less than half of individuals with depression (Mental Health America, 2014a). Even if depression is identified, only about 25% of patients receive treatment consistent with current guidelines (Unutzer et al., 2013). The U.S. Preventive Services Task Force recommends screening for depression in the general adult population (USPSTF, 2016). It is important that all health care professionals receive adequate education about depression in older adults.

Racial, Ethnic, and Cultural Considerations

Studies have consistently found that older racial and ethnic minorities are less likely to be diagnosed with depression than their white counterparts but are also less likely to get treated (Akincigil et al., 2012; Woodward et al., 2013). Hispanic adults aged 50 and older are reported to experience more depression than white, non-Hispanic adults; black, non-Hispanic adults; or other, non-Hispanic adults. Gender differences are also present in depression prevalence, and older women suffer depression at twice the rate of older men (Hall & Reynolds, 2014).

Differences in the prevalence of major depressive disorder and other mental disorders may be due to differences in the presentation of self-reported symptoms or other aspects of cultural context (Box 24.3). The new criteria in the *DSM-5* addressing culturally based explanatory models will assist in better understanding differences in presentation, help-seeking behavior, and provision of more culturally appropriate treatment for all individuals. Racial, ethnic, and gender differences in mental illness, as well as differences within racial groups, have not received adequate attention in the United States (see Chapter 2).

Consequences

Depression is a common and serious medical condition second only to heart disease in causing disability and harm to an individual's health and quality of life. Depression and depressive symptomatology are associated with negative consequences, such as delayed recovery from illness and surgery, excess use of health services, cognitive impairment, exacerbation of coexisting medical illnesses, malnutrition, decreased quality of life, and increased suicide and non–suicide-related deaths (Abbasi & Burke, 2014; Alexopoulos, 2014; Sacuiu et al., 2016). It is highly likely that nurses will encounter a large number of older people with depressive symptoms in all settings. Recognizing depression and enhancing access to appropriate mental health care are important nursing roles to improve outcomes for older people.

Etiology

The causes of depression in older adults are complex and must be examined in a biopsychosocial framework. Factors of health, gender, developmental needs, socioeconomics, environment, personality, losses, and functional decline are all significant to the development of depression in later life. Depression can occur for the first time in late life or can be part of a long-standing mood disorder with onset in earlier years (Harvath & McKenzie, 2012). Compared with patients with early-life depression, older patients with late-onset major depression have less frequent family history of mood disorders. Biologic causes, such as neurotransmitter imbalances, have a strong association with many depressive disorders in late life. This may be a factor in the high incidence of depression in individuals with neurological conditions such as stroke, Parkinson's disease, and Alzheimer's disease (Abbasi & Burke, 2014; Alexopoulos, 2014).

High rates of depression are seen in individuals with dementia, and depression is also a risk factor for dementia, particularly early-onset, recurrent, severe depression (Morimoto et al., 2014). Serious symptoms of depression occur in up to 50% of older adults with Alzheimer's disease, and major depression occurs in about 25% of cases. Depression in individuals with Alzheimer's disease may be due to an awareness of progressive decline, but research suggests that there may be a biological connection between depression and Alzheimer's disease as well (Harvath & McKenzie, 2012). Among patients who have suffered a cerebral vascular accident, the incidence of major depressive disorder is approximately 25%, with rates being close to 40% in patients with Parkinson's disease.

Medical disorders and medications can also result in depressive symptoms (Boxes 24.11 and 24.12). Other important factors influencing the development of depression are alcohol abuse, loss of a spouse or partner, loss of social supports, lower income level, caregiver stress (particularly caring for a person with dementia), and gender. Some common risk factors for depression are presented in Box 24.13.

BOX 24.11 Medical Conditions and Depression

Cancers
Cardiovascular disorders
Endocrine disorders, such as thyroid problems and diabetes
Metabolic and nutritional disorders, such as vitamin B_{12} deficiency, malnutrition, diabetes
Neurological disorders, such as Alzheimer's disease, stroke, and Parkinson's disease
Viral infections, such as herpes zoster and hepatitis
Vision and hearing impairment

BOX 24.12 Medications and Depression

Antihypertensives	Anticholesteremics
Angiotensin-converting enzyme (ACE) inhibitors	Antibiotics
	Analgesics
Methyldopa	Corticosteroids
Reserpine	Digoxin
Guanethidine	L-Dopa
Antiarrhythmics	

❖ IMPLICATIONS FOR GERONTOLOGICAL NURSING AND HEALTHY AGING

◆ Assessment

Making the diagnosis of depression in older people can be challenging, and symptoms of depression present differently in older people. Older people who are depressed report more somatic complaints such as insomnia, loss of appetite, weight loss, memory loss, and chronic pain. It is often difficult to distinguish somatic complaints from the physical symptoms associated with chronic illness. In medically ill individuals, assessment should focus on nonsomatic complaints such as sadness, helplessness, hopelessness, difficulty making decisions, and irritability (Avari et al., 2014). Hypochondriasis is also common, as are constant complaining and criticism, which may actually be expressions of depression. Older depressed individuals also have a higher rate of psychotic and severe depression with more weight loss and decreased appetite (Abbasi & Burke, 2014).

Decreased energy and motivation, lack of ability to experience pleasure, increased dependency, poor grooming and difficulty completing activities of daily living (ADLs), withdrawal from people or activities enjoyed in the past, decreased sexual interest, and a preoccupation with death or "giving up" are also signs of depression in older people. Feelings of guilt and

BOX 24.13 Risk Factors for Depression

- Chronic medical illnesses, disability, functional decline
- Alzheimer's disease and other dementias
- Bereavement
- Caregiving
- Female (2 : 1 risk)
- Socioeconomic deprivation
- Family history of depression
- Previous episode of depression
- Admission to long-term care or other change in environment
- Medications
- Alcohol or substance abuse
- Living alone
- Widowhood

worthlessness, seen in younger depressed individuals, are less frequently seen in older people.

Individuals often present with complaints of memory problems and a cognitive impairment of recent onset that mimics dementia but subsides upon remission of depression (previously called pseudodementia). It is important to note that a large percentage of these patients progress into irreversible dementia within 2 to 3 years, so recognition and treatment of depression are important. It is essential to differentiate between dementia and depression, and older people with memory impairment should be evaluated for depression. Symptoms such as agitated behavior and repetitive verbalizations in persons with dementia may be an indicator of depression (see Chapter 25).

Comprehensive assessment involves a systematic and thorough evaluation using a depression screening instrument, interview, psychiatric and medical history, physical (with focused neurological exam), functional assessment, cognitive assessment, laboratory tests, medication review, determination of iatrogenic or medical causes, and family interview as indicated (Avari et al., 2014). Assessment for depressogenic medications, for alcohol and substance abuse, and for related comorbid physical conditions that may contribute to or complicate treatment of depression must also be included (Box 24.14).

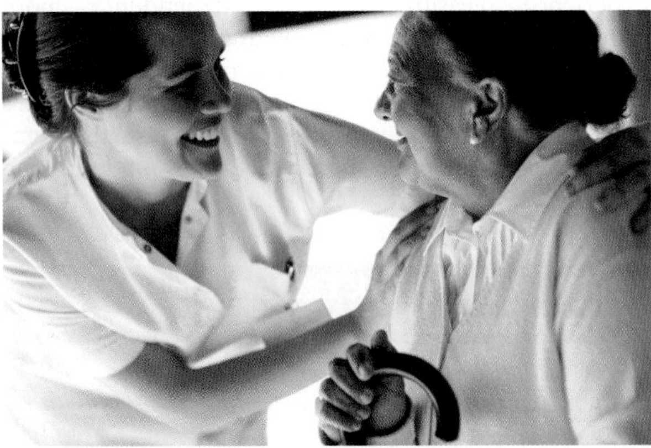

Creating hopeful environments in which meaningful activities and supportive relationships can be enjoyed is an important nursing role in the treatment of depression. (© iStock.com/Yuri.)

BOX 24.14 Tips for Best Practice

Assessment of Depression

- Utilize a depression screening tool (GDS or Cornell if cognitive impairment).
- Assess for suicidal thoughts.
- Investigate somatic complaints and look for underlying acute or chronic stressful events.
- Investigate sleep patterns, changes in appetite or weight, socialization pattern, level of physical activity, and substance abuse (past and present).
- Ask direct questions about psychosocial factors that may influence depression: elder abuse, poor environmental conditions, and changes in the patient role after death or disability of a spouse/partner.
- Obtain psychiatric and medical histories.
- Perform a physical exam including a focused neurological exam.
- Complete a functional assessment (pay close attention to changes in ADL function).
- Perform a cognitive assessment; depressed patients may show little effort during examination, answer "I don't know," and have inconsistent memory loss and performance during exam.
- Conduct a medication review (assessment for medications that may cause depressive symptoms).
- Ask about psychotic symptoms (delusions, hallucinations) and symptoms of bipolar disorder.
- Perform laboratory work as appropriate to rule out other causes of symptoms (e.g., TSH, T_4, serum B_{12}, vitamin D, folate, complete blood count, urinalysis).
- Utilize family/significant others in obtaining key information to correlate patient's symptoms with others' observations; always assess and interview patient first.

From Avari J, Yuen G, AbdelMalak B, et al: Assessment and management of late-life depression, *Psychiatr Ann* 44(3):131–137, 2014; Campbell J, Resnick B, Warshaw G: Alcoholism. In Ham R, Sloane P, Warshaw G, et al, editors: *Primary care geriatrics*, ed 6, pp 365–371, Philadelphia, 2014, Elsevier.

Screening of all older adults for depression should be incorporated into routine health assessments across the continuum of care—in hospitals, primary care, long-term care, home care, and community-based settings. The Geriatric Depression Scale (GDS), a self-report scale, was developed specifically for screening older adults and has been tested extensively in a number of settings (see Chapter 8, Table 8-3). It is only appropriate for cognitively intact individuals and those with mild to moderate cognitive impairment. The Cornell Scale for Depression in Dementia (CSD-D) is recommended for the assessment of depression in individuals with severe cognitive impairment and includes an interview with an informant followed by an attempted interview with the individual with dementia. If he or she is unable to respond to the questions, many can be completed through observation. The instrument takes about 20 minutes to administer. Additional research is needed to develop and validate a depression screening instrument that will accurately detect depression symptoms across varying levels of dementia (Brown et al., 2015).

◆ Interventions

The goals of depression treatment in older adults are to decrease symptoms, reduce relapse and recurrence, improve function and quality of life, and reduce mortality and health care costs (Harvath & McKenzie, 2012). When compared with younger individuals, older people demonstrate comparable treatment response rates, although they may have higher rates of relapse following treatment. As a result, treatment may need to be longer to prevent recurrences (Abbasi et al., 2014). If depression is diagnosed, treatment should begin as soon as possible and appropriate follow-up should be provided. Depressed people are usually unable to follow through on their own and without appropriate treatment and monitoring may be candidates for deeper depression or suicide. Interventions are individualized and are based on history, severity of symptoms, concomitant illnesses, and level of disability.

◆ Nonpharmacological Approaches

Current evidence shows that both cognitive-behavioral therapy (CBT) and second-generation antidepressants have similar effectiveness but the medications are more likely to cause harm than the utilization of CBT alone. The American College of Physicians recommends that clinicians choose between either CBT or second-generation antidepressants to treat patients with major depressive disorder after discussing treatment effects, adverse effect profiles, cost, accessibility, and preferences with the patient (Garthlehner et al., 2016).

Other types of nonpharmacological treatment that have been found to be helpful in depression include family and social support, education, grief management, exercise, humor, spirituality, CBT, brief psychodynamic therapy, interpersonal therapy, reminiscence, life review therapy (see Chapter 4), problem-solving therapy, and complementary therapy (e.g., tai chi) (Abbasi & Burke, 2014; Chan et al., 2014; DeKeyser & Jacobs, 2014). The development of effective, simplified, and accessible psychotherapeutic approaches, including telephone or Internet-based programs, is important.

Despite evidence-based guidelines calling for combined pharmacological and psychotherapeutic treatment, and the fact that older adults often prefer psychotherapy to psychiatric medications, psychological interventions are often not offered as an alternative treatment of depression (American Psychological Association, 2014). Reasons for this include time, reimbursement constraints, and a limited well-trained geriatric mental health workforce (McGovern et al., 2014).

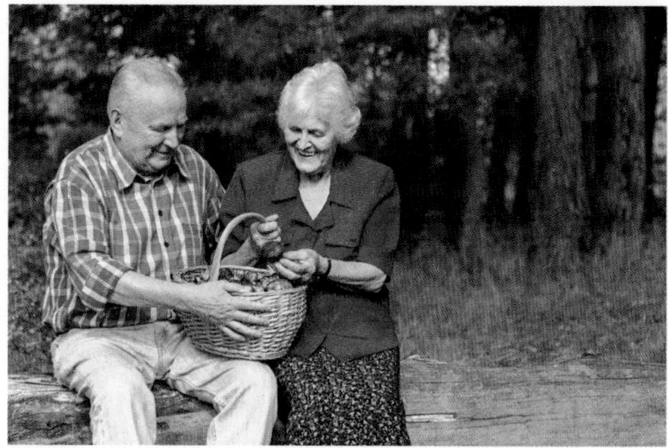

Elders enjoying an activity together. (© iStock.com/FredFroese.)

◆ ***Collaborative care.*** Few older adults with mental health disorders receive care from mental health specialists and most prefer treatment in primary care settings. More than 70 randomized controlled trials have shown collaborative care, an evidence-based approach for integrating physical and behavioral health services in primary care, is more effective and cost-efficient than usual care across diverse practice settings and patient populations (Hall & Reynolds, 2014; Unutzer et al., 2013). Some research suggests that collaborative care may improve ethnic and economic disparities in the diagnosis and treatment of depression (Hall & Reynolds, 2014).

Collaborative care models include a primary care provider (PCP, an MD or NP), care management staff (often nurses), and a psychiatric consultant working in an interprofessional team. Care managers are trained to provide evidence-based care coordination, brief behavioral interventions/psychotherapy, and treatment support initiated by the PCP, such as medications. The psychiatric consultant, either through face-to-face or by telemedicine consult, advises the team and provides guidance on patients who present diagnostic challenges or who are not yet showing improvement (Hall & Reynolds, 2014; Unutzer et al., 2013).

◆ Pharmacological Approaches

Choice of medication depends on comorbidities, drug side effects, and the type of effect desired. People with agitated depression and sleep disturbances may benefit from medications with a more sedating effect, whereas those who are not eating may do better taking medications that have an appetite-stimulating effect. There are more than 20 antidepressants approved by the FDA for the treatment of depression in older adults.

The most commonly prescribed antidepressants are the selective serotonin reuptake inhibitors (SSRIs). These agents work selectively on neurotransmitters in the brain to alleviate depression. The SSRIs are generally well tolerated in older people. Many are now available in both tablet and oral concentrate forms for easier use. Side effects are manageable and usually resolve over time; most cause initial problems with nausea, vomiting, dizziness, dry mouth, or sedation. Hyponatremia can also occur. If sexual dysfunction occurs, it will resolve only with discontinuation; therefore, if the person is or plans to become sexually active, a different drug may be necessary.

For those who do not respond to an adequate trial of SSRIs, there is another group of antidepressants that combines the inhibition of both serotonin and norepinephrine reuptake inhibitors (SNRIs) (e.g., venlafaxine [Effexor]). These also may be preferred by those who are engaged in or who anticipate sexual activity because they are less likely to have sexual side effects. One of the atypical antidepressants, such as bupropion (Wellbutrin) or trazodone, may also be used. In the context of reducing polypharmacy, Wellbutrin also reduces nicotine dependency, and trazodone is sedating—for the person who has difficulty getting to or staying asleep.

Since the development of the SSRIs and SNRIs, the older monoamine oxidase (MAO) inhibitors and tricyclic antidepressants are no longer indicated because of their high side effect profile including risk for falls. If depression is immobilizing, psychostimulants may be used but cardiac function must be monitored closely because there are limited data on safe use in the older adult (Abbasi & Burke, 2014).

All antidepressant medications must be closely monitored for side effects and therapeutic response. Side effects can be especially problematic for older people with comorbid conditions and complex drug regimens. There is a wide range of antidepressant medications, and several may have to be evaluated. Only about one-third of depressed older adults achieve remission with any single agent (McGovern et al., 2014). Similar to other medications for older people, doses should be lower at first (50% of the target does) and titrated as indicated while adequate treatment effect is ensured.

A patient who has responded to antidepressant treatment should continue treatment for approximately 1 year after a first depressive episode because recurrence rates are high after earlier discontinuation. After a second or third episode, treatment should be extended after remission and some may require lifelong treatment. Often, older people may be resistant to take medication for depression, and it is helpful to stress that although there may be circumstances precipitating the depression, the final effect is a biochemical one that medications can correct (Abbasi & Burke, 2014).

◆ Other Treatments

Electroconvulsive therapy (ECT) is considered an excellent, safe therapy for older people with depression that is resistant to other treatments and for patients at risk for serious harm because of psychotic depression, suicidal ideation, or severe malnutrition. ECT results in a more immediate response in symptoms and is also a useful alternative for frail older people with multiple comorbid conditions who are unable to tolerate antidepressant treatment. ECT is much improved, but older people will need a careful explanation of the treatment because they may have many misconceptions.

Rapid transcranial magnetic stimulation (rTMS) is a treatment approved in 2008 by the FDA to treat major depressive disorder in adults for whom medication was not effective or tolerated. The treatment consists of administering brief magnetic pulses to the brain by passing high currents through an electromagnetic coil adjacent to the patient's scalp. The targeted magnetic pulses stimulate the circuits in the brain that are underactive in patients with depression with the goal of restoring normal function and mood. For most patients, treatment is administered in 30- to 40-minute sessions over a period of 4 to 6 weeks. The effectiveness of the treatment is still being evaluated in older adults (Abbasi & Burke, 2014). Box 24.15 presents suggestions for families and professionals caring for older adults with depression.

SUICIDE

Even though the suicide rates in older people have been decreasing over the past 8 years, the rate of suicide among older adults in most countries is higher than that for any other age group—and the suicide rate for white males 85 years and older is the highest of all—four times the national age-adjusted rate (Abbasi & Burke, 2014). Older widowers are thought to be the most vulnerable because they have often depended on their wives to maintain the comforts of home and the social network of family and friends. Despite these statistics, there is little research on suicide ideation and behavior among older adults. Women in all countries have much lower suicide rates, possibly because of greater flexibility in coping skills based on multiple roles that women fill throughout their lives.

In most cases, depression and other mental health problems, including anxiety, contribute significantly to suicide risk. Common precipitants of suicide include

BOX 24.15 Tips for Best Practice

Family and Professional Support for Depression

- Provide relief from discomfort of physical illness.
- Enhance physical function (i.e., regular exercise and/or activity; physical, occupational, recreational therapies).
- Develop a daily activity schedule that includes pleasant activities.
- Increase opportunities for socialization and enhance social support.
- Provide opportunities for decision-making and the exercise of control.
- Focus on spiritual renewal and rediscovery of meanings.
- Reactivate latent interests, or develop new ones.
- Validate depressed feelings as aiding recovery; do not try to bolster the person's mood or deny his or her despair.
- Help the person become aware of the presence of depression, the nature of the symptoms, and the availability of effective treatments.
- Emphasize depression as a medical, not mental, illness that must be treated like any other disorder.
- Provide easy-to-use educational materials to older adults and family members, such as those available through NIMH.
- Involve family in patient teaching, particularly younger family members who may have different life experiences related to depression and its treatment.
- Provide an accepting atmosphere and an empathic response.
- Demonstrate faith in the person's strengths.
- Praise any and all efforts at recovery, no matter how small.
- Assist in expressing and dealing with anger.
- Do not stifle the grief process; grief cannot be hurried.
- Create a hopeful environment in which self-esteem is fostered and life is meaningful.

physical or mental illness, death of a spouse or partner, substance abuse, and chronic pain (Abbasi & Burke, 2014; Draper, 2014). One of the major differences in suicidal behavior in the old and the young is the lethality of method. Eight out of 10 suicides for men older than 65 were with firearms. Older people rarely threaten to commit suicide; they just do it.

Many older adults who die by suicide reached out for help before they took their own life. Seventy percent visited a physician within 1 month before death; 40% visited within 1 week of the suicide, and 20% visited the physician on the day of the suicide (American Psychological Association, 2014). Depression is frequently missed, and older people with suicide ideation or with other mental health concerns often present with somatic complaints. The statistics suggest that opportunities for assessment of suicidal risk are present, but the need for intervention is not seen as urgent or even recognized. Consequently, it is very important for providers in all settings to inquire about recent life events, implement depression screening for all older people, evaluate for anxiety disorders, assess for suicidal thoughts and ideas based on depression assessment, and recognize warning signs and risk factors for suicide.

❖ IMPLICATIONS FOR GERONTOLOGICAL NURSING AND HEALTHY AGING

◆ Assessment

Older people with suicidal intent are encountered in many settings. It is our professional obligation to prevent, whenever possible, an impulsive destruction of life that may be a response to a crisis or a disintegrative reaction. The lethality potential of an elder must always be assessed when elements of depression, disease, and spousal loss are evident. Any direct, indirect, or enigmatic references to the ending of life must be taken seriously and discussed. In the nursing home setting, the Minimum Data Set (MDS) (see Chapter 8) includes screening for suicide risk and mandates that long-term care facilities have effective protocols for managing suicide risk (O'Riley et al., 2013).

The most important consideration for the nurse is to establish a trusting and respectful relationship with the person. Because many older people have grown up in an era when suicide bore stigma and even criminal implications, they may not discuss their feelings in this area. It is also important to remember that in older people, typical behavioral clues—such as putting personal affairs in order, giving away possessions, and making wills and funeral plans—are indications of maturity and good judgment in late life and cannot be construed as indicative of suicidal intent. Even statements such as "I won't be around long" or "I'm ready to die" may be only a realistic appraisal of the situation in old age.

If there is suspicion that the elder is suicidal, use direct and straightforward questions such as the following:

- Have you ever thought about killing yourself?
- How often have you had these thoughts?
- How would you kill yourself if you decided to do it?

SAFETY ALERT

Always ask direct questions of the patient and family about suicide risks and suicide ideation.

◆ Interventions

It is important to have a suicide protocol in place that clearly defines how the nurse will intervene if a positive response is obtained from any of the preceding questions. The person should never be left alone for any period of time until help arrives to assist and care for him or her. Patients at high risk should be hospitalized, especially if they have current psychological stressors and/or access to lethal means. Patients at moderate risk may be treated as outpatients provided they have adequate social support and no access to lethal means. Patients at low risk should have a full psychiatric evaluation and be followed up carefully.

Suicide is a taboo topic for most of us, and there is a lingering fear that the introduction of the topic will be suggestive to the patient and may incite suicidal action. Precisely the opposite is true. By introducing the topic, we demonstrate interest in the individual and open the door to honest human interaction and connection on the deep levels of psychological need. It is the nature of our concern and our ability to connect with the alienation and desperation of the individual that will make a difference. Working with isolated, depressed, and suicidal elders challenges the depths of nurses' ingenuity, patience, and self-knowledge.

BOX 24.16 *Healthy People 2020*

Substance Abuse Objectives for Adults

- Increase the proportion of persons who need alcohol and/or illicit drug treatment and received specialty treatment for abuse or dependence in the past year.
- Increase the proportion of persons who are referred for follow-up care for alcohol problems, drug problems after diagnosis, or treatment for one of these conditions in a hospital emergency department.
- Increase the number of Level I and Level II trauma centers and primary care settings that implement evidence-based alcohol Screening and Brief Intervention (SBI).
- Reduce the proportion of adults who drank excessively in the previous 30 days.
- Reduce average alcohol consumption.
- Reduce the past-year nonmedical use of prescription drugs (pain relievers, tranquilizers, stimulants, sedatives, any psychotherapeutic drug).
- Decrease the number of deaths attributable to alcohol.

From U.S. Department of Health and Human Services, Office of Disease Prevention and Health Promotion: *Healthy People 2020,* 2012. Available at http://www.healthypeople.gov/2020.

SUBSTANCE USE DISORDERS

Substance use disorders among older adults are a growing public health concern. With the aging of the baby boomer generation, the number of adults older than age 50 with substance abuse problems is projected to double by 2020 (CDC, 2013). The baby boomer generation has had more exposure to alcohol and illegal drugs in their youth and has a more lenient attitude about substance abuse. Additionally, psychoactive drugs became more readily available for dealing with anxiety, pain, and stress. The use of illicit drugs, such as cocaine, heroin, and marijuana, is becoming more prevalent, and baby boomer marijuana users will triple in the next decades (Wang & Andrade, 2013). Box 24.16 presents *Healthy People 2020* objectives for substance abuse in adults.

Alcohol Use Disorder

Prevalence and Characteristics

In the United States, alcohol use disorders are reported in 11% of adults aged 54 to 64 years and about 6.7% of those older than 65 years. Two-thirds of elderly alcoholics are early-onset drinkers (alcohol use began at age 30 or 40), and one-third are late-onset drinkers (use began after age 60). Late-onset drinking may be related to situational events such as illness, retirement, or death of a spouse and includes a higher number of women (Campbell et al., 2014). Most severe alcohol abuse is seen in people ages 60 to 80 years, not in those older than 80 years.

Alcoholism is the third most prevalent psychiatric disorder (after dementia and anxiety) among older men. The prevalence of alcohol abuse among older adults who are hospitalized for general medical and surgical procedures and institutionalized elders is approximately 18%. Alcohol-related problems in the elderly often go unrecognized, although the residual effects of alcohol abuse complicate the presentation and treatment of many chronic disorders of older people.

Gender Issues

Although men (particularly older widowers) are four times more likely to abuse alcohol than women, the prevalence in women may be underestimated. The number and impact of older female drinkers are expected to increase over the next 20 years as the disparity between men's and women's drinking decreases. Women of all ages are significantly more vulnerable to the effects of alcohol misuse, including faster progression to dependence and earlier onset of adverse consequences. Even low-risk drinking levels (no more than one standard drink per day) can be hazardous for older women. Older women also experience unique barriers to detection of and treatment for alcohol problems. Health care providers often assume that older women do not drink problematically, so they do not screen for alcohol abuse. Often alcohol abuse in women is undetected until consequences are severe (Wang & Andrade, 2013).

Physiology

Older people, especially females, develop higher blood alcohol levels because of age-related changes (increased body fat, decreased lean body mass, and total body water content) that alter absorption and distribution of alcohol. Decreases in hepatic metabolism and kidney function also slow alcohol metabolism and elimination. A decrease in the level of the gastric enzyme alcohol dehydrogenase results in slower metabolism of alcohol and higher blood levels for a longer time. Risks of gastrointestinal ulceration and bleeding related to alcohol use may be higher in older people because of the decrease in gastric acidity that occurs in aging (Nogueira et al., 2013).

Consequences

The health consequences of long-term alcohol use disorder include cirrhosis of the liver, cancer, immune system disorders, cardiomyopathy, cerebral atrophy, dementia, and delirium. Effects of alcohol on cognitive function are receiving greater attention, and a recent study reported that middle-aged men who drink more than 2.5 standard drinks a day are more likely to experience faster decline in all cognitive areas, especially memory (Sabia et al., 2014). It is estimated that 10% of dementia is alcohol related (Campbell et al., 2014).

Other effects of alcohol in older people include urinary incontinence, which results from rapid bladder filling and diminished neuromuscular control of the bladder; gait disturbances, from alcohol-induced cerebellar degeneration and peripheral neuropathy; depression; functional decline, increased risk for injury; and sleep disturbances and insomnia. Alcohol misuse has also been implicated as a major factor in morbidity and mortality as a result of trauma, including falls, drownings, fires, motor vehicle crashes, homicide, and suicide (U.S. Preventive Services Task Force, 2013).

Alcohol use also exacerbates conditions such as osteoporosis, diabetes, hypertension, and ulcers. The rate of hospitalization of older adults for alcohol-related conditions is similar to those admitted for myocardial infarction (Flores, 2016). Many drugs that elders use for chronic illnesses cause adverse effects when combined with alcohol (Box 24.17). All older people should be given precise instructions regarding the interaction of alcohol with their medications.

BOX 24.17 Medications Interacting With Alcohol

Analgesics
Antibiotics
Antidepressants
Antipsychotics
Benzodiazepines
H_2-receptor antagonists
Nonsteroidal anti-inflammatory drugs (NSAIDs)
Herbal medications (echinacea, valerian)
Acetaminophen taken on a regular basis, when combined with alcohol, may lead to liver failure
Alcohol diminishes the effects of oral hypoglycemics, anticoagulants, and anticonvulsants

Alcohol Guidelines for Older Adults

The possible health benefits of alcohol in moderation have been reported in the literature (reduced risk of coronary artery disease, ischemic stroke, Alzheimer's disease, and vascular dementia). As a result, older people may not perceive alcohol use as potentially harmful, but clinically significant adverse effects can occur in some individuals consuming as little as two to three drinks per day over an extended period. A drink is defined as 5 ounces of wine, 12 ounces of beer, or 1.5 ounces of 80-proof distilled spirits or liquor.

Because of the increased risk of adverse effects from alcohol use, the National Institute of Alcohol Abuse and Alcoholism defines "at-risk drinking" for men and women aged 65 years and older as more than one drink per day. The American Geriatrics Society guidelines indicate that two or more drinks on a usual drinking day within the past 30 days is considered "at-risk drinking" and five or more drinks on the same occasion as "binge drinking" (Wang & Andrade, 2013). Health professionals must share information with older people about safe drinking limits and the deleterious effects of alcohol intake.

❖ IMPLICATIONS FOR GERONTOLOGICAL NURSING AND HEALTHY AGING

◆ Assessment

Reasons for the low rate of alcohol detection among older adults by health care professionals include poor symptom recognition, inadequate knowledge about screening instruments, lack of age-appropriate diagnostic criteria for abuse in older people, and ageism. The diagnosis may be missed in three out of four older hospitalized patients with alcohol dependence (Campbell et al., 2014). Alcohol-related problems may be overlooked in older people because they do not disrupt their lives or are not clearly linked to physical disorders. Health care providers may also be pessimistic about the ability of older people to change long-standing problems.

The U.S. Preventive Services Task Force (2013) recommends that clinicians in primary care screen adults 18 years and older for alcohol misuse. Screening should be a part of health visits for people older than the age of 60 years in primary, acute, and long-term care settings. Although alcohol is the drug most often used among older adults, assessment should include all substances used (recreational drugs, prescription, nicotine, and OTC medications) (Snyder & Platt, 2013). The Hartford Institute of Geriatric Nursing recommends that the Short Michigan Alcoholism Screening Test–Geriatric Version be used with older adults because it is more age appropriate than other instruments (Campbell et al., 2014) (Table 24.1). A single question can also be used for alcohol screening: "How many times in the past year have you had 5 or more drinks in a day (if a man), or 4 or more drinks (if you are a woman older than 65 years of age)?" If the individual acknowledges drinking that much, follow-up assessment is indicated.

Assessment of depression is also important because depression is often comorbid with alcohol abuse. Alcohol and depression screenings should be offered routinely at health fairs and other sites where older people may seek health information. A medication review should be conducted, and screening should be done both before prescribing any new medications that may interact with alcohol and as needed after life-changing events. Alcohol abuse should be suspected in an older person who presents with a history of falling, unexplained bruises, or medical problems associated with alcohol abuse problems.

Alcoholism is a disease of denial and not easy to diagnose, particularly in older people with psychosocial and functional decline from other conditions that may mask decline caused by alcohol. Early signs such as weight loss, irritability, insomnia, and falls may not be recognized as indicators of possible alcohol problems and may be attributed to "just getting older." Box 24.18 presents signs and symptoms that may indicate the presence of alcohol problems in older adults.

Alcohol users often reject or deny the diagnosis, or they may take offense at the suggestion of it. Feelings of shame or disgrace may make elders reluctant to disclose a drinking problem. Families of older people with substance abuse disorders, particularly their adult children, may be ashamed of the problem and choose not to address it. Health care providers may feel helpless over alcoholism or uncomfortable with direct questioning or may approach the person in a judgmental manner. A caring and supportive approach that provides a safe and open atmosphere is the foundation for the therapeutic relationship. It is always important to search for the pain beneath the behavior.

◆ Interventions

Alcohol problems affect physical, mental, spiritual, and emotional health. Interventions must address quality of life in all of these spheres and be adapted to meet the unique needs of the older adult. Abstinence from alcohol

TABLE 24.1 Short Michigan Alcoholism Screening Test—Geriatric Version (SMAST-G)

	Yes (1)	No (0)
1. When talking with others, do you ever underestimate how much you drink?		
2. After a few drinks, have you sometimes not eaten, or been able to skip a meal, because you didn't feel hungry?		
3. Does having a few drinks help decrease your shakiness or tremors?		
4. Does alcohol sometimes make it hard for you to remember parts of the day or night?		
5. Do you usually take a drink to relax or calm your nerves?		
6. Do you drink to take your mind off your problems?		
7. Have you ever increased your drinking after experiencing a loss in your life?		
8. Has a doctor or nurse ever said they were worried or concerned about your drinking?		
9. Have you ever made rules to manage your drinking?		
10. When you feel lonely, does having a drink help?		
TOTAL SMAST-G SCORE* (1–10)		

*Scoring: 2 or more "Yes" responses indicate an alcohol problem.
From The Regents of the University of Michigan, Ann Arbor, 1991, University of Michigan Alcohol Research Center.

BOX 24.18 Signs and Symptoms of Potential Alcohol Problems in Older Adults

Anxiety
Irritability (feeling worried or "crabby")
Blackouts
Dizziness
Indigestion
Heartburn
Sadness or depression
Chronic pain
Excessive mood swings
New problems making decisions
Lack of interest in usual activities
Falls
Bruises, burns, or other injuries
Family conflict, abuse
Headaches
Incontinence
Memory loss
Poor hygiene
Poor nutrition
Insomnia
Sleep apnea
Social isolation
Out of touch with family or friends
Unusual response to medications
Frequent physical complaints and physician visits
Financial problems

Adapted from National Institute on Alcohol Abuse and Alcoholism: *Older adults and alcohol problems: Participant handout,* 2005. Available at http://www.niaaa.nih.gov; Geriatric Mental Health Foundation: *Substance abuse and misuse among older adults: Prevention, recognition, and help,* 2006. Available at http://www.gmhfonline.org.

is seen as the desired goal, but a focus on education, alcohol reduction, and reducing harm is also appropriate. Increasing the awareness of older adults about the risks and benefits of alcohol consumption in the context of their own situation is an important goal. Treatment and intervention strategies include cognitive-behavioral approaches, individual and group counseling, medical and psychiatric approaches, referral to Alcoholics Anonymous, family therapy, case management and community and home care services, and formalized substance abuse treatment. Treatment outcomes for older people have been shown to be equal to or better than those for younger people (Campbell et al., 2014). Providing education about alcohol use to older people and their families and referring to community resources are important nursing roles and essential to best practices.

Unless the person is in immediate danger, a stepped-care intervention approach beginning with brief interventions followed by more intensive therapies, if necessary, should be used. The U.S. Preventive Services Task Force (2013) recommends brief counseling interventions to reduce alcohol use for adults. Brief intervention is a time-limited, patient-centered strategy focused on changing behavior and assessing patient readiness to change. Sessions can range from one meeting of 10 to 30 minutes to four or five short sessions. The goals of brief intervention are to (1) reduce or stop alcohol consumption and (2) facilitate entry into formalized treatment if needed. Research results indicate that this type of intervention, with counseling by nurses in primary care settings, is effective for reducing alcohol consumption, and older people may be more likely to accept treatment given by their primary care provider.

Long-term self-help treatment programs for elders show high rates of success, especially when social outlets are emphasized and cohort supports are available. A significant concern is the lack of programs designed specifically for older people, particularly older women, whose concerns are very different from those of a younger population who abuse drugs or alcohol. Health status, availability of transportation, and mobility impairments may further limit access to treatment. Development of treatment sites in senior centers and assisted living facilities and telemedicine programs would increase accessibility. Additional resources are presented in Box 24.7.

Acute Alcohol Withdrawal

When there is significant physical dependence, withdrawal from alcohol can become a life-threatening emergency. Detoxification should be done in an inpatient setting because of the potential medical complications and because withdrawal symptoms in older adults can be prolonged. Older people who drink are at risk of experiencing acute alcohol withdrawal if admitted to the hospital for treatment of acute illnesses or emergencies. All patients admitted to acute care settings should be screened for alcohol use and assessed for signs and symptoms of alcohol-related problems. Older people with a long history of consuming excess alcohol, previous episodes of acute withdrawal, and/or a history of prior detoxification are at increased risk of acute alcohol withdrawal.

Symptoms of acute alcohol withdrawal vary but may be more severe and last longer in older people. Minor withdrawal (withdrawal tremulousness) begins 6 to 12 hours after a patient has consumed the last drink.

Symptoms include tremor, anxiety, nausea, insomnia, tachycardia, and increased blood pressure and frequently may be mistaken for common problems in older adults. Major withdrawal is seen 10 to 72 hours after cessation of alcohol intake, and symptoms include vomiting, diaphoresis, hallucinations, tremors, and seizures.

Delirium tremens (DTs) is the term used to describe alcohol withdrawal delirium; it usually occurs 24 to 72 hours after the last drink but may occur up to 10 days later. DTs occur in 5% of patients with acute alcohol withdrawal and are considered a medical emergency, with a mortality rate from respiratory failure and cardiac dysrhythmia as high as 15%. Other signs and symptoms include confusion, disorientation, hallucinations, hyperthermia, and hypertension. The Clinical Institute Withdrawal Assessment (CIWA) scale is recommended as a valid and reliable screening instrument (https://www.merckmanuals.com/medical-calculators/CIWA.htm) (Letizia & Reinboltz, 2005). Recommended treatment is the use of short-acting benzodiazepines at one-half to one-third the normal dose around-the-clock or as needed during withdrawal. The use of oral or intravenous alcohol to prevent or treat withdrawal is not established.

Other interventions include assessing mental status, monitoring vital signs, and maintaining fluid balance without overhydrating. Calm and quiet surroundings, no unnecessary stimuli, consistent caregivers, frequent reorientation, prevention of injury, and support and caring are additional suggested interventions. Nutritional assessment is indicated, as well as addition of a multivitamin containing folic acid, pyridoxine, niacin, vitamin A, and thiamine (Campbell et al., 2014; Letizia & Reinboltz, 2005).

Other Substance Abuse Concerns

A more common concern seen among older people is the misuse and abuse of prescription psychoactive medications. Dependence on sedative, hypnotic, or anxiolytic drugs, often prescribed for anxiety or insomnia, and taken for many years with resulting dependence, is especially problematic for older women, who are more likely than men to receive prescriptions for these drugs (IOM, 2012).

Some of the reasons for the abuse of psychoactive prescription medications may be inappropriate prescribing and ineffective monitoring of response and follow-up. In many instances, older people are given prescriptions for benzodiazepines or sedatives because of complaints of insomnia or nervousness, without adequate assessment for depression, anxiety, or other conditions that may be causing the symptoms. Older people may not be informed of the side effects of these medications, including interactions with alcohol, dependence, and withdrawal symptoms. More importantly, conditions such as anxiety and depression may not be recognized and treated appropriately (Wang & Andrade, 2013). Opioids are ranked second only to benzodiazepines among abused prescription drugs in the older adult population (Naegle, 2012). Abuse and addiction to prescription opioid pain medications is a major concern, and a new federal effort is being proposed to combat this growing issue in the United States (Pugh, 2016). Chapter 18 discusses pain management.

❖ IMPLICATIONS FOR GERONTOLOGICAL NURSING AND HEALTHY AGING

Risk, prevention, assessment, and treatment of alcohol and substance abuse have not been sufficiently studied among older people. Diagnostic criteria to identify alcohol and prescription drug misuse among older adults, particularly older women and culturally and ethnically diverse elders, also need further investigation. Nurses in contact with older adults in all settings must be competent in assessment for mental health disorders as well as in screening, assessment, and counseling about the use of alcohol and prescribed, illicit, and OTC drug use. Providing education to older people and their families and referring to specialists and community resources are also important nursing roles and essential to best practices.

KEY CONCEPTS

- The prevalence of mental health disorders is expected to increase significantly with the aging of the baby boomers.
- Mental health disorders are underreported and underdiagnosed among older adults. Somatic complaints are often the presenting symptoms of mental health disorders, making diagnosis difficult.
- The incidence of psychotic disorders with late-life onset is low among older people, but psychotic manifestations can occur as secondary symptoms in a variety of disorders, the most common being Alzheimer's disease.
- Psychotic symptoms in Alzheimer's disease necessitate different assessment and treatment than do long-standing psychotic disorders.
- Anxiety disorders are common in late life and re-establishing feelings of adequacy and control is the heart of crisis resolution and stress management.
- Depression remains underdiagnosed and undertreated in the older population and is considered a significant public health issue. Depression in older adults can be effectively treated. Unfortunately, it is often neglected or assumed to be a condition of aging

that one must "learn to live with." An important nursing intervention is assessment of depression.

- Suicide is a significant problem among older men, particularly widowers. Many persons considering suicide are seen by the health care professional with physical complaints shortly before they commit suicide, and assessment of depression and suicidal intent is important.
- Substance abuse, particularly alcohol, and misuse of prescription drugs are often underrecognized and undertreated problems of older adults, particularly older women. Screening and appropriate assessment and intervention are important in all settings.
- Treatment outcomes for substance abuse for older people are equal to or better than those for younger people.
- Further research is needed to fully understand the cultural and ethnic differences in mental health concerns, as well as appropriate assessment and treatment in culturally and ethnically diverse older people.

ACTIVITIES AND DISCUSSION QUESTIONS

1. Discuss the three most common mental health disturbances that elders are likely to experience and describe appropriate assessment and treatment.
2. What is likely to be different in the appearance of depression in a person who is 70 years old compared to its appearance in a person who is 20 years old?
3. Describe a time when you were depressed, and discuss the feelings you experienced. What did you do about it?
4. Ask classmates who are from a different race or cultural group how they view depression.
5. What behaviors are indicative of suicidal intent in an older adult?
6. With a partner, assess for suicidal intent using the questions posed in the text.
7. What type of teaching would you provide to an older adult related to the use of alcohol and medications?

REFERENCES

Abbasi O, Burke W: Depression. In Ham R, Sloane P, Warshaw G, et al, editors: *Primary care geriatrics*, ed 6, Philadelphia, 2014, Elsevier, pp 214–226.

Agency for Healthcare Research and Quality: *Certain therapies and medications improve outcomes of adults with post-traumatic stress disorder. Research Activities*, July 2013. Available at http://www.ahrq.gov/news/newsletters/research-activities/13jul/0713RA3.html. Accessed February 2016.

Akincigil A, Olfson M, Siegel M, et al: Racial and ethnic disparities in depression care in community-dwelling elderly in the United States, *Am J Public Health* 102(2):319–328, 2012.

Alexopoulos G: Clinical and neurobiological findings, treatment developments in late-life depression, *Psychiatr Ann* 44(3): 126–129, 2014.

American Psychiatric Association: *Diagnostic and statistical manual of mental disorders*, ed 5, Arlington, VA, 2013, Author.

American Psychological Association: *Mental and behavioral health and older Americans*, 2014. Available at http://www.apa.org/about/gr/issues/aging/mental-health.aspx. Accessed February 2016.

Avari J, Yuen G, AbdelMalak B, et al: Assessment and management of late-life depression, *Psychiatr Ann* 44(3):131–137, 2014.

Baxter A, Patton G, Scott K, et al: Global epidemiology of mental disorders: What are we missing? *PLoS ONE* 2013. doi: 10.1371/journal.pone.0065514.

Bludau J: Second institutionalization: Impact of personal history on patients with dementia, *Caring Ages* 3(5):3–4, 2002.

Bottche M, Kuwert P, Knaevelsrud C: Posttraumatic stress disorder in older adults: An overview of characteristics and treatment approaches, *Int J Geriatr Psychiatry* 27(3):230–239, 2012.

Brenes G, Danhauer S, Lyles M, et al: Telephone-delivered psychotherapy for rural-dwelling older adults with generalized anxiety disorder: Study protocol of a randomized controlled trial, *BMC Psychiatry* 14:34, 2014.

Brown E, Raue P, Halpert K: Depression detection in older adults with dementia, *J Gerontol Nurs* 41(11):15–21, 2015.

Bryant C, Mohlman J, Gum A, et al: Anxiety disorders in older adults: Looking to *DSM5* and beyond, *Am J Geriatr Psychiatry* 21(9):872–876, 2013.

Byers A, Yaffe K, Covinsky K, et al: High occurrence of mood and anxiety disorders among older adults, *Arch Gen Psychiatry* 67:489–496, 2010.

Campbell J, Resnick B, Warshaw G: Alcoholism. In Ham R, Sloane P, Warshaw G, et al, editors: *Primary care geriatrics*, ed 6, Philadelphia, 2014, Elsevier, pp 365–371.

Carson V, Yambor S: Managing patients with bipolar disorder at home, *Home Healthc Nurse* 30(5):280–291, 2012.

Catic A: Nonpharmacological management of behavioral and psychological symptoms in long-term care residents, *Ann Longterm Care* 23(11):2015. Available at http://www.annalsoflongtermcare.com/article/nonpharmacologic-management-behavioral-and-psychological-symptoms-dementia-long-term-care. Accessed January 2016.

Center for Medicare Advocacy: *Medicare and mental health*, 2014. Available at http://www.medicareadvocacy.org/medicare-and-mental-health. Accessed February 2016.

Centers for Disease Control and Prevention: Suicide among adults aged 35–64 years—United States, 1999–2010, *MMWR Morb Mortal Wkly Rep* 62(17):321–325, 2013.

Chan M, Leong K, Heng B, et al: Reducing depression among community-dwelling older adults using life-story review: A pilot study, *Geriatr Nurs* 35:105–110, 2014.

Chopra M, Zhang H, Kaiser A, et al: PTSD is a chronic, fluctuating disorder affecting the mental quality of life in older adults, *Am J Geriatr Psychiatry* 22(1):86–96, 2014.

Christianson S, Marren J: *Impact of Event Scale-Revised (IES-R)*, New York, 2013, Hartford Institute for Geriatric Nursing.

Clapp J: The diagnosis and treatment of post-traumatic stress disorder in older adults, *Ann Longterm Care* 24(2):12–16, 2016.

Clapp J, Beck J: Treatment of PTSD in older adults: Do cognitive-behavioral interventions remain viable? *Cogn Behav Pract* 19(1):126–135, 2012.

Clifford K, Duncan N, Heinrich K, et al: Update on managing generalized anxiety disorder in older adults, *J Gerontol Nurs* 41(4):10–20, 2015.

Collier E, Sorrell J: Schizophrenia in older adults, *J Psychosoc Nurs Ment Health Serv* 49(11):17–20, 2011.

Crowe M, Whitehead L, Wilson L, et al: Disorder-specific psychosocial interventions for bipolar disorder—A systematic review of the evidence for mental health nursing practice, *Int J Nurs Stud* 47:896–908, 2010.

DeKeyser F, Jacobs J: The effect of humor on elder mental and physical health, *Geriatr Nurs* 35(3):205–211, 2014.

Dols A, Rhebergen D, Beckman A, et al: Psychiatric and medical comorbidities: Results from a bipolar elderly cohort study, *Am J Geriatr Psychiatry* 22:1066–1074, 2014.

Draper B: Suicidal behaviour and suicide prevention in later life, *Maturitas* 79:179–183, 2014.

Eells K: The use of music and singing to help manage anxiety in older adults, *Ment Health Pract* 17(5):10–17, 2014.

Flores D: *Geriatric gems and palliative pearls: Alcohol use among older adults*, University of Texas Health Science Center at Houston. Available at http://www.uth.tmc.edu/HGEC/GemsAndPearls/index.html. Accessed February 2016.

Foundation for Psychocultural Research: *DSM-5 on culture: A significant advance*, 2013. Available at http://thefprorg.wordpress.com/2013/06/27/dsm-5-on-culture-a-significant-advance. Accessed February 2016.

Friedman M, Furst L, Gellis Z, et al: Anxiety disorders in older adults, *Social Work Today* 13(4):10, 2013.

Garthlehner G, Gaynes B, Amick H, et al: Comparative benefits and harms of antidepressants, psychological, complementary, and exercise treatments for major depression: An evidence report for a clinical practice guideline from the American College of Physicians, *Ann Intern Med* published online 9 Feb 2016. doi: 10.7326/M15-1813.

Grabowski D, Aschbrenner K, Rome V, et al: Quality of mental health care for nursing home residents: A literature review, *Med Care Res Rev* 67(6):627–656, 2010.

Hall C, Reynolds C: Late-life depression in the primary care setting: Challenges, collaborative care, and prevention, *Maturitas* 2014. Available at http://www.maturitas.org/article/S0378-5122(14)00195-9/fulltext. Accessed February 2016.

Hampton L, Daubresse M, Chang H-Y, et al: Emergency department visits by adults for psychiatric medication adverse effects, *JAMA Psychiatry* 2014. doi: 10.1001/jamapsychiatry.2014.436. [Epub ahead of print].

Harvath T, McKenzie G: Depression in older adults. In Boltz M, Capezuti E, Fulmer T, et al, editors: *Evidence-based geriatric nursing protocols for best practice*, ed 4, New York, 2012, Springer, pp 135–162.

Hendrie H, Tu W, Tabbey R, et al: Health outcomes and cost of care among older adults with schizophrenia: A 10-year study using medical records across the continuum of care, *Am J Geriatr Psychiatry* 22(5):427–435, 2014.

Hildon Z, Montgomery S, Blane D, et al: Examining resilience of quality of life in the face of health-related and psychosocial adversity at older ages: What is "right" about the way we age? *Gerontologist* 50:36–47, 2009.

Institute of Medicine (IOM): *The mental health and substance use workforce for older adults: In whose hands?* 2012. Available at http://nationalacademies.org/hmd/reports/2012/the-mental-health-and-substance-use-workforce-for-older-adults.aspx. Accessed September 2016.

Jeste D, Maglione J: Treating older adults with schizophrenia: Challenges and opportunities, *Schizophr Bull* 39(5):966–968, 2013.

Jimenez D, Bartels S, Cardenas V, et al: Cultural beliefs and mental health treatment preferences of ethnically diverse older adult consumers in primary care, *Am J Geriatr Psychiatry* 20(6):533–542, 2012.

Jimenez D, Cook B, Bartels S, et al: Disparities in mental health service use of racial and ethnic minority elderly adults, *J Am Geriatr Soc* 61:18–25, 2013.

Kaiser A, Wachen J, Potter C, et al: *Posttraumatic stress symptoms among older adults: A review*, 2014a. Available at http://www.ptsd.va.gov/professional/PTSD-overview/index.asp. Accessed February 2016.

Kaiser A, Wachen J, Potter C, et al: *PTSD assessment and treatment in older adults*, 2014b. Available at http://www.ptsd.va.gov/professional/treatment/older. Accessed February 2016.

Katz C, Stein M, Sareen J: Anxiety disorders in the *DSM-5:* New rules on diagnosis and treatment, *Mood Anxiety Disord Rounds* 2(3):2013. Available at http://www.moodandanxietyrounds.ca/crus/144-010%20English.pdf. Accessed February 2016.

Khouzam H: Posttraumatic stress disorder: Psychological and spiritual interventions, *Consultant* 53(10):720–725, 2013.

Kim G, Parton J, DeCoster J, et al: Regional variations of racial disparities in mental health service use among older adults, *Gerontologist* 53(4):618–626, 2012.

Letizia M, Reinboltz M: Identifying and managing acute alcohol withdrawal in the elderly, *Geriatr Nurs* 26(3):176–183, 2005.

Leutwyler H, Wallhagen M: Understanding physical health of older adults with schizophrenia: Building and eroding trust, *J Gerontol Nurs* 36(5):38–45, 2010.

McGovern A, Kiosses D, Raue P, et al: Psychotherapies for late-life depression, *Psychiatr Ann* 44(3):147–152, 2014.

Meesters P: Late-life schizophrenia: Remission, recovery, resilience, *Am J Geriatr Psychiatry* 22(5):423–426, 2014.

Mental Health America: *Depression in older adults*, 2014a. Available at http://www.mentalhealthamerica.net/conditions/depression-older-adults. Accessed February 2016.

Morimoto S, Kanellopoulos T, Alexopoulos G: Cognitive impairment in depressed older adults: Implications for prognosis and treatment, *Psychiatr Ann* 44(3):138–142, 2014.

Murphy K: The ups and downs of bipolar disorder, *Am J Nurs* 11(4):44–50, 2013.

Naegle M: Substance misuse and alcohol use disorders. In Boltz M, Capezuti E, Fulmer T, et al, editors: *Evidence-based geriatric nursing protocols for best practice*, ed 4, New York, 2012, Springer, pp 516–537.

National Institute of Mental Health: *Post-traumatic stress disorder (PTSD)*, 2014a. Available at http://www.nimh.nih.gov/health/

topics/post-traumatic-stress-disorder-ptsd/index.shtml#part1. Accessed February 2016.

National Institute of Mental Health: Senior Health: *Depression*, 2014b. Available at http://nihseniorhealth.gov/depression/aboutdepression/01.html. Accessed February 2016.

Nogueira E, Neto A, Cauduro M, et al: Prevalence and patterns of alcohol misuse in a community-dwelling elderly sample in Brazil, *J Aging Health* 25:1340–1357, 2013.

O'Riley A, Nadorff M, Conwell Y, et al: Challenges associated with managing suicide risk in long-term care facilities, *Ann Longterm Care* 21(6):28–34, 2013.

Osterweil N: Older adults with schizophrenia can achieve remission, *Clin Psychiatry News*, 2012. Available at http://www.clinicalpsychiatrynews.com/single-view/older-adults-with-schizophrenia-can-achieve-remission/ded3b0fff74af27314348d657b26309c.html. Accessed February 2016.

Pugh T: Obama seeks $1.1 billion to fight heroin and opioid addiction, *McClatchy DC*, 2016. Available at http://www.mcclatchydc.com/news/politics-government/white-house/article58008678.html. Accessed February 2016.

Resnick B, Inguito P: The resilience scale: Psychometric properties and clinical applicability in older adults, *Arch Psychiatr Nurs* 25(1):11–20, 2011.

Reuben D, Ganz D, Roth C, et al: Effect of nurse practitioner comanagement on the care of geriatric conditions, *J Am Geriatr Soc* 61(6):857–867, 2013.

Sabia S, Elbaz A, Britton A, et al: Alcohol consumption and cognitive decline in early old age, *Neurology* 82(4):332–339, 2014.

Sacuiu S, Insel P, Mueller S, et al: Chronic depressive symptomatology in mild cognitive impairment is associated with frontal atrophy rate which hastens conversion to Alzheimer's dementia, *Am J Geriatr Psychiatry* 24(2):128–135, 2016.

Smith M, Haedtke C, Shibley D: Evidence-based practice guideline: Late-life depression detection, *J Gerontol Nurs* 41(2):18–25, 2015.

Snyder M, Platt L: Substance use and brain reward mechanisms in older adults, *J Psychosoc Nurs Ment Health Serv* 51(7):15–20, 2013.

Splete H: Mentally ill eclipse residents with dementia, *Caring Ages* 10(12):11, 2009.

Thorp S, Ayers C, Nuevo R, et al: Meta-analysis comparing different behavioral treatments for late-life anxiety, *Am J Geriatr Psychiatry* 17:105–115, 2009.

Uher R, Payne J, Pavlova B, et al: Major depressive disorder in *DSM-5:* Implications for clinical practice and research of changes from *DSM-IV*, *Depress Anxiety* 31:459–471, 2014.

Unutzer J, Harbin H, Schoenbaum M, et al: *The collaborative care model: An approach for integrating physical and mental health care in Medicaid health homes* (Health Home Resource Center brief), May 2013. Available at http://www.medicaid.gov/State-Resource-Center/Medicaid-State-Technical-Assistance/Health-Homes-Technical-Assistance/Downloads/HH-IRC-Collaborative-5-13.pdf. Accessed February 2016.

U.S. Department of Health and Human Services (USDHHS), Office of Disease Prevention and Health Promotion: *Healthy People 2020*, 2012. Available at http://www.healthypeople.gov/2020. Accessed May 12, 2015.

U.S. Department of Veterans Affairs, Office of Research and Development: *Heart-mind mystery, VA Research Currents*, Feb 28, 2014. Available at http://www.research.va.gov/currents/spring2014/spring2014-1.cfm. Accessed February 2016.

U.S. Preventive Services Task Force (USPSTF): *Alcohol misuse: Screening and behavioral counseling interventions in primary care*, 2013. Available at http://www.uspreventiveservicestaskforce.org/uspstf12/alcmisuse/alcmisusefinalrs.htm. Accessed February 2016.

U.S. Preventive Services Task Force (USPSTF): *Depression in adult screening*, 2016. Available at http://www.uspreventiveservicestaskforce.org/Page/Document/draft-recommendation-statement115/depression-in-adults-screening1%20#Pod3. Accessed February 2016.

van der Aa H, van Rens G, Comijs H, et al: Stepped-care to prevent depression and anxiety in visually impaired older adults—Design of a randomized controlled trial, *BMC Psychiatry* 13:209, 2013.

van Kessel G: The ability of older people to overcome adversity: A review of the resilience concept, *Geriatr Nurs* 34(2):122–127, 2012.

Wang Y, Andrade L: Epidemiology of alcohol and drug use in the elderly, *Curr Opin Psychiatry* 26(4):343–348, 2013.

Warren B: How culture is assessed in the *DSM-5*, *J Psychosoc Nurs Ment Health Serv* 51(4):40–45, 2013.

Wetherell J, Jeste D: Older adults with schizophrenia, *Elder Care* 3(2):8–11, 2011.

Woodward A, Taylor R, Abelson J, et al: Major depressive disorder among older African-Americans, Caribbean Blacks, and non-Hispanic Whites: Secondary analysis of the national survey of American life, *Depress Anxiety* 30:589–597, 2013.

World Health Organization (WHO): *Mental Health Gap Action Programme: Scaling up care for mental, neurological, and substance abuse disorders*, 2014. Available at http://www.who.int/mental_health/mhgap/en. Accessed February 2016.

25

Care of Individuals With Neurocognitive Disorders

Theris A. Touhy

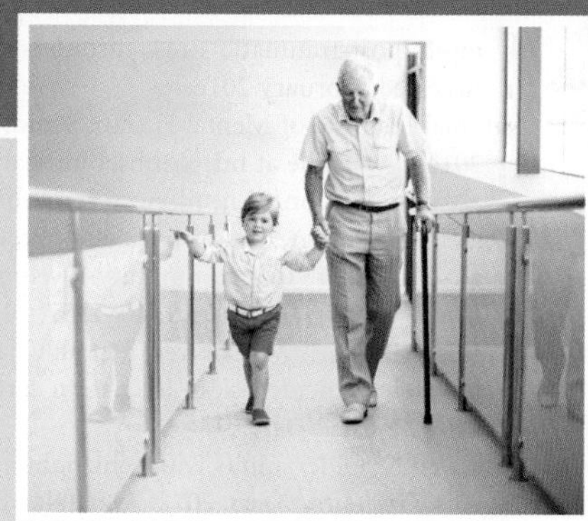

 evolve.elsevier.com/Touhy/gerontological

LEARNING OBJECTIVES

Upon completion of this chapter, the reader will be able to:

- Identify the characteristics of delirium and differentiate between delirium and mild and major neurocognitive disorders (dementia) and depression.
- Discuss prevention, treatment, and nursing interventions for individuals with delirium.
- Describe nursing models of care for persons with mild and major neurocognitive disorders.
- Discuss common concerns in care of persons with major neurocognitive disorders (communication, behavior, personal care, safety, nutrition) and nursing interventions.

THE LIVED EXPERIENCE

The Alzheimer's patient asks nothing more than a hand to hold, a heart to care, and a mind to think for them when they cannot; someone to protect them as they travel through the dangerous twists and turns of the labyrinth. These thoughts must be put on paper now. Tomorrow they may be gone, as fleeting as the bloom of night jasmine beside my front door.

Diana Friel McGowin, who was diagnosed with Alzheimer's disease when she was 45 years old (McGowin, 1993, p. viii)

This chapter focuses on care of older adults with mild and major neurocognitive disorders (dementia) and delirium with an emphasis on nursing interventions. The term dementia has been replaced with mild and major neurocognitive disorders (NCDs) in the *DSM-5* (American Psychiatric Association, 2013), but the terms *dementia* and *cognitive impairment* will also be used in this chapter. Chapter 23 provides information about neurocognitive disorders including classification, etiology, disease-specific information, and pharmacological treatment. Cognitive function in aging is discussed in Chapter 4 and cognitive screening instruments in Chapter 8.

NEUROCOGNITIVE DISORDER: DELIRIUM

Although delirium is common in older adults, it often is unrecognized, which increases the risk of functional decline, mortality, and health care costs (Inouye et al., 2014). Nurses play a key role in early identification and implementation of interventions aimed at reducing delirium and associated risks. Depression, delirium, and the mild and major neurocognitive disorders (dementia) are called the *three D's* of cognitive impairment because they occur frequently in older adults. These important geriatric syndromes are not a normal consequence of aging, although incidence increases with age. Because cognitive and behavioral changes characterize all *three D*'s, it can be difficult to diagnose delirium, delirium superimposed on mild or major neurocognitive disorder (dementia) (DSD), or depression (see Chapter 24).

Differences Among Delirium, Dementia (Mild and Major Neurocognitive Disorder), and Depression

Delirium is an acute decline in cognitive function and attention and represents brain failure (American Geriatrics Society, 2014). Symptoms develop over a short period of time (usually hours to days) and tend to fluctuate over the course of the day, often worsening at night. People often experience reduced ability to focus, sustain, or shift attention, which leads to cognitive or perceptual disturbances (O'Mahony et al., 2011). Perceptual disturbances are often accompanied by delusional (paranoid) thoughts and behavior and hallucinations. Box 25.1 presents the symptom requirements for a diagnosis of delirium from the *DSM-5* (American Psychiatric Association, 2013). In contrast, mild and major and mild neurocognitive disorder typically has a gradual onset and a slow, steady pattern of decline without alterations in consciousness.

These disorders represent serious pathological alterations and require assessment and interventions. However, a change in cognitive function in older adults is often seen as "normal" and not investigated. Any change in mental status in an older person requires appropriate assessment. Knowledge about cognitive function in aging and appropriate assessment and evaluation are keys to differentiating these three syndromes. Table 25.1 presents the clinical features and the differences in cognitive and behavioral characteristics in delirium, mild and major neurocognitive disorders, and depression.

Etiology

The exact pathophysiological mechanisms involved in the development and progression of delirium remain uncertain. One single cause or mechanism is not likely, but rather emerging evidence supports the theory of complex interaction of biological factors leading to the disruption of neuronal networks (Inouye et al., 2014). Delirium results from the interaction of predisposing factors (e.g., vulnerability on the part of the individual attributable to predisposing conditions, such as underlying cognitive impairment, functional impairment, depression, acute illness, sensory impairment) and precipitating factors/insults (e.g., medications, procedures, restraints, iatrogenic events, sleep deprivation, bladder catheterization, pain, and environmental factors). A highly vulnerable older individual requires a lesser amount of precipitating factors to develop delirium (Inouye et al., 2014; Voyer et al., 2010). The causes of delirium are potentially reversible; therefore accurate assessment and diagnosis are critical. Delirium is given many labels: acute confusional state, acute brain syndrome, confusion, reversible dementia, metabolic encephalopathy, and toxic psychosis.

BOX 25.1 Symptom Requirements for Delirium Diagnosis

- Disturbance in attention and awareness
- Disturbance develops over a short period of time (usually a few hours to a few days) and represents a change from baseline attention and awareness
- At least one additional disturbance in cognition (e.g., memory deficit, disorientation, language, visuospatial, perception)
- Evidence that the disturbance is a direct physiological consequence of another medical condition, substance abuse, toxin exposure, or multiple conditions

Incidence and Prevalence

Delirium is a prevalent and serious disorder that occurs in older adults across the continuum of care. Among medical inpatients, delirium is present on admission to the hospital in 10% to 31% of older patients. During hospitalization, 11% to 42% of older adults develop delirium. The highest incidence rates have been in intensive care units and in postoperative and palliative care areas (Inouye et al., 2014; Tullmann et al., 2012). Up to 80% of patients in the intensive care unit (ICU) develop delirium and 5% to 50% of older patients develop delirium after an operation (American College of Surgeons/NSQIP/American Geriatrics Society, 2014; American Geriatrics Society, 2014; Bledowski & Trutia, 2013).

In subacute settings, a 16% delirium rate in patients newly admitted to subacute care has been reported. More than 50% of these patients are still delirious 1 month after admission (Marcantonio et al., 2010). The prevalence of delirium in the community is low (about 1% to 2%), but the development of delirium often leads to an emergency department visit, where the prevalence is about 8% to 17% of all older adults and 40% of nursing home residents (Inouye et al., 2014).

Delirium Superimposed on Mild and Major Neurocognitive Disorders (Dementia)

Older patients with mild and major neurocognitive disorders are three to five times more likely to develop delirium, and it is less likely to be recognized and treated than delirium in a cognitively intact individual. Dementia superimposed on dementia (DSD) can accelerate the trajectory of cognitive decline in individuals and is associated with high mortality among hospitalized older

TABLE 25.1 Differentiating Delirium, Depression, and Dementia

Characteristic	Delirium	Depression	Dementia
Onset	Sudden, abrupt	Recent, may relate to life change	Insidious, slow, over years and often unrecognized until deficits are obvious
Course over 24 hr	Fluctuating, often worse at night	Fairly stable, may be worse in the morning	Fairly stable, may see changes with stress
Consciousness	Reduced	Clear	Clear
Alertness	Increased, decreased, or variable	Normal	Generally normal
Psychomotor activity	Increased, decreased, or mixed Sometimes increased, other times decreased	Variable, agitation or retardation	Normal, may have apraxia or agnosia
Duration	Hours to weeks	Variable and may be chronic	Years
Attention	Disordered, fluctuates	Little impairment	Generally normal but may have trouble focusing
Orientation	Usually impaired, fluctuates	Usually normal; may answer "I don't know" to questions or may not try to answer	Often impaired, may make up answers or answer close to the right thing or may confabulate but tries to answer
Speech	Often incoherent, slow or rapid, may call out repeatedly or repeat the same phrase	May be slow	Difficulty finding word, perseveration
Affect	Variable but may look disturbed, frightened	Flat	Slowed response, may be labile

Modified from Sendelbach S, Guthrie PF, Schoenfelder DP: Acute confusion/delirium, *J Gerontol Nurs* 35(11):11–18, 2009.

individuals. Changes in the mental status of older adults with dementia are often attributed to underlying dementia, or "sundowning," and not investigated. Despite its prevalence, DSD has not been well investigated, and there are only a few relevant studies in either the hospital or the community setting (Inouye et al., 2014).

Recognition of Delirium

Delirium is a medical emergency and one of the most significant geriatric syndromes. However, it is often not recognized by health care practitioners. A comprehensive review of the literature suggested that "nurses are missing key symptoms of delirium and appear to be doing superficial mental status assessments" (Steis & Fick, 2008, p. 47). Factors contributing to the lack of recognition of delirium among health care professionals include inadequate education about delirium, limited use of formal assessment methods, a view that delirium is not as essential to the patient's well-being in light of more serious medical problems, and ageist attitudes (Kuehn, 2010a,b; Waszynski & Petrovic, 2008).

Cognitive changes in older people are often labeled as confusion, are frequently accepted as part of normal aging, and are rarely questioned. If the nurse believed that confusion was normal in older adults, he or she would be less likely to recognize symptoms of delirium as a medical emergency necessitating attention and intervention. Confusion in a child or younger adult would be recognized as a medical emergency, but confusion in older adults may be accepted as a natural occurrence, "part of the older person's personality" (Dahlke & Phinney, 2008, p. 46). Failure to recognize delirium, identify the underlying causes, and implement timely interventions contributes to the negative sequelae associated with the condition (Kuehn, 2010a,b; Tullmann et al., 2012).

Risk Factors for Delirium

There are many predisposing and precipitating factors for delirium (Box 25.2). The risk of delirium increases with the number of risk factors present. Among the most predictive risk factors are age greater than 65 years, mild or major neurocognitive disorders (NCDs), poor vision or hearing, functional deficits, infection, acute illness, alcohol or drug abuse, laboratory or electrolyte abnormalities, and respiratory insufficiency (American Geriatrics Society, 2014). Unrelieved or inadequately treated pain significantly increases the risk of delirium. Invasive equipment, such as nasogastric tubes, intravenous (IV) lines, catheters, and restraints, also contributes to delirium by interfering with normal feedback mechanisms of the body.

BOX 25.2 Precipitating Factors for Delirium

- Age greater than 65 years
- Cognitive impairment
- Severe illness or comorbidity burden
- Hearing or vision impairment
- Current hip fracture
- Presence of infection
- Inadequately controlled pain
- Polypharmacy and use of psychotropic medications (benzodiazepines, anticholinergics, antihistamines, antipsychotics)
- Depression
- Alcohol use
- Sleep deprivation or disturbance
- Renal insufficiency
- Aortic procedures
- Anemia
- Hypoxia or hypercarbia
- Poor nutrition
- Dehydration
- Electrolyte abnormalities
- Poor functional status
- Immobilization or limited mobility
- Risk of urinary retention or constipation
- Use of invasive equipment, restraints

Data from American Geriatrics Society: *Clinical practice guidelines for postoperative delirium in older adults,* 2014.

BOX 25.3 What Causes Delirium?*

Dementia
Electrolytes
Lungs, liver, heart, kidney, brain
Infection
Rx (polypharmacy, psychotropics)
Injury, pain, stress
Unfamiliar environment
Metabolic

*There is usually more than one cause.

Anticholinergic medications, sedative-hypnotics, and meperidine contribute considerably to delirium risk (American Geriatrics Society, 2012). The Beers Criteria for potentially inappropriate medication use in older adults (see Chapter 9) is a resource for potential problem medications. A mnemonic representing causes of delirium can be found in Box 25.3.

Clinical Subtypes of Delirium

Delirium is categorized according to the level of alertness and psychomotor activity. The clinical subtypes are hyperactive, hypoactive, and mixed. Box 25.4 presents the characteristics of each of these clinical subtypes. Because of the increased severity of illness and the use of psychoactive medications, hypoactive delirium may be more prevalent in the intensive care unit (ICU). Although the negative consequences of hyperactive delirium are serious, the hypoactive subtype may be more often missed and is associated with a worse prognosis because of the development of complications such as aspiration, pulmonary embolism, pressure ulcers, and pneumonia.

BOX 25.4 Types of Delirium

Hypoactive Delirium

- Quiet or "pleasantly confused"
- Reduced activity
- Lack of facial expression
- Passive demeanor
- Lethargy
- Inactivity
- Withdrawn and sluggish state
- Limited, slow, and wavering vocalizations

Hyperactive Delirium

- Excessive alertness
- Easy distractibility
- Increased psychomotor activity
- Hallucinations, delusions
- Agitation and aggressive actions
- Fast or loud speech
- Wandering, nonpurposeful repetitive movement
- Verbal behaviors (yelling, calling out)
- Removing tubes
- Attempting to get out of bed
- Unpredictable fluctuations between hypoactivity and hyperactivity

Consequences of Delirium

Delirium has serious consequences and is a "high priority nursing challenge for all nurses who care for older adults" (Tullmann et al., 2008, p. 113). Delirium is a terrifying experience for the individual and his or her family, and significant others and people often think the patient is "going crazy." Delirium is associated with increased length of hospital stay and hospital readmissions, need for increased services after discharge, and increased morbidity, mortality, and institutionalization, independent of age, coexisting illnesses, or illness severity (Balas et al., 2012). Box 25.5 presents resources for delirium including video descriptions of delirium by patients.

BOX 25.5 Resources for Best Practice

Delirium and Dementia

Advancing Excellence in America's Nursing Homes: Resources for professionals to improve dementia care

American College of Surgeons/NSQIP/American Geriatrics Society: *Optimal perioperative management of the geriatric patient,* 2014: Excellent resource for delirium prevention and treatment and other geriatric syndromes

American Geriatrics Society: Clinical Practice Guidelines for Postoperative Delirium in Older Adults, 2014

Centers for Medicare and Medicaid Services (CMS.gov): National Partnership to Improve Dementia Care in Nursing Homes; Hand in Hand: A Training Series for Nursing: Educational program for staff on how to employ nonpharmacological alternatives in caring for individuals with BPSDs

European Delirium Association: Patient Experiences of Delirium: Teaching Video

Hartford Institute for Geriatric Nursing: Delirium: Nursing Standard of Practice Protocol: Prevention, early recognition, and treatment; Assessment and management of delirium in older adults with dementia; CAM, CAM ICU

Hartford Institute for Geriatric Nursing: Dementia Series; Home Safety Inventory for Older Adults with Dementia; Eliminating the use of antipsychotic medications – it can't be done without professional nurses

Hospital Elder Life Program (HELP): Program materials, Family-HELP program, The Family Confusion Assessment Method (FAM-CAM)

ICU Delirium and Cognitive Impairment Study Group: Patient and Family Report: Memories from the ICU

ICU-DIARY.org: Informal network for all health care workers interested in the ICU diary

Nursing Home Toolkit: Promoting Positive Behavioral Health: http://www.nursinghometoolkit.com/

Person-centered matters: Making life better for someone living with dementia. https://www.youtube.com/watch?feature=player_embedded&v=5R3idi0e1eg

Society of Critical Care Medicine: Clinical practice guidelines for the management of pain, agitation, and delirium in adult patients in ICU

Although the majority of hospital inpatients recover fully from delirium, a substantial minority will never recover or recover only partially. Each episode of delirium increases vulnerability of the brain, which further enhances the risk of dementia (Inouye et al., 2014). The persistence of delirium after discharge may interfere with the ability to manage chronic conditions and contribute to poor outcomes (Hain et al., 2012). Further research is needed to determine the reasons for the long-term poor outcomes, whether characteristics of the delirium itself (subtype or duration) influence prognosis, and how the long-term effects might be decreased.

❖ IMPLICATIONS FOR GERONTOLOGICAL NURSING AND HEALTHY AGING

◆ Assessment

◆ Cognitive Assessment

Whenever there is a change in cognitive status, it is essential that a comprehensive cognitive assessment be performed to identify reversible conditions that may be the cause of an individual's symptoms. An important aspect of this is differentiating delirium, dementia, and depression (see Table 25.1). Older adults should be routinely and regularly assessed for cognitive function in all settings, and nurses must have the skills to recognize cognitive impairment and monitor cognitive functioning. "Assessment of cognitive function is the first and most critical step in a cascade of strategies to prevent, reverse, halt, or minimize cognitive decline" (Braes et al., 2008, p. 42).

Assessing cognitive function can be challenging. Some of the reasons for this include the complexity of cognitive assessment and the existence of several conditions with overlapping symptoms (dementia, depression, delirium). Other reasons include the often atypical presentation of illness in older people and the belief, on the part of health care professionals as well as older people, that alterations in cognitive functioning are part of the "normal" aspects of aging (see Chapter 4).

◆ Assessment of Delirium

Prevention of delirium is the first step in caring for vulnerable older adults. Identification of high-risk patients and risk factors, prompt and appropriate assessment, and continued surveillance are the cornerstones of delirium prevention. Delirium is preventable in up to 40% of patients (American Geriatrics Society, 2014). Nurses play a pivotal role in the identification of risk factors and signs and symptoms of delirium, and it is imperative that they accurately report patients' mental status to the health care team so that causative factors can be identified and treated.

SAFETY ALERT

Older adults with risk factors should be screened for delirium upon admission to the hospital, when transitioning from one area of care to another, and before discharge to other care settings or home. Individuals with unresolved delirium at discharge should be screened again at 3 months and monitored closely until the delirium has resolved (Lindquist et al., 2011).

Assessment begins with a thorough history and identification of key diagnostic features. Several instruments can be used to assess the presence and severity of delirium. To detect changes, it is very important to determine the person's baseline cognitive status. If the person cannot tell you this, family members or other caregivers who are with the patient can be asked to provide this information. Family members and other caregivers know the person well and will notice subtle changes in behavior. They can give information about whether or not these behaviors are normal for this person. If the patient is alone, the responsible party or the institution transferring the patient can provide this information by phone.

Do not assume the person's current mental status represents his or her usual state, and do not attribute altered mental status to age alone or assume that dementia is present. All older patients, regardless of their current cognitive function, should have a formal assessment to identify possible delirium when admitted to the hospital.

The Mini-Mental State Exam-2 (MMSE-2) is considered a general test of cognitive status that helps identify mental status impairment. Although the MMSE-2 alone is not adequate for diagnosing delirium, it represents a brief, standardized method to assess mental status and can provide a baseline from which to track changes (see Chapter 8). Several delirium-specific assessment instrument are available, such as the Confusion Assessment Method (CAM) (Inouye et al., 1990) (http://www.hospitalelderlifeprogram.org) recommended by the Hartford Institute for Geriatric Nursing (Box 25.5) and the NEECHAM Confusion Scale (Neelon et al., 1996). An ultrabrief two-item bedside test for delirium is currently under development and evaluation (Fick et al., 2015).

The CAM-ICU is another instrument specifically designed to assess delirium in an intensive care population and has recently been validated for use in critically ill, nonverbal patients who are on mechanical ventilation. The Family Confusion Assessment Method (FAM-CAM) (Steis et al., 2012) can be used to identify symptoms based on reports from family members (Box 25.5). Assessment using the CAM or NEECHAM should be conducted on admission to the hospital, throughout the hospitalization for all patients identified at risk for delirium, and for all patients who exhibit signs and symptoms of delirium or develop additional risk factors (Steis & Fick, 2008). Many acute care settings have made the CAM a part of the electronic medical record.

Once a patient is identified as having delirium, reassessment should be conducted every shift. Documenting specific objective indicators of alterations in mental status rather than using the global, nonspecific term confusion will lead to more appropriate prevention, detection, and management of delirium and its negative consequences. Findings from assessment using a validated instrument are combined with nursing observation, chart review, and physiological findings. Delirium often has a fluctuating course and can be difficult to recognize, so assessment must be ongoing and include multiple data sources.

Individuals should also undergo assessments before discharge and an appropriate follow-up plan should be established. The following assessments are recommended:

- Nutrition (Mini Nutritional Assessment)
- Cognition (Mini-Mental State Exam)
- Ambulation ability (Timed Get Up and Go Test)
- Functional status
- Presence of delirium (CAM) (American College of Surgeons/NSQIP/American Geriatrics Society, 2014).

◆ Interventions

◆ Nonpharmacological Approaches

Because the etiology of delirium is multifactorial, interventions that are multicomponent and address more than one risk factor are more likely to be effective (American Geriatrics Society, 2014; Reston & Schoelles, 2013). Interprofessional approaches to prevention of delirium seem to show the most promising results, but continued research is needed to evaluate what type of approach has the most beneficial effect in specific clinical settings. A person-centered approach to care, rather than a disease-focused approach, can yield the best outcomes (Box 25.6).

BOX 25.6 Taking a Person-Centered Approach to Delirium

Mr. M., an 81-year-old male, was admitted to an acute care facility 2 days ago because of a change in his behavior. The admitting diagnoses were dehydration and acute kidney injury. Suddenly one day he became agitated and yelled loudly. The nurse caring for him was busy with an unstable patient in the next bed, so her first response was to medicate Mr. M. with an antianxiety medication. The clinical practice specialist just happened to be present and recalled the risks for delirium and that nonpharmacological approaches were best. She quickly suggested to the nurse: "Let's move him out of this room to a quieter area." This simple change in environment was effective in reducing Mr. M.'s agitation, and for the next few days before discharge, he remained calm. This exemplar demonstrates the importance of working together to reduce the use of pharmacological interventions in individuals with delirium.

From Candice Hickman, MSN, RN, Clinical Practice Specialist.

A well-researched program of delirium prevention in the acute care setting, the Hospital Elder Life Program (HELP) (Inouye et al., 1999), focuses on managing six risk factors for delirium: cognitive impairment, sleep deprivation, immobility, visual impairments, hearing impairments, and dehydration. An interprofessional team of geriatric specialists, including nurses, takes a multifaceted approach to maintain cognitive and physical function for high-risk older adults, maximize independence at discharge, assist with transitions, and prevent unnecessary readmissions. Trained volunteers are also utilized in the HELP program. The program is used in more than 200 hospitals in the United States and internationally (see Box 25.5).

Most of the interventions in the HELP program can be considered quite simple and part of good nursing care. Interventions include the following: offering herbal tea or warm milk instead of sleeping medications, keeping the ward quiet at night by using vibrating beepers instead of paging systems, removing catheters and other devices that hamper movement as soon as possible, encouraging mobilization, assessing and managing pain, and correcting hearing and vision deficits. Fall risk–reduction interventions should be implemented (see Chapter 15). Interventions monitored by an interprofessional team have been found to reduce the incidence of delirium about 30% to 40% in a number of high-quality studies (Box 25.7) (American Geriatrics Society, 2014).

BOX 25.7 Tips for Best Practice

Prevention of Delirium

- Sensory enhancement (ensuring glasses, hearing aids, listening amplifiers)
- Mobility enhancement (ambulating at least twice a day if possible)
- Bedside presence of a family member whenever possible
- Cognitive orientation and therapeutic activities (tailored to the individual)
- Pain management
- Cognitive stimulation (if possible, tailored to individual's interests and mental status)
- Simple communication standards and approaches to prevent escalation of behaviors
- Nutritional and fluid repletion enhancement
- Sleep enhancement (sleep hygiene, nonpharmacological sleep protocol)
- Medication review and appropriate medication management
- Adequate oxygenation
- Prevention of constipation
- Minimize the use of invasive medical devices, restraints, or immobilizing devices
- Pay attention to environmental noise, light, temperature
- Normalize the environment (provide familiar items, routines, clocks, calendars)
- Minimize the number of room changes and interfacility transfers

Adapted from American College of Surgeons NSQIP and American Geriatrics Society: *Optimal perioperative management of the geriatric patient.* Available at https://www.facs.org/~/media/files/quality%20programs/geriatric/acs%20nsqip%20geriatric%202016%20guidelines.ashx; and American Geriatrics Society: *Clinical Practice Guidelines for Postoperative Delirium in Older Adults,* 2014. Available at http://www.sciencedirect.com/science/article/pii/S1072751514017931. Accessed February 2016.

◆ Pharmacological Approaches

Antipsychotic drugs are routinely used to treat delirium even though the U.S. Food and Drug Administration has not approved their use for treating the condition. The American Geriatrics Society guidelines suggest avoiding use of these medications as a part of the routine care of individuals with delirium. A recent systematic review and meta-analysis evaluating the effectiveness of antipsychotics for the prevention or treatment of delirium concluded that current evidence does not support the use of these medications. Limited use of antipsychotics may be considered if the patient's life or safety is at risk because of severe agitation. Non–drug treatments, discussed previously, are first-line treatment for delirium (Neufeld et al., 2016).

Caring for individuals with delirium can be a challenging experience. Communication with patients with delirium can be difficult, and disturbing behaviors, such as removing intravenous (IV) lines or attempting to get out of bed, disrupt medical treatment and compromise safety. It is important for nurses to realize that behavior is an attempt to communicate something and express needs. The patient with delirium feels frightened and out of control. The calmer and more reassuring the nurse is, the safer the patient will feel. Box 25.8 presents some communication strategies that are helpful in caring for people experiencing delirium and Chapter 15 discusses interventions for safety and restraint-free care.

CARE OF INDIVIDUALS WITH MILD AND MAJOR NEUROCOGNITIVE DISORDERS

Nurses provide direct care for people with dementia in the community, hospitals, and long-term care facilities. They also work with families and staff, teaching best practice approaches to care and providing education and support. With the rising incidence of dementia, nurses will play an even larger role in the design and

BOX 25.8 Tips for Best Practice

Communicating With a Person Experiencing Delirium

- Know the person's past patterns.
- Look at nonverbal signs, such as tone of voice, facial expressions, and gestures.
- Speak slowly.
- Be calm and patient.
- Face the person and keep eye contact; get to the level of the person rather than standing over him or her.
- Explain all actions.
- Smile.
- Use simple, familiar words.
- Allow adequate time for response.
- Repeat if needed.
- Tell the person what you want him or her to do rather than what you do not want him or her to do.
- Give one-step directions; use gestures and demonstration to augment words.
- Reassure person's safety.
- Keep caregivers consistent.
- Assume that communication and behavior are meaningful and an attempt to tell us something or express needs.
- Do not assume that the person is unable to understand or is demented.

implementation of evidence-based practice and provision of education, counseling, and supportive services to individuals with dementia and their caregivers.

The overriding goals in caring for older adults with dementia are to maintain function and prevent excess disability, structure the environment and relationships to maintain stability, compensate for the losses associated with the disease, and create a therapeutic milieu that nurtures the personhood of the individual and maintains quality of life. Box 25.9 presents an overview of general nursing intervention principles in the care of persons with dementia.

Nutrition, activities of daily living (ADLs), maintenance of health and function, safety, communication, behavioral changes, caregiver needs and support, and quality of life are the primary care concerns for patients, families, and staff caring for individuals with mild and major NCDs. Five common care concerns and nursing interventions are discussed in the remainder of this chapter: communication, behavior concerns, ADL care, wandering, and nutrition. Caregiving for individuals with NCDs is discussed in Chapter 27, and other care concerns such as falls and incontinence are discussed in earlier chapters of this book.

BOX 25.9 General Nursing Interventions in Care of Persons With Dementia

- Address safety.
- Structure daily living to maximize remaining abilities.
- Monitor general health and impact of dementia on management of other medical conditions.
- Provide meaningful activities and relationships to enhance quality of life.
- Support advance care planning and advance directives.
- Educate caregivers in the areas of problem-solving, resources access, long-range planning, emotional support, and respite care.

From Evans L: *Complex care needs in older adults with common cognitive disorders.* Available at http://www.hartfording.org/uploads/file/gnec_state_of_science_papers/gnec_dementia.pdf.

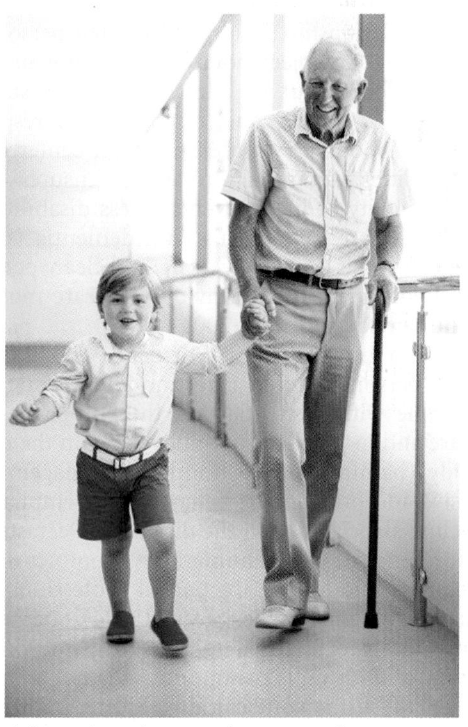

Maintaining function and preventing unnecessary decline are important. (© iStock.com/Squaredpixels.)

Person-Centered Care

Irreversible NCDs have no cure, and although new medications offer hope for improved function, the most important treatment for the disease is competent and compassionate person-centered care. Person-centered care is one of the six major aims in the redesign of the U.S. health care system and considers "what matter most" to individuals. Long ago, Mary Opal Wolanin, a gerontological nursing pioneer, suggested that nurses are not as interested in the neurofibrillary tangles in the brain as they are in trying to smooth out the environmental and relational tangles the person and his or her loved ones experience. "Since Alzheimer's affects mind and personality, as well as physical function, there is a great danger that the person can become obscured by the disease, defined by symptoms rather than by her or his unique spirit and continuing sense of self" (Sifton, 2001, p. iv). The focus in person-centered care is not on what we need to do to the person but on the person himself or herself and how to enhance well-being and quality of life.

Gerontological nurses know that the person, not the disease, is always the focus of care, and they practice from a belief that the person with dementia is still a whole person, someone who can think, feel, learn, grow, and be in a relationship (Touhy, 2004). "The person with dementia is not an object, not a vegetable, not an empty body, not a child, but an adult, who, given support, might exercise choices and respond to a respectful approach" (Woods, 1999, p. 35). Person-centered care fosters abilities, supports limitations, ensures safety, enhances quality of life, prevents excess disability, and offers hope. Care for persons with dementia is more than keeping their bodies alive, safe, and clean; performing tasks; and managing behavior—the care must also nourish their souls (Touhy, 2004).

There is a growing body of evidence on the importance of person-centered care and therapeutic work with people with dementia, but the emphasis in the literature and in practice continues to be on the care of the body (bathing, feeding) and the management of aggressive and problematic behavior. The emphasis on the decline associated with the disease, the catastrophic behaviors, and the loss of humanness promotes despair, hopelessness, and fear on the part of professional caregivers, patients, and families (Touhy, 2004). Special skills and attitudes are required to nurse the person with dementia, and caring is paramount. It is not an area of nursing that "just anyone can do" (Splete, 2008, p. 11). The overarching principles of person-centered dementia care and resources are presented in Box 25.10.

BOX 25.10 Principles of Person-Centered Dementia Care

- Individuals can live fully with dementia.
- The quality of life for individuals living with dementia is derived not only from the care and support they receive, but also in how others perceive their value.
- Being meaningfully engaged and having purpose and value as are vital to well-being as physical health.
- Respect, dignity, and providing choices in daily life are foundational to person-centered care and are basic human rights.

Adapted from Love K, Femia E: Helping individuals with dementia live more fully through person-centered practices, *J Gerontol Nurs* 41(11):9–14, 2015.

BOX 25.11 Patient's Descriptions of Communication Difficulties

Hain et al., 2014, p. 85

"I forget words. Sometimes it doesn't mean much and other times it means a great deal. I have learned ways to avoid making mistakes like shaking hands when I don't remember the person's name, joking, looking at their faces for a reaction."

Hain et al., 2010

"There are a range of things you want to say over and over because I think it was a word that was important to say and I'll forget…I hope that what I am saying makes sense."

COMMUNICATION

The experience of losing cognitive and expressive abilities is both frightening and frustrating. In early stages of NCD people may experience mild difficulty communicating. As the disease progresses, memory, speech, and communication also decline. Older adults experiencing NCDs have difficulty expressing their personhood in ways easily understood by others. Identifying receptive and expressive abilities can help the nurse design patient-specific interventions addressing communication challenges. However, the need to communicate and the need to be treated as a person remain despite memory and communication impairments. No group of patients is more in need of supportive relationships with skilled, caring health care providers. People with cognitive and communication impairments "depend on their relationship with and trust of others to provide emotional support, solve problems, and coordinate complex activities" (Buckwalter et al., 1995, p. 15).

Communication with older adults experiencing NCDs requires special skills and patience. Caregivers experience frustration and anxiety when their attempts to communicate with the person who has cognitive limitations are unsuccessful (Williams & Tappen, 2008). NCDs affect both receptive and expressive communication and alter the way people speak. Early in the disease, word finding is difficult (anomia), and remembering the exact facts of a conversation is challenging (Box 25.11). The person may wander from the topic of conversation and introduce seemingly unrelated topics. The person may fail to pick up on humor or sarcasm or abstract ideas in conversation. Nonverbal and behavioral responses become especially important as a way of communication as verbal skills become more limited.

As the disease progresses, verbal output may become less frequent although the grammar and sounds of the language being spoken remain relatively intact. Williams and Tappen (2008) remind us that even in the later stages of NCDs, the person may understand more than you realize and still needs opportunities for interaction and caring communication, both verbal and nonverbal. Often, health care providers do not communicate with older adults with major NCDs, or they limit communication only to task-focused topics.

To effectively communicate with a person experiencing an NCD, it is essential to believe that the person is trying to communicate something that is important. It is critical that nurses recognize various ways a person with dementia may communicate by knowing the person. The best thing we can do is discover what the person is trying to communicate and intervene according to needs. However jumbled it may seem, the person is attempting to tell us something. It is our responsibility as professionals to understand and know how to respond. The person cannot change his or her communication; we must change ours.

Nurses can overcome barriers to communication by taking a person-centered approach. A person-centered framework encourages coming to know the person by taking time to find out the individual's story: "Who am I?" In some cases people are unable to disclose a lifetime of memories, but taking the time to determine their background and making time to be present can contribute to effective communication. A person with NCD, like anyone else, values being recognized as important enough for the nurse to care to listen or pay attention to what is being communicated.

Evidence-Based Communication Strategies

Classic research conducted by Ruth Tappen of Florida Atlantic University (Boca Raton, FL) and colleagues (Tappen et al., 1997, 1999) provided insight into communication strategies that were helpful in creating and maintaining a therapeutic relationship with people with mild and major NCDs. The findings challenged some of the commonly held beliefs about communication with persons with NCDs; for example, avoiding the use of open-ended questions and keeping communication focused only on simple topics, task-oriented topics, and questions that can be answered with yes or no responses. Suggestions for specific communication strategies effective in various nursing situations were derived from the research (Box 25.12).

Use of these strategies will enhance communication and development of meaningful relationships to nurture the personhood of individuals with NCDs. Communication strategies differ depending on the purpose of communication (e.g., performing ADLs, encouraging expression of feelings). Approaches to communication must be adapted not only to the person's ability to understand but also to the purpose of the interaction. What is appropriate for assessment may be a barrier to conversation that is designed to facilitate expression of concerns and feelings (Williams & Tappen, 2008).

Reality Orientation

In the past, structured programs of reality orientation (RO) (orienting the person to the day, date, time, year, weather, upcoming holidays) were often used in long-term care facilities and chronic psychiatric units as a way to stimulate interaction and enhance memory. This intervention is still often noted as being of benefit to persons with NCDs. However, it has been found that structured RO may place unrealistic expectations on persons and may be distressing when persons cannot respond to these questions. Families and professional caregivers can often be heard asking people to name relatives, state their birth year, and remember other current facts. One can imagine how upsetting and demoralizing this might be to a person unable to remember these answers.

This does not imply that we should not provide orienting information to the person about daily activities, time of day, and other important events, but the information should be offered without the expectation that the person will remember the answers. Caregivers can provide orienting information as part of general conversation (e.g., "It's quite warm for December 10, but it will be a beautiful day for our lunch date").

Rather than structured RO, a better approach is to determine the person's time frame (where the person is in his or her own world) rather than trying to bring the person's time frame into yours. For example, if the individual insists that he or she needs to leave the house to meet the school bus, it is more helpful to ask the individual to talk about the times he or she did this activity rather than informing the person that his or her children are grown and do not ride the school bus.

Validation therapy, developed by Naomi Feil in the 1980s, involves following the person's lead and responding to feelings expressed rather than interrupting to supply factual data. Helping families and caregivers to understand validation therapy can assist in enhancing quality time with their loved ones. See Box 25.5 for links to a video beautifully illustrating this approach.

BOX 25.12 Four Useful Strategies for Communicating With Individuals Experiencing Cognitive Impairment

1. **Simplification Strategies (Useful With ADLs)**
   - Give one-step directions.
   - Speak slowly.
   - Allow time for response.
   - Reduce distractions.
   - Interact with one person at a time.
   - Give clues and cues as to what you want the person to do. Use gestures or pantomime to demonstrate what it is you want the person to do—for example, put the chair in front of the person, point to it, pat the seat, and say, "Sit here."
2. **Facilitation Strategies (Useful in Encouraging Expression of Thoughts and Feelings)**
   - Establish commonalities.
   - Share self.
   - Allow the person to choose subjects to discuss.
   - Speak as if to an equal.
   - Use broad openings, such as "How are you today?"
   - Employ appropriate use of humor.
   - Follow the person's lead.
3. **Comprehension Strategies (Useful in Assisting With Understanding of Communication)**
   - Identify time confusion. *(In what time frame is the person operating at the moment?)*
   - Find the theme. *(What connection is there between apparently disparate topics?)* Recognize an important theme, such as fear, loss, or happiness.
   - Recognize the hidden meanings. *(What did the person mean to say?)*
4. **Supportive Strategies (Useful in Encouraging Continued Communication and Supporting Personhood)**
   - Introduce yourself, and explain why you are there. Reach out to shake hands, and note the response to touch.
   - If the person does not want to talk, go away and return later. Do not push or force.
   - Sit closely, and face the person at eye level.
   - Limit corrections.
   - Use multiple ways of communicating (gestures, touch).
   - Search for meaning.
   - Know the person's past life history as well as daily life experiences and events.
   - Remember there is a person behind the disease.
   - Recognize feelings, and respond.
   - Treat the person with respect and dignity.
   - Show interest through body posture, facial expression, nodding, and eye contact. Assume a pleasant, relaxed attitude.
   - Attend to vision and hearing losses.
   - Do not try to bring the person to the present or use reality orientation. Go to where the person is, and enjoy the conversation.
   - When leaving, thank the person for his or her time and attention as well as information.
   - Remember that the quality, not the content or quantity, of the interaction is basic to therapeutic communication.

ADLs, Activities of daily living.

❖ IMPLICATIONS FOR GERONTOLOGICAL NURSING AND HEALTHY AGING

Care and communication that respect and value the dignity and the worth of every person, and use of research-based communication techniques, will enhance communication and personhood. "Gerontological nurses who are sensitive to communication and interaction patterns can assist both formal and informal caregivers in using more personal verbal and nonverbal communication strategies that are humanizing and show respect for the person. Similarly, they can monitor and try to change object-oriented communication approaches, which are not only insensitive and dehumanizing but also often lead to diminished self-image and angry, agitated responses on the part of the patient with cognitive impairment" (Buckwalter et al., 1995, p. 15).

BEHAVIOR CONCERNS AND NURSING MODELS OF CARE

Behavior and psychological symptoms of dementia (BPSDs) may present in up to 98% of individuals with NCDs at some point in the disease trajectory. These symptoms cause a great deal of distress to the person and the caregivers and often precipitate institutionalization (Kales et al., 2014; Kolanowski et al., 2013). Family caregivers of individuals with challenging behavioral conditions experience more stress than other caregivers and receive little or no guidance on how to deal with these conditions (Reinhard et al., 2014) (see Chapter 27). These symptoms occur in all types of dementia and include anxiety, depression, hallucinations, delusions, aggression, screaming, sleep disturbances, restlessness, agitation, and resistance to care.

BPSDs appear to be a consequence of multiple, but sometimes modifiable, interacting factors. These factors are both external and internal and result in part from heightened vulnerability to the environment as cognitive function declines. BPSDs should be viewed as a form of communication that is meaningful (rather than problematic) and is the individual's best attempt to communicate a variety of unmet needs (Kolanowski & Van Haitsma, 2013).

Several nursing models of care are helpful in recognizing and understanding the behavior of individuals with NCDs and can be used to guide practice and assist families and staff in providing care from a more person-centered framework. The *Progressively Lowered Stress Threshold (PLST)* model and the *Need-Driven Dementia-Compromised Behavior (NDDB)* model focus on "the close interplay between person, context, and environment. These models propose that behavior is used to communicate or express, in the best way the person has available, unmet needs (physiological, psychosocial, disturbing environment, uncomfortable social surroundings) and/or difficulty managing stress as the disease progresses" (Evans & Kurlowicz, 2007, p. 7).

The Progressively Lowered Stress Threshold Model

The progressively lowered stress threshold (PLST) model (Hall & Buckwalter, 1987; Hall, 1994) was one of the first models used to plan and evaluate care for people with NCDs in every setting. The PLST model categorizes symptoms of NCDs into four groups: (1) cognitive or intellectual losses, (2) affective or personality changes, (3) conative or planning losses that cause a decline in functional abilities, and (4) loss of the stress threshold, causing behaviors such as agitation or catastrophic reactions. Symptoms such as agitation are a result of a progressive loss of the person's ability to cope with demands and stimuli when the person's stress threshold is exceeded. Some examples of stressors that may trigger these symptoms are presented in Box 25.13.

Using this model, care is structured to decrease the stressors and provide a safe and predictable environment. Positive outcomes from use of the model include improved sleep; decreased sedative and tranquilizer use; increased food intake and weight; increased socialization; decreased episodes of aggressive, agitated, and disruptive behaviors; increased caregiver satisfaction with care; and increased functional level (DeYoung et al., 2003; Hall & Buckwalter, 1987).

Need-Driven Dementia-Compromised Behavior Model

The need-driven dementia-compromised behavior (NDDB) model (Algase et al., 2003; Kolanowski, 1999; Richards et al., 2000) is a framework for the study and understanding of behavioral symptoms of dementia. All behaviors have meaning and are a form of communication, particularly as verbal communication becomes more limited. Rather than behavior being viewed as disruptive, it is viewed as having meaning and expressing needs. Behavior reflects the interaction of background factors (cognitive changes as a result of dementia, gender, ethnicity, culture, education, personality, responses to stress) and proximal factors (physiological needs such as hunger or pain, mood, physical environment [e.g., light, noise, temperature]) with social environment (e.g., staff stability and mix, presence of others) (Richards et al., 2000).

Optimal care is provided by manipulating the proximal factors that precipitate behavior and by maximizing strengths and minimizing the limitations of the background factors. It is important for caregivers to identify and address the unmet need(s) that arise from both sets of factors rather than ignore the call for help and attempt to control the behavior with the use of sedating drugs (Dettmore et al., 2009). For instance, sleep disruptions are common in people with dementia. If the person is not getting adequate sleep at night, agitated or aggressive behavior during the day may signal the need for

BOX 25.13 Conditions Precipitating Behavioral Symptoms in Persons With Dementia

- Communication deficits
- Pain or discomfort
- Acute medical problems
- Sleep disturbances
- Perceptual deficits
- Depression
- Need for social contact
- Hunger, thirst, need to toilet
- Loss of control
- Misinterpretation of the situation or environment
- Crowded conditions
- Changes in environment or people
- Noise, disruption
- Being forced to do something
- Fear
- Loneliness
- Psychotic symptoms
- Fatigue
- Environmental overstimulation or understimulation
- Depersonalized, rushed care
- Restraints
- Psychoactive drugs

more rest. Interventions to modify proximal factors interfering with sleep, such as noise, frequent awakenings during the night, and daytime boredom, can help meet the need for rest and sleep and decrease agitation or aggression.

❖ IMPLICATIONS FOR GERONTOLOGICAL NURSING AND HEALTHY AGING

◆ Assessment

The focus must be on understanding that behavioral expressions communicate distress, and the response is to investigate the possible sources of distress and intervene appropriately. There are many possible reasons for BPSDs. After ruling out medical problems (e.g., pneumonia, dehydration, impaction, infection/sepsis, fractures, pain, or depression) as a cause of behavior, continued assessment to identify why distressing symptoms are occurring is important. Conditions such as constipation or urinary tract infections (UTIs) can cause great distress for cognitively impaired individuals and may lead to marked changes in behavior. Pain and discomfort are also common reasons for changes in behavior (striking out, resistance to care) (Cohen-Mansfield, 2013). After careful assessment of other possible causes of pain or discomfort, treatment with a trial of analgesics should be considered.

The need for socialization, support, and stimulation to address boredom can also contribute to changes in behavior (Cohen-Mansfield, 2013). "For the individual with late-stage dementia, a good deal of their discomfort comes from non-physiological sources, for example, from difficulty sorting out and negotiating everyday life activities" (Kovach, 1999, p. 412).

Putting yourself in the place of the person with an NCD and trying to see the world from his or her eyes will help you understand his or her behavior. Box 25.14 presents an example of seeing the world from the eyes of the individual with dementia. Questions of what, where, why, when, who, and what now are important components of the assessment of behavior. Box 25.15 presents a framework for asking questions about the possible meanings and messages behind observed behavior. Asking caregivers to play back the situation "as if in a movie" is often helpful in eliciting details and understanding the circumstances associated with the problematic behavior. Except in late-stage NCDs, when verbal communication may be problematic, the perspective of the individual should be elicited to determine what he or she can describe about the situation. It is also important to understand what aspect of the behavior is most problematic or distressing for the individuals and the caregiver and the treatment goal (Kales et al., 2014).

BOX 25.14 Understanding Behavior: Seeing Through the Eyes of the Person With Dementia

You are asleep in the chair at home when suddenly you are awakened by a person you have never seen before trying to undress you. Then he or she puts you naked into a hard, cold chair and wheels you down a hallway. Suddenly cold water hits you in the face and the person is touching your private areas. You don't understand why the person is trying to do this to you. You are embarrassed, frightened, cold, and angry. You hit and scream at this person and try to get away.

BOX 25.15 Framework for Asking Questions About the Meaning of Behavior

What?
What is being sought? What is happening? Does the behavior have a physical or emotional component or both? What are the person's responses? What would be done if the person was 20 years old instead of 80? What is the behavior saying? What is the emotion being expressed?

Where?
Where is the behavior occurring? What environmental triggers are involved?

When?
When does the behavior most frequently occur, for example, after activities of daily living (ADLs), during family visits, or at mealtimes?

Who?
Who is involved, for example, other residents, caregivers, or family?

Why?
What happened before, for example, poor communication, tasks too complicated, physical or medical problem, or person being rushed or forced to do something? Has this occurred before and why?

What Now?
What approaches and interventions (physical, psychosocial) are needed? What changes are needed and by whom? Who else might know something about the person or the behavior or approaches? Communicate to all and include in plan of care.

Adapted from Hellen C: Can you provide care for residents with difficult behaviors? *Alzheimers Care Q* 1(4):4, 2000; Ortigara A: Understanding the language of behaviors, *Alzheimers Care Q* 1(4):91, 2000.

TABLE 25.2 Examples of Behavior and Environmental Modification Strategies for Managing BPSDs

Behavior	Strategy
Hearing voices	Evaluate hearing or adjust amplification of hearing aids. Assess quality and severity of symptoms. Determine whether they present an actual threat to safety or function. Assess noise around patient's room (e.g., staff talking in hallway).
Aggression	Determine and modify underlying causes of aggression (e.g., pain, caregiver interaction, being forced to do something). Teach caregiver not to confront individual, use distraction, observe facial expression and body posture, leave individual alone if safe, return later for the task (e.g., bathing). Create a calmer, more soothing environment.
Repetitive questioning	Respond with a calm, reassuring voice. Use calm touch for reassurance. Place warm water bottle covered with soft fleece cover on the lap or abdomen (Fitzsimmons et al., 2014). Inform individual of events only as they occur. Structure daily routines. Involve person in meaningful activities.

Adapted from Kales H, Gitlin L, Lyketsos C, et al: Management of neuropsychiatric symptoms of dementia in clinical settings: Recommendations from a multidisciplinary expert panel, *J Am Geriatr Soc* 62:762–769, 2014.

Use of a behavioral log or diary over a 2- to 3-day period to track when the behavior occurs, the circumstances, and the response to interventions is recommended and required in skilled nursing facilities. The Behave-AD, the Cohen-Mansfield Agitation Inventory, and the Neuropsychiatric Inventory for Nursing Homes are examples of reliable instruments that can be used in assessment. Table 25.2 presents examples of some common behaviors and possible strategies.

◆ Interventions

◆ Pharmacological Approaches

All evidence-based guidelines endorse an approach that begins with comprehensive assessment of the behavior and possible causes followed by the use of nonpharmacological interventions as a first line of treatment except in emergency situations when BPSDs could lead to imminent danger or compromise safety (American Geriatrics Society, 2014; Centers for Medicare and Medicaid Services, 2013; Kales et al., 2014). Despite these recommendations, antipsychotic medications to treat BPSDs are often given as the first-line response in nursing homes, hospitals, and ambulatory care centers without appropriate determination of whether there is a medical, physical, functional, psychological, psychiatric, social, or environmental cause of the behaviors (Gordon, 2014). Often, these drugs are prescribed in response to frustration and helplessness on the parts of both professionals and loved ones, in addition to inadequate knowledge of BPSDs in dementia and nonpharmacological interventions (Kales et al., 2014).

SAFETY ALERT

Do not use antipsychotics as your first choice to treat behavioral and psychological symptoms of dementia (BPSDs). People with dementia often exhibit aggression, resistance to care, and other challenging or disruptive behaviors. In such instances, antipsychotic medications are often prescribed, but they provide limited benefit and can cause serious harm, including stroke and premature death. Use of these drugs should be limited to cases where nonpharmacological measures have failed and patients pose an imminent threat to themselves or others. Identifying and addressing causes of behavior change can make drug treatment unnecessary (American Geriatrics Society, 2015).

Pharmacological approaches may be considered, in addition to nonpharmacological approaches, if there has been a comprehensive assessment of reversible causes of behavior (Box 25.16); the person presents a danger to self or others; nonpharmacological interventions have not been effective; and the risk/benefit profiles of the medications have been considered. If used, these medications should be given for the shortest period of time, monitored closely for side effects, and be subject to gradual dose reduction and re-review (CMS, 2013) (see Chapter 9).

In 2012, the Centers for Medicare and Medicaid Services (CMS) launched a nationwide public-private initiative to improve dementia care (Partnership to Improve Dementia Care in Nursing Homes). The mission of the Partnership is to enhance the use of nonpharmacological approaches and person-centered dementia care practices. One of the first initiatives was to reduce the use of unnecessary antipsychotic medications to address behavioral expressions in dementia care. Since 2011, there has been a decrease of 28.2% in use of antipsychotic medication in nursing homes (excluding residents diagnosed with schizophrenia,

BOX 25.16 Investigating Causes of Behavior

- What was the person trying to communicate through the behavior; what were the possible reasons for the person's behavior that led to the initiation of the medication?
- What other approaches and interventions were attempted before the use of the antipsychotic medication?
- Was the family or representative contacted before initiating the medication?
- Were personal needs not being met appropriately or sufficiently, such as hunger, thirst, or constipation?
- Was there fatigue, lack of sleep, or change in sleep patterns that may make the person more likely to misinterpret environmental cues, resulting in anxiety, aggression, or confusion?
- Were there environmental factors involved, for example, noise levels that could be causing or contributing to discomfort or misinterpretation of noises such as overhead pagers or alarms, causing delusions or hallucinations?
- Was there a mismatch between the activities or routines selected and the resident's cognitive and other abilities to participate in those activities/routines?

From Berkowitz C: Dust off your policies and procedures: CMS releases updates to SOM Appendix PP, *Florida Health Care Association, PULSE*, January 2015.

Huntington's disease, or Tourette's syndrome) to a national prevalence of 17.0% in the fourth quarter of 2015. The new national goal is to reduce the use of these medications by 30% by the close of 2016 (CMS, 2016). The American Psychiatric Association has issued practice guidelines for antipsychotic use in dementia (American Psychiatric Association, 2016). Use of antipsychotic drugs is now a quality indicator in the 5-Star rating system for nursing homes (see Chapter 6). A targeted dementia care–focused survey is also now in pilot testing across the country as part of an effort to improve all aspects of care of individuals with dementia residing in nursing homes (U.S. Department of Health and Human Services, 2015).

◆ Nonpharmacological Approaches

Nonpharmacological approaches tend to view behavior as stemming from unmet needs, environmental overload, and interactions of individual, caregiver, and environmental factors. The goals of nonpharmacological treatment are prevention, symptom relief, and reduction of caregiver distress (Kales et al., 2014). These approaches are resident-centered and include interventions such as meaningful activities tailored to the individual's personality and interests, validation therapy, social contact (real or simulated), animal-assisted therapy, exercise, sensory stimulation, art therapy, reminiscence, Montessori-based activities, environmental design (e.g., special care units, homelike environments, gardens, safe walking areas), changes in mealtime and bathing environments, consistent staffing assignments, bright light therapy, aromatherapy, massage, music, relaxation, distraction, nonconfrontational interaction, and pain management (Fitzsimmons et al., 2014; Gitlin et al., 2013; Gordon, 2014; Kolanowski et al., 2013).

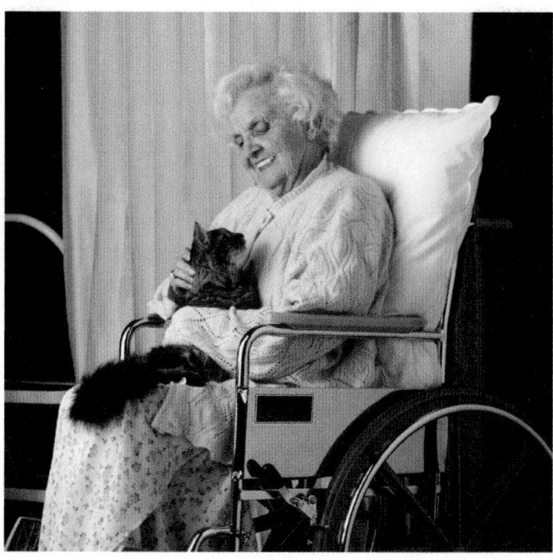

A nursing home resident enjoying pet therapy. (Courtesy Corbis.)

There is a large amount of literature on nonpharmacological interventions, and these approaches are recommended in the culture change movement (see Chapter 6). In general, these interventions have shown promise for improving quality of life for persons with dementia despite a lack of rigorous evaluation (Kales et al., 2014). Continued attention must be paid to translating these interventions into real-world practice. Pleasant sensory stimulation and relaxation methods such as bright light therapy, music therapy, Snoezelen (a relaxation technique popular in Europe), and massage have been studied most extensively, and there is good evidence for their effectiveness (Zimmerman et al., 2012). Other therapies with strong support include cognitive training/stimulation, physical exercise, and music (Burgener et al., 2015). Use of iPads to both prevent and address agitation in individuals with dementia holds interesting possibilities. Although further research is needed related to the types of applications and programs that are effective, preliminary findings suggested that even individuals with severe

BOX 25.17 Taking a Person-Centered Approach to BPSDs

Dr. A. was a retired cardiovascular surgeon with a history of dementia; he currently resided in a nursing home and was becoming increasingly agitated. Members of the interprofessional team expressed concerns about his behavior and the request for antipsychotic medications. Ivy, the director of nursing, knew about a new program using iPads for resident-family communication. Taking a person-centered approach, she knew this man was a physician who was now in a medical facility where he was the one receiving care. Upon the recommendation from nursing, the recreational therapist downloaded cardiovascular procedure videos and placed headphones on Dr. A.'s head. Within a brief time, a transformation took place. He became calm and appeared to enjoy the videos. Coming to know the person and recognizing his background led to nonpharmacological approaches to treat BPSD, thus avoiding the use of antipsychotic medication.

From Ivy Gordon-Thompson, RN, MSN, Director of Nursing, John Knox Village, Pompano Beach, FL.

cognitive impairment were able to interact with the device, and episodes of agitation and restlessness were reduced (Ross et al., 2015). Box 25.17 presents an exemplar on use of the iPad to calm agitation behavior. Practical guidance for implementing nonpharmacological approaches that emerged from focus groups with direct care providers is presented in Box 25.18.

Gerontological nurse researcher Ann Kolanowski co-led an expert panel that developed an on-line nursing home toolkit: *Promoting Positive Behavioral Health: A Non-pharmacologic Toolkit for Senior Living Communities* (Kolanowski & van Haitsma, 2013). The toolkit provides many resources for nurses, other caregivers, and families, including behavior assessment tools, clinical decision-making algorithms, and evidence-based approaches to ameliorate or prevent BPSDs.

CMS also has an on-line training tool specifically for nursing homes that teaches staff how to employ nonpharmacological alternatives in caring for individuals with BPSDs: Hand in Hand program (Box 25.5). Health care providers and family caregivers can benefit from training in approaches for behavioral concerns, and behavioral health programs must be better integrated with medical care for individuals with dementia.

PROVIDING CARE FOR ACTIVITIES OF DAILY LIVING

The losses associated with dementia interfere with the person's communication patterns and ability to understand and express thoughts and feelings. Perceptual disturbances and misinterpretations of reality contribute to fear and misunderstanding. Often, bathing and the provision of other ADL care, such as dressing, grooming, and toileting, are the cause of much distress for both the person with dementia and the caregiver.

BOX 25.18 Practical Guidance for Nonpharmacological Approaches

- Human behaviors are a dynamic, moving target; all of us have good and bad days and what works on one day may not work the next; it can be really difficult to pinpoint "what set someone off" on any given day.
- It is all about trial and error; there is no magic bullet.
- Foster a mind-set of "Let's try it and see what happens." Always have a backup approach if a given approach is not successful. One trial of an approach may not be sufficient; try again another day. Interview and observe what a "successful" direct care provider is doing and saying.
- Individualizing (tailoring) the approach to a given person is critical to success. Get to know the person's preferences, past history. Come to know the person as a unique individual.
- Relax the "rules." There is no right or wrong way to perform an activity if the individual is safe.
- Understand that behaviors are not intentional or done "in spite" but are a consequence of the person's inability to initiate or comprehend steps of a task or its purpose.

From CMS: Center for Clinical Standards and Quality/Survey & Certification Center, 2013.

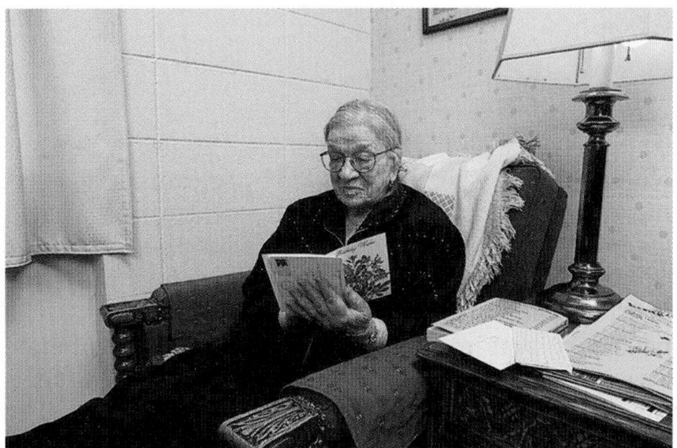

Meaningful activities provide cognitive stimulation. (From Sorrentino SA, Gorek B: *Mosby's textbook for long-term care assistants,* ed 5, St Louis, 2007, Mosby.)

Bathing

Bathing is an essential aspect of everyday life that most people enjoy. However, bathing and care for ADLs can

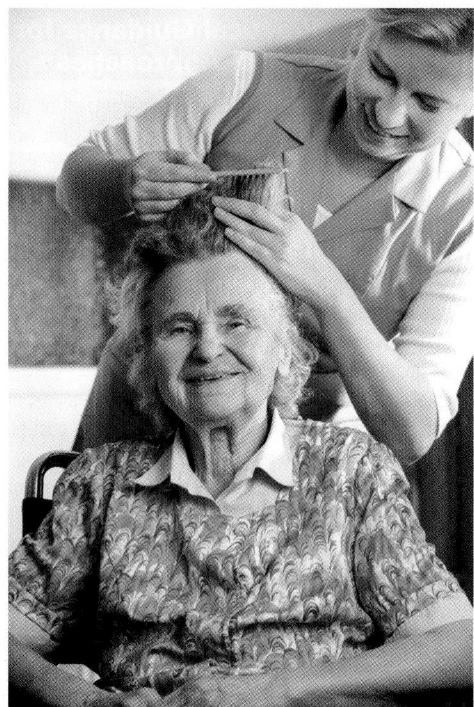
ADL care enhances self-esteem. (© iStock.com/AlexRaths.)

BOX 25.19 Techniques for Bathing Without a Battle

1. Rethink the bathing experience.
   - Make the experience comfortable and pleasurable.
   - Consider what makes the individual feel good.
   - Determine preferred methods for bathing (bath, shower, bathe at sink).
   - Do not be in a hurry.
2. Use approach techniques such as "let's go get freshened up for the day" and avoid bathing terminology (e.g., "it's time for your bath") to create a more positive environment.
   - Tell person it is time to get freshened up and try not to ask "do you want a bath?" because the answer may be no.
3. Have the room ready.
   - Keep the room warm and low-lit.
   - Hand-held showerhead wets one area at a time.
   - Have a large towel or blanket to preserve dignity and keep person warm.
4. Begin bathing least sensitive area first.
   - Wash legs and feet first, followed by arms, trunk, perineum area, and face last.
   - Give the individual a washcloth to assist in bathing.
5. Save washing hair until last or do separately.
6. Use distraction techniques.
   - Consider using music or singing songs that the person likes.
   - Consider having the person hold a towel or something to provide distraction.
7. Consider a towel bath for those who may not respond to the above strategies.

be perceived with fright as a personal attack by persons with dementia who may respond by screaming or striking out (Box 25.13). In institutional settings, a rigid focus on tasks or institutional care routines, such as a shower three mornings each week, can contribute to the distress and precipitate distressing behaviors. The behaviors that may be exhibited are not deliberate attacks on caregivers by a violent person, but rather a way to express self in an uncertain situation. The message is, in the words of Rader and Barrick: "Please find another way to keep me clean, because the way you are doing it now is intolerable" (2000, p. 49).

IMPLICATIONS FOR GERONTOLOGICAL NURSING AND HEALTHY AGING

Assessment and Interventions

In research conducted in nursing homes, Rader and Barrick (2000) have provided comprehensive guidelines for bathing people with dementia in ways that are pleasurable and decrease distress. Asking the question "What is the easiest, most comfortable, least frightening way for me to clean the person right now?" guides the choice of interventions (Rader & Barrick, 2000, p. 42). *Bathing Without a Battle* is an approach that can be used to create a better bathing experience for people with dementia (Box 25.19). Another innovative approach being investigated in Sweden is caregiver singing and the use of background music during ADL care in nursing homes. Caregivers play and sing familiar songs during care routines. When compared to usual care practices, this approach enhanced the expression of positive moods and emotions, increased the mutuality of communication, and reduced aggression and resistive care behaviors (Hammar et al., 2011).

The use of music and other sound stimulation can contribute to improved health and well-being and is easily implemented in long-term care facilities. This cost-effective intervention includes use of CD players, iPads, personalized playlists, sing-a-long or music-making groups, group or individual music therapy, recreational music activities, and background music (Clements-Cortes & Bartel, 2015).

WANDERING

Wandering associated with dementia is one of the most difficult management problems encountered in home and institutional settings. One in five people with dementia wanders. Wandering is a complex behavior and is not well understood. Wandering is defined as "a syndrome of dementia-related locomotion behavior having a frequent, repetitive, temporally disordered and/or spatially disoriented nature that is manifested in lapping, random and or pacing patterns, some of which is associated with eloping, eloping attempts or getting lost unless accompanied" (Algase et al., 2007, p. 696).

Risk factors for wandering include visuospatial impairments, anxiety and depression, poor sleep patterns, unmet needs, and a more socially active and outgoing premorbid lifestyle (Futrell et al., 2014; Lester et al., 2012). Wandering frequency tends to increase as cognitive function decreases (Futrell et al., 2014). There is a need for more research and evidence-based interventions to understand this behavior.

Wandering presents safety concerns in all settings. Wandering behavior affects sleeping, eating, safety, and the caregiver's ability to provide care, and it also interferes with the privacy of others. The behavior can lead to falls, elopement (leaving the home or facility), injury, and death (Futrell et al., 2010; Rowe et al., 2010). The stimulus for wandering arises from many internal and external sources. Wandering can be considered a rhythm, intrinsically and extrinsically driven. Box 25.20 presents insight into the behavior of wandering from the perspective of individuals with dementia.

BOX 25.20 Patient Perspectives on Wandering Behavior

Davis, 1989, p. 96

"Wandering and restlessness is one of the by-products of Alzheimer's disease ... When the darkness and emptiness fills my mind, it is totally terrifying ... Thoughts increasingly haunt me. The only way I can break the cycle is to move."

Henderson, 1998

"Very often, I wander around looking for something which I know is very pertinent, but then after a while I forget all about what it was I was looking for. When I'm wandering around, I'm trying to touch base with—anything, actually. If anything appeared I'd probably enjoy it, or look at it or examine it and wonder how it got there. I feel very foolish when I'm wandering around not knowing what I'm doing and I'm not always quite sure how to do any better. It's not easy to figure out what the heck I'm looking for."

❖IMPLICATIONS FOR GERONTOLOGICAL NURSING AND HEALTHY AGING

◆ Assessment and Interventions

Careful assessment of physical problems that may trigger wandering, such as acute illness, exacerbations of chronic illness, fatigue, medication effects, need to urinate, and constipation, is important. Unmet needs or pain can increase wandering (Futrell et al., 2014). Wandering behaviors can be predicted through careful observation and awareness of the person's patterns. For example, if the person with dementia starts wandering or trying to leave the home in the afternoon every day, meaningful activities such as music, exercise, and refreshments can be provided at this time. Research suggests that wandering may be less likely to occur when the person is involved in social interaction.

There are also several instruments to assess risk for wandering, and nurse researcher May Futrell and colleagues (2010, 2014) developed an evidence-based protocol for wandering. There are a number of assistive technology devices and programs that can enhance the safety of persons who wander (see Chapter 20). The Hartford Institute for Geriatric Nursing has a Home Safety Inventory for Older Adults with Dementia (Box 25.5). Box 25.21 presents other suggested interventions.

Wandering behavior may also result in people with dementia going outside and getting lost, a phenomenon studied by nurse researcher Meredith Rowe (2003). All people with dementia should be considered capable of getting lost. Caregivers must prevent people with dementia from leaving homes or care facilities unaccompanied, register the person in the Alzheimer's Association Safe Return program, and have a plan of action in case the person does become lost.

In care facilities, "a risk-management approach needs to include (1) identification of the wanderer; (2) a wandering prevention program; (3) an elopement response plan when patients are missing; and (4) staff mobilization around the problem" (Futrell et al., 2014, p. 22). Rowe also suggests that police must respond rapidly to requests for searches, and the general public should be informed about how to recognize and assist people with dementia who may be lost (Rowe, 2003).

NUTRITION

Older adults with dementia are particularly at risk for weight loss and inadequate nutrition. Weight loss often becomes a considerable concern in late-stage dementia. Some of the factors predisposing individuals with dementia to nutritional inadequacy include lack of awareness of the need to eat, depression, loss of

BOX 25.21 Tips for Best Practice

Interventions for Wandering or Exiting Behaviors

- Face the person and make direct eye contact (unless this is interpreted as threatening).
- Gently touch the person's arm, shoulders, back, or waist if he/she does not move away from a door or other exit.
- Call the person by his or her formal name (e.g., Mr. Jones).
- Listen to what the person is communicating verbally and nonverbally; listen to the feelings expressed.
- Repeat specific words or phrases, or state the need or emotion (e.g., "You need to go home; you're worried about your husband.").
- If such repetition fails to distract the person, accompany him or her, talking calmly, repeating phrases and the emotion you identify.
- Provide orienting information only if it calms the person. If it increases distress, stop talking about the present situations. Do not "correct" the person or belittle his or her agenda.
- At intervals, redirect the person toward the facility or his home by suggesting: "Let's walk this way now" or "I'm so tired, let's turn around."
- If orientation and redirection fail, continue to walk, allowing the person control but ensuring safety.
- Make sure you have a backup person, but he or she should stay out of eyesight of the person.
- Have someone call for help if you are unable to redirect. Usually the behavior is time limited because of the person's attention span and the security and trust between you and the person.

Adapted from Rader J et al: How to decrease wandering, a form of agenda behavior, *Geriatr Nurs* 6(4):196–199.

independence in self-feeding, agnosia, apraxia, vision impairments (deficient contrast sensitivity), wandering, pacing, and behavior disturbances. Weight loss increases risk for infection, pressure wound development and poor wound healing, and hospitalization, and is associated with higher mortality and morbidity. Nurses, as members of interprofessional teams, play a significant role in assessing nutrition in persons with dementia. Chapter 10 discusses nutritional needs and interventions in depth.

❖ IMPLICATIONS FOR GERONTOLOGICAL NURSING AND HEALTHY AGING

◆ Assessment and Interventions

Assessment includes evaluation of nutrition status and identification of eating and feeding problems through observation of meals. The Mini Nutritional Assessment (MNA) is an easy tool to identify those at risk (see Chapter 10). Collaborating with a dietitian to perform a clinical examination that yields information regarding potential or real nutritional deficits is an excellent way to develop strategies to minimize or improve the nutritional status of persons with dementia.

One of the best strategies for managing poor intake is establishing a routine so that the older person does not have to remember time and places for eating. Caregivers should continue to serve foods and fluids that the person likes and has always eaten. Nutrient-dense foods (e.g., peanut butter, protein bars, yogurt) are preferred. Attention to mealtime ambience is important, and the person should be able to take as much time as needed to eat the food. Food should be available 24 hours a day, and the person should be allowed to follow his or her accustomed eating schedule (e.g., late breakfast, early dinner). Other suggestions to enhance food intake for individuals with dementia are presented in Box 25.22.

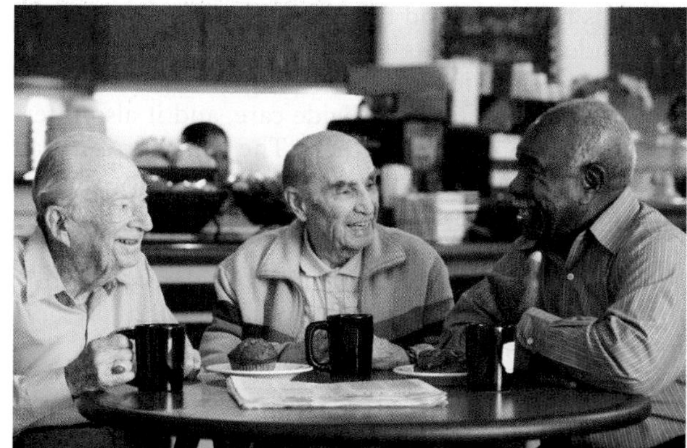

A pleasurable dining experience can enhance intake. (© iStock.com/monkeybusinessimages.)

NURSING ROLES IN THE CARE OF PERSONS WITH DEMENTIA

Caregiving for someone with dementia by family members, or formal caregivers, requires special skills, knowledge of evidence-based practice, and a deep understanding of the person. Rader and Tornquist (1995) reflect on the knowledge required and provide a view of caregiving roles that is quite useful and understandable for all caregivers. The authors have found that nursing assistants and family caregivers can truly relate to the practical wisdom in these words.

- **Magician role:** To understand what the person is trying to communicate both verbally and nonverbally, we must be a magician who can use our

BOX 25.22 Tips for Best Practice

Improving Intake for Individuals With Dementia

- Serve only one dish at a time.
- Provide only one utensil at a time.
- Consider using a "spork" (combination spoon-fork).
- Serve finger foods such as fried chicken, chicken strips, pizza in bite-size pieces, fish sticks, sandwiches.
- Serve soup in a mug.
- Remove any hot items or items that should not be eaten.
- Cut up foods before serving.
- Sit next to the person at his or her level.
- Demonstrate eating motions that the person can imitate.
- Use hand-over-hand feeding technique to guide self-feeding.
- Use verbal cueing and prompting (e.g., take a bite, chew, swallow).
- Use gentle tone of voice, and avoid scolding or demeaning remarks.
- Provide verbal encouragement to participate in eating by talking about food taste and smell.
- Offer small amounts of fluid between bites.
- Help person focus on the meal at hand; turn off background noise, remove clutter from the table.
- Avoid patterned dishes or table coverings.
- Use red plates/glasses/cups; food intake may increase when food is served with high-contrast tableware.
- Use unbreakable dishes that will not slide around.
- Serve smaller, more frequent meals rather than expecting the person to complete a big meal.

Data from Dunne T, Neargarder S, Cipolloni P, et al: Visual contrast enhances food and liquid intake in advanced Alzheimer's disease, *Clin Nutr* 23(4):533–538, 2004; Spencer P: *How to solve eating problems common to people with Alzheimer's and other dementias*. Retrieved June 1, 2015, from https://www.caring.com/articles/alzheimers-eating-problems.

magical abilities to see the world through the eyes, the ears, and the feelings of the person. We know how to use tricks to change an individual's behavior or prevent it from occurring and causing distress.

- **Detective role:** The detective looks for clues and cues about what might be causing distress and how it might be changed. We have to investigate and know as much about the person as possible to be a good detective.
- **Carpenter role:** By having a wide variety of tools and selecting the right tools for the job, we build individualized plans of care for each person.
- **Jester role:** Many people with dementia retain their sense of humor and respond well to the appropriate use of humor. This does not mean making fun of the person but rather sharing laughter and fun. "Those who love their work and do it well employ good doses of humor as part of the care of others, as well as for self-care" (Rader & Barrick, 2000, p. 42). The jester spreads joy, is creative, energizes, and lightens the burdens (Laurenhue, 2001; Rader & Barrick, 2000).

Fig. 25.1 presents a nursing situation that one nurse experienced in caring for a patient with dementia who was being admitted to a nursing home. Written from the perspective of the nurse and his knowledge of the patient, the story provides insight into important nursing responses, such as providing person-centered care, implementing therapeutic communication, and establishing meaningful relationships. It is a lovely example of expert gerontological nursing for individuals with dementia and a fitting way to end this chapter.

KEY CONCEPTS

- Nurses must advocate for thorough assessment of any elder who appears to be experiencing cognitive decline and inability to function in important aspects of life.
- Delirium results from the interaction of predisposing factors (e.g., vulnerability on the part of the individual attributable to predisposing conditions such as cognitive impairment, severe illness, sensory impairment) and precipitating factors/insults (e.g., medications, procedures, restraints).
- Delirium is characterized by fluctuating levels of consciousness, sometimes in a diurnal pattern, and frequent misperceptions and illusions. It is often unrecognized and is attributed to age or dementia. People with dementia are more susceptible to delirium. Knowledge of risk factors, preventive measures, and treatment of underlying medical problems is essential to prevent serious consequences.
- Acute illness (e.g., UTIs, respiratory tract infections), medications, and pain are frequently the causes of delirium in older people. Individuals with dementia are highly susceptible to delirium.
- It is essential to view all behavior as meaningful and an expression of needs. The focus must be on understanding that behavioral expressions communicate distress and the response is to investigate the possible source of distress and intervene appropriately.
- Fear, discomfort, unfamiliar surroundings and people, illness, fatigue, depression, need for autonomy and control, caregiver approaches and communication, and environmental stressors are frequent precipitants of behavioral symptoms.

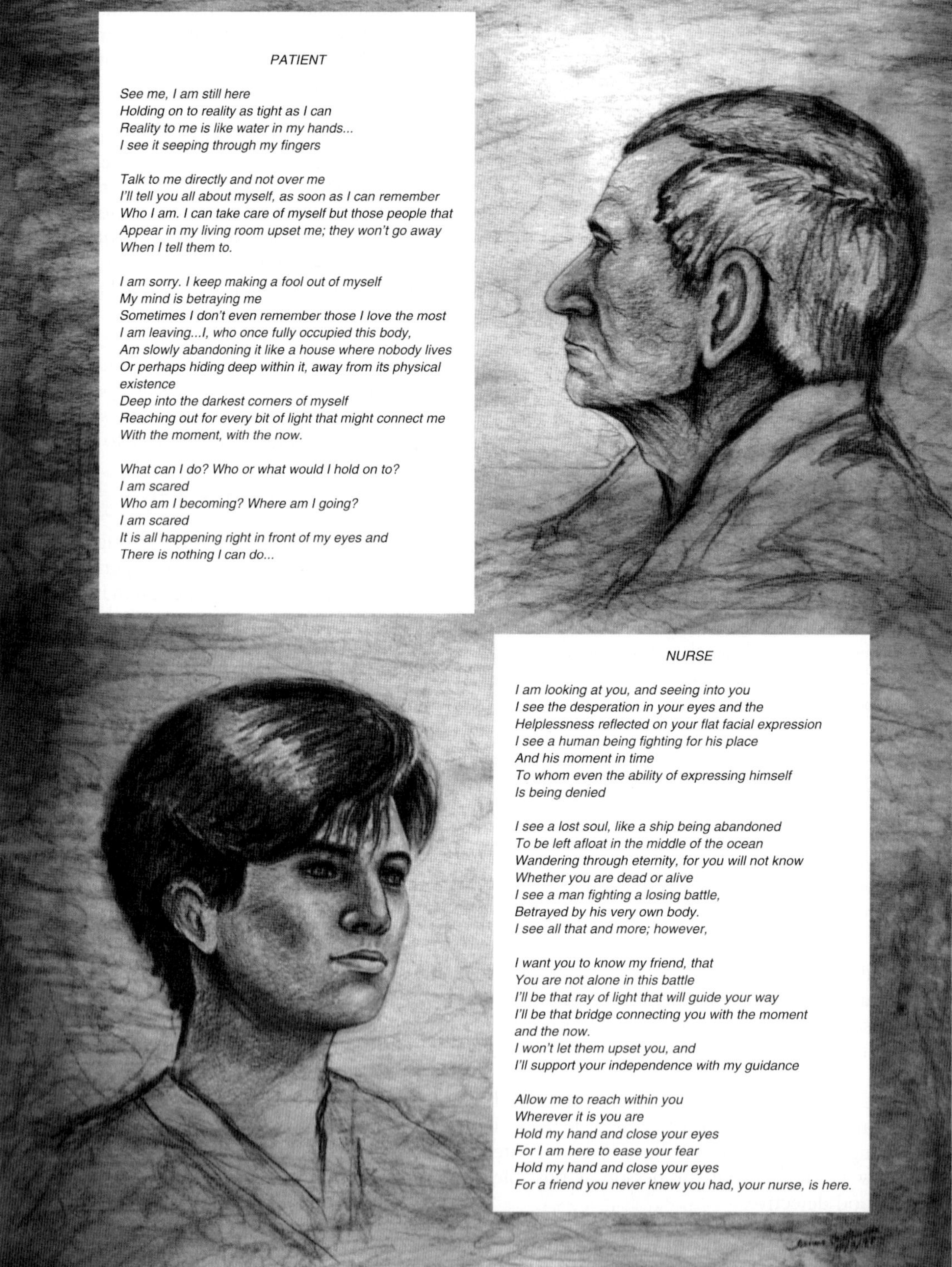

FIGURE 25.1 Nurse and person. (Copyright © 1998 by Jaime Castaneda, Lake Worth, FL.)

- All evidence-based guidelines endorse an approach that begins with comprehensive assessment of BPSDs and possible causes followed by use of nonpharmacological interventions as a first-line treatment, except in emergency situations when symptoms could lead to imminent danger or compromise safety.
- Individuals with cognitive impairment respond best to calmness and patience, adaptations of communication techniques, and environments and relationships that enhance function, support limitations, ensure safety, and provide opportunities for a meaningful quality of life. Because cognitively impaired persons may be unable to express their feelings and needs in ways that are easily understood, the gerontological nurse must always try to understand the world from their perspective.

ACTIVITIES AND DISCUSSION QUESTIONS

1. What are the differences between delirium, dementia, and depression?
2. What are some of the risk factors for development of delirium?
3. Discuss communication strategies useful for the person experiencing delirium.
4. Why is it important to ensure that the person experiencing any change in mental status receives a thorough assessment and evaluation?
5. Brainstorm with fellow students how it would feel to be bathed by a total stranger.
6. The nursing assistants in a nursing home complain to you that Mr. G. hit them when they were trying to give him his required twice-weekly shower. How might you assist them in meeting Mr. G.'s need for bathing?
7. A family caregiver tells you that his or her loved one keeps trying to leave the house to find the children. What are some strategies you might share with the caregiver to deal with this situation?

REFERENCES

Algase DL, Beel-Bates C, Beattie ERA: Wandering in long-term care, *Ann Longterm Care* 11:33–39, 2003.

Algase DL, Moore DH, Vanderweerd C, et al: Mapping the maze of terms and definitions in dementia-related wandering, *Aging Ment Health* 11:686–698, 2007.

American College of Surgeons/NSQI/American Geriatrics Society: *Optimal perioperative management of the geriatric patient*, 2014. Available at https://www.facs.org/~/media/files/quality%20programs/geriatric/acs%20nsqip%20geriatric%202016%20guidelines.ashx. Accessed February 2016.

American Geriatrics Society: AGS updated Beers Criteria for potentially inappropriate medication use in older adults, *J Am Geriatr Soc* 60(4):616–631, 2012.

American Geriatrics Society: *Clinical practice guidelines for postoperative delirium in older adults*, 2014.

American Geriatrics Society: *Ten things physicians and patients should question*, April 23, 2015. Available at http://www.choosingwisely.org/societies/american-geriatrics-society/. Accessed February 2016.

American Psychiatric Association: *Diagnostic and statistical manual of mental disorders*, ed 5, Washington, DC, 2013, Author.

American Psychiatric Association Guideline Writing Group: *New practice guidelines on antipsychotic use in dementia*, 2016. Available at http://psychiatryonline.org/doi/book/10.1176/appi.books.9780890426807.

Balas M, Rice M, Chaperon C, et al: Management of delirium in critically ill older adults, *Crit Care Nurse* 32(4):15–26, 2012.

Bledowski J, Trutia A: A review of pharmacologic management and prevention strategies for delirium in the intensive care unit, *J Lifelong Learning Psychiatry* XI(4):568–575, 2013.

Braes T, Milisen K: Foremen M: Assessing cognitive function. In Capezuti E, Zwicker D, Mezey M, et al, editors: *Evidence-based geriatric nursing protocols for best practice*, ed 3, New York, 2008, Springer, pp 122–134.

Buckwalter K, Gerdner L, Hall G, et al: Shining through: The humor and individuality of persons with Alzheimer's disease, *J Gerontol Nurs* 21:11–16, 1995.

Burgener S, Jao Y-L, Anderson J, et al: Mechanism of action for nonpharmacological therapies for individuals with dementia: Implications for practice and research, *Res Gerontol Nurs* 2015. doi: 10.3928/19404921-20150429-02.

Centers for Medicare and Medicaid Services: *Center for Clinical Standards and Quality/Survey and Certification Group (Memo)*, May 14, 2013. Available at http://www.cms.gov/Medicare/Provider-Enrollment-and-Certification/SurveyCertificationGenInfo/Downloads/Survey-and-Cert-Letter-13-35.pdf. Accessed May 19, 2015.

Centers for Medicare and Medicaid Services: *National partnership to improve dementia care in nursing homes: Antipsychotic medication use trend update*, February 2016. Available at http://www.leadingageny.org/providers/nursing-homes/survey-clinical-and-quality/antipsychotic-drug-use-in-nursing-homes-trend-update/. Accessed February 2016.

Clements-Cortes A, Bartel L: Sound stimulation in patients with Alzheimer's disease, *Ann Longterm Care* 23(5):10–16, 2015.

Cohen-Mansfield J: Nonpharmacologic treatment of behavioral disorders in dementia, *Curr Treat Options Neurol* 15(6):765–785, 2013.

Dahlke S, Phinney A: Caring for hospitalized older adults at risk for delirium: The silent, unspoken piece of nursing practice, *J Gerontol Nurs* 34:41–47, 2008.

Davis R: *My journey into Alzheimer's disease*, Wheaton, IL, 1989, Tyndale House.

Dettmore D, Kolanowski A, Boustani M: Aggression in persons with dementia: Use of nursing theory to guide clinical practice, *Geriatr Nurs* 30:8–17, 2009.

DeYoung S, Just G, Harrison R: Decreasing aggressive, agitated, or disruptive behavior: Participation in a behavior management unit, *J Gerontol Nurs* 28:22–31, 2003.

Evans L, Kurlowicz L: *Complex care needs in older adults with common cognitive disorders, Section A: Assessment and management of dementia*, 2007. Available at http://hartfordign.org/uploads/File/gnec_state_of_science_papers/gnec_delirium.pdf. Accessed February 2016.

Fick D, Inouye S, Guess J, et al: Preliminary development of an ultrabrief two-item bedside test for delirium, *J Hosp Med* 2015. doi: 10.1002/jhm2418.

Fitzsimmons S, Barba B, Stump M: Sensory and nurturing pharmacological interventions for behavioral and psychological symptoms of dementia, *J Gerontol Nurs* 40(11):9–15, 2014.

Futrell M, Mellilo K, Remington R, et al: Evidence-based practice guideline: Wandering, *J Gerontol Nurs* 36:6–16, 2010.

Futrell M, Mellilo K, Remington R, et al: Evidence-based practice guideline: Wandering, *J Gerontol Nurs* 40(11):16–23, 2014.

Gitlin L, Mann W, Vogel W, et al: A non-pharmacologic approach to address challenging behaviors of veterans with dementia: Description of the tailored activity program—VA randomized trial, *BMC Geriatr* 13:96, 2013.

Gordon M: When should antipsychotics for the management of behavioral and psychological symptoms of dementia be discontinued?, *Ann Longterm Care* 22(4):2014. Available at: http://www.annalsoflongtermcare.com/article/antipsychotics-discontinued-management-behavioral-psychological-symptoms-dementia. Accessed February 2016.

Hain D, Tappen R, Diaz S, et al: Cognitive impairment and medication self-management errors in older adults discharged home from a community hospital, *Home Healthc Nurse* 30(4):246–254, 2012.

Hain D, Touhy T, Engstrom G: What matters most to carers of people with mild to moderate dementia as evidence for transforming care, *Alzheimers Care Today* 11:162–171, 2010.

Hain D, Touhy T, Sparks D, et al: Using narratives of individuals and couples living with early dementia to guide practice, *JNPARR* 4(2):82–93, 2014.

Hall GR: Caring for people with Alzheimer's disease using the conceptual model of progressively lowered stress threshold in the clinical setting, *Nurs Clin North Am* 29:129–141, 1994.

Hall GR, Buckwalter KC: Progressively lowered stress threshold: A conceptual model for care of adults with Alzheimer's disease, *Arch Psychiatr Nurs* 1:399–406, 1987.

Hammar LM, Emami A, Engstrom G, et al: Communicating through caregiver singing during morning care situations in dementia care, *Scand J Caring Sci* 25(1):160–168, 2011.

Henderson C: *Partial view: An Alzheimer's journal*, Dallas, TX, 1998, Southern Methodist Press.

Inouye SK, Bogardus ST Jr, Charpentier PA, et al: A multicomponent intervention to prevent delirium in hospitalized older patients, *N Engl J Med* 340:669–676, 1999.

Inouye SK, van Dyck CH, Alessi CA, et al: Clarifying confusion: The Confusion Assessment: A new method for detection of delirium, *Ann Intern Med* 113:941–948, 1990.

Inouye SK, Westendorp RG, Saczynski JS: Delirium in elderly people, *Lancet* 383:911–922, 2014.

Kales H, Gitlin L, Lyketsos C, et al: Management of neuropsychiatric symptoms of dementia in clinical settings: Recommendations from a multidisciplinary panel, *J Am Geriatr Soc* 62:762–769, 2014.

Kolanowski A: An overview of the need-driven dementia-compromised behavior model, *J Gerontol Nurs* 25:7–9, 1999.

Kolanowski A, Van Haitsma K: *Promoting positive behavioral health: A non-pharmacologic toolkit for senior living communities*, 2013. Available at http://www.nursinghometoolkit.com. Accessed February 2016.

Kolanowski A, Resnick B, Beck C, et al: Advances in nonpharmacological interventions, 2011–2012, *Res Gerontol Nurs* 6(1):5–8, 2013.

Kovach C: Assessment and treatment of discomfort for people with late-stage dementia, *J Pain Symptom Manage* 18(6):412–419, 1999.

Kuehn B: Delirium often not recognized or treated despite serious long-term consequences, *JAMA* 304:389–390, 2010a.

Kuehn B: Questionable antipsychotic prescribing remains common despite serious risks, *JAMA* 303:1582–1584, 2010b.

Laurenhue K: Each person's journey is unique, *Alzheimers Care Q* 2:79–83, 2001.

Lester P, Garite A, Kohen I: Wandering and elopement in nursing homes, *Ann Longterm Care* 20(3):32–36, 2012.

Lindquist I, Go L, Fleisher J, et al: Improvements in cognition following hospital discharge of community dwelling seniors, *J Gen Intern Med* 26(7):765–770, 2011.

Marcantonio E, Bergmann M, Kiely D, et al: Randomized trial of a delirium abatement program for postacute skilled nursing facilities, *J Am Geriatr Soc* 58:1019–1026, 2010.

McGowin DF: *Living in the labyrinth: A personal journey through the maze of Alzheimer's*, New York, 1993, Dell.

Neelon VJ, Champagne MT, Carlson JR, et al: The NEECHAM confusion scale: Construction, validation and clinical testing, *Nurs Res* 45:324–330, 1996.

Neufeld K, Yue J, Robinson T, et al: Antipsychotic medication for prevention and treatment of delirium in hospitalized adults: A systematic review and meta-analysis, *J Am Geriatr Soc* 2016. doi: 10.1111/jgs.14076.

O'Mahony R, Murthy L, Akunne A, et al: Synopsis of the National Institute for Health and Clinical Excellence guideline for prevention of delirium, *Ann Intern Med* 154:746–751, 2011.

Rader J, Barrick A: Ways that work: Bathing without a battle, *Alzheimers Care Q* 1:35–49, 2000.

Rader J, Tornquist E: *Individualized dementia care*, New York, 1995, Springer.

Reinhard S, Samis S, Levine C: *Family caregivers providing complex chronic care to people with cognitive and behavioral health conditions*, Insight on the Issues 93, August 2014, AARP Public Policy Institute. Available at http://www.aarp.org/home-family/caregiving/info-2014/family-caregivers-providing-complex-chronic-care-cognitive-behavioral-AARP-ppi-health.html. Accessed February 2016.

Reston JT, Schoelles KM: In-facility delirium prevention programs as a patient safety strategy: A systematic review, *Ann Intern Med* 158(5 Pt 2):375–380, 2013.

Richards K, Lambert C, Beck C: Deriving interventions for challenging behaviors from the need-driven dementia-compromised behavior model, *Alzheimers Care Q* 1:62–72, 2000.

Ross L, Ramirez S, Bhatt A, et al: *Tables devices (IPad) for control of behavioral symptoms in older adults with dementia*, Presented at the American Association for Geriatric Psychiatry (AAGP) 2015 Annual Meeting, March 31, 2015.

Rowe MA: People with dementia who become lost, *Am J Nurs* 103:32–39, 2003.

Rowe MA, Kairalla JA, McCrae CS: Sleep in dementia caregivers and the effect of a nighttime monitoring system, *J Nurs Scholarsh* 42:338–347, 2010.

Sifton C: Life is what happens while we are making plans, *Alzheimers Care Q* 2:iv, 2001.

Splete H: Nurses have special strategies for dementia, *Caring Ages* 9:11, 2008.

Steis M, Fick D: Are nurses recognizing delirium?, *J Gerontol Nurs* 34:40–48, 2008.

Steis M, Evans L, Hirschman K, et al: Screening for delirium using family caregivers: Convergent validity of the Family Confusion Assessment Method and interviewer-rated Confusion Assessment Method, *J Am Geriatr Soc* 60(11):2121–2126, 2012.

Tappen R, Williams-Burgess C, Edelstein J, et al: Communicating with individuals with Alzheimer's disease: Examination of recommended strategies, *Arch Psychiatr Nurs* 11:249–256, 1997.

Tappen R, Williams C, Fishman S, et al: Persistence of self in advanced Alzheimer's disease, *Image J Nurs Sch* 31:121–125, 1999.

Touhy T: Dementia, personhood and nursing: Learning from a nursing situation, *Nurs Sci Q* 17:43–49, 2004.

Tullmann D, Fletcher K, Foreman M: Boltz M, Capezuti E, Fulmer T, et al, editors: *Evidence-based geriatric nursing protocols for best practice*, ed 4, New York, 2012, Springer.

Tullmann D, Mion L, Fletcher K, et al: Delirium prevention, early recognition and treatment. In Capezuti E, Zwicker D, Mezey M, et al, editors: *Evidence-based geriatric nursing: protocols for best practice*, ed 3, New York, 2008, Springer.

U.S. Department of Health and Human Services, Centers for Medicare and Medicaid Services: *Focused dementia care survey tools*, November 2015. Available at https://www.cms.gov/Medicare/Provider-Enrollment-and-Certification/SurveyCertificationGenInfo/Downloads/Survey-and-Cert-Letter-16-04.pdf. Accessed February 2016.

Voyer P, Richard S, Doucet L, et al: Examination of the multifactorial model of delirium among long-term care residents with dementia, *Geriatr Nurs* 31:105–114, 2010.

Waszynski C, Petrovic K: Nurses' evaluation of the Confusion Assessment Method: A pilot study, *J Gerontol Nurs* 34:49–56, 2008.

Williams C, Tappen R: Communicating with cognitively impaired persons. In Williams C, editor: *Therapeutic interaction in nursing*, ed 2, Boston, 2008, Jones & Bartlett.

Woods B: Dementia challenges assumptions about what it means to be a person, *Generations* 13:39, 1999.

Zimmerman S, Anderson W, Brode S, et al: *Comparison of characteristics of nursing homes and other residential long-term care settings for people with dementia* (Comparative Effectiveness Review no. 79, AHRQ publication no. 12[13]-EHC127-EF), Rockville, MD, 2012, Agency for Healthcare Research and Quality.

26

Relationships, Roles, and Transitions

Theris A. Touhy

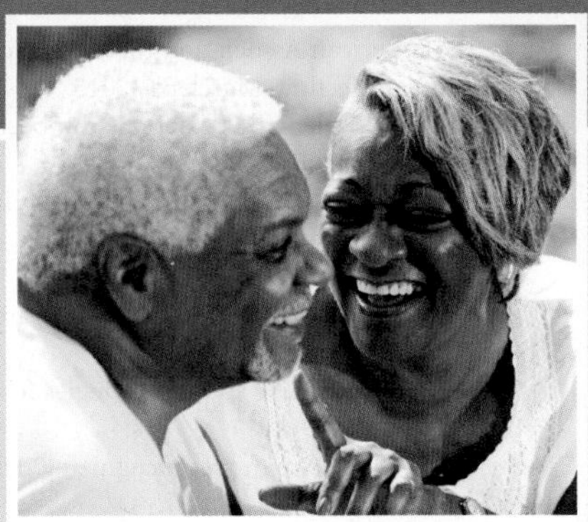

 evolve.elsevier.com/Touhy/gerontological

LEARNING OBJECTIVES

Upon completion of this chapter, the reader will be able to:

- Explain the issues involved in adapting to transitions and role changes in later life.
- Discuss changes in family structure and functions in today's society.
- Examine family relationships in later life.
- Discuss nursing responses with older adults experiencing transitions.
- Discuss intimacy and sexuality in late life and appropriate nursing responses.

THE LIVED EXPERIENCE

It is so irritating when Madge tries to help me do things. After all, I have lived 85 years and have done very well. I think she wants to put me away somewhere. I wish she would just leave me alone. I'm sure I could manage if she just wouldn't interfere.

John, the father

I just can't stand watching as my father becomes weaker and is unable to do the things he always did so naturally and well. Yesterday he got lost on his way to the market. He was always my guide and protector. I knew I could count on him no matter what. It makes me feel sort of alone in the world.

Madge, the daughter

LATER LIFE TRANSITIONS

This chapter examines the various relationships, roles, and transitions that characteristically play a part in later life. The transitions of retirement, widowhood, and widowerhood and the concepts of family structure and function, as well as intimacy and sexuality, are examined. Nursing responses to support older adults in maintaining fulfilling roles and relationships and adapting to transitions are discussed. Transition to becoming a caregiver or recipient of care is discussed in Chapter 27.

Retirement

Every culture has mechanisms for retiring their elders. Although retirement patterns differ across the world, in industrialized nations, as well as in many developing nations, the expectation is that older workers will cease full-time career job employment and be entitled to economic support (McNamara & Williamson, 2013). However, whether that support will be adequate, or even available, is a growing concern worldwide. In the United States and many European countries and Australia, the problems are emerging as the generation born after

World War II moves into retirement. Developing countries face similar issues with the growth of the older population combined with decreasing birth rates. Governments may not be able to afford retirement systems to replace the tradition of children caring for aging parents. Most countries are not ready to meet what is projected to be one of the defining challenges of the twenty-first century (Jackson et al., 2013).

Retirement, as we formerly knew it, has changed. The transitions are blurring, and the numerous patterns and styles of retiring have produced more varied experiences in retirement. Older adults are increasingly interested in part-time opportunities and other activities to stay busy and productive with age (National Institute on Aging, National Institutes of Health, U.S. Department of Health and Human Services, 2015). Retirement is no longer just a few years of rest from the rigors of work before death. It is a developmental stage that may occupy 30 or more years of one's life and involve many stages. Some individuals will be retired longer than they worked.

Retirees are living longer, and declining birth rates mean there will be fewer workers to support them. Countries are scaling down retirement benefits and raising the age to start collecting them. Individuals can expect to work longer before retirement, continue to work after they retire, or not retire at all (Board of Governors of the Federal Reserve System, 2015). Some individuals continue to work because of economic need, whereas others have a desire to remain involved and productive. Obviously, health and financial status affect decisions and abilities to work or engage in new work opportunities.

The Great Recession and the declining economy have contributed to a rising level of economic risk facing retirees. Many Americans are not financially prepared for retirement, with almost one-third of working adults without savings or a pension, including nearly one-fourth of those older than 45 (Board of Governors of the Federal Reserve System, 2015). Single senior households, mostly women, are at even greater financial vulnerability (Polivka, 2012).

Special Considerations in Retirement

In the United States, retirement security depends on the "three-legged stool" of Social Security pensions, savings, and investments (Stanford & Usita, 2002). Older people with disabilities, those who have lacked access to education or who have held low-paying jobs with no benefits, and those not eligible for Social Security are at increased economic risk during retirement years. Non-white older persons, women—especially widows and those divorced or never married—immigrants, and gay and lesbian men and women often face greater challenges related to adequate income and benefits in retirement. Unmarried women, particularly African Americans, face the most negative prospects for retirement now and for at least the next 20 years (Hooyman & Kiyak, 2011).

Inadequate coverage for women in retirement is common because their work histories have been sporadic and diverse. Women often retire earlier than anticipated because of family needs. Whereas most men have always worked outside the home, it is only within the past 30 years that this has been the expectation of women. Therefore large cohort differences exist. Traditionally, the variability of women's work histories, including interrupted careers, and the residuals of sexist pension policies, Social Security inequities, and low-paying jobs created hazards for adequacy of income in retirement. The scene is gradually changing in many respects, but the gender bias remains (see Chapter 7).

Retirement Planning

Current research suggests that retirement has positive effects on life satisfaction and health, although this may vary depending on the individual's circumstances. However, approximately 61% of retirees report that they found the retirement transition to be very satisfying (National Institute on Aging, National Institutes of Health, U.S. Department of Health and Human Services, 2015). Decisions to retire are often based on financial resources; attitudes toward work, family roles, and responsibilities; the nature of the job; access to health insurance; chronological age; health; and self-perceptions of ability to adjust to retirement. Retirement planning is advisable during early adulthood and essential in middle age. However, people differ in their focus on the past, present, and future and their realistic ability to "put away something" for future needs.

Retirement preparation programs are usually aimed at employees with high levels of education and occupational status, those with private pension coverage, and government employees. Thus the people most in need of planning assistance may be those least likely to have any available, let alone the resources for an adequate retirement. Individuals who are retiring in poor health, minorities, women, those in lower socioeconomic levels, and those with the least education may experience greater concerns in retirement and may need specialized counseling and targeted education efforts.

❖ IMPLICATIONS FOR GERONTOLOGICAL NURSING AND HEALTHY AGING

Successful retirement adjustment depends on socialization needs, energy levels, health, adequate income, variety of interests, amount of self-esteem derived from

BOX 26.1 Predictors of Retirement Satisfaction

- Good health
- Functional abilities
- Adequate income
- Suitable living environment
- Strong social support system characterized by reciprocal relationships
- Decision to retire involved choice, autonomy, adequate preparation, higher-status job before retirement
- Retirement activities that offer an opportunity to feel useful, learn, grow, and enjoy oneself
- Positive outlook, sense of mastery, resilience, resourcefulness
- Good marital or partner relationship
- Sharing similar interests to spouse/significant other

Data from Hooyman N, Kiyak H: *Social gerontology: A multidisciplinary perspective,* ed 9, Boston, 2011, Allyn & Bacon.

work, presence of intimate relationships, social support, and general adaptability (Box 26.1). Talking with clients older than age 50 about retirement plans, providing anticipatory guidance about the transition to retirement, identifying those who may be at risk for lowered income and health concerns, and referring to appropriate resources for retirement planning and support are important nursing interventions. Additionally, the period of preretirement and retirement may be an opportune time to enhance the focus on health promotion and illness/injury prevention.

It is important to build on the strengths of the individual's life experiences and coping skills and to provide appropriate counseling and support to assist individuals to continue to grow and develop in meaningful ways during the transition from the work role. In ideal situations, retirement offers the opportunity to pursue interests that may have been neglected while fulfilling other obligations. However, for too many individuals, retirement presents challenges that affect both health and well-being, and nurses must be advocates for policies and conditions that allow all older people to maintain quality of life in retirement.

Death of a Spouse or Life Partner

Losing a spouse or other life partner after a long, close, and satisfying relationship is the most difficult adjustment one can face, aside from the loss of a child. This loss is a stage in the life course that can be anticipated but seldom is considered. Spousal bereavement in later life is a high probability for women and, while less common among men, still a significant event.

BOX 26.2 Common Widower Bereavement Reactions

- Search for the lost mate
- Neglect of self
- Inability to share grief
- Loss of social contacts
- Struggle to view women as other than wife
- Erosion of self-confidence and sexuality
- Protracted grief period

The death of a life partner is essentially a loss of self. The mourning is as much for oneself as for the individual who has died. A core part of oneself has died with the partner, and even with satisfactory grief resolution, that aspect of self will never return. Even those widows and widowers who reorganize their lives and invest in family, friends, and activities often find that many years later they still miss their "other half" profoundly.

With the loss of the intimate partner, several changes occur simultaneously in almost every domain of life and have a significant impact on well-being: physical, psychological, social, practical, and economic. Individuals who have been self-confident and resilient seem to fare best (Bennett & Soulsby, 2012). The transitional phase of grief, if handled appropriately, leads to the confirmation of a new identity, the end of one stage of life, and the beginning of another.

Gender differences on widowhood are found in the literature. Bereaved husbands may be more socially and emotionally vulnerable. Suicide risk is highest among men older than 80 years of age who have experienced the death of a spouse (see Chapter 24). Widowers adapt more slowly than widows to the loss of a spouse and often remarry quickly. Loneliness and the need to be cared for are factors influencing widowers to pursue new partners. Having associations with family and friends, being members of a church community, and continuing to work or engage in activities can all be helpful in the adjustment period following the death of a wife. Common bereavement reactions of widowers are listed in Box 26.2 and should be discussed with male clients.

❖ IMPLICATIONS FOR GERONTOLOGICAL NURSING AND HEALTHY AGING

◆ Assessment

Losing a spouse can have serious physical and mental health consequences. There is an elevated risk of morbidity and mortality, particularly in the early bereavement period (DiGiacomo et al., 2013). The likelihood of a heart attack or stroke doubles in the critical 30-day period after a partner's death. The risk seems likely to be the result of adverse physiological responses associated with acute grief (Carey et al., 2014). The bereavement period is also associated with an elevated risk of multiple psychiatric disorders, particularly if the death was unexpected (Keyes et al., 2014). This is an important time for nurses to assess the health status of the individual and provide interventions to assist in coping. However, the risks of effects of spousal bereavement and increasing age on health, particularly chronic issues, remain elevated even among those long past the event (10+ years), so ongoing surveillance and assessment are indicated (Das, 2013).

Feelings of the bereaved one are not orderly or progressive; they are conflicted, ambivalent, suicidal, full of rage, and often suspicious. Bereaved individuals may exhibit personality disorganization that would be considered mentally aberrant or frankly psychotic under other circumstances. Some people handle grief with less apparent decompensation. Grief reactions must be accepted as personally valid and useful evidences of healing. deVries (2001) discusses the signs of ongoing bonds and connections with the deceased (e.g., dreaming of the deceased, ongoing daily communication, "checking in") that persist long after death and counsels professionals to reexamine the idea that there is a timetable for "resolution" of grief. Maintaining bonds with the deceased is considered normal and healthy (Bennett & Soulsby, 2012).

◆ Interventions

Nurses will interact with bereaved older people in many settings. Knowing the stages of transition to a new role as a widow or widower will be useful in determining interventions, although each individual is unique in this respect. Individuals respond to losses in ways that reflect the nature and meaning of the relationships, as well as the unique characteristics of the bereaved. Patterns of adjustment are presented in Box 26.3. With adequate support, reintegration can be expected in 2 to 4 years. People with few familial or social supports may need professional help to get through the early months of grief in a way that will facilitate recovery.

To support the grieving person, it is necessary to extend one's own self to reconnect the bereaved person with a world of warmth and caring. No one nurse or family member can accomplish this task alone. Hundreds of small, caring gestures build strength and confidence in the grieving person's ability and willingness to survive. Additional information about dying, death, and grief can be found in Chapter 28.

BOX 26.3 Patterns of Adjustment to Widowhood

Stage 1: Reactionary (First Few Weeks)

Early responses of disbelief, anger, indecision, detachment, and inability to communicate in a logical, sustained manner are common. Searching for the mate, visions, hallucinations, and depersonalization may be experienced.

Intervention: Support, validate, be available, listen to individual talk about mate, reduce expectations.

Stage 2: Withdrawal (First Few Months)

Depression, apathy, physiological vulnerability; movement and cognition are slowed; insomnia, unpredictable waves of grief, sighing, and anorexia occur.

Intervention: Protect individual against suicide, monitor health status, and involve in support groups.

Stage 3: Recuperation (Second 6 Months)

Periods of depression are interspersed with characteristic capability. Feelings of personal control begin to return.

Intervention: Support accustomed lifestyle patterns that sustain and assist individual to explore new possibilities.

Stage 4: Exploration (Second Year)

Individual begins new ventures, testing suitability of new roles; anniversaries, holidays, birthdays, and date of death may be especially difficult.

Intervention: Prepare individual for unexpected reactions during anniversaries. Encourage and support new trial roles.

Stage 5: Integration (Fifth Year)

Individual will feel fully integrated into new and satisfying roles if grief has been resolved in a healthy manner.

Intervention: Assist individual to recognize and share own pattern of growth through the trauma of loss.

RELATIONSHIPS IN LATER LIFE

Friendships

Friends are often a significant source of support in late life and can promote health and well-being (Blieszner, 2014). The number of friends may decline, but the majority of older adults have at least one close friend with whom they maintain close contact, share confidences, and can turn to in an emergency. The social network may narrow as one ages with intimate personal relationships being maintained and the more instrumental relationships discontinued (van Groenou et al., 2013).

Friendships can be sustaining in the face of overwhelming circumstances. Personality characteristics

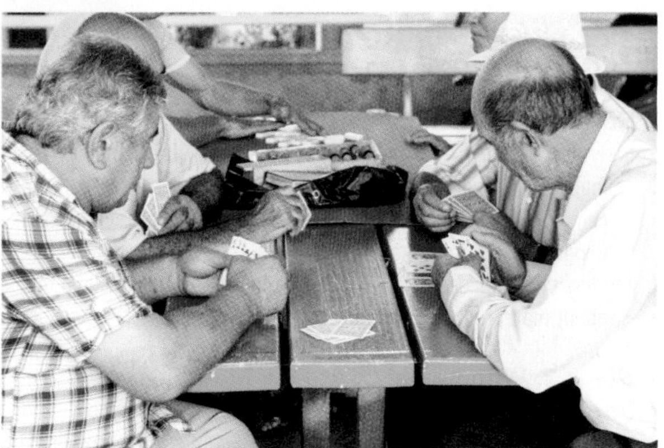

Friends play an important role in the lives of older adults. (By Michal Osmenda from Brussels, Belgium [CC BY 2.0 http://creativecommons.org/licenses/by/2.0], via Wikimedia Commons.)

between friends are compatible because the relationships are chosen and caring is shared without obligation. Trust, demonstrations of caring, and mutual problem solving are important aspects of the friendships. Friends may share a lifelong perspective or may bring a totally new intergenerational viewpoint into one's life. Late-life friendships often develop out of changing situations, such as relocation to retirement or assisted living communities, widowhood, and involvement in volunteer pursuits. As desires and pursuits change, some friendships evolve that the person never would have considered in his or her youth.

Considering the obvious importance of friendship, it seems to be a neglected area of exploration and a seldom considered resource for professionals working with older people. Because close friendships have such influence on the sense of well-being of elders, anything done to sustain them or assist in building new friendships and social networks will be helpful. Internet access and social media offer new opportunities to interact with friends or even to form new friendships (Blieszner, 2014) (see Chapter 4). Generally, women tend to have more sustaining friendships than do men, and this factor contributes to resilience, a characteristic linked to successful aging (Hooyman & Kiyak, 2011) (see Chapter 24).

Nurses may include questions about the individual's friendships and their importance and availability in their assessment of older adults. Although friendships do provide much support, they are also a further source of grief in old age. The loss of friends through death occurs often, and nurses must appreciate the nature of this loss. Encouraging intergenerational friendships and linking older adults to resources for social participation and meaningful activities are important interventions.

FAMILIES

The idea of family evokes strong impressions of whatever an individual believes the typical family should be. Because everyone comes from a family, these impressions have powerful symbolic meanings. However, in today's world, the definition of family is in a state of flux. As recently as 100 years ago, the norm was the extended family made up of parents, their grown children, and the children's children, often living together and sharing resources, strengths, and challenges.

As cities grew and adult children moved in pursuit of work, parents did not always come along, and the nuclear family evolved. The norm in the United States became two parents and their two children (nuclear family), or at least that was the norm in what has been considered mainstream America. This pattern was not as common among ethnically diverse families, where the extended family is often the norm. However, families are changing, and today only about 19% of U.S. households are composed of nuclear families (United States Census Bureau, 2013).

Baby boomers are more likely to live alone than previous generations, and the number of single-person households is increasing. Other countries are also experiencing changes in family composition, and even values, as the numbers of older citizens increase and the younger members of society become more mobile and move away from their home (Batiashvili & Gerzmava, 2013). A decrease in fertility rates has reduced family size, and American families are smaller today than ever before. The high divorce and remarriage rate results in households of blended families of children from previous marriages and the new marriage.

The new modern family includes single-parent families, blended families, gay and lesbian families, domestic partnerships, and childless families. Fewer families altogether are common. Older people without families, either by choice or by circumstance, have created their own "families" through communal living with siblings, friends, or others. Indeed, it is not unusual for childless persons residing in long-term care facilities to refer to the staff as their new "family."

Multigenerational Families

In the United States, multigenerational families have grown by approximately 60% since 1990 and 1 in 6 Americans live in a multigenerational ("multigen") household (Generations United, 2014). Multigenerational families are more common among other cultures, but the growth of multigenerational households in the

United States has accelerated during the economic downturn. This growing trend is expected to continue and has benefits for older family members, as well as younger ones (Generations United, 2011). "Multigen" remodeling or new home building to accommodate intergenerational families is an increasing trend. Box 26.4 presents tips when planning to add an older person to the household.

Family Relationships

Family members, however they are defined, form the nucleus of relationships for the majority of older adults and their support system if they become dependent. A long-standing myth in society is that families are alienated from their older family members and that families have abandoned their care to institutions. Nothing could be further from the truth. Family relationships remain strong in old age, and most older people have frequent contact with their families. Most older adults possess a large intergenerational web of significant people, including sons, daughters, stepchildren, in-laws, nieces, nephews, grandchildren, and great-grandchildren, as well as partners and former partners of their offspring. Families provide the majority of care for older adults. Changes in family structure will have a significant impact on the availability of family members to provide care for older people in the future.

As families change, the roles of the members or the expectations of one another may change as well. Grandparents may assume parental roles for their grandchildren if their children are unable to care for them; or grandparents and older aunts and uncles may assume temporary caregiving roles while the children, nieces, and nephews work. Adult children of any age may provide limited or extensive caregiving to their own parents or aging relatives who may become ill or

BOX 26.4 Tips for Best Practice

Adding an Older Person to the Household

Questions to Ask

- What are the needs of the new member and of the family?
- Where will space be allotted for the new member?
- How will the new member be included in existing family patterns?
- How will responsibilities be shared?
- What resources in the community will assist in the adjustment phase?
- Is the environment safe for the new member?
- How will family life change with the added member, and how does the family feel about it?
- What are the differences in socialization and sleeping patterns?
- What are the older person's strong needs and expectations?
- What are the older person's skills and talents?

Modifications That May Need to Be Made

- Arrange private or semiprivate living quarters if possible.
- Regularly schedule visits to other relatives to give each family time for respite and privacy.
- Arrange adult day health programs and senior activities for the older person to help keep contact with members of his or her own generation. Consider how the older person will feel about giving up familiar surroundings and friends.

Potential Areas of Conflict

- Space: especially if someone has given up his or her space to the older relative.
- Possessions: older people may want to move possessions into the house; others may not find them attractive or may insist on replacing them with new things.
- Entertaining: times when old and young feel the need or desire to exclude the other from social events.
- Responsibilities and chores: the older person may feel useless if he or she does nothing and may feel in the way if he or she does something.
- Expenses: increased cost of home maintenance, food, clothing, and recreation may not be shared appropriately.
- Vacations: whether to go together or alone; young persons may feel uneasy not taking the older person out and may feel resentful if they must.
- Childrearing: disagreement over childrearing policies.
- Childcare: grandparental babysitting may be welcomed by family and resented by older person, or, if not allowed, older person may feel lack of trust in capability.

Ways to Decrease Areas of Conflict

- Respect privacy.
- Discuss space allocations.
- Discuss the older person's furnishings before move.
- Make it clear in advance when social events include everyone or exclude someone.
- Make clear decisions about household tasks; all should have responsibility geared to ability.
- Have the older person pay a share of expenses and maintain a separate phone to reduce strain and increase feelings of independence.

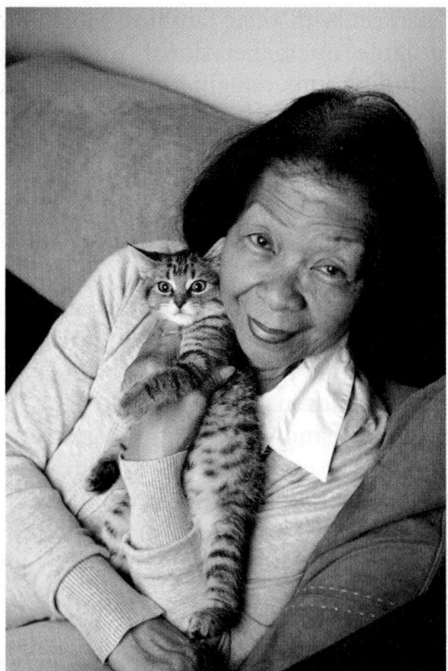

Pets are a part of the family and are particularly beneficial to older adults. They provide companionship, comfort, and caring. (© iStock.com/michellegibson.)

impaired. A spouse, sibling, or grandchild may become a caregiver as well (see Chapter 27).

Close-knit families are more aware of the needs of their members and work to resolve problems and find ways to meet the needs of members, even if they are not always successful. Emotionally distant families are less available in times of need and have greater potential for conflict. If the family has never been close and supportive, it will not magically become so when members grow older. Resentments long buried may emerge and produce friction or psychological pain. Long-submerged conflicts and feelings may return if the needs of one family member exceed those of the others.

In coming to know the older adult, the gerontological nurse comes to know the family as well, learning of their special gifts and their life challenges. The nurse works with the elder within the unique culture of his or her family of origin, present family, and support networks, including friends.

Types of Families

Traditional Couples

The marital or partnered relationship in the United States is a critical source of support for older people, and nearly 55% of the population age 65 and older is married and lives with a spouse. Although this relationship is often the most binding if it extends into late life, the chance of a couple going through old age together is exceedingly slim. Women older than age 65 are three times as likely as men of the same age to be widowed. Men who survive their spouse into old age ordinarily have multiple opportunities to remarry if they wish. Even among the oldest-old, the majority of men are married. A woman is less likely to have an opportunity for remarriage in late life. Often, older couples live together but do not marry because of economic and inheritance reasons.

The needs, tasks, and expectations of couples in late life differ from those in earlier years. Some couples have been married more than 60 or 70 years. These years together may have been filled with love and companionship or abuse and resentment, or anything in between. However, in general, marital status (or the presence of a long-time partner) is positively related to health, life satisfaction, and well-being (Korporaal et al., 2013).

For all couples, the normal physical and sociological circumstances in late life present challenges. Some of the issues that strain many of these relationships include (1) the deteriorating health of one or both partners; (2) limitations in income; (3) conflicts with children or other relatives; (4) incompatible sexual needs; and (5) mismatched needs for activity and socialization.

Divorce. In the past, divorce was considered a stigmatizing event. Today, however, it is so common that a person is inclined to forget the ostracizing effects of divorce from 60 years ago. The divorce rate among people 50 years of age and older has doubled in the past 20 years. Older couples are becoming less likely to stay in an unsatisfactory marriage, and with the aging of the baby boomers, divorce rates will continue to rise. Health care professionals must avoid making assumptions and be alert to the possibility of marital dissatisfaction in old age. Nurses should ask, "How would you describe your marriage?"

Long-term relationships are varied and complex, with many factors forming the glue that holds them together. Marital breakdown may be more devastating in old age because it is often unanticipated and may occur concurrently with other significant losses. Nurses and other health care professionals must be concerned with supporting a client's decision to seek a divorce and with assisting him or her in seeking counseling in the transition. Divorce will initiate a grieving process similar to the death of a spouse, and a severe disruption in coping capacity may occur until the individual adjusts to a new life. The grief may be more difficult to cope with because no socially sanctioned patterns have been established. In addition, tax and fiscal policies favor married couples, and many divorced older women are at a serious economic disadvantage in retirement.

Nontraditional Couples

As the variations in families grow, so do the types of coupled relationships. Among the types of couples we see today are lesbian, gay, bisexual, and transgender (LGBT) couples. Although the number of LGBT people of any age has remained elusive given the reluctance many have about disclosing their status, an estimated 1.5 million Americans more than 60 years of age are LGB with projections that this figure is likely to double by 2030 (Caceres & Frank, 2016). There are no clear population estimates of LGB individuals globally and little information on transgender individuals. There is also a dearth of information and research on the aging experience of older LGBT individuals (Caceres & Frank, 2016; Cloyes, 2016). Much more knowledge of cohort, cultural, and generational differences among age groups is needed to understand the dramatic changes in the lives of LGBT individuals in family lifestyles.

Most LGBT adults older than age 60 are single because the ability to legally marry is a recent occurrence. Many have been part of a live-in couple at some time during their life, but as they age, they are more likely to live alone. Gay and bisexual men older than age 50 are twice as likely to live alone as heterosexual men of the same age, while older lesbian and bisexual women are about one-third more likely to live alone. Approximately one-third of the lesbians "come out" after age 50. Many lesbians married, raised children, divorced, and led double lives.

In the case of transgender people, medical providers for many years required candidates for sex reassignment surgery to divorce their spouses, move to a new place, and construct a false personal history consistent with their new gender expression. These practices resulted in transgender people losing even more of their social and personal support systems than might otherwise have been the case (SAGE & MAP, 2010).

It is important to recognize that there are considerable differences in the experiences of younger LGBT individuals when compared with those who are older. Older LGBT individuals did not have the benefit of antidiscrimination laws and support for same-sex partners and are more likely to have kept their relationships hidden than those who grew up in the modern-day gay liberation movement. Transgender and bisexual individuals are less likely to "be out" (American Society on Aging and MetLife, 2010).

Some LGBT individuals may have developed social networks of friends, members of their family of origin, and the larger community, but many lack support. Because many LGBT couples may have no or fewer children, they will have fewer caregivers as they age. The continued legal and policy barriers faced by LGBT elders contribute to the challenges for those in domestic partnerships as they age. Increasing numbers of same-sex couples are choosing to have families, and this will call for greater understanding of these "new" types of families, young and old. Organizations that serve LGBT elders in the community need to enhance outreach and support mechanisms to enable them to maintain independence and age safely and in good health. Box 26.5 presents resources for LGBT elders.

Elders and Their Adult Children

In adulthood, relationships between the generations become increasingly important for most people. Older

BOX 26.5 Resources for Best Practice

LGBT Resources

Lavender Health: Site maintained by a team of nurses – educational resources and PPT presentations on LGBT health issues and best practices for LGBT communities.

Lesbian and Gay Aging Issues Network (LGAIN): A constituent group of the American Society on Aging that works to raise awareness about the concerns of LGBT elders and the unique barriers they encounter in gaining access to housing, health care, long-term care, and other needed services.

National Resource Center of LGBT Aging: Technical assistance resource center aimed at improving the quality of services and supports offered to LGBT older adults.

Services and Advocacy for Gay, Lesbian, Bisexual, and Transgender Elders (SAGE)

Sexuality and Aging

Administration on Aging: Older Adults and HIV Toolkit

CDC: Guide to Taking a Sexual History

The Center for Older Adult Sexuality: Policy and guidelines for sexual expression among individuals with dementia in long-term care.

Hartford Institute for Geriatric Nursing: Issues regarding sexuality, Protocol: Sexuality in the Older Adult: See Assessment series for video illustrating use of PLISSIT model

HIV/Age.org: Resources, research

HIV Wisdom for Older Women

National Institute on Aging: Sexuality in later life; Sexuality and older people

National Institute on Aging, National Institutes of Health: Intimacy and sexuality: Resources for caregivers, Sample policies on sexual expression among individuals with dementia in long-term care facilities.

parents enjoy being told about the various activities and successes of their offspring, and these adult children begin to see aspects of themselves that have developed from their parents. At times, the relationships may become strained because the younger adults are more concerned with their own spouses, partners, and children. The parents are no longer central to their lives, though offspring may be central to the lives of their parents. The most difficult situations occur when the elder parents are openly critical or judgmental about the lives of their offspring. In the best of situations, adult children shift to the role of friend, companion, and confidant to the elder, a concept known as filial maturity.

By and large, elders and their children have relationships that are reciprocal in nature and characterized by affection and mutual support. These relationships are both the most important and potentially the most conflicted. Family resources are shared from birth and usually in some way until and after death. These resources may be tangible, such as money, belongings, and housing. Intangible resources may include advice, support, guidance, and day-to-day assistance with life. Elders provide a family history perspective, models for growing old, assistance with grandchildren, a sense of continuity, and a philosophy of aging.

Most older people see their children on a regular basis, and even children who do not live close to their older parents maintain close connections, so "intimacy at a distance" can occur (Hooyman & Kiyak, 2011; Silverstein & Angelli, 1998). Approximately 50% of older people have daily contact with their adult children; nearly 80% see an adult child at least once a week; and more than 75% talk on the phone at least weekly with an adult child (Hooyman & Kiyak, 2011).

Never-Married Older Adults

Approximately 5% of women and 4% of men today have never married. Older people who have lived alone most of their lives often develop supportive networks with siblings, friends, and neighbors. Never-married older adults may demonstrate resilience to the challenges of aging as a result of their independence and may not feel lonely or isolated. Furthermore, they may have had longer lifetime employment and may enjoy greater financial security as they age. Single older adults will increase in the future because being single is increasingly more common in younger years.

Grandparents

The role of grandparenting, and increasingly great-grandparenthood, is experienced by most older adults. The numbers of grandparents are at record highs and still growing at more than twice the overall population growth rate. There were an estimated 65 million grandmothers and grandfathers in 2010. By 2020, they are projected to reach 80 million, at which time they will be nearly one-in-three adults (MetLife, 2011). Sixty-eight percent of individuals born in 2000 will have four grandparents alive when they reach 18; and 76% will have at least one grandparent at 30 years of age (Hooyman & Kiyak, 2011). Great-grandparenthood will become more common in the future in light of projections of a healthier aging.

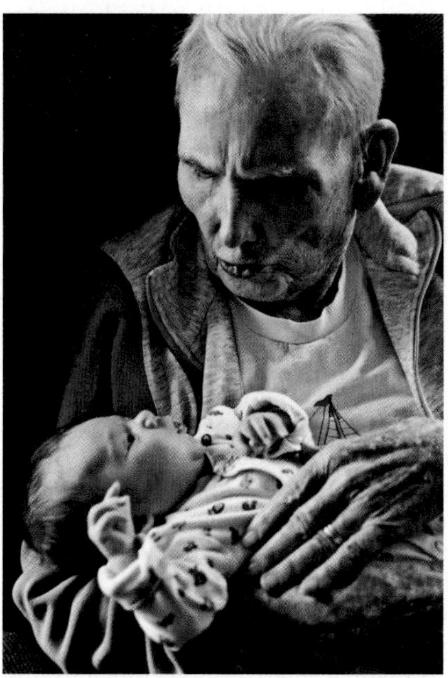

The author's grandson and his maternal great-grandfather. (Photo courtesy Ben Aronoff, Fogline Studios.)

As the term implies, the "grands" are a step beyond parents in their concerns, exposure, and responsibility. The majority of grandparents derive great emotional satisfaction from their grandchildren. Historically, the emphasis has been on the progressive aging of the grandparent as it affects the relationship with the grandchild, but little has been said about the effects of the growth and maturation of the grandchild on the relationship. Many young adults who have had close contact with their grandparents report that this relationship was very meaningful in their lives. Growing numbers of adult grandchildren are assisting in caregiving for grandparents.

The age, vitality, and proximity of both grandchild and grandparent produce a kaleidoscope of possible

BOX 26.6 A Grandmother as Seen by an 8-Year-Old Child

"A grandmother is a woman who has no children of her own. That is why she loves other people's children."

"Grandmothers have nothing to do. They are just there: when they take us for a walk they go slowly, like caterpillars along beautiful leaves. They never say, 'Come on, faster, hurry up!'"

"Everyone should try to have a grandmother, especially those who don't have a TV."

From *Ageing in Focus,* March 2006.

activities and interactions as both progress through their aging processes. Approximately 80% of grandparents see a grandchild at least monthly, and nearly 50% do so weekly. Geographic distance does not significantly affect the quality of the relationship between grandparents and their grandchildren. The Internet is increasingly being used by distant grandparents as a way of staying involved in their grandchildren's lives and forging close bonds (Hooyman & Kiyak, 2011).

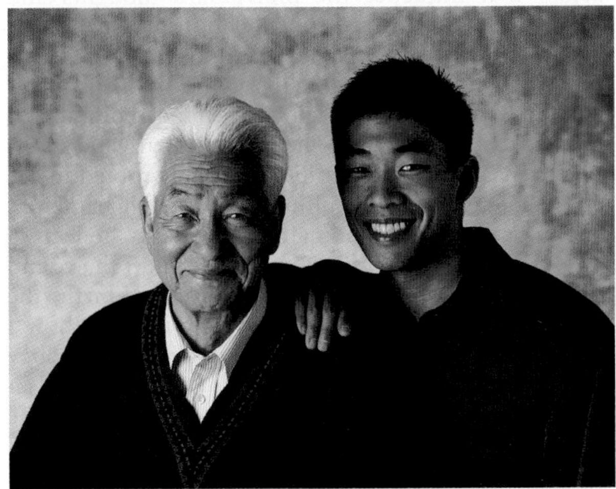

Grandparenting is an important role for elders. (Copyright © Getty Images.)

Younger grandparents typically live closer to their grandchildren and are more involved in childcare and recreational activities (Box 26.6). Older grandparents with sufficient incomes may provide more financial assistance and other types of instrumental help. Grandparent-headed households are one of the fastest growing U.S. family groups, and this phenomenon is taking place in other countries as well (Hadfield, 2014). Approximately 2.5 million grandparents are responsible for raising their grandchildren (Legacy Project, 2014). This phenomenon is discussed in Chapter 27.

Siblings

Late-life sibling relationships are poorly understood and have been neglected by researchers. As individuals age, they often have more contact with siblings than they did in the years when family and work demands were more pressing. About 80% of older people have at least one sibling, and they are often strong sources of support in the lives of never-married older persons, widowed persons, and those without children. For many elders, these relationships become increasingly important because they have a long history of memories and are of the same generation and similar backgrounds.

Sibling relationships become particularly important when they are part of the support system, especially among single or widowed elders living alone. The strongest of sibling bonds is thought to be the relationship between sisters. When blessed with survival, these relationships remain important into late old age. Service providers should inquire about sibling relationships of past and present significance.

The loss of siblings has a profound effect in terms of awareness of one's own mortality, particularly when those of the same gender die. When an elder reaches the age of the sibling who died, the reaction can be quite disruptive. Not only is grieving activated, but also rehearsal for one's own death may occur. In some cases in which an elder sibling survives younger ones, there may be not only a deep grief but also pangs of guilt: "Why them and not me?" (see Chapter 28).

Fictive Kin

Fictive kin are nonblood kin who serve as "genuine fake families," as expressed by Virginia Satir. These nonrelatives become surrogate family and take on some of the instrumental and affectional attributes of family. Fictive kin are important in the lives of many elders, especially those with no close or satisfying family relationships and those living alone or in institutions. Fictive kin includes both friends and, often, paid caregivers. Primary care providers, such as nursing assistants, nurses, or case managers, often become fictive kin. Professionals who work with older people need to recognize the instrumental and emotional support, as well as the mutually satisfying relationships, that occur between friends, neighbors, and other fictive kin who assist older adults who are dependent.

INTIMACY

Although intimacy is often thought of in the context of sexual performance, it encompasses more than sexuality and includes five major relational components: commitment, affective intimacy, cognitive intimacy, physical intimacy, and interdependence (Youngkin, 2004). It is a warm, meaningful feeling of joy. Intimacy includes the need for close friendships; relationships with family, friends, and formal caregivers; spiritual connections; knowing that one matters in someone else's life; and the ability to form satisfying social relationships with others (Steinke, 2005; Syme, 2014). Intimacy needs change over time, but the need for intimacy and satisfying social relationships remains an important component of healthy aging.

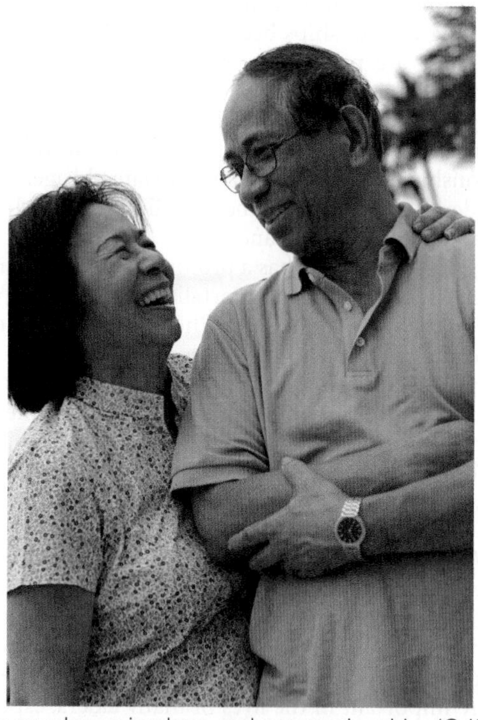

Older couples enjoy love and companionship. (© iStock .com/DanielBendjy.)

SEXUALITY

Sexuality is a state of physical, emotional, mental, and social well-being in relation to sexuality; it is not merely the absence of disease, dysfunction, or infirmity. It is a central aspect of being human and encompasses sex, gender identities and roles, sexual orientation, eroticism, pleasure, intimacy, and reproduction (World Health Organization, 2014).

As a major aspect of intimacy, sexuality includes the physical act of intercourse, as well as many other types of intimate activity. It includes components such as sexual desire, activity, attitudes, body image, gender-role activity, and sexual self-esteem (Syme, 2014; Zeiss & Kasl-Godley, 2001). Sexuality provides the opportunity to express passion, affection, admiration, and loyalty. It can also enhance personal growth and communication. Sexuality also allows a general affirmation of life (especially joy) and a continuing opportunity to search for new growth and experience.

Sexuality, similar to food and water, is a basic need, yet it goes beyond the biological realm to include social, psychological, and moral dimensions (Waite et al., 2009) (Fig. 26.1). The constant interaction among these spheres of sexuality works to produce harmony. The linkage of the four dimensions composes the holistic quality of an individual's sexuality. "Historically, sexuality has been perceived more narrowly in a biomedical context, with emphasis placed on the sexual response cycle, hetero-normative behaviors (e.g., penile-vaginal intercourse), and heterosexist and ageist assumptions" (Syme, 2014, p. 36). A holistic view better reflects the philosophy of healthy aging for all individuals. *Healthy People 2020* goals related to sexual health are presented in Box 26.7.

The social sphere of sexuality is the sum of cultural factors that influence the individual's thoughts and actions related to interpersonal relationships, as well as sexuality related to ideas and learned behavior. Television, radio, literature, and the more traditional sources of family, school, and religious teachings combine to influence social sexuality. The belief of that which constitutes masculine and feminine is deeply rooted in the individual's exposure to cultural factors (see Chapter 2).

The psychological domain of sexuality reflects a person's attitudes, feelings toward self and others, and learning from experiences. Beginning with birth, the individual is bombarded with cues and signals of how a person should act and think about the use of "dirty words" or body parts. Conversation is self-censored in the presence of or in discussion with certain people. The moral aspect of sexuality, the "I should" or "I shouldn't,"

BOX 26.7 *Healthy People 2020*

Goals for Sexual Health

- Improve the health, safety, and well-being of lesbian, gay, bisexual, and transgender (LGBT) individuals.
- Promote healthy sexual behaviors, strengthen community capacity, and increase access to quality services to prevent sexually transmitted diseases (STDs) and their complications.
- Prevent human immunodeficiency virus (HIV) infection and its related illness and death.

Data from U.S. Department of Health and Human Services, Office of Disease Prevention and Health Promotion: *Healthy People 2020,* 2012. Available at http://www.healthypeople.gov/2020.

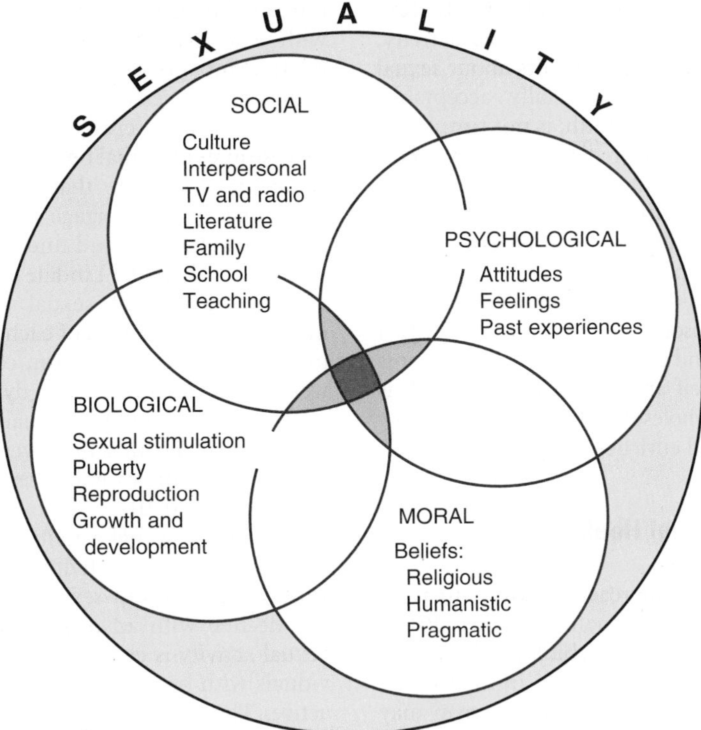

FIGURE 26.1 Interrelationship of dimensions of sexuality.

makes a difference that is based in religious and cultural beliefs or in a pragmatic or humanistic outlook.

The final dimension, biological sexuality, is reflected in physiological responses to sexual stimulation, reproduction, puberty, and growth and development. Because of the interrelatedness, these dimensions affect each other directly or indirectly whenever an aspect of sexuality is out of harmony.

Sexuality is a vital aspect to consider in the care of the older person regardless of the setting. Sexuality exists throughout life in one form or another in everyone. All older people have a need to express sexual feelings, whether the individuals are healthy and active or whether they are frail. Sexuality is linked with the person's personality and identity and has a significant role in promoting better life adaptation (Bach et al., 2013; Steinke, 2013). Sex and intimacy cannot be ignored since adults are living longer and healthier lives and engaging in a variety of intimate and sexual behaviors (Syme, 2014).

SEXUAL HEALTH

The World Health Organization defines sexual health as a state of physical, emotional, mental, and social well-being related to sexuality (2014). Sexual health is a realistic phenomenon that includes four components: personal and social behaviors in agreement with individual gender identity; comfort with a range of sexual role behaviors and engagement in effective interpersonal relations with both sexes in a loving relationship or

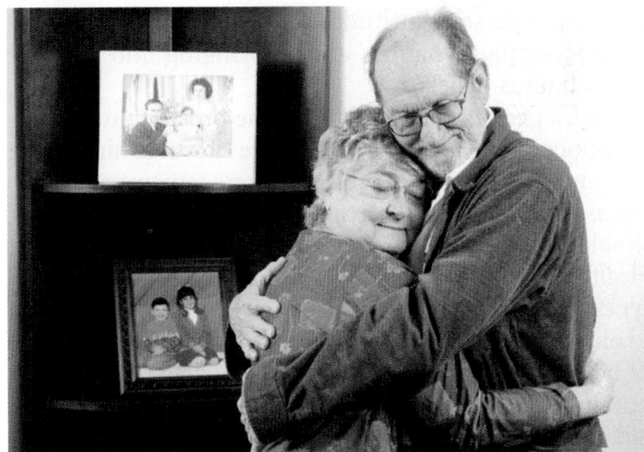

Love and affection are important to older persons. (From Sorrentino SA, Gorek B: *Mosby's textbook for long-term care assistants,* ed 5, St Louis, 2007, Mosby.)

long-term commitment; response to erotic stimulation that produces positive and pleasurable sexual activity; and the ability to make mature judgments about sexual behavior that is culturally and socially acceptable. "Sexual health, as with physical health, is not simply the absence of sexual dysfunction or disease, but, rather a state of sexual well-being that includes a positive approach to a sexual relationship and anticipation of a pleasurable experience without fear, shame, or coercion" (Rheaume & Mitty, 2008, p. 342).

These interpretations address the multifaceted nature of the biological, psychosocial, cultural, and spiritual components of sexuality and imply that sexual behavior is the capacity to enhance self and others. Sexual health is individually defined and wholesome if it leads to intimacy (not necessarily coitus) and enriches the involved parties.

Factors Influencing Sexual Health

Expectations

Older adults are becoming increasingly open in their attitudes and beliefs about sexuality (Syme, 2014). However, a large number of cultural, biological, psychosocial, and environmental factors can influence the sexual behavior of older adults. The older person may be confronted with barriers to the expression of his or her sexuality by reflected attitudes, health, culture, economics, opportunity, and historical trends. Factors affecting a person's attitudes on intimacy and sexuality include family dynamics and upbringing and cultural and religious beliefs.

Older people often internalize the broad cultural proscriptions of sexual behavior in late life that hinder the continuance of sexual expression. There remains a prevailing assumption that as we age, we become sexually undesirable, incapable of sex, or asexual (DiNapoli et al., 2013). Health care professionals are not immune to these stereotypes and may assume sexual issues are of lesser concern to older adults and neglect to address this important aspect of healthy aging. Much sexual behavior stems from incorporating other people's reactions. Older people do not feel old until they are faced with the fact that others around them consider them old. Similarly, older adults do not feel asexual until they are continually treated as such.

An often quoted statement by Alex Comfort (1974) sums it up nicely: "In our experiences, old folks stop having sex for the same reasons they stop riding a bicycle—general infirmity, thinking it looks ridiculous, no bicycle."

Activity Levels

For both heterosexual and homosexual individuals, research supports that liberal and positive attitudes toward sexuality, greater sexual knowledge, satisfaction with a long-term relationship or a current intimate relationship, good social networks, psychological well-being, and a sense of self-worth are associated with greater sexual interest, activity, and satisfaction. Both early studies of sexual behavior in older adults and more recent ones indicate that most elders continue to be interested in sex, engage in a variety of sexual and intimate behaviors, and find their sexual lives satisfying (Lindau et al., 2007; Lindau & Gavrilova, 2010).

Determinants of sexual activity and functioning include the interaction of each partner's sexual capacity, physical health, motivation, conduct, and attitudes, as well as the quality of the dyadic relationship (Waite et al., 2009). Having a sexual partner, frequent intercourse, good health, a low level of stress, and the absence of financial worries enhances a happy sexual relationship (Fisher, 2010).

Patterns of sexual activity in earlier years are a major predictor of sexual activity in later life, and individuals with higher levels of sexual activity in middle age show less decline with advanced age (Kennedy et al., 2010). Sexual activity is closely tied to overall health, and individuals with better health are more likely to be sexually active. The most common reason for sexual inactivity among heterosexual couples is the male partner's health. Men are more sexually active than women, most likely because women live longer and may not have a partner.

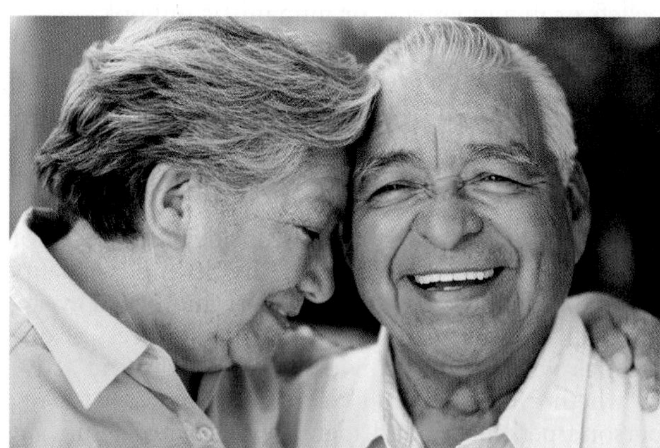

Sexuality is an important need in late life and affects pleasure, adaptation, and a general feeling of well-being. (© iStock.com/Aldo Murillo.)

Cohort and Cultural Influences

The era in which a person was born influences attitudes about sexuality. Women in their eighties today may have been strongly influenced by the prudish Victorian atmosphere of their youth and may have experienced difficult marital adjustments and serious sexual problems early in their marriages. Sexuality was not openly expressed or discussed, and this was a time when "pleasurable sex was for men only; women engaged in sexual activity to satisfy their husbands and to make babies" (Rheaume & Mitty, 2008, p. 344). These kinds of experiences shape beliefs and knowledge about sexual expression, as well as comfort with sexuality, particularly for older women. It is important to come to know and understand the older person within his or her social and cultural background and not make judgments based on one's own belief system.

The next generation of older people (baby boomers) has experienced other influences, including more liberal attitudes toward sexuality, the women's movement, a higher number of divorced adults, the human immunodeficiency virus (HIV) epidemic, and increased numbers of LGBT couples, that will affect their views and attitudes as they age. The baby boomers and beyond, as they find themselves experiencing sexuality beyond the age they had assigned to their elders, may alter current perceptions. Most of what is known about sexuality in aging has been gained through research with well-educated, healthy, white older adults. Further research is needed among culturally, socially, and ethnically diverse older people; those with chronic illness; and LGBT older people.

Biological Changes With Age

Acknowledgment and understanding of the age changes that influence sexual physiology, anatomy, and the stages of sexual response may partially explain alteration in sexual behavior to accommodate these changes and facilitate continued pleasurable sex. Characteristic physiological changes during the sexual response cycle do occur with aging, but these vary among individuals depending on general health factors. The changes occur abruptly in women starting with menopause but more gradually in men, a phenomenon called andropause (Kennedy et al., 2010).

The "use it or lose it" phenomenon applies here: the more sexually active the person is, the fewer changes he or she is likely to experience in the pattern of sexual response. Changes in the appearance of the body (wrinkles, sagging skin) may also affect the older person's security about his or her sexual attractiveness (Arena & Wallace, 2008). Table 26.1 summarizes physical changes in the sexual response cycle.

Older people who do not understand the physical changes that affect sexual activity become concerned that their sex life is approaching its natural conclusion with the onset of menopause or, for men, when they discover a change in the firmness of their erection or the decreased need for ejaculation with each orgasm or when the refractory period is extended between episodes of intercourse. A major nursing role is to provide information about these changes, as well as appropriate assessment and counseling within the context of the individual's needs.

SEXUAL DYSFUNCTION

Sexual dysfunction is defined as impairment in normal sexual functioning and can have many causes, both physical and psychological. Sexual disorders in older people have not been well studied, but generally, the following four categories are described: hypoactive sexual desire disorder; sexual arousal disorder; orgasmic disorder; and sexual pain disorders (Arena & Wallace, 2008).

Male Dysfunction

Erectile dysfunction (ED) is the most prevalent sexual problem in men. ED is defined as the inability to achieve and sustain an erection sufficient for satisfactory sexual intercourse in at least 50% or more attempts. When discussing ED with older men, it is important to provide education about normal age-related changes as well. Older men require more physical penile stimulation and a longer time to achieve erection, and the duration of orgasm may be shorter and less intense (Rheaume & Mitty, 2008).

An erection is governed by the interaction among the hormonal, vascular, and nervous systems. A problem in any of these systems can cause ED. Of course, multiple causes exist for this problem in older men. Nearly one-third of ED is a complication of diabetes. Alcoholism, medications, depression, and prostate cancer and treatment are also causes of ED in older men. The new nerve-saving microsurgical techniques used for prostatectomies often spare erectile function.

Anxiety and relationship issues are additional causes of ED, and, as Rheaume and Mitty (2008) note, some men may have widower's syndrome (difficulty achieving erection because they harbor guilt about pursuing a sexual relationship after the death of their spouse). Testosterone levels have little to do with ED but can have a major effect on libido (sexual desire).

The use of phosphodiesterase inhibitors such as sildenafil (Viagra), vardenafil (Levitra), and tadalafil (Cialis) has revolutionized treatment for ED regardless of cause. Contraindications to the use of these medications include use of nitrate therapy, heart failure with low blood pressure, certain antihypertensive regimens, and other medications and cardiovascular conditions (see Chapter 9).

Before the availability of these medications, intracavernosal injections with the drugs papaverine and

TABLE 26.1 Physical Changes in Sexual Response in Old Age

Female	Male
Excitation Phase	
Diminished or delayed lubrication (1 to 3 minutes may be required for adequate amounts to appear)	Less intense and slower erection (but can be maintained longer without ejaculation)
Diminished flattening and separation of labia majora	Increased difficulty regaining an erection if lost
Disappearance of elevation of labia majora	Less vasocongestion of scrotal sac
Decreased vasocongestion of labia minora	Less pronounced elevation and congestion of testicles
Decreased elastic expansion of vagina (depth and breadth)	
Breasts not as engorged	
Sex flush absent	
Plateau Phase	
Slower and less prominent uterine elevation or tenting	Decreased muscle tension
Nipple erection and sexual flush less often	No color change at coronal edge of penis
Decreased capacity for vasocongestion	Slower penile erection pattern
Decreased areolar engorgement	Delayed or diminished erectile and testicular elevation
Labial color change less evident	
Less intense swelling or orgasmic platform	
Less sexual flush	
Decreased secretions of Bartholin's glands	
Orgasmic Phase	
Fewer number and less intense orgasmic contractions	Decreased or absent secretory activity (lubrication) by Cowper's gland before ejaculation
Rectal sphincter contraction with severe tension only	Fewer penile contractions
	Fewer rectal sphincter contractions
	Decreased force of ejaculation (approximately 50%) with decreased amount of semen (if ejaculation is long, seepage of semen occurs)
Resolution Phase	
Observably slower loss of nipple erection	Vasocongestion of nipples and scrotum slowly subsides
Vasocongestion of clitoris and orgasmic platform	Very rapid loss of erection and descent of testicles shortly after ejaculation
	Refractory time extended (time required before another erection ranges from several to 24 hours, occasionally longer)

phentolamine, vasoactive agents that reduce resistance of arteriolar and cavernosal smooth muscle tissue of the penis, were used. Penile implants of the semirigid, adjustable-malleable, or hinged and inflatable types are available when impotence does not respond to other treatments or is irreversible. The hinged and inflatable types, which are inserted in the testicular area, are the most popular. Another alternative is the vacuum pump device, which works by creating a vacuum that draws blood into the penis, causing an erection. Vacuum pumps are available in manual and battery-operated versions and may be covered by Medicare if deemed medically necessary.

Female Dysfunction

Female dysfunction is considered "persistent impediment to a person's normal pattern of sexual interest, response, or both" (Kaiser, 2000, p. 1174). Female sexual function can be influenced by factors such as culture, ethnicity, emotional state, age, and previous sexual experiences, as well as age-related changes in sexual response. Frequency of intimacy depends more on the age, health, and sexual function of the partner or the availability of a partner, rather than on their own sexual capacity.

Postmenopausal changes in the urinary or genital tract as a result of lower estrogen levels can make sexual activity less pleasurable (Rheaume & Mitty, 2008). Dyspareunia, resulting from vaginal dryness and thinning of the vaginal tissue, occurs in one-third of women older than age 65. In many instances, using water-soluble lubricants such as K-Y Jelly, Astroglide, Slip, and HR lubricating jelly during foreplay or intercourse can resolve the difficulty. Topical low-dose estrogen creams, rings, or pills that are introduced into the vagina may also help to plump tissues and restore lubrication, with less absorption than oral hormones (Kennedy et al., 2010; Rheaume & Mitty, 2008).

Women can experience arousal disorders resulting from drugs such as anticholinergics, antidepressants, and chemotherapeutic agents and from lack of lubrication from radiation, surgery, and stress. Orgasmic disorders also may result from drugs used to treat depression. Unlike ED, studies of vascular insufficiency are less clear in women with sexual dysfunction. Prolapse of the uterus, rectoceles, and cystoceles can be surgically repaired to facilitate continued sexual activity. Urinary incontinence (UI) is another condition that may affect sexual activity for both men and women. Appropriate assessment and treatment are important because many causes of UI are treatable (see Chapter 12).

ALTERNATIVE SEXUAL LIFESTYLES: LESBIAN, GAY, BISEXUAL, AND TRANSGENDER

Discrimination in health and social systems affects gays, lesbians, bisexuals, and transgender individuals of all ages. Older individuals may be even more at risk for discrimination as a result of lifelong experiences with marginalization and oppression. They may have been shunned by family or friends, religious organizations, and the medical community; ridiculed or physically attacked; or labeled as sinners, perverts, or criminals.

It was not until 1973 that homosexuality was removed from the *Diagnostic and Statistical Manual of Mental Disorders* (Institute of Medicine, 2011; Jablonski et al., 2013; Lim et al., 2014). Gay and lesbian older people face the "double stigma" of being both old and homosexual, with lesbians facing the triple threat of being women, being old, and having a different sexual orientation (Agronin, 2004; Jablonski et al., 2013).

As a result of lifelong discrimination and negative experiences with health care agencies and personnel, LGBT older adults are much less likely than their heterosexual peers to access needed health and social services or identify themselves as gay or lesbian to health care providers (SAGE & MAP, 2010). As a result, they are at greater risk for poorer health than their heterosexual counterparts. LGBT older adults are more likely than their heterosexual counterparts to experience poor health and aging outcomes, including chronic illnesses. They are also more likely to have serious mental health issues (Cloyes, 2016). Among LGBT individuals, transgender older adults have the most difficulty accessing health care and are more likely to experience financial barriers, receive inferior care, and be denied health care (Jablonski et al., 2013).

❖ IMPLICATIONS FOR GERONTOLOGICAL NURSING AND HEALTHY AGING

◆ Assessment

Health care providers may assume that their LGBT patients are heterosexual and neglect to obtain a sexual history, discuss sexuality, or be aware of their particular medical needs. Providers receive little education and training in the needs of this population and may lack sensitivity when caring for older LGBT individuals (Cloyes, 2016; Jablonski et al., 2013; Lim et al., 2014). Sensitivity is of utmost importance when attempting to obtain a health history. Using open-ended questions such as "Who is most important to you?" or "Do you have a significant other?" is much better than asking "Are you married?" Asking individuals if they consider themselves as primarily heterosexual, homosexual, bisexual, or transgender is also better and conveys recognition of sexual variety. If the patient identifies as transgender, it is important to ask how the individual wants to be addressed.

Euphemisms are frequently used for a life partner (e.g., roommate, close friend). An older lesbian woman in a health care situation may refer to herself indirectly by saying "people like us." Nurses need to be more aware of these nuances and try to understand the fear of discovery that is apparent in the older gay man and lesbian woman. These elders are of a generation in which they were, and may still be, closeted because of the homophobic experiences they had throughout their younger years.

◆ Interventions

Better support and care services for LGBT individuals by care providers should include working through homophobic attitudes and discomfort discussing sexuality, learning about special issues facing LGBT individuals, and becoming aware of resources in the community specific to this population. When caring for transgender older adults, it is important to use discretion and sensitivity when obtaining medical and surgical histories and performing physical examinations (Caceres & Frank, 2016; Jablonski et al., 2013).

Facilities or agencies in the community need to be assessed from the perspective of the client, patient, or resident who may be gay, lesbian, bisexual, or transgender. It is important that service providers create programs that are inclusive and culturally appropriate for all individuals. LGBT older adults fear discrimination and mistreatment from service providers across a range of settings. "The need to go back into the closet to protect oneself while receiving home health services, or when transitioning from community to residential living, is a recurring theme within studies of LGBT older adults' views on long-term care" (Cloyes, 2016, p. 54). LGBT specific retirement communities and long-term care facilities are emerging in certain parts of the country. It is important for providers of aging services to implement programs to increase awareness of the needs of LGBT elders and reduce discrimination, especially in light of the anticipated increase in older LGBT individuals. Other resources are presented in Box 26.5.

INTIMACY AND CHRONIC ILLNESS

Chronic illnesses and their related treatments may bring many challenges to intimacy and sexual activity. Physical capacity may be affected by illness and psychological factors (anxiety, depression) affect sexual activity (Steinke, 2013). Often, patients and their partners are given little or no information about the effect of illnesses on sexual activity or strategies to continue sexual activity within functional limitations. Individuals want and need information on sexual functioning, and health care professionals need to become more knowledgeable and more actively involved in sexual counseling.

Table 26.2 presents suggestions for individuals with chronic illness. Timing of intercourse (mornings or when energy level is highest), oral or anal sex, masturbation, appropriate pain relief, and different sexual positions are all strategies that may assist in continued sexual activity. There is no consensus on what kind of position the individual should assume for sexual activity, but a lesser amount of energy is expended with the person on the bottom during use of the missionary position. Alternative positions may require less energy and may be more comfortable depending on the situation (Fig. 26.2) (Kennedy et al., 2010; Steinke, 2013; Steinke et al., 2013).

INTIMACY AND SEXUALITY IN LONG-TERM CARE FACILITIES

Research is needed on sexuality in residential care facilities and nursing homes, but surveys suggest that a significant number of older people living in these

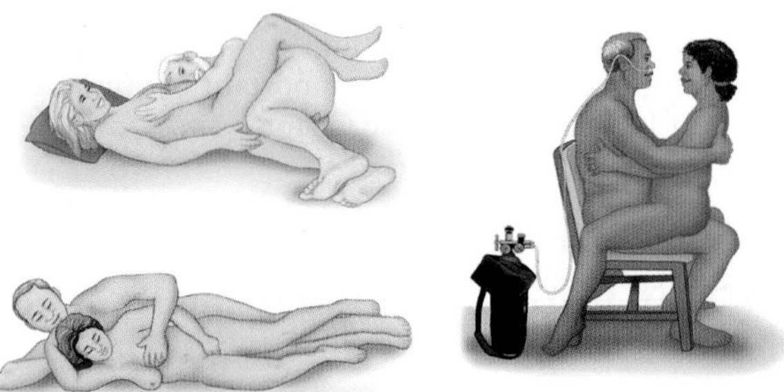

FIGURE 26.2 Adaptations of sexual positions for individuals with chronic illness.

TABLE 26.2 Chronic Illness and Sexual Function: Effects and Interventions

Condition	Effects/Problems	Interventions
Arthritis	Pain, fatigue, limited motion Steroid therapy may decrease sexual interest or desire	Advise patient to perform sexual activity at time of day when less fatigued and most relaxed Suggest use of analgesics and other pain-relief methods before sexual activity Encourage use of relaxation techniques before sexual activity, such as a warm bath or shower, application of hot packs to affected joints Advise patient to maintain optimal health through a balance of good nutrition, proper rest, and activity Suggest that he or she experiment with different positions, use pillows for comfort and support Recommend use of a vibrator if massage ability is limited Suggest use of water-soluble jelly for vaginal lubrication

TABLE 26.2 Chronic Illness and Sexual Function: Effects and Interventions—cont'd

Condition	Effects/Problems	Interventions
Cardiovascular disease	Most men have no change in physical effects on sexual function; one-fourth may not return to pre–heart attack function; one-fourth may not resume sexual activity Women do not experience sexual dysfunction after heart attack Fear of another heart attack or death during sex Shortness of breath	Encourage counseling on realistic restrictions that may be necessary **Post–myocardial infarction (MI):** Those able to engage in mild to moderate physical activity without symptoms can generally resume sexual activity; those with a complicated MI may need to resume sexual activity gradually over a longer period of time Avoid large meals several hours before sex Avoid anal sex Instruct patient and spouse on alternative positions to avoid strain and allow for unrestricted breathing Stop and rest if chest pain is experienced, take nitroglycerin if prescribed, and seek emergency treatment for sustained chest pain **Post–coronary artery bypass graft or pacemaker or internal cardiac defibrillator (ICD) insertion:** Avoid strain or direct pressure on device/incision Individuals with poorly controlled dysrhythmias should not engage in sexual activity until the condition is well managed Instruct individual that ICD could fire with sex, although uncommon; a change in device setting may be needed
Cerebrovascular accident (stroke)	Depression May or may not have sexual activity changes Often erectile disorders occur Change in role and function of partners Decreased physical endurance, fatigue Mobility and sensory deficits Perceptual and visual deficits Communication deficits Cognitive and behavioral deficits Fear of relapse or sudden death	Encourage counseling Instruct patient to use alternative positions Suggest use of a vibrator if massage ability is limited Suggest use of pillows for positioning and support Suggest use of water-soluble jelly for lubrication Suggest alternate forms of sexual expression acceptable to the individuals
Chronic obstructive pulmonary disease (COPD)	No direct impairment of sexual activity, although affected by coughing, exertional dyspnea, positions, and activity intolerance Medications may lead to erectile difficulties	Encourage patient to plan sexual activity when energy is highest Instruct patient to use alternative positions; use ample pillows for support and elevate the upper body, or use a sitting upright position; avoid any pressure on the chest Advise patient to plan sexual activity at time medications are most effective Suggest use of oxygen before, during, or after sex, depending on when it provides the most benefit Teach partner to observe for breathing difficulty and allow time for change of positions and time to catch breath when needed

Continued

TABLE 26.2 Chronic Illness and Sexual Function: Effects and Interventions—cont'd

Condition	Effects/Problems	Interventions
Diabetes	Sexual desire and interest unaffected Neuropathy and/or vascular damage may interfere with erectile ability; about 50% to 75% of men have erectile disorders; a small portion have retrograde ejaculation Some men regain function if diagnosis of diabetes is well accepted, if diabetes is well controlled, or both Women have less sexual desire and vaginal lubrication Decrease in orgasms/absence of orgasm can occur; less frequent sexual activity; local genital infections	Recommend possible candidates for penile prosthesis Suggest use of alternative forms of sexual expression Recommend immediate treatment of genital infections
Cancers		
Breast	No direct physical affect; there is a strong psychological effect: loss of sexual desire, body-image change, depression/reaction of partner	Refer to support groups, sex therapists, counselors Encourage open expression of sexual concerns
Prostate	Incontinence can occur following surgery Erectile dysfunction Psychological effects Use of nerve-sparing surgery causes less dysfunction	Kegel exercises and routine toileting Use of phosphodiesterase inhibitors Provide information related to sexual functioning/continence
Most other cancers	Men and women may lose sexual desire temporarily Men may have erectile dysfunction; dry/retrograde ejaculation Women may have vaginal dryness, dyspareunia Both men and women may experience anxiety, depression, pain, nausea from chemotherapy, radiation, hormone therapy, and nerve damage from pelvic surgery	New sexual positions may be helpful; explore alternative sexual activities

settings might choose to be sexually active if they had privacy and a sexual partner (Messinger-Rapport et al., 2003). Intimacy and sexuality among residents includes the opportunity to have not only coitus but also other forms of intimate expressions, such as hugging, kissing, hand holding, and masturbation. Wallace (2003) commented that the sexual needs of older adults in long-term care facilities should be addressed with the same priority as nutrition, hydration, and other well-accepted needs. The institutionalized older person has the same rights as noninstitutionalized elders to engage in or refrain from sexual activity.

Attitudes about intimacy and sexuality among long-term care staff and, often, family members may reflect general societal attitudes that older people do not have sexual needs or that sexual activity is inappropriate. Families may have difficulty understanding that their older relative may want to have a new relationship. Nursing home staff generally have limited knowledge of late-life sexuality and may view residents' sexual acts as problems rather than as expressions of the need for love and intimacy (DiNapoli et al., 2013). Reactions may include disapproval, discomfort, and embarrassment, and caregivers may explicitly or implicitly discourage or deny intimacy needs.

Privacy is a major issue in nursing homes that can prevent fulfillment of intimacy and sexual needs. Suggestions for providing privacy and an atmosphere accepting of sexual activity include offering the availability of a private room, not interrupting when doors are closed and sexual activity is taking place, allowing residents to have sexually explicit materials in their rooms, and providing adaptive equipment, such as side rails or trapezes and double beds. In one facility where one of the authors (T.T.) worked, the staff would assist one of the female residents to be freshly showered, perfumed, and in a lovely nightgown when she and her partner wanted to have sexual relations.

Interventions

Staff, family, and resident education programs to promote awareness, provide education on sexuality and intimacy in later life, involve residents in discussions of sexuality, and discuss interventions to respond to residents' needs are important in long-term care settings. Staff education should include the opportunity to discuss personal feelings about sexuality, changes associated with aging, the impact of diseases and medications on sexual function, sexual expression among same-sex residents, as well as role-playing and skill training in sexual assessment and intervention (DiNapoli et al., 2013).

INTIMACY, SEXUALITY, AND DEMENTIA

Intimacy and sexuality remain important in the lives of persons with dementia and their partners throughout the illness. Intimacy and sexuality may "serve as a nonverbal form of communication and intimacy when other cognitive skills and functions have declined" (Agronin, 2004, p. 13). Yet sexual behavior between life partners when one has dementia is not often addressed, and individuals with dementia may be viewed as asexual. Nurses need to have an awareness of the sexual needs of the individual with dementia and the individual's partner and be comfortable discussing this area with both persons. Robinson and Davis (2013) suggest asking the question: "How has dementia affected your sexual relationship?" (Robinson & Davis, 2013, p. 35).

As dementia progresses, particularly in persons living in long-term care facilities, intimacy and sexuality issues may present challenges, especially regarding the impaired person's ability to consent to sexual activity, and require accurate assessment and documentation. Inappropriate sexual behavior (exposing oneself, masturbating in public, or making inappropriate sexual advances or sexual comments) may also occur in long-term care settings. These behaviors are most distressing to staff and to other residents. Sexual inappropriateness (sexual disinhibition) is one of the least understood aspects of dementia. Individuals with subtypes of dementia that include frontal lobe impairment (Pick's disease and alcoholic dementia) may exhibit more sexually inappropriate behavior (Balasubramaniam et al., 2013).

These kinds of behavior may be triggered by unmet intimacy needs or may be symptoms of an underlying physical problem, such as a urinary tract or vaginal infection. The lack of privacy in nursing homes may lead to sexually inappropriate behavior in public areas. Social cues such as explicit television shows may also precipitate behaviors. Bodily contact, such as when bathing residents, may be misinterpreted as a sexual act or romantic advance.

Rheaume and Mitty (2008) suggest that an interdisciplinary sexual assessment to determine the underlying need that the person is expressing and how it might be addressed is important. Encouraging family and friends to touch, hug, kiss, and hold hands when visiting may help to meet touch and intimacy needs and decrease inappropriate sexual behavior. Also, allowing the person to stroke a pet or hold a stuffed animal may be helpful. Similar to other behavior symptoms in individuals with dementia, nonpharmacological interventions are first-line treatment for behaviors related to sexual needs. Aggressive or violent behavior may require limit setting, working with the resident and family, providing for sexual expression in a nonharmful manner, and initiating pharmacological treatment if indicated (Messinger-Rapport et al., 2003). Staff will need opportunities for discussion and assistance with interventions.

Sexuality among nursing home residents with dementia is a sensitive topic, and there are no national guidelines for determining sexual consent capacity among individuals with severe dementia (DiNapoli et al., 2013). Determination of a cognitively impaired person's ability to consent to participation in a sexual activity involves concepts of voluntary participation, mental competence, and an understanding of the risks and benefits. The Hebrew Home in Riverdale, New York, initiated model sexual policies in 1995. The recently updated policies are valuable resources on intimacy, sexuality, and sexual behavior for older people with dementia (National Institute on Aging, National Institutes of Health, 2015) (Box 26.5).

HIV/AIDS AND OLDER ADULTS

An increasingly significant trend in the global HIV epidemic is the growing number of people aged 50 years and older who are living with HIV. This trend is occurring in both developed and developing countries. In the United States, nearly 37% of people with HIV are older than age 50. Predictions are that this figure could rise to 70% by 2020 (Fig. 26.3) (HIVAge.org, 2014; HIVAge.org, 2016). In major metro areas, more than half of all those living with HIV are age 50 and older. The racial/ethnic disparities in HIV/AIDS among older people parallel trends among all age groups, with higher rates among African Americans and Hispanics/Latinos. Fourteen percent of gay or bisexual men are HIV positive (Jablonski et al., 2013). Women older than age 60 make up one of the fastest-growing risk groups, and 70% of older HIV-positive women are African American or Hispanic/Latina (Greene et al., 2013). Most got the virus

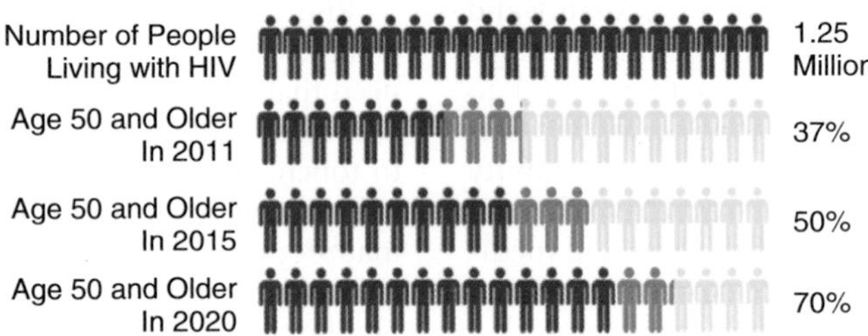

FIGURE 26.3 HIV and older adults. Data estimations are based on CDC surveillance data. (From http://hiv-age.org. Used with permission from S.E. Karpiak, PhD.)

from sex with infected partners (CDC, 2016; HIV Wisdom for Older Women, 2010).

Although rates of HIV/AIDS have remained relatively stable in younger age groups, the number of older people infected with the virus is growing. The largest increase in HIV diagnoses from 2008 to 2010 was among people ages 65 and older (Baron-Faust, 2013; CDC, 2016). The incidence is expected to continue to increase as more individuals become infected later in life, and those who were infected in early adulthood live longer as a result of advances in disease treatment.

The compromised immune system of an older individual makes him or her even more susceptible to HIV or AIDS than a younger person. Older women who are sexually active are at high risk for HIV/AIDS (and other sexually transmitted infections) from an infected partner, resulting, in part, from normal age changes of the vaginal tissue—a thinner, drier, friable vaginal lining that makes viral entry more efficient (CDC, 2016; UNAIDS, 2013).

Studies show that sexually active older men and women do not routinely use condoms, thus increasing their risk of sexually transmitted diseases. Recently widowed or divorced individuals may not understand the need for practicing safe sex because they do not worry about an unwanted pregnancy and may not understand the risk of sexually transmitted diseases (Johnson, 2013). Box 26.8 presents some other risk factors.

BOX 26.8 Risk Factors for HIV

- You are sexually active and do not use a latex or polyurethane condom.
- You do not know your partner's drug and sexual history. Questions you should ask: "Has your partner been tested for HIV/AIDS?" "Has he or she had a number of different sexual partners?" "Has your partner ever had unprotected sex with someone or shared needles?" "Has he or she injected drugs or shared needles with someone else?" Drug users are not the only people who might share needles. People with diabetes who inject insulin or draw blood to test glucose level might share needles.
- You have had a blood transfusion or operation in a developing country at any time.
- You have had a blood transfusion in the United States between 1978 and 1985.

From National Institute on Aging: *HIV, AIDS, and older people*, 2009. Available at http://www.nia.nih.gov/sites/default/files/hiv_aids_and_older_people.pdf. Accessed June 2016.

Assessment

Physicians, nurse practitioners, and other health professionals need to increase their knowledge of HIV in older adults and become comfortable taking a complete sexual history and talking about sex with all older adults. A thorough sex and drug use/assessment screening should be conducted with attention to HIV risk factors (Johnson, 2013). The idea that elders are not sexually active limits health care providers' objectivity to recognize HIV/AIDS as a possible diagnosis.

AIDS in older adults has been called the "Great Imitator" because many of the symptoms, such as fatigue, weakness, weight loss, and anorexia, are common to other disease conditions and may be attributed to normal aging. Additionally, older people may blame possible symptoms on aging or be reluctant to seek testing or share symptoms because of the stigma they associate with the disease (National Institute on Aging, 2009). Older adults living with HIV/AIDS are thought to experience a "double stigma" of being both old and HIV/AIDS-positive (National Resource Center on LGBT Aging, 2011).

Most U.S. guidelines recommend HIV testing among high-risk groups regardless of age, but routine screening recommendations differ and some have a cut-off age of 65 years. Medicare covers annual screenings for HIV for those who are at increased risk and those who ask for the test. Also covered is annual screening for those who are at increased risk for sexually transmitted infections (STIs). A home HIV test system is made by the Home Access Health Corporation and is the only system approved by the FDA. It is available at retail pharmacies (National Institute on Aging, 2009).

Interventions

Lack of awareness about HIV in older people results in older people diagnosed with HIV infection late in the course of their disease, meaning a late start to treatment, possibly more damage to their immune system, and poorer prognoses than younger individuals (CDC, 2016; UNAIDS, 2013). HIV-infected adults may also be at increased risk of geriatric syndromes that complicate their treatment and face higher rates of cardiovascular disease, diabetes, hypertension, and cancer (HIVAge.org, 2014). Some research has reported more cognitive deficits in individuals with HIV, and this may be due to the systemic inflammation that also promotes neuroinflammation (Jablonski et al., 2013).

Antiretroviral therapy (ART) can be more complicated if there are chronic illnesses, comorbidities, and polypharmacy (Kazer, 2012). Long-term effects of antiretroviral therapy are also not well studied. However, there is no evidence that response to therapy is different in older people than in younger individuals and some data suggest that older individuals may be more adherent to ART. Presently, guidelines for care of adults 60 to 80 years of age with HIV are somewhat limited because this population has not been studied in clinical trials or pharmacokinetic trials (Greene et al., 2013).

Misinformation about HIV is more common in older adults, and they may know less about the disease than younger individuals (Kazer et al., 2013; UNAIDS, 2013). Educational materials and programs aimed at older adults need continued development. They should include information about what HIV/AIDS is and how it is (and is not) transmitted, risk-reduction counseling, symptoms of which to be aware, and the treatments that are available.

Jane Fowler, director of the National HIV Wisdom for Older Women program (WOW), suggests that HIV/AIDS educational campaigns and programs are not targeted to older individuals and asks, "How often does a wrinkled face appear on a prevention poster?" (HIV Wisdom for Older Women, 2010). The National Institute on Aging provides an HIV/AIDS toolkit with resources designed specifically for education of older people (see Box 26.5).

❖ IMPLICATIONS FOR GERONTOLOGICAL NURSING AND HEALTHY AGING

Nurses have multiple roles in the area of sexuality and older people. The nurse is a facilitator of a milieu that is conducive to the person asking questions and expressing his or her sexuality. The nurse is also an educator and provides information and guidance to those who need it. Some older people remain or want to remain sexually active, whereas others do not see this as an important part of their life. Nurses should open the door to discussions of sexual concerns in a nonjudgmental manner, helping those who want to continue to be sexually active, and making it clear that stopping sex is an acceptable option for others.

◆ Assessment

Sexuality and intimacy are crucial to healthy aging, and the way these are expressed among older adults is changing, particularly with the aging of the baby boomers and upcoming generations. When promoting healthy aging, nurses must consider increasingly open attitudes toward sexuality, dating and developing new relationships, the challenges of facilitating intimacy in residential settings, and the importance of promoting sexual health and safe sex practices (Syme, 2014). Being aware of one's own feelings about sexuality and attitudes toward intimacy and sexuality in older people of all sexual preferences is important. Only after confronting one's own attitudes, values, and beliefs can the nurse provide support without being judgmental.

Anticipation of problems in older individuals' sexual experiences can ward off anxiety, misconceptions, and an arbitrary cessation of sexual pleasure. Validation of the normalcy of sexual activity and a discussion of the physiological changes that occur either with age or as a result of illness are important. Adaptations that will promote sexual function for individuals with chronic illness should be provided. Screening for HIV/AIDS and other sexually transmitted diseases and education about safe sexual practices are also important (Box 26.9) (Johnson, 2013).

In addition, the myth that elders do not engage in sexual activity must be put to rest. After age 50, only 38% of U.S. men and 22% of U.S. women report discussing sexual activity with their health care provider, and only about one-fourth of U.S. adults, without obvious risk for HIV acquisition, are screened for HIV (Greene et al., 2013). When questions about sexual issues are asked or when the older adult is examined, the nurse needs to be particularly cognizant of the era and culture in which the individual has lived to understand the factors affecting conduct. The CDC provides a guide to taking a sexual history (Box 26.5).

BOX 26.9 Tips for Best Practice

Screening for Sexually Transmitted Infections Among Older Adults

- Adults who are sexually active should talk to their health care provider about STI testing.
- All adults should be tested at least once for HIV.
- All sexually active older women with risk factors such as new or multiple sex partners or who live in communities with a high burden of disease should be screened annually for chlamydia and gonorrhea.
- Screening is recommended at least once a year for syphilis, chlamydia, gonorrhea, and HIV for all sexually active gay men, bisexual men, and other men who have sex with men.

From Johnson B: Sexually transmitted infections and older adults, *J Gerontol Nurs* 39(11):53–60, 2013.

BOX 26.10 PLISSIT Model

P—**Permission** from the client to initiate sexual discussion
LI—Providing the **Limited Information** needed to function sexually
SS—Giving **Specific Suggestions** for the individual to proceed with sexual relations
IT—Providing **Intensive Therapy** surrounding the issues of sexuality for the clients (may mean referral to specialist)

Compiled from Annon J: The PLISSIT model: A proposed conceptual scheme for behavioral treatment of sexual problems, *J Sex Educ Ther* 2:1–15, 1976; Wallace M: Best practices in nursing care to older adults: Sexuality, *Dermatol Nurs* 15:570–571, 2003; Youngkin EQ: The myths and truths of mature intimacy, *Adv Nurse Pract* 12:45–48, 2004.

A medication review is essential because many medications affect sexual functioning. Often, medications are prescribed to both older men and women without attention to the sexual side effects. If medications that affect sexual function are necessary, adjustment of doses, use of alternative agents, and prescription of antidotes to reverse the sexual side effects are important.

The PLISSIT Model (Annon, 1976) is a helpful guide for discussion of sexuality (Box 26.10). Youngkin (2004) provides suggestions for use of the PLISSIT Model with older people:

- **Permission:** Obtain permission from the client to initiate sexual discussion. Allow the person to discuss concerns related to sexual issues, and gather information about what might have changed in the person's life to affect sexual needs and response. Questions such as the following can be used: "What concerns or questions do you have about fulfilling your sexual needs?" or "In this era of HIV and other sexually transmitted infections, I ask all my patients about sexual practices and concerns. Are there any questions I can answer for you?"
- **Limited Information:** Provide the limited information to function sexually (Wallace, 2003). Offer teaching about the normal age-associated changes that affect sexual performance or how illness may affect sexuality. Encourage the person to learn more about the concern from books and other sources.
- **Specific Suggestions:** Offer suggestions for dealing with problems such as lubricants for atrophic vaginitis; use of condoms to prevent sexually transmitted infections; proper use of ED medications; how to communicate sexual and other needs; ways to increase comfort with coitus or ways to be intimate without coital relations.
- **Intensive Therapy:** Refer as appropriate for complex problems that require specialist intervention.

◆ Interventions

Interventions will vary depending on the needs identified from the assessment data. Following a comprehensive assessment, interventions may center on the following categories: (1) education regarding age-associated change in sexual function; (2) compensation for age-associated changes and effects of chronic illness; (3) effective management of acute and chronic illness affecting sexual function; (4) provision of education on HIV and STIs and reduction of risk factors; (5) removal of barriers associated with fulfilling sexual needs; and (6) special interventions to promote sexual health in cognitively impaired older adults (Arena & Wallace, 2008) (Box 26.5).

KEY CONCEPTS

- The ability to successfully negotiate transitions and develop new and gratifying roles in later life depends on personal and environmental supports, timing, clarity of expectations, personality, and degree of change required.
- Retirement is no longer just a few years of rest from the rigors of work before death. It is a developmental stage that may occupy 30 or more years of one's life and involve many stages. Some individuals will be retired longer than they worked.
- Preretirement planning and postretirement follow-up significantly affect positive adaptation to the transition.

- Elders and their family members carry a long history. Current family dynamics must be understood within the context of family history.
- Loss of a spouse is the role change that has the greatest potential for life disruption, and nursing support can make a positive difference in the transition.
- Sexuality is love, sharing, trust, and warmth, as well as physical acts. Sexuality provides an individual with self-identity and affirmation of life.
- Generally speaking, medications, ill health, and lack of a partner affect sexual activity as one ages.
- Further research is needed to promote knowledge and understanding of the sexual health of LGBT older adults.
- The major role of the nurse in enhancing the sexual health of older adults in the community or in long-term care settings is education and counseling about sexual function and adaptations for age-related changes and chronic conditions; prevention of HIV/AIDS and STDs in sexually active individuals; and the maintenance of sexuality for health, well-being, and pleasure.
- AIDS awareness and the practice of safe sex among older adults is still lacking. Older adults and health professionals may not consider older adults at risk for AIDS or STDs even though the incidence of these diseases in the older population is rapidly increasing.

ACTIVITIES AND DISCUSSION QUESTIONS

1. Discuss your position in the family and how that has affected your relationship with siblings and parents.
2. Write a brief essay discussing the ways in which your grandparents have affected your life.
3. With a classmate, role-play how you would conduct a review of systems in the area of sexual health with an older adult.
4. What would be the most important factors to consider when providing education about sexuality and sexual health?
5. What resources are available for older LGBT individuals in your community?

REFERENCES

Agronin M: Sexuality and aging: An introduction, *CNS Longterm Care* 3:12–13, 2004.

American Society on Aging and MetLife: *Still out, still aging,* 2010. Available at https://www.metlife.com/assets/cao/mmi/publications/studies/2010/mmi-still-out-still-aging.pdf. Accessed March 2016.

Annon J: The PLISSIT model: A proposed conceptual scheme for behavioral treatment of sexual problems, *J Sex Educ Ther* 2:1–15, 1976.

Arena J, Wallace M: Issues regarding sexuality. In Capezuti E, Swicker D, Mezey M, et al, editors: *Evidence-based geriatric nursing protocols for best practice*, ed 3, New York, 2008, Springer, pp 629–648.

Bach L, Mortimer J, Vandeweerd C, et al: The association of physical and mental health with sexual activity in older adults in a retirement community, *J Sex Med* 10(11):2671–2678, 2013.

Balasubramaniam M, Clark L, Jensen T, et al: Medroxyprogesterone acetate treatment for sexually inappropriate behavior in a patient with frontotemporal dementia, *Ann Longterm Care* 21(11):30–36, 2013.

Baron-Faust R: *HIV/AIDS in older adults: Rising, and unchecked,* 2013. Available at http://www.rheumatologynetwork.com/articles/hivaids-older-adults-rising-and-unchecked. Accessed May 2014.

Batiashvili G, Gerzmava O: Administration on Aging, Global comparison of formal and informal caregiving, *Eur Sci J* 2:89–97, 2013.

Bennett K, Soulsby L: Well-being in bereavement, *Illn Crises Loss* 20(4):321–337, 2012.

Blieszner R: The worth of friendships: Can friends keep us happy and healthy? *Generations* 38(1):24–30, 2014.

Board of Governors of the Federal Reserve System: *Report of the economic well-being of households in 2015.* Available at https://www.federalreserve.gov/econresdata/2016-economic-well-being-of-us-households-in-2015-retirement.htm. Accessed September 2016.

Caceres B, Frank M: Successful ageing in lesbian, gay and bisexual older people: A concept analysis, *Int J Older People Nurs* 2016. doi: 10.1111/opn.12108.

Carey I, Shah S, DeWilde S, et al: Increased risk of acute cardiovascular events after partner bereavement, *JAMA* 174(4):598–605, 2014.

Centers for Disease Control and Prevention: *HIV among older Americans,* 2016. Available at http://www.cdc.gov/hiv/risk/age/olderamericans. Accessed March 2016.

Cloyes K: Seeing silver in the spectrum: LGBT older adult health, aging, and gerontological nursing research, *Res Gerontol Nurs* 9(12):54–57, 2016.

Comfort A: Sexuality in old age, *J Am Geriatr Soc* 22:440–442, 1974.

Das A: Spousal loss and health in late life: Moving beyond emotional trauma, *J Aging Health* 25:221–242, 2013.

deVries B: Grief: Intimacy's reflection, *Generations* 25:75–80, 2001.

DiGiacomo M, Lewis J, Nolan M, et al: Health transitions in recently widowed women: A mixed methods study, *BMC Health Serv Res* 13:143, 2013.

DiNapoli E, Breland G, Allen R: Staff knowledge and perceptions of sexuality and dementia of older adults in nursing homes, *J Aging Health* 25:1087–1105, 2013.

Fisher L: *Sex, romance and relationships: AARP survey of midlife and older adults,* May 2010. Available at http://assets.aarp.org/rgcenter/general/srr_09.pdf. Document 1. Accessed September 2016.

Generations United: *Family matters: multigenerational families in a volatile economy,* 2011. Available at http://www.gu.org/RESOURCES/Publications/FamilyMattersMultigenerationalFamilies.aspx. Accessed September 2016.

Generations United: *What is a multigenerational household?* 2014. Available at http://www2.gu.org/OURWORK/Multigenerational/MultigenerationalHouseholdInformation.aspx. Accessed March 2016.

Greene M, Justice A, Lampiris H, et al: Management of human immunodeficiency virus infection in advanced age, *JAMA* 309(13):1387–1405, 2013.

Hadfield J: The health of grandparents raising grandchildren, *J Gerontol Nurs* 40(4):32–42, 2014.

HIVAge.org: *Geriatric syndromes are common among HIV-infected adults,* April 4, 2014. Available at http://hiv-age.org/2014/04/04/geriatric-syndromes-common-among-older-hiv-infected-adults. Accessed March 2016.

HIVAge.org: *Older adults dominate the USA HIV/AIDS epidemic,* September 12, 2016. Available at http://hiv-age.org/2016/09/12/older-adults-dominate-usa-hivaids-epidemic/. Accessed September 2016.

HIV Wisdom for Older Women: *Things you should know about HIV and older women,* 2010. Available at http://www.hivwisdom.org/facts.html. Accessed March 2016.

Hooyman N, Kiyak H: *Social gerontology: A multidisciplinary perspective,* ed 9, Boston, 2011, Allyn & Bacon.

Institute of Medicine: *The health of lesbian, gay, bisexual, and transgender people: Building a better foundation for better understanding,* 2011. Available at http://nationalacademies.org/HMD/Reports/2011/The-Health-of-Lesbian-Gay-Bisexual-and-Transgender-People.aspx. Accessed September 2016.

Jablonski R, Vance D, Beattie E: The invisible elderly: Lesbian, gay, bisexual, and transgender older adults, *J Gerontol Nurs* 39(11):46–52, 2013.

Jackson L, Howe N, Tobias P: *The global aging preparedness index,* ed 2, Washington, DC, 2013, Center for Strategic and International Studies. Available at http://csis.org/publication/global-aging-preparedness-index-second-edition. Accessed September 2016.

Johnson B: Sexually transmitted infections and older adults, *J Gerontol Nurs* 39(11):53–60, 2013.

Kaiser FE: Sexual dysfunction in men; sexual dysfunction in women. In Beers MH, Berkow R, editors: *The Merck manual of geriatrics,* ed 3, Whitehouse Station, NJ, 2000, Merck.

Kazer M: Issues regarding sexuality. In Boltz M, Capezuti E, Fulmer T, et al, editors: *Evidence-based geriatric nursing protocols for best practice,* ed 4, New York, 2012, Springer, pp 500–515.

Kazer M, Grossman S, Kerins G, et al: Validity and reliability of the Geriatric Sexual Inventory, *J Gerontol Nurs* 39(11):40–45, 2013.

Kennedy G, Martinez M, Garo N: Sex and mental health in old age, *Prim Psychiatry* 17:22–30, 2010.

Keyes K, Pratt C, Galea S, et al: The burden of loss: Unexpected death of a loved one and psychiatric disorders across the life course in a national study, *Am J Psychiatry* 171:864–871, 2014.

Korporaal M, van Groenou M, Tilburg T: Health problems and marital satisfaction among older couples, *J Aging Health* 25:1279–1298, 2013.

Legacy Project: *Grandparents today,* 2014. Available at http://www.tcpnow.com/guides/gptoday.html. Accessed March 2016.

Lim F, Brown D, Justin K, et al: Addressing health care disparities in the lesbian, gay, bisexual, and transgender population, *Am J Nurs* 114(6):24–34, 2014.

Lindau S, Gavrilova N: Sex, health, and years of sexually active life gained due to good health: Evidence from two US populations based cross sectional surveys of ageing, *BMJ* 340:c810, 2010. Available at http://www.bmj.com/content/340/bmj.c810. Accessed September 2016.

Lindau S, Schumm L, Laumann E, et al: A study of sexuality and health among older adults in the United States, *N Engl J Med* 357:762–774, 2007.

McNamara T, Williamson J: What can other countries teach us about retirement? *Generations* 37(1):33–37, 2013.

Messinger-Rapport BJ, Sandhu SK, Hujer ME: Sex and sexuality: Is it over after 60? *Clin Geriatr* 11:45–53, 2003.

MetLife: *Report on American grandparents,* New York, 2011, MetLife Mature Market Institute.

National Institute on Aging: *HIV, AIDS, and older people,* 2009. Available at http://www.nia.nih.gov/health/publication/hiv-aids-and-older-people. Accessed March 2016.

National Institute on Aging, National Institutes of Health, U.S. Department of Health and Human Services: *Intimacy and sexuality resources for dementia caregivers,* 2015. Available at https://www.nia.nih.gov/alzheimers/intimacy-and-sexuality-resources-dementia-caregivers. Accessed March 2016.

National Resource Center on LGBT Aging: *HIV/AIDS and older adults: Fact versus fiction,* 2011. Available at http://www.lgbtagingcenter.org/resources/resource.cfm?r=322. Accessed March 2016.

Polivka L: A future out of reach? The growing risk in the U.S. retirement security system, *Generations* 36(2):12–17, 2012.

Rheaume C, Mitty E: Sexuality and intimacy in older adults, *Geriatr Nurs* 29:342–349, 2008.

Robinson K, Davis S: Influence of cognitive decline on sexuality in individuals with dementia and their caregivers, *J Gerontol Nurs* 39(11):31–36, 2013.

Services and Advocacy for Gay, Lesbian, Bisexual, and Transgender Elders (SAGE), Movement Advancement Project (MAP): *Improving the lives of LGBT older adults,* 2010. Available at http://www.lgbtmap.org/policy-and-issue-analysis/improving-the-lives-of-lgbt-older-adults. Accessed March 2016.

Stanford P, Usita P: Retirement: Who is at risk? *Generations* 26:45, 2002.

Steinke E: Intimacy needs and chronic illness, *J Gerontol Nurs* 31:40–50, 2005.

Steinke E: Sexuality and chronic illness, *J Gerontol Nurs* 39(11):18–27, 2013.

Steinke E, Jaarsma T, Barnason S, et al: Sexual counseling for individuals with cardiovascular disease and their partners: A consensus statement from the American Heart Association and the ESC Council on Cardiovascular Nursing and Allied Professions (CCNAP), *Circulation* 128:2075–2096, 2013. Available at https://circ.ahajournals.org/content/early/2013/07/29/CIR.0b013e31829c2e53. Accessed March 2016.

Syme M: The evolving concept of older adult sexual behavior and its benefits, *Generations* 38(1):35–41, 2014.

United Nations (UNAIDS): *HIV and aging,* 2013. Available at http://www.unaids.org/sites/default/files/media_asset/20131101_JC2563_hiv-and-aging_en_0.pdf. Accessed March 2016.

U.S. Census Bureau: *American families and living arrangements,* 2013. Available at http://www.census.gov/hhes/families. Accessed March 2016.

U.S. Department of Health and Human Services: *LGBT health and well-being,* 2015. Available at http://www.hhs.gov/lgbt. Accessed March 2016.

van Groenou M, Hoogendijk E, van Tilburg T: Continued and new personal relationships in later life: Differential effects of health, *J Aging Health* 25:274–295, 2013.

Waite L, Laumann E, Das A, et al: Sexuality: Measures of partnerships, practices, attitudes, and problems in the National Social Life, Health and Aging Study, *J Gerontol B Psychol Sci Soc Sci* 64(Suppl 1):i56–i66, 2009.

Wallace M: Best practices in nursing care to older adults: Sexuality, *Dermatol Nurs* 15:570–571, 2003.

World Health Organization: *Sexual and reproductive health: Defining sexual health,* 2014. Available at http://www.who.int/reproductive health/topics/sexual_health/sh_definitions/en. Accessed March 2016.

Youngkin EQ: The myths and truths of mature intimacy, *Adv Nurse Pract* 12:45–48, 2004.

Zeiss A, Kasl-Godley J: Sexuality in older adults' relationships, *Generations* 25:18, 2001.

27

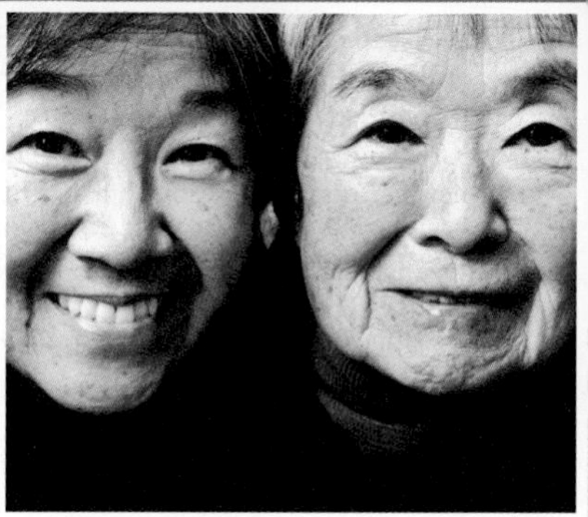

Caregiving

Theris A. Touhy

evolve.elsevier.com/Touhy/gerontological

LEARNING OBJECTIVES

Upon completion of this chapter, the reader will be able to:

- Identify the range of caregiving situations and the potential challenges and opportunities of each.
- Differentiate between abuse and neglect.
- Define the nurse's role in the prevention of elder mistreatment.
- Discuss nursing responses with older adults and their families experiencing caregiver roles.

THE LIVED EXPERIENCE

There are four kinds of people in the world: those who have been caregivers, those who are currently caregivers, those who will be caregivers, and those who will need caregivers.

Rosalyn Carter quoted in Alzheimer's Reading Room (2013)

CAREGIVING

Gerontological nurses are most likely to encounter elders with their family and friends in situations relating to caregiving of some kind. Family members and other unpaid caregivers provide the majority of care for older adults in the United States. About 34.2 million Americans have provided unpaid care to an adult age 50 or older in the last 12 months (Family Caregiver Alliance, 2016). The most common caregiver arrangement is that of an adult female child providing care to an older female parent (Messecar, 2012).

Among individuals older than 70 years of age who require care, whites are more likely to receive help from spouses; Hispanics are more likely to receive help from their adult children; and African Americans are the most likely to receive help from a nonfamily member (Messecar, 2012). However, family caregiving has become a normative experience (similar to marriage, working, or retirement) for many of America's families and cuts across racial, ethnic, and social class distinctions. Box 27.1 presents some statistics on caregiving.

Caregiving is considered a major public health issue across the globe, and attention to the physical and mental health of caregivers is receiving increased attention (Columbo et al., 2011; Shahly et al., 2013). *Healthy People 2020* goals include reducing the proportion of unpaid caregivers of older adults who report an unmet need for caregiver support services.

Current trends suggest that the use of paid, formal care by older persons in the community has been decreasing, while their sole reliance on family caregivers has been increasing (Family Caregiver Alliance, 2016). The need for family caregivers will increase substantially, but the number of family caregivers who are available to provide care is decreasing substantially as well. In the

BOX 27.1 Facts About Caregiving

- Family caregivers are children (41.3%), spouses (38.4%), and other family and friends (20.4%).
- Approximately 75% of all caregivers are female with an average age of 49 years. The number of male caregivers is smaller but increasing, and continued research is needed to address their unique needs. Among spousal caregivers 75 years and older, both sexes provide equal amounts of care.
- The average duration of a caregiver's role is 4 years.
- 1.4 million children 8 to 18 years of age provide care for an adult relative, and 73% are caring for a parent or grandparent.
- Hispanic (non-white, non–African American) caregivers have the highest reported prevalence of caregiving at 21%. Caregiver prevalence rates among other racial/ethnic groups are Asian-American, 20.3%; African American, 19.7%; white, 16.9%.
- Hispanic (non-white, non–African American) and African American caregivers experience higher burdens from caregiving and spend more time caregiving on average than white or Asian-American peers.
- 70% of working caregivers suffer work-related difficulties attributable to their caregiving roles.
- Caregiving can have serious negative effects on mental and physical health. Approximately 40% to 70% of caregivers have clinically significant symptoms of depression.
- Caregiving can also present financial burdens, and women who are family caregivers are 2.5 times more likely than noncaregivers to live in poverty.

Data from Family Caregiver Alliance: *Caregiver Statistics: Demographics,* 2016. Available at https://www.caregiver.org/caregiver-statistics-demographics. Accessed March 2016.

BOX 27.2 Resources for Best Practice

Administration on Aging, National Center on Elder Abuse: Information on abuse and neglect in diverse populations

Alzheimer's Association: EssentiALZ – Caregiving resources, e-learning workshops, DVDs, on-line care training for dementia care and certification for professionals

Caregiver Action Network: Resources, education

Caregiver Preparedness Scale: https://consultgeri.org/try-this/general-assessment/issue-28.pdf

Family Caregiver Alliance: Resources, education

Hartford Institute for Geriatric Nursing: Family Caregiving Standard of Practice Protocol; Detection of Elder Mistreatment Nursing Standard of Practice Protocol; Modified Caregiver Strain Index

National Alliance for Caregiving: International resources and best practices in caregiving

United Hospital Fund: Next Step in Care: Family Caregivers and Health Care Professionals Working Together: Guides and information for caregivers

United States, informal care provided by caregivers is universally recognized as the foundation of the long-term care system. Informal caregivers basically provide free services to care recipients (Mast, 2013). In 2015, these services were valued at $522 billion per year. This is more than the value of paid home care and total Medicaid spending in the same year (Chari et al., 2015). Without family caregivers, the present level of long-term care could not be sustained.

Some suggest that the conception of caregiving is different among the baby boomer generation. Although they recognize their responsibility to care for ill family members, they view themselves as partners in the organization of care and want to negotiate and set limits to the amount and kind of care they wish to undertake. Baby boomer caregivers and upcoming generations will expect more support and formal assistance from national and local agencies in a coordinated long-term care network (Mast, 2013).

Impact of Caregiving

Although caregiving is a means to "give back" to a loved one and can be a source of joy, it is also stressful. "Caregiving is a very complex issue, and assuming a caregiving role is a time of transition that requires a restructuring of one's goals, behaviors, and responsibilities. It requires taking on something new, but it is also about loss—of what was and what could have been" (Lund, 2005, p. 152). Caregivers are considered to be "the hidden patient" (Schulz & Beach, 1999, p. 2216). Family caregiving has been associated with increased levels of depression and anxiety, poorer self-reported physical health, compromised immune function, higher rates of insomnia, increased alcohol use, and increased mortality (Newell et al., 2012; Mast, 2013; Sorrell, 2014).

Caregiver burden is defined as the negative psychological, economic, and physical effects of caring for a person who is impaired. Whereas not all caregivers experience stress and caregiver burden, the circumstances that are more likely to cause problems with caregiving include competing role responsibilities (e.g., work, home), advanced age of the caregiver, high-intensity caregiving needs, insufficient resources, financial difficulty, poor self-reported health, living in the same household with the care recipient, dementia of the care recipient, length of time caregiving, and prior relational conflicts between the caregiver and care recipient. The Modified Caregiver Strain Index (Box 27.2) can be used to assess caregiver stress. Unrelieved caregiver stress increases the potential

BOX 27.3 Tips for Best Practice

Reducing Caregiver Stress

- Educate yourself about the disease or medical condition.
- Contact the appropriate disease-related organization to learn about resources and education and support groups to help you adapt to the challenges you encounter.
- Find a health care professional who understands the disease.
- Consult with other experts to help plan for the future (legal, financial).
- Tap your social resources for assistance.
- Take time for relaxation and exercise.
- Use community resources.
- Maintain your sense of humor.
- Explore religious beliefs and spiritual values.
- Participate in pleasant, nurturing activities such as reading a good book, taking a warm bath.
- Seek supportive counseling when you need it.
- Identify and acknowledge your feelings; you have a right to ALL of them.
- Set realistic goals.
- Attend to your own health care needs.

From U.S. Department of Health and Human Services Administration on Aging, National Family Caregiver Support Program Resources: *Taking care of yourself,* 2014. Available at http://www.acl.gov/NewsRoom/Publications/Index.aspx Accessed June 2016.

for abuse and neglect, which are discussed later in this chapter (Newell et al., 2012). Box 27.3 presents further information on caregiver stress.

The positive benefits of caregiving have been given more attention in recent years, but further research is needed to help understand what factors influence how caregivers perceive the experience. Positive benefits of caregiving may include enhanced self-esteem and well-being, personal growth and satisfaction, and finding or making meaning through caregiving (Sorrell, 2014). Caregiving is perceived as rewarding if the caregiver feels needed and useful, has a close and reciprocal relationship with the care recipient, and has an adequate support network (Mast, 2013).

Family caregivers are undertaking more and more complex medical and nursing tasks of the kind and complexity once provided only in hospitals, often with significant difficulty and little preparation. It is common for caregivers to provide ostomy, wound, and incontinence care; administer intravenous fluids, injections, and other medications; and manage ventilators and tube feeding—tasks that can "make nursing students tremble" (Reinhard et al., 2012, p. 4). Most caregivers are not prepared for the many responsibilities they face and receive no formal instruction in caregiving activities (Montgomery, 2013). Lack of preparedness can greatly increase the caregiver's stress (Messecar, 2012). Caregivers who have a positive relationship with the care recipient (mutuality) and are prepared for caregiving experience less stress and find caregiving more meaningful (Ching-Tzu et al., 2014). The Preparedness for Caregiving Scale (Archbold et al., 1990) (Box 27.2) can be used to determine caregiver needs.

Spousal Caregiving

Eighty percent of persons who live with spouses with disabilities provide care for them. An older spousal caregiver may have significant health problems that are neglected in deference to the greater needs of the incapacitated partner. The disabled spouse may need physical care that is beyond the capabilities of the spousal caregiver. Spousal caregivers provide more intensive, time-consuming care than other family caregivers, as much as 56 hours of care per week on average. They are also less likely to receive assistance from other family members.

Older spouses are at greater risk for negative consequences and often take on greater burdens than they can reasonably handle and wait longer for outside help, using formal services as a last resort. Spousal caregivers are more prone to loneliness and depression and have a 63% greater chance of dying than people of the same age who are not caring for spouses (Ostwald, 2009). More wives than husbands provide care, but this is expected to change as the life expectancy for men increases.

Older spouses caring for disabled partners also face many role changes. Older women may need to learn to drive, manage money, or make decisions by themselves. Male caregivers may need to learn how to cook, shop, do laundry, and provide personal care to their wives. Spousal caregivers also deal with the added responsibilities of caregiving while at the same time dealing with the anticipated loss of their spouse.

Nurses should be alert to situations in which health care personnel may be able to provide support services and resources that make it possible for an individual to assume new responsibilities without being totally overwhelmed. Adult day programs, respite care services, or periodic assistance from a home health aide or homemaker may make it possible for the couple to continue to live together. It is important to pay attention to the physical and mental health needs of the caregiver, as well as the care recipient.

Caring for Individuals With Dementia

More than 70% of individuals with dementia live at home, and family and friends provide nearly 75% of their care. Approximately two-thirds of the caregivers are women and 34% are age 65 or older. These caregivers provide more hours of help than caregivers of other older people and also provide care for a longer time, on average, than caregivers of older adults with other conditions. Compared with caregivers of people without dementia, twice as many caregivers of people with dementia indicate substantial negative aspects of caregiving, including financial, emotional, and physical difficulties. Sixty percent rated the emotional stress of caregiving as high or very high, and approximately 40% suffer from depression.

Factors that increase the stress of caregiving include grief over the multiple losses that occur, the physical demands and duration of caregiving, and resource availability. Demands are intensified if the care recipient demonstrates behavioral disturbances and impairments in activities of daily living (ADLs) and instrumental activities of daily living (IADLs) (Alzheimer's Association, 2016a; Ching-Tzu et al., 2014). The rising numbers of individuals with dementia, issues related to caregiving, and health care costs of dementia are public health concerns across the globe. Chapters 23 and 25 discuss dementia in depth.

Aging Parents Caring for Developmentally Disabled Children

Although we tend to think of caregivers as middle-aged adults caring for elders, an unknown number of elders are caring for their middle-aged children who are physically and mentally disabled. In the past century, developmentally disabled children usually died before reaching adulthood; now, with improved care, they are surviving. For the first time in history, individuals with developmental disabilities are outliving their parents. Planning for their future is an area posing challenges for older people and for service providers internationally (Ryan et al., 2014).

Often, the burden of caring for a developmentally disabled child has been carried by parents for their entire adult life and will end only with the death of the parent or the adult child. Parental caregivers who are aging face changes in their financial resources and health that affect their continued caregiving ability. A majority of these caregivers worry how their child will receive care if they develop a debilitating illness or die.

In the United States, the Planned Lifetime Assistance Network (PLAN), available in some states through the National Alliance for the Mentally Ill, provides lifetime assistance to individuals with disabilities whose parents or other family members are deceased or can no longer provide for their care. The Alzheimer's Association and other aging organizations offer education and support programs for both parents and their developmentally disabled adult children in some communities. There is a continued need for the development of both in-home and community options for developmentally disabled adults who are aging (Ryan et al., 2014).

Grandparents Raising Grandchildren

Around the world, an increasing number of grandparents are raising grandchildren in households without a biological parent. More than 2.5 million grandparents are providing primary care (custodial grandparents) for grandchildren in the United States, and grandparent-headed households are one of the fastest-growing U.S. family groups (Hadfield, 2014). In the United States, 1 out of every 10 children lives with a grandparent, and 41% of those children are being raised primarily by that grandparent.

More than two-thirds of grandparent primary caregivers are younger than 60 years of age, and 62% are female. Nearly one in five is living below the poverty line (Hadfield, 2014). The phenomenon of grandparents serving as primary caregivers is more common among African Americans and Hispanics than whites, but the increase in grandparent primary caregiving across the past decade has been much more pronounced among whites (a 19% increase) (Hadfield, 2014).

The reasons grandparents take a child into the home without his or her parents vary among countries, groups, and individuals. Many grandparents have become, by default, the primary caregivers of grandchildren because the parents are unable to provide the care needed as a result of child abuse, teen pregnancy, imprisonment, joblessness, military deployment, drug and alcohol addictions, illness, death, and other social problems.

Research is lacking related to the effect of grandparent caregiving on health status, but existing literature suggests that there are economic, health, and social challenges inherent in this role. Single non-white women caring for their grandchildren appear to be the highest risk group for depression (Hadfield, 2014). Often, crisis situations precipitate the decision, and time for preparation is not available. In many cases, grandparents assume care so that their grandchildren's care is not taken over by the public care system (del Bene, 2010). The unexpected career of caregiving for grandchildren and the "off timing" of this family role transition contribute to the challenges faced (Musil et al., 2011).

As with other types of caregiving, there are both blessings and burdens, and caregivers' experiences will be unique (Hadfield, 2014). However, for many grandparents the challenges may include limited income and financial support through the welfare system, lack of informal support systems, loss of leisure activities in retirement, and shame or guilt related to their children's inability to parent. Physical and mental stressors appear

BOX 27.4 Tips for Best Practice

Interventions With Grandparent Caregivers

- Early identification of at-risk grandparents
- Comprehensive assessment of physical, psychosocial, and environmental factors affecting those in the caregiving role for grandchildren
- Anticipatory guidance and counseling about child growth and development and other child-raising issues
- Referral to resources for support, counseling, and financial assistance
- Advocacy for policies supportive of grandparents who have assumed a caregiving role

to be greater when grandparents are raising a chronically ill or special-needs child or a child with behavioral problems, or experiencing chronic illness themselves (del Bene, 2010; Hooyman & Kiyak, 2011).

Interventions

Routine screening and monitoring of the psychological distress of primary care grandparents and offering support, advice, and referral to reduce stressors are important. Health care institutions, schools, and churches are potential sites where grandparents could access needed information and support (Van Etten & Gautam, 2012). Education and training programs and support groups are valuable resources that should be available in communities. Nurses can be instrumental in developing and conducting these types of interventions. The National Family Caregiver Support Program (NFCSP), under the Older Americans Act program, provides support services, education and training, counseling, and respite care. Nurses can refer the grandparents to their local Area Agency on Aging to inquire about available resources. Suggestions for nursing interventions are presented in Box 27.4.

Long-Distance Caregiving

Because of the increasing mobility of today's global society, more children move away for education or employment and do not return home. When the parent needs help, it must be provided "long distance." Approximately 15% of all caregivers are long-distance caregivers, and this number is projected to double by 2020. Long-distance caregivers have the highest annual expense compared to co-resident caregivers and are more likely to report emotional distress than caregivers residing with the care recipient or residing less than 1 hour away (Family Caregiver Alliance, 2016).

Issues that need to be considered in long-distance caregiving include identifying a local person who will be available quickly in emergency situations; identifying reliable individuals or services that will provide daily monitoring if necessary; identifying acceptable facilities for assisted living or nursing home care if that becomes necessary; determining which family member is most likely to be free to travel to the elder if needed; and ensuring that legalities regarding advance directives, a will, and power of attorney (for health care and financial) have been established.

A profession and industry have emerged to assist the geographically distant family member to ensure that an older relative will receive care. This profession is made up of geriatric care managers, some of whom are nurses or social workers. A care manager can be hired to do everything a family member would do if able, from being available in an emergency, to helping with estate planning, to making arrangements for a move to a nursing home. These services are available primarily to those who are able to pay for them because they are not covered by private insurance, Medicare, or any public agencies. Although these services are expensive, they may be far less expensive than alternative living arrangements or institutional placement (see Chapter 5).

Similar services may be available for persons with very low incomes by asking the local Area Agency on Aging about local "Community Care for the Elderly" programs. When incomes are too high to qualify for Medicaid and too low to pay for private care managers, the persons and their families must do the best they can. Long-distance care then depends on the goodness of neighbors, local friends, and apartment managers and frequent trips by the long-distance caregiver to the elder.

❖ IMPLICATIONS FOR GERONTOLOGICAL NURSING AND HEALTHY AGING

◆ Caregiver Assessment

Caregiver assessment should be a part of the routine delivery of health and long-term care services. Caregiver assessment is a systematic process of gathering information about a caregiving situation to identify the specific problems, strengths, and resources of the family caregiver; the caregiver's ability to contribute to the needs of the care recipient; the needs and preferences of both the care recipient and the caregiver; and ways the health care team can help the person providing care.

Caregiver assessment should be conducted by a health care or social service professional and should approach the care issues from the caregiver's perspective and culture. An important component of the assessment is providing the caregiver with the opportunity to talk to someone about his or her circumstances and be involved in developing the plan of care. Talking with someone who understands caregiving issues and who listens to the family member's concerns can improve outcomes for both the caregiver and the care recipient (Feinberg, 2012). A resource for a nursing standard of practice protocol for family caregiving can be found in Box 27.2.

◆ Interventions

In designing interventions to support caregiving, a partnership model that combines the nurse's professional expertise with the caregiver's knowledge of the family member is recommended (Box 27.5). Given the range of caregiving situations and the uniqueness of each, interventions must be tailored to individual needs (Messecar, 2012). "There is no single, easily implemented and consistently effective method for eliminating the stresses and/or strain of being a caregiver" (Messecar, 2012, p. 479). Tailored multicomponent interventions designed to match a specific target population seem to have the most positive outcomes on caregiver burden and stress—for example, groups designed to assist caregivers caring for individuals with early-stage dementia or those with Parkinson's disease. Interventions include risk assessment, education about caregiving and stress, needed care skills, caregiver health and home safety, support groups, linkages to ongoing support, counseling, resource identification, relief/respite from daily care demands, and stress management (Messecar, 2016; Sorrell, 2014).

Education provided by nurses to help prepare the caregiver for the caregiving role, particularly at the time of discharge from the hospital or nursing home, can help to prevent role strain and lessen burden (Sorrell, 2014). When the nurse works with a family from a different culture that may have rituals and routines unfamiliar to him or her, the nurse needs to be particularly careful to respect these differences. The nurse can work with the family to make the best use of their strengths, whatever they may be. Each family member can be valued for what he or she brings to the situation. Service providers need to enhance cultural competence and design programs that are culturally acceptable (see Chapter 2).

Linking caregivers to community resources, such as respite care, adult day programs, and financial support resources, is important. Respite care allows the caregiver to take a break from caregiving for various periods of time. Respite care may be provided in institutions, in the home, or in other community settings. Nurses should be aware of respite care resources in their communities, and the local Area Agency on Aging can provide information on respite care and other caregiver services. These interventions, when available, can alleviate much of the stress of caregiving but are utilized infrequently or very late in the course of caregiving in the United States (Mast, 2013). Many countries in Europe offer generous respite care services as part of the long-term care system.

BOX 27.5 Tips for Best Practice

Nursing Actions to Create and Sustain a Partnership With Caregivers

- Surveillance and ongoing monitoring
- Coaching: helping caregivers apply knowledge and develop skills
- Teaching: providing information and instruction
- Providing accurate and complete information about services; determine with the family referrals for services based on needs and preferences of caregiver and care recipient; mutually determine with the family services that are affordable, acceptable, and logistically feasible
- Fostering partnerships: fostering communication and collaboration between the caregiver and the care recipient and between them and the nurse
- Providing psychosocial support: attending to psychosocial well-being; help the caregiver and family identify effective coping strategies
- Coordinating: orchestrating the work of other health care team members and the activities of the caregiver

Data from Eilers J, Heermann JA, Wilson ME, et al: Independent nursing actions in cooperative care, *Oncol Nurs Forum* 32:849–855, 2005; Mast M: To use or not to use: A literature review of factors that influence family caregivers' use of support services, *J Gerontol Nurs* 39(1):20–28, 2013; Schumacher K, Beck CA, Marren JM: Family caregivers: Caring for older adults, working with their families, *Am J Nurs* 106:40–49, 2006.

◆ Special Considerations for Caregivers of Individuals With Dementia

Therapeutic programs for both individuals and their caregivers should be individualized to meet the varied and changing needs over the course of the illness. The voice of the individual with Alzheimer's disease (AD) needs to be heard, and he/she should be included in activities and support groups. Programs should be offered both in the community and in long-term care and assisted living facilities (Annals of Long-Term Care, 2015). On-line psychoeducational interventions for caregivers offer flexibility and can overcome the barriers of geographic distance and availability (Gaugler et al., 2015). The Alzheimer's Association is a valuable resource for both in-person and on-line support group formats.

Access to a knowledgeable provider who can follow the individual and family throughout the course of the illness is essential and leads to improved outcomes and less distress (Hain et al., 2010). The current model of primary care does not adequately address the complexities of dementia care, and most caregivers do not receive adequate support to help them with dementia-related problems throughout the course of the illness (Jennings et al., 2015). Collaborative care management programs for the treatment of AD, often led by advanced practice nurses with expertise in dementia, have been shown to improve quality of care, decrease the incidence of behavioral and psychological symptoms, and decrease caregiver stress (Callahan et al., 2006; Jennings et al., 2015; Reuben et al., 2013).

Interventions with caregivers must always consider the great variability in family structures, resources, traditions, and history. The range of adaptations is enormous, and the goal is always to restore the balance of the system to the greatest extent possible and support caregivers in their caring. The family can be visualized as a mobile structure with many parts, and when one part is touched, each part shifts to regain the balance. The intrusion of professionals in a family system will temporarily unbalance the system and may provide an opportunity to restore the balance in a healthier manner, sometimes by adding an element or increasing the weight of one or decreasing the weight of another. Further research is needed to provide the foundation for nursing interventions with family caregivers, particularly among racially and ethnically diverse families and nontraditional families. Resources for caregiving are presented in Box 27.2.

ELDER MISTREATMENT

Elder mistreatment is a complex phenomenon that includes elder abuse and neglect. It is the infliction of actual harm, or a risk for harm, to vulnerable older persons through the action or behavior of others (American Psychological Association [APA], 2012). It is a universal problem and occurs in all educational, racial, cultural, religious, and socioeconomic groups, in any family configuration and in every setting. It is one of the most unrecognized and underreported social problems today.

Although there are no reliable statistics available related to the prevalence on a worldwide basis, the World Health Organization estimates that up to 4% to 6% of those older than age 60 have been or will be mistreated (World Health Organization [WHO], 2012). In the United States, approximately 1 in 10 older adults has experienced some form of elder abuse. Estimates are that only 7% of abuse cases are ever reported to authorities (Family Caregiver Alliance, 2016).

In order for mistreatment to occur, the perpetrator and a vulnerable elder must have a trusting relationship of some kind. This may be as simple as a salesperson (financial exploitation) or as complex as a long-time caregiver such as a spouse or a child. Most abuse (90%) occurs in the home setting and is committed by adult children or spousal caregivers (National Center on Elder Abuse [NCEA], 2016). Abusers can be men or women, of any age, race, or socioeconomic status. Individuals with dementia are especially vulnerable to mistreatment because the disease may prevent them from reporting abuse or recognizing it. They may also be vulnerable to strangers who take advantage of their cognitive impairment (Alzheimer's Association, 2016b). The risk factors for one to become an abuser or be abused are often interconnected (Box 27.6).

Mistreatment at the hands of formal caregivers occurs as well. When a number of different providers are giving care, monitoring becomes especially difficult. Situations of increased potential for formal caregiver abuse include those in which there is inadequate supervision of patient care, poor coordination of services, inadequate staff training, theft and fraud, drug and alcohol abuse by staff, tardiness and absenteeism, unprofessional and criminal conduct, and inadequate record keeping. The nurse

BOX 27.6 More Likely to Mistreat and Be Mistreated

More Likely to Abuse or Neglect

- Family member
- One with emotional or mental illnesses
- One who is abusing alcohol or other substances
- History of family violence
- Cultural acceptance of interpersonal violence
- Caregiver frustration
- Social isolation
- Impaired impulse control of caregiver

More Likely to Be Abused or Neglected

- Cognitive impairment, especially with aggressive features
- Dependent on abuser
- Physically or mentally frail
- Having abused the caregiver earlier in life
- Women either living alone or living in a household with family members
- Having been abused in the past
- Behavior that is considered aggressive, demanding, or unappreciative
- Living in an institutional setting
- Feeling deserving of abuse because of own inadequacies

Adapted from Sehgal SR, Mosqueda L: Mistreatment and neglect. In Ham RJ, Sloane D, Warshaw GA, editors: *Primary care geriatrics: A case-based approach*, ed 6, pp 360–364, Philadelphia, 2014, Elsevier.

should pay particular attention to the person who is alone with a formal caregiver for extended periods of time, with no support from others and no opportunities for respite for the caregiver.

Resident-to-resident elder mistreatment (inappropriate, disruptive, or hostile behavior among nursing home residents) is a sizable and growing problem. Among nursing home residents, reports are that 19.8% have experienced resident-to-resident mistreatment. Specific types of mistreatment include cursing, screaming, or yelling at another person; physical incidents such as hitting, kicking, or biting; and sexual incidents. These incidents are likely to cause emotional and/or physical harm and are stressful to staff. Further research is needed to develop prevention and management interventions. All residents have the right to be protected from abuse and mistreatment, and the facility is required to ensure the safety of all residents and investigate reports of abuse (Segelken & Young, 2016; The National Consumer Voice for Quality Long-Term Care, 2016) (see Chapter 6).

Abuse

Abuse is intentional and may be physical, psychological, medical, financial, or sexual. Many states have reporting statutes that require certain persons, including nurses, who become aware of abuse, neglect, or exploitation to report it to the appropriate authorities. The designated authority can be found in each state's laws (NCEA, 2016). Many factors interfere with the identification of those who are mistreated (Box 27.7). It is further complicated by varying cultural perspectives on abuse and expectations of elder care. Financial exploitation is common and often difficult to detect since there are no external signs of mistreatment. Changes in banking practices, access to a bank account by an unauthorized person, failure to pay medical or other bills, unexpected changes in a will, or the disappearance of personal items are all evidence of possible financial exploitation.

BOX 27.7 Factors Influencing Identification of Abuse of Older Adults

- Cultural or societal tolerance of violence, especially against women
- Shame and embarrassment
- Fear of retaliation
- Fear of institutionalization
- Social isolation
- Unacceptability of emotional expression, especially that of fear or distress

Adapted from Sehgal SR, Mosqueda L: Mistreatment and neglect. In Ham RJ, Sloane D, Warshaw GA, et al, editors: *Primary care geriatrics: A case-based approach,* ed 6, pp 360–364, Philadelphia, 2014, Elsevier.

Impact of Elder Abuse

The abuse of elders has effects that are more far-reaching than is usually discussed. Those subjected to even minimal abuse have been found to have a 300% higher risk for death than those who have never been abused (Family Care Alliance, 2016). In addition, older adults who have been victims of violence have more health problems than other older adults, including increased bone or joint problems, digestive problems, depression or anxiety, chronic pain, hypertension, and cardiovascular disease (Dyer et al., 2000).

Neglect

Neglect is a form of mistreatment resulting from the failure of action by a caregiver or through one's own behavior or choices. Neglect of self and neglect by caretakers are often difficult to define because they are intertwined with energy, lifestyle, and resources. Nurses are particularly challenged by issues of self-neglect when the ethical principle of beneficence (do good) counters that of autonomy (self-determination) (Zorowitz, 2014). In either case, the needs of the individual may not become known until there is a medical crisis when the person's unmet needs become visible to others.

Neglect by a Caregiver

Neglect by a caregiver requires a socially (formally or informally) recognized role and responsibility of a person to provide care to a vulnerable other. Neglect is most often passive mistreatment, such as an act of omission. It is not only the failure to provide the goods and services—such as food, medication, medical treatment, and personal care—necessary for the well-being of the frail elder, but also the failure or inability to recognize the responsibility to provide such goods and services. Neglect is active when care is withheld deliberately and for malicious reasons (Quinn & Tomita, 2003). In some cases this level of neglect would be considered abuse as well. Neglect by caregivers occurs for many reasons (Box 27.8).

Self-Neglect

Self-neglect is a behavior in which people fail to meet their own basic needs in the manner in which the average person would in similar circumstances. It generally manifests itself as a refusal to, or failure to, provide themselves with adequate safety, food, water, clothing, shelter, personal hygiene, or health care. It may be due to diminished capacity, but it also may be the result of a long-standing lifestyle, homelessness, or alcoholism or other substance abuse. It is important for the nurse to remember that there are many mentally competent people who understand the consequences of their

BOX 27.8 Possible Reasons for Neglect by Caregivers

Caregiver personal stress and exhaustion
Multiple role demands
Caregiver incompetence
Unawareness of importance of the neglected care
Financial burden of caregiving limiting resources available
Caregivers' own frailty and advanced age
Unawareness of community resources available for support and respite

decisions and make conscious and voluntary decisions to engage in acts that threaten their health or safety as a matter of personal choice. There are both ethical and legal questions as to how much health care professionals can and should intervene in these situations.

❖ IMPLICATIONS FOR GERONTOLOGICAL NURSING AND HEALTHY AGING

◆ Elder Mistreatment

When working with frail and vulnerable elders, nurses must always be vigilant and sensitive to the signs and symptoms of mistreatment. In addition to the obvious indicators of physical abuse (e.g., unexplained bruises), the nurse looks for more subtle signs (Box 27.9). For the person who is clearly competent and refuses assessment, this cannot be done. For a person with unmet needs or other signs of abuse or neglect, as well as questionable capacity, intervention is required.

A full and specialized assessment includes the immediate determination of the person's safety. Further assessment of mistreatment involves a number of very sensitive components and tools developed by experts in the field that may be very useful (Box 27.2). Assessment of mistreatment in the cross-cultural setting is especially difficult; however, helpful guidelines can be found at the National Center on Elder Abuse through the Administration on Aging (http://www.ncea.acl.gov). Because of the sensitive nature of such an assessment, specialized training is recommended for all gerontological nurses.

BOX 27.9 Signs of Mistreatment

The first signs that further evaluation may be necessary are if the histories given by the (usually cognitively intact) elder and the caregiver are inconsistent or the caregiver refuses to leave the elder alone with the nurse. Although it is always important to ask the elder if he or she is a recipient of abuse/shame/suffering/family disharmony/moral cruelty, one cannot assume that this will be acknowledged. Although there is more than one category of abuse and abuse combined with neglect, the following specific signs would be included:

Physical Abuse

- Unexplained bruising or lacerations in unusual areas in various stages of healing
- Fractures inconsistent with functional ability

Sexual Abuse

- Bruises or scratches in the genital or breast area
- Fear or an unusual amount of anxiety related to either routine or necessary exam of the anogenital area
- Torn undergarments or presence of blood

Medical Abuse

- Caregiver repeatedly requesting procedures that are not recommended and not desired by elder

Medical Neglect

- Unusual delay between the beginning of a health problem and when help is sought
- Repeated missed appointments without reasonable explanations

Psychological Abuse

- Caregiver does all of the talking in a situation, even though the elder is capable
- Caregiver appears angry, frustrated, or indifferent while the elder appears hesitant or frightened
- Caregiver or the care recipient aggressive toward one another or the nurse

Neglect by Self or Caregiver

- Weight loss
- Uncharacteristically neglected grooming
- Evidence of malnutrition and dehydration
- Fecal/urine smell
- Inappropriate clothing to the situation or weather
- Insect infestation

◆ Mandatory Reporting

In most states and U.S. jurisdictions, licensed nurses are "mandatory reporters," that is, persons who are required to report suspicions of abuse to the state, usually to a group called Adult Protective Services (APS) (National Adult Protective Services Association [NAPSA], 2014). The standard for reporting is one of reasonable belief; that is, the nurse must have a reasonable belief that a vulnerable person either has been or is likely to be abused, neglected, or exploited.

Usually these reports are anonymous. If the nurse believes the elder to be in immediate danger, the police

BOX 27.10 Tips for Best Practice

Prevention of Elder Mistreatment

- Make professionals aware of potentially abusive situations.
- Help families develop and nurture informal support systems.
- Link families with support groups.
- Teach families stress management techniques.
- Arrange comprehensive care resources.
- Provide counseling for troubled families.
- Encourage the use of respite care and day care.
- Obtain necessary home health care services.
- Inform families of resources for meals and transportation.
- Encourage caregivers to pursue their individual interests.

are notified. How the nurse accomplishes this varies with the work setting. In hospitals and nursing homes, suspicions of abuse are often reported first internally to the facility social worker. In the home care setting, the report is made to the nursing supervisor. It would be very unusual for the nurse not to approach this subject through his or her employer. However, the nurse who is a neighbor, friend, or privately paid caregiver may be under obligation to make the report directly. In the nursing home or licensed assisted living facility, the nurse has the additional resource of calling the state long-term care ombudsman for help.

If the abuse is triggered by the stress of caregiving, nurses can be very proactive and help all involved take action to lessen the stress. Interventions to assist caregivers are discussed in the first part of this chapter and Box 27.10 presents Tips for Best Practice to prevent mistreatment.

KEY CONCEPTS

- Family members and other unpaid caregivers provide 80% of care for older adults in the United States.
- Grandparents are increasingly assuming primary caregiving roles with grandchildren.
- Caregiving activities are one of the most major social issues of our time, as well as a significant global public health problem.
- Nursing interventions with caregivers include risk assessment, education about caregiving and stress, needed care skills, caregiver health and home safety, support groups, linkages to ongoing support, counseling, resource identification, relief/respite from daily care demands, and stress management.
- Elder mistreatment is an umbrella term that covers abuse, neglect, exploitation, and abandonment.
- Most abuse (90%) occurs in the home setting and is committed by adult children or spousal caregivers. Nursing interventions can assist in mitigating the stress and burden of caregiving.

ACTIVITIES AND DISCUSSION QUESTIONS

1. What do you think your role will be when your parent or parents need help?
2. What would you find most difficult in regard to assisting your older parent/grandparent?
3. You are preparing an 81-year-old woman for discharge following a stroke. Her husband will be the caregiver. What teaching might you provide to prepare him for the caregiving role?

REFERENCES

Alzheimer's Association: *Alzheimer's disease facts and figures*, 2016a. Available at http://www.alz.org/documents_custom/2016-facts-and-figures.pdf. Accessed April 2016.

Alzheimer's Association: *Abuse*, 2016b. Available at https://www.alz.org/care/alzheimers-dementia-elder-abuse.asp. Accessed April 2016.

Alzheimer's Reading Room: *Quote of the day*, 2013. Available at http://www.alzheimersreadingroom.com/2009/11/quote-of-day-caregivers.html. Accessed April 2015.

American Psychological Association (APA): *Elder abuse and neglect: In search of solutions*, 2012. Available at http://www.apa.org/pi/aging/resources/guides/elder-abuse.aspx?item=1. Accessed April 2015.

Annals of Long-Term Care: *Providing support for residents with dementia and their families*, August 20, 2015. Available at http://www.annalsoflongtermcare.com/content/providing-support-residents-dementia-and-their-families. Accessed April 2016.

Archbold P, Stewart B, Greenlick M, et al: Mutuality and preparedness as predictors of role strain, *Res Nurs Health* 13:376–385, 1990.

Callahan C, Boustani M, Unversagt F, et al: Effectiveness of collaborative care for older adults with Alzheimer's disease in primary care, *JAMA* 295:2148–2157, 2006.

Chari A, Engberg J, Ray K, et al: The opportunity costs of informal elder-care in the United States, *Health Serv Res* 50(3):S71–S82, 2015.

Ching-Tzu Y, Hsin-Yun L, Yea-Ing L: Dyadic relational resources and role strain in family caregivers of persons living with dementia at home: A cross-sectional survey, *Int J Nurs Stud* 51(4):593–602, 2014.

Columbo F, Llena-Nozal A, Mercier J, et al: *Help wanted? Providing and paying for LTC, OECD Health Policy Studies*, OECD Publishing, 2011. Available at http://dx.doi.org/10.1787/9789264097759-en. Accessed April 2015.

del Bene S: African American grandmothers raising grandchildren: A phenomenological perspective of marginalized women, *J Gerontol Nurs* 36:32–40, 2010.

Dyer CB, Pavlik VN, Murphy KP, et al: The high prevalence of depression and dementia in elder abuse or neglect, *J Am Geriatr Soc* 48:205–208, 2000.

Family Caregiver Alliance: *Caregiver statistics: Demographics*, 2016. Available at https://www.caregiver.org/caregiver-statistics-demographics. Accessed March 2016.

Feinberg L: *Assessing family caregiver needs: Policy and practice considerations*. Fact Sheet no. 258, June 2012, AARP Public Policy Institute. Available at http://www.caregiving.org/wp-content/uploads/2010/11/AARP-caregiver-fact-sheet.pdf. Accessed April 2016.

Gaugler J, Hobday J, Robbins J, et al: CARES dementia care for families, *J Gerontol Nurs* 41(10):18–24, 2015.

Hadfield J: The health of grandparents raising grandchildren, *J Gerontol Nurs* 40(4):32–42, 2014.

Hain D, Touhy T, Engstrom G: What matters most to carers of people with mild to moderate dementia as evidence for transforming care, *Alzheimers Care Today* 11:162–171, 2010.

Hooyman N, Kiyak H: *Social gerontology: A multidisciplinary perspective*, ed 9, Boston, 2011, Allyn & Bacon.

Jennings L, Reuben D, Evertson K: Unmet needs of caregivers of individuals referred to a dementia care program, *J Am Geriatr Soc* 63(2):282–289, 2015.

Lund M: Caregiver, take care, *Geriatr Nurs* 26:152–153, 2005.

Mast M: To use or not to use: A literature review of factors that influence family caregivers' use of support services, *J Gerontol Nurs* 39(1):20–28, 2013.

Messecar D: Family caregiving. In Boltz M, Capezuti E, Fulmer T, et al, editors: *Evidence-based geriatric nursing protocols for best practice*, ed 4, New York, 2012, Springer, pp 469–499.

Messecar D: Family caregiving. In Boltz M, Capezuti E, Fulmer T, et al, editors: *Evidence-based geriatric nursing protocols for best practice*, ed 5, New York, 2016, Springer.

Montgomery A: *No disrespect: How family caregivers can improve care transitions*. MediCaring.org, May 23, 2013. Available at http://medicaring.org/2013/05/23/no-disrespect-how-family-caregivers-can-improve-care-transitions/. Accessed April 2016.

Musil C, Gordon N, Warner C, et al: Grandmothers and caregiving to grandchildren: Continuity, change, and outcomes over 24 months, *Gerontologist* 51(1):86–100, 2011.

National Adult Protective Services Association (NAPSA): *About NAPSA*, 2014. Available at http://www.napsa-now.org/about-napsa/. Accessed November 25, 2014.

National Center on Elder Abuse (NCEA), Administration on Aging: *Statistics/data*, 2016. Available at http://www.ncea.aoa.gov/library/data/#problem. Accessed April 2016.

Newell R, Dowd O, Netinho S, et al: Stress among caregivers of chronically ill older adults: Implications for nursing practice, *J Gerontol Nurs* 38(9):18–29, 2012.

Ostwald S: Who is caring for the caregiver? Promoting spousal caregiver's health, *Fam Community Health* 32:S5–S14, 2009.

Quinn M, Tomita SK: *Elder abuse and neglect: Causes, diagnoses and intervention strategies*, ed 3, New York, 2003, Springer.

Reinhard S, Levine C, Samis S: *Home Alone: Family caregivers providing complex chronic care*, Oct. 2012. Available at http://www.aarp.org/content/dam/aarp/research/public_policy_institute/health/home-alone-family-caregivers-providing-complex-chronic-care-rev-AARP-ppi-health.pdf. Accessed March 2016.

Reuben D, Evertsonn L, Wenger N, et al: The UCLA Alzheimer's and Dementia Care Program for Comprehensive, Coordinated, Patient-centered care: Preliminary data, *J Am Geriatr Soc* 61(12):2214–2218, 2013.

Ryan A, Taggart L, Truesdale-Kennedy M, et al: Issues in caregiving for older people with intellectual disabilities and their ageing family carers: A review and commentary, *Int J Older People Nurs* 9(3):217–226, 2014.

Schulz R, Beach SR: Caregiving as a risk factor for mortality: The caregiver health effects study, *JAMA* 262:2215–2219, 1999.

Segelken R, Young J: *Elder-to-elder abuse is common in nursing homes, Cornell Chronicle*, May 10, 2014. Available at http://www.news.cornell.edu/stories/2014/11/elder-elder-abuse-common-nursing-homes. Accessed April 2016.

Shahly V, Chatterji S, Gruber M, et al: Cross-national differences in the prevalence and correlates of burden among older family caregivers in the World Health Organization World Mental Health Surveys, *Psychol Med* 43(4):865–879, 2013.

Sorrell J: Moving beyond caregiver burden, *J Psychosoc Nurs Ment Health Serv* 52(3):15–18, 2014.

The National Consumer Voice for Quality Long-Term Care: *What is resident mistreatment?* Available at http://theconsumervoice.org/uploads/files/issues/rrm-brochure-508-compliant.pdf. Accessed April 2016.

Van Etten D, Gautam R: Custodial grandparents raising grandchildren: Lack of legal relationship is a barrier for services, *J Gerontol Nurs* 38(6):18–22, 2012.

World Health Organization (WHO): *World elder abuse awareness day*, 2012. Available at http://www.un.org/en/events/elderabuse. Accessed April 2015.

Zorowitz RA: Ethics. In Ham RJ, Sloane D, Warshaw GA, et al, editors: *Primary care geriatrics: A case-based approach*, ed 6, Philadelphia, 2014, Elsevier, pp 77–91.

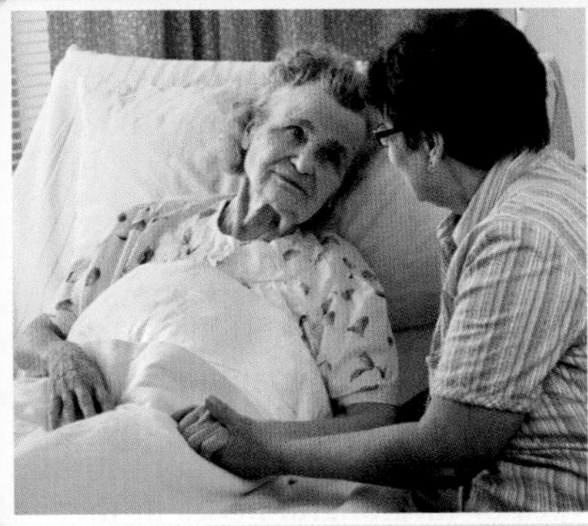

28

Loss, Death, and Palliative Care

Kathleen Jett

evolve.elsevier.com/Touhy/gerontological

LEARNING OBJECTIVES

Upon completion of this chapter, the reader will be able to:

- Differentiate between loss and grief.
- Explain the different types of grief and the dynamics of the grieving process.
- Explain the characteristics required of the nurse to be able to effectively care for those who are grieving.
- Propose palliative measures when comfort is the goal of care.
- Explain the role and responsibility of the nurse in assisting persons with advance care planning.
- Explain the difference between passive and active euthanasia.

THE LIVED EXPERIENCE

When we were in our sixties my friends and I met over cards, went on trips, and experienced all the joys of retirement. We didn't have much time to worry about aches and pains. In our seventies we had less time to play because we were busy visiting one another in the hospital or nursing home. In our eighties we met frequently again, but it was usually at our friends' funerals, leaving little time for cards or travel. Now that I am in my nineties hardly any of my friends are still alive; you know it gets kind of lonely, so you just have to make new younger friends!

Theresa, age 93

Life is like a pinwheel, a thing of beauty and change. Loss, like the wind, sets it in motion, beginning the life-changing process of grieving. Throughout one's life the winds of loss will gently stir recurrent episodes of grief through sights, sounds, smells, anniversary dates, and other triggers. The arms of the pinwheel suggest movement by the bereaved, reaching out of the experience of grief by surrendering through resting, or lowering one's defenses toward life and reaching out to others and rejoining life through change. Each gust of wind may generate a resurgence of grief, but the pinwheel will never lose its beauty.

Loss, dying, and death are universal, incontestable events of the human experience. Some loss is associated with the normal changes with aging, such as the loss of flexibility in the joints (see Chapter 3). Some is related to the normal changes in everyday life and life transitions, such as moving and retirement. Other losses are those of loved ones through death. Some deaths are considered normative and expected, such as older parents and friends. Other deaths are considered non-normative and unexpected, such as the death of adult children or grandchildren.

Regardless of the type of loss, each one has the potential to trigger grief and a process we call bereavement or mourning. Grieving and mourning are usually used synonymously. However, grieving is an individual's emotional response to a loss, and mourning is an active and evolving process that includes those behaviors used to incorporate the loss experience into one's life after the loss. Mourning behaviors are strongly influenced by social and cultural norms that prescribe the appropriate ways of both reacting to the loss and coping with it (Chow et al., 2007; Gerdner et al., 2007). For example, in much of the world, widows are expected to wear black after the death of their husbands; but in India the traditional dress is a white sari. There is no single way to grieve or respond to loss; each person grieves in his or her own way.

Although there are cultural expectations related to grief due to death, there are no guidelines for behavior when the loss is of another type. For example, an individual who moves to a nursing home (loses one's home) or who retires (willingly or unwillingly) may be very sad, irritable, and forgetful. The person may be suspected of developing dementia when he or she is actually grieving. When the losses accumulate in quick succession, a state of bereavement overload may result. The griever may become temporarily incapacitated and require careful and skilled support and guidance.

Gerontological nurses need to have basic knowledge of the morning rituals of those who receive their care and how to comfort and care for grievers, including one another. Additional knowledge and skills are related to care of the dying person and his or her survivors including those needed to provide quality care. And finally nurses caring for the dying must be comfortable with their own mortality. In this chapter we hope to provide the basic information necessary to promote effective grieving, peaceful dying, and good and appropriate deaths.

GRIEF WORK

Researchers have tried for years to understand the grieving process (grief work), resulting in a number of models and theories to explain and predict the human response. Pioneer thanatologist (one who studies the dying process) Elisabeth Kübler-Ross is best known for describing what became known as the stages of dying (1969). Other early theorists included Rando (1995), Corr and colleagues (2000), and the early work of Doka (2002). Each of these scholars described successful grieving as movement through predictable stages, phases, or tasks until one eventually was able to "let go" of that which was lost (Hall, 2011). The models have strongly influenced what caregivers and society in general have been taught about the grieving process.

Newer approaches have described grief work as more of a circular process in which a continued attachment to that which has been lost, at some level, is "normal" (Hall, 2011). Although the theories are intended to describe physical death and related grief, we propose that these same models can serve as a framework for understanding other types of meaningful losses in the lives of older adults.

A Loss Response Model

Jett's Loss Response Model (LRM) is influenced by the systems' work of nurse theorist Dr. Betty Newman (Alward, 2010), and the writing of nurse Barbara Giacquinta (1977), psychiatrist Avery Weisman (1979), and thanatological scholars Doka (2002) and Neimeyer and Sands (2011). It can be used to improve the understanding of grieving and to assist nurses in caring and comforting those who have experienced, or are experiencing, a loss of any kind. The framework is provided from which nursing interventions can be easily developed.

The grievers are part of a greater system that is striving to maintain equilibrium (Fig. 28.1). However, the impact of the loss (or the anticipation of it) results in disequilibrium or instability within the system. The loss seems unreal and the system is in chaos; the grievers are emotionally and functionally compromised (functional disruption). Common, simple activities, such as dressing, that normally take a few minutes may take much longer. Deciding which clothing to wear may seem too complex a task. Even as the tasks are accomplished, the person may complain of feeling distracted, restless, "at loose ends," and numb. Men who complained of numbness have been found to have higher cortisol levels (i.e., indicators of physiological stress) than women (Richardson et al., 2013).

As the system attempts to stabilize and grievers attempt to make sense of the chaos and integrate the loss into their lives, they search for meaning, asking such questions as the following: What did I do to have to leave my home? Could I have done more? Why did this happen to us (me)? How will we survive the loss? In reacting to the loss of a child or a grandchild, thoughts of "why wasn't it me?" are common. Searching for meaning is difficult, and as it is done, others are informed of the loss.

Each time the story is repeated, emotions are engaged in ways that are consistent with the griever's culture and personality. The expression of emotions can be quite

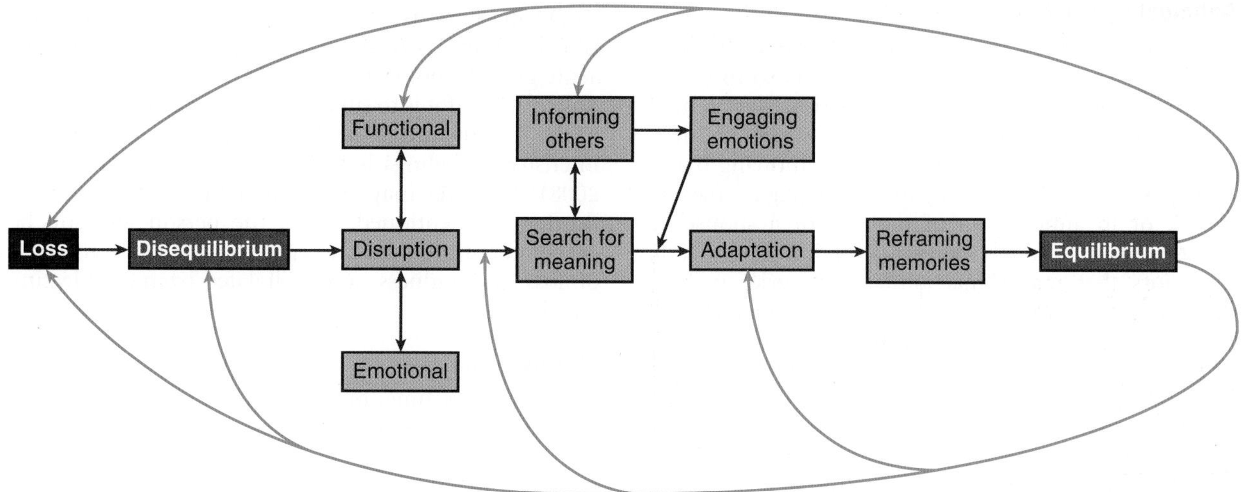

FIGURE 28.1 The Loss Response Model and cyclical loss.

powerful: anger, frustration, or even relief. Nurses can and do listen to the stories about the loss over and over again. Each time the story is slightly different as the meaning is incorporated into the person's life. These discussions can be a dress rehearsal of sorts as the person prepares to tell outsiders of the loss (e.g., "I can't drive anymore"). While acute grief may be triggered at each telling the intensity lessens and the duration shortens.

As roles and circumstances in which persons find themselves change, adaptation is necessary. Adaptation is a process in which the system changes in order to survive. For example, when a person is no longer able to do a task because of loss of ability, someone else must step in to perform it; when the elder patriarch dies, it may be a cultural expectation that the eldest son assumes his father's roles and responsibilities.

Finally, if the system is to survive, it must redefine itself. This is accomplished not by forgetting or ignoring the loss but by reframing memories. In the case of a death, family portraits and reunions will still be possible, just different from how they were before, and new memories can and will be made. Similarly, if celebrations had always been at the home of the elder (eliciting the sights, smells, and memories of childhood), the elder's move to a nursing home will prevent this custom. Adaptation leads to the development of new memories when the celebrations are held at the home of another, such as that of a child. The system can return to a new but different steady state. The nurse serves as a role model who displays the behavioral qualities of responsiveness, authenticity, commitment, and competence—that is, caring.

The Loss Response Model is cyclical and especially applicable to those with multiple underlying chronic conditions and multiple losses as are common in later life. At any point in the movement toward stabilization new disturbances may lead to renewed instability. The grievers are finding ways to adapt to the functional disruption related to one loss when another occurs. A home has been rearranged to make it safe for the person who has suffered a stroke when she falls and breaks her hip, necessitating a nursing home stay, either short-term or permanent, because of the combined losses.

Types of Grief

Grieving takes enormous amounts of physical and emotional energy. It is the hardest thing anyone can do and may be especially hard for older adults who must simultaneously face other challenges discussed throughout this text. Emotions can be intense, and this intensity may manifest as confusion, depression, or preoccupation with thoughts of the deceased or the loss. This reaction may be mistaken for other conditions, such as dementia, when it probably is a type of delirium, a temporary change in mental status or something that requires careful assessment and care (see Chapter 25). The gerontological nurse is most likely to work with elders who are experiencing anticipatory grief, acute grief, or chronic grief. A fourth type, disenfranchised grief, may be hidden, but when it occurs it is nonetheless significant.

Anticipatory Grief

Anticipatory grief is the emotional response to a loss before it actually occurs, a dress rehearsal, so to speak. The nurse observes this grief in preparation for potential loss, such as losing belongings (e.g., selling of a home), moving (e.g., into a nursing home), or knowing that a body part or function is going to change (e.g., a mastectomy), or in anticipation of the loss of a spouse or oneself either through dementia or through death. Behaviors that may signal anticipatory grief include preoccupation with the loss, unusually detailed planning, or a sudden change in attitude toward the thing or person to be lost (Lewis & McBride, 2004). End-of-life communication has been found to be associated with anticipatory grief and improved bereavement-related outcomes (Metzger & Gray, 2008).

If the loss is certain but no one can say when it will occur, or if it does not occur when or as expected, those awaiting the actual loss or death may become irritable, hostile, or impatient; not because they want the loss to occur but in response to the emotional ups and downs of the waiting. Researchers Glaser and Strauss (1968) described this as an "interruption in the sentimental order" of nursing units. When this occurs, no one, including care staff, quite knows how to behave. It may be easier to cope with anticipated losses when they occur at an expected time or in an expected manner.

Anticipatory grief can result in the phenomenon of premature detachment from an individual who is dying or detachment of the dying person from the environment. Pattison (1977) called the premature withdrawal of others sociological death, and the premature withdrawal of the person, psychological death. In either case, the person who is dying is no longer involved in day-to-day activities of living and essentially suffers a premature death.

Acute Grief

Acute grief is a crisis. It has a definitive syndrome of somatic, psychological, and spiritual symptoms of distress that occur in waves lasting varying periods of time. These symptoms may occur every time the loss is acknowledged, when others are informed, or even when another person offers condolences. They may lead to preoccupation with the loss similar to daydreaming and is accompanied by a sense of unreality. Depending on the situation, feelings of self-blame or guilt may also be acute and manifest themselves as hostility or anger toward friends, depression, or withdrawal. The intense stress of acute grief may lead to significant declines in physical health and the manifestation of depressive symptoms (Utz et al., 2012). A formerly bad relationship may be idealized and confusing to others.

During periods of acute grief functional disruption is at its peak. Fortunately, the signs and symptoms of acute grief do not last forever. The system has to find a way to adapt if it is to survive. Acute grief is most intense in the months immediately following the loss with the intensity of feelings lessening over time (Taylor et al., 2008). A griever may cry in the first months any time the loss is mentioned. Later, the person will still be grieving, but the tears are replaced with a surging sense of loss and sadness, and still later by more fleeting reactions.

Shadow Grief

Grieving takes time, but over the months, the intense pain of the acute period of impact lessens as memories are reframed. But the old memories never go away completely. There are often moments of intermittent sadness referred to as shadow grief (Horacek, 1991). It may temporarily inhibit some function but is considered a normal response. Although most often discussed in the context of perinatal death, a type of shadow death can occur at any age. It may be triggered by anniversary dates (birthdays, holidays, anniversaries) or by sensory stimuli, such as the smell of perfume, a color, or a sound (Carr et al., 2014) (Box 28.1).

Complicated Grief

Shadow grief is a type of chronic grief that is considered healthy and restorative. Yet for others, such as survivors of major tragedies, war, rape, abuse, and other horrific events, the "shadows" may be debilitating and are now recognized as posttraumatic stress. This is a form of complicated grief regardless of the age of the person.

Complicated grief also comes in the form of acute grief that does not significantly lessen over the months and even years after the loss. Obstacles of one form or another interfere with the evolution toward the reestablishment of equilibrium of the system; stability is elusive. The memories resist being reframed. Issues of guilt, anger, and ambivalence toward the person who has died are factors that will impede the grieving process until

BOX 28.1 The Carved Birds

One day as I was browsing at an art show, I came across a booth of carved birds, a favorite design of my beloved mother. I turned to remark to her. Except she was not there: she had died 15 years earlier in my home. Sadness passed over me like a cloud, and I wished she were there—I would buy her one as a special gift. Instead, I turned to my husband and shared reminiscences as I had done before. As the wind blows, so do the clouds pass.

these issues are resolved. Reactions are exaggerated and memories are experienced as if they are fresh, over and over again.

Signs of possible complicated grief include excessive and irrational anger, outbursts in social settings, and insomnia that lingers for an extended time or surfaces months or years later, or a grief episode that triggers a major depressive episode. The families who have had a loved one who has committed suicide have been found to be among those who have a greater risk for complicated and chronic grief (Sveen & Walby, 2008). This type of grief necessitates the professional intervention of a grief counselor, a psychiatric nurse practitioner, or a psychologist who has skills at helping grieving elders and their loved ones.

Disenfranchised Grief

Disenfranchised grief is experienced by persons whose loss cannot be openly acknowledged or publicly mourned. The grief is socially disallowed or unsupported (Doka, 2002). The person does not have a socially recognized right to be perceived or function as a griever. In other words, a relationship is not recognized; the loss is not sanctioned, or the griever is not recognized or cannot be made public. Disenfranchised grief has frequently been associated with domestic partnerships in which the family of the deceased does not acknowledge the partner or in secret relationships in which the involved party cannot tell others of the meaning or depth of the attachment. Disenfranchised grief can also occur in situations of family discord in which a member of the family is considered the "black sheep." Older adults can experience disenfranchised grief when persons close to them do not understand the full meaning of a loss, such as when others perceive the death of an elder from Alzheimer's disease as a blessing and fail to support the griever or caregiver who has struggled for years with anticipatory grief and now must cope with the acute grief of the actual death (Doka, 2002; Paun & Farran, 2011).

Factors Affecting Coping With Loss

To cope effectively with loss is to have the ability to move from a state of chaos to one of stability; to disequilibrium to renewed equilibrium, if only for a moment. It is to find meaning in the loss and be able to find a way to reframe memories. Many factors affect the ability to cope with loss and grief (Box 28.2).

Psychiatrist Avery Weisman described those who are more likely to effectively deal with loss as "good copers"; that is, individuals or families who have successfully navigated through crises in the past (1979, pp. 42–43). In other words, they can acknowledge the loss and try to make sense of it. They can maintain composure when necessary, can generally use good judgment, and can remain optimistic and appropriately hopeful without denying the loss. Good copers seek guidance when it is needed.

On the contrary, those who cope less effectively have few, if any, of these abilities. They tend to be more rigid, pessimistic, and demanding. They are more likely to be dogmatic and expect perfection in themselves and others. Ineffective copers are more likely to live alone, socialize little, and have few close friends or have an ineffective support network. They may have a history of mental illness, or have guilt, anger, or ambivalence toward the person who has died or that which has been lost. The person is more likely to have unresolved past conflicts or be facing the loss at the same time as secondary life stressors. In some cases the person will have fewer opportunities as a result of the loss. Those at special risk for significantly adverse effects of grief are older spouses and life partners of any kind. Intense grief may cause a temporary decrease in cognitive function that can be misinterpreted as dementia, isolating the griever (Ward et al., 2007). They are the elders who are most in need of the expert interventions of grief counselors and skilled, sensitive gerontological nurses.

BOX 28.2 Factors Influencing Grieving

Physical

Number of concurrent medical conditions
Use of sedatives (delays, but does not lessen grief)
Nutritional state
Exercise
Mental health

Emotional

Unique nature and meaning of loss
Coping strategies, personality, and maturity
Previous experience with loss or death
Sex-role conditioning
Immediate circumstances surrounding loss
Timeliness of the loss
Perception of preventability (sudden vs. expected)
Number, type, and quality of secondary losses

Social

Individual support systems
Sociocultural, ethnic, religious expectations, and rituals

Modified from Beare PG, Myers JL: *Adult health nursing,* ed 3, St Louis, MO, 1998, Mosby.

❖ IMPLICATIONS FOR GERONTOLOGICAL NURSING AND HEALTHY AGING

Like good copers, good gerontological nurses must be flexible, practical, resourceful, and abundantly optimistic. Nurses introduce themselves, establish rapport, and learn the cultural rules regarding the situation. The nurse fosters the griever's movement from disequilibrium to a new, albeit modified, steady state (Box 28.3).

The goal of the nurse is not to prevent grief but to support those who are grieving. Although that which has been lost can never be replaced, the potential long-term detrimental effects can be lessened. Working with grieving elders is part of the normal workday of gerontological nurses, who are professional grievers in their own way. It is one of the few areas in nursing where small actions can make a large difference in the quality of life for the person to whom we provide care.

BOX 28.3 Tips for Best Practice

Helping Grievers Move Through the Impact of Loss to the Reestablishment of Equilibrium

Functional Disruption
- Provide functional assistance

Searching for Meaning
- Provide reliable sources of information (e.g., websites).
- Inform appropriate providers of the person's need for information and make sure the person receives it.
- Engage in active listening.

Engaging Emotions
- "Give permission" to express emotions.
- Offer physical presence.
- Offer to locate usual sources of support during times of crisis (e.g., minister, tribal elder).
- Engage in active listening.

Informing Others
- Offer physical presence.
- Engage in active listening.

Adaptation
- Identify meaningful events influenced by the loss.
- Help find new ways of replacing that which has been lost.
- Offer discussions of how the loss has affected life.
- Engage in active listening.

Reframing Memories
- Offer to discuss mechanisms to develop new memories without denying connection with that or with whom has been lost.
- Encourage reminiscence.
- Facilitate opportunities for culturally based and desired bereavement rituals.
- Assure grievers that stability will return.
- Engage in active listening.

◆ Assessment

The goal of the grief assessment is to differentiate those who are likely to cope effectively from those who are at risk for ineffective coping so that appropriate interventions can be planned. A grief assessment is based on knowledge of the mourning process and the subsequent grieving. Data are obtained through observation of behavior of the individual and are assessed within the context of the person's culture (Goldstein et al., 2004).

A thorough grief assessment includes questions about recent significant life events, life or spiritual values, and relationship to that which has been lost. How many other stressful or demanding events or circumstances are occurring in the griever's life? This information will help determine who is most at risk for complicated grieving. The more concurrent stressors in the person's life, the more he or she will need grief specialists. The nurse determines what stress management techniques have been used in the past, and whether they were helpful (e.g., meditation) or potentially harmful (e.g., substance use or abuse). Was the griever's identity closely tied to that which is lost, such as a lifelong athlete who is faced with never walking again? If the loss is of a partner, how was the relationship? The loss of an abusive or controlling partner may liberate the survivor, who may feel guilty for not feeling the amount of grief that is expected. For many older women of today who have been dependent financially on their spouses, death may leave them impoverished, significantly complicating their grief. Knowing more about the loss and the effect of the loss on the elder's life will enable the nurse to construct and implement appropriate and caring responses.

◆ Interventions

For the new nurse who is confronted with a person's grief for the first time, there may be discomfort, fear, and insecurity. The tendency is to be sympathetic rather than empathetic. Questions arise in one's mind: What do I say? Should I be cheerful or serious? Should I talk about or even mention the dead person's name?

Nursing interventions, especially when elders are in crisis, begin with the gentle establishment of rapport. Nurses introduce themselves and explain the nature of their roles (e.g., charge nurse, staff nurse, medication nurse) and the times they have available. If it is the time of impact (e.g., just after a new serious diagnosis, at the death of a family member, or upon becoming a new but resistant resident of a long-term care facility), the most we can do is to provide support and a safe environment and ensure that basic needs, such as meals, are met. The nurse can soften the despair by fostering *reasonable* hope, such as, "You will make it through this time, one moment at a time, and I will be here to help."

Nurses make a significant contribution to the family in fostering even momentary stability by knowing what questions to ask at the time of death, such as the following: What cultural or familial rituals are important right now? Is there anyone who should be called at this time (see informing others below)? Would a spiritual advisor be a support for you right now? Have funeral arrangements already been made; if not, who can help you with this? Had he or she made his or her wishes known for this time?

Nurses observe for functional disruption and offer support and direction. They may have to help the family decide what needs to be done immediately and find ways to do it—either the nurse offers to complete the task or the nurse finds a friend or family member who can step in so the disruption does not have any deleterious effects (Box 28.4).

As grievers search for meaning, they may need help finding what they are looking for if this is possible. Sometimes it is information about a disease, a situation, or a person. Sometimes it is a spiritual search and help in finding a source of comfort such as a priest, rabbi, or medicine woman or man or a place of peace, such as the chapel or mosque. Often what is needed most is someone to listen to the "whys" and "hows"—questions that cannot be answered.

Sometimes nurses offer to contact others for those who are grieving, thinking that this is something that will help. However, it is far more therapeutic for grievers to be the ones who inform others because it helps the loss become part of their new reality. The nurse can offer to find a phone number or hold the griever's hand during the conversation or just "be there" when the news is being shared. In this way the nurse can be available to provide support when the griever's emotions engage and move toward wellness and equilibrium.

As the elder moves forward in adapting to the loss, such as a move from home to a nursing home, the nurse can talk with the person about what was most valued about living at home and what habits were comforting, and find ways to incorporate these in a new way into the new environment. If the elder does not have access to a kitchen and always had a cup of tea before bed, this can become part of the individualized plan of care.

Memories are reframed so that they can account for the loss without diminishing the value of that which has been lost, thus minimizing the risk for complicated grief (Maccallum & Bryant, 2011). Nurses can help elders reframe their memories and move toward equilibrium through seemingly simple interventions that can make a very big difference. The grandmother who had always hosted her eldest daughter's birthday party can still do that even if she is now a resident in a long-term care facility. When the nurse has the information about this important ritual, she or he can help the person reserve a private space, send out invitations, and have the birthday party as always, just reframed in that it is catered by the facility in the elder's new "home."

The nurse knows that at any point in the movement toward equilibrium a new loss can occur and the cycle begins again or moves back to an earlier point, and movement forward starts afresh (Fig. 28.1).

BOX 28.4 Functional Disruption: The Dirty Dishes

During a visit to the home of a woman who was in the last months of her life and getting progressively weaker so she could hardly stand, I noticed that there was a stack of dirty dishes in the sink. Her husband sat watching TV. Using the best therapeutic conversation I learned in nursing school I asked about the dishes. They both started crying. He said he did not know how to load the dishwasher—she had always done it and she did not know how to tell him they needed to be done. My "nursing intervention" that day was a lesson on using a dishwasher.

Countercoping

Avery Weisman (1979) described the work of health care professionals related to grief as "countercoping." Although he was speaking of working with people with cancer, it is equally applicable to working with people who are grieving for any loss and for families coping with the pending or past loss. "Countercoping is like counterpoint in music, which blends melodies together into a basic harmony. The patient copes; the therapist [nurse] countercopes; together they work out a better fit" (Weisman, 1979, p. 109). Weisman suggests four very specific types of interventions or countercoping strategies: (1) clarification and control, (2) collaboration, (3) directed relief, and (4) cooling off.

Clarification and control. The nurse helps griever(s) cope with loss by helping them confront it by getting or receiving information, considering alternatives, and finding a way to make the grief manageable. The nurse helps persons resume control by encouraging them to avoid acting on impulse. It may be necessary to say, "No, this is probably not a good time to make any major decisions."

Collaboration. The nurse collaborates by encouraging grievers to share stories with others and repeat the stories as often as is necessary as they "talk it out." The nurse as a collaborator is more directive than usual; it may be acceptable to say, "Yes—this is a good time to talk."

Directed relief. Some temporary directed relief may be necessary, especially during acute grief. Catharsis may be helpful. In many instances it is the nurse who encourages the griever to cry or otherwise express feelings such as hurt or anger, which is culturally acceptable to the griever. The nurse may have to say something like, "Expressing your feelings might help." Activity may also be recommended as a natural extension of feelings. Intense physical activity gives one emotional relief. In some cultures, people may tear their clothes or cut their hair. Today, there are numerous ways of acting out feelings—from throwing things, to taking a walk, to expressing feelings through creative works.

Cooling off. From time to time grievers might need to be encouraged to temporarily avoid active mourning through diversions that worked in the past during times of stress, especially when things have to be done or decisions have to be made. The nurse may need to suggest new tactics that may prove helpful. Although there is considerable cultural variation, cooling off also means encouraging the person to modulate emotional extremes at times and to think about ways to make sense of the loss, to build a new sense of self-esteem after the loss, and to help reestablish life patterns.

In all interventions related to grief, the nurse must have skills in therapeutic communication. Active listening is greatly preferable to giving advice. When listening, the nurse soon discovers that it is often not the actual loss that is of utmost concern, but rather the fear associated with the loss. If the nurse listens carefully to both the stated and the implied, what will be heard may be expressions such as the following: "How will I go on?" "What will I do now?" "What will become of me?" "What will happen to my loved ones, pets, etc.?" "I don't know what to do." "How could he (she) do this to me?" Because the nurse knows adaptation of some kind will ultimately occur, such comments may seem exaggerated or melodramatic, but to the one who is acutely grieving there seems to be no end. The person cannot yet look ahead and know that the despair and other acute feelings will ever lessen. Like good copers, good gerontological nurses must be flexible, practical, resourceful, and abundantly optimistic.

DYING, DEATH, AND PALLIATIVE CARE

Many people have said that death is not the problem; it is the dying that takes the work. This is true for all involved: the person who is dying, the loved ones, and the professional caregivers, including nurses. Dying is both a challenging life experience and a private one. A major question arises when considering dying and death in late life today: When is a person with multiple chronic or repeated acute or progressive health problems considered to be "dying"? Both treatable chronic conditions and those associated with an irreversible terminal condition often occur at the same time, more so as we age (Goldstein & Morrison, 2014).

How people deal with their own dying is often a reflection of the way they responded to earlier losses and stressors. Most people probably die as they have lived; that is, the manner in which one faces dying is an expression of personality, circumstances, illness, and culture (National Cancer Institute [NCI], 2013). Although not all older adults have had fulfilling lives or have a sense of completion, transcendence, or self-actualization (see Chapter 26), they often consider their own deaths around the age of their parents as "normal." If dying occurs after a particularly prolonged or painful illness, it is sometimes rationalized as a relief, at least in part. At the same time, the deaths of persons subjected to catastrophic events, such as murder or as the result of terrorist acts are neither reliefs nor socially acceptable.

Although the signs and symptoms attributed to terminal conditions may appear obvious, they can easily be confused with frailty and exacerbations of chronic diseases in later life. Anxiety, depression, restlessness, and agitation are behaviors that are frequently categorized as manifestations of confusion or dementia but may also be responses to the inability to express feelings that death is near. Ensuring that the person remains comfortable, whether the condition is acute, near the end of life, or anywhere in between, is the work of the nurse and other members of the caring team.

The Family

Today's older adults are usually members of multigenerational and complex networks. Those considered "family" are increasingly including friends, ex-spouses and partners, step-grandchildren, and fictive kin (those considered family as a result of affective bonds). Although children may be geographically distant, some degree of filial ties exist (see Chapter 26). When an elder becomes seriously or terminally ill and cannot uphold his or her role or obligation, the family balance or dynamics are significantly altered (functional disruption). For example, new arrangements are needed when an elder who has been providing child care or meal preparation is no longer able to do so. This change may cause considerable familial distress, as will the need for elder care when day-to-day help seems impossible because of the work demands and schedules of adult children. Depending on the role the individual has in the family/friend constellation, while changes may not occur at the time of diagnosis, they will as frailty advances (see Chapters 26 and 27). Adult children begin to see their own mortality through the death of their parents as a new family is established.

The idea that family members can remain involved with the dying person may be a source of constant conflict as they anticipate and plan for life without the dying family member. This change requires enormous energy by family members who are already burdened with their own anticipatory grief, daily living, and, in many cases, raising their own children and possibly grandchildren. A number of adaptive tasks may facilitate the reestablishment of equilibrium following the loss of a family member.

Family members learn, sometime early on, that reframing memories will be necessary to separate their own identities from that of the patient and learn to tolerate the reality that another family member will die while they live. The ability of the family to support, love, and provide intimacy may lead to exhaustion, impatience, anger, and a sense of futility if the dying is prolonged. Family members may be grieving differently than each other, hindering communication when it is needed the most. As the illness worsens, physical disability increases, and the patient's needs intensify, so may the family members' feelings of helplessness and frustration.

The family may feel extremely pressured to provide very personal care during the final days of a relative's life. They may feel caught between experiencing the present and remembering the person as he or she was, between pushing for more interventions with the potential to extend the dying and allowing a natural death to occur. Nurses often hear families lament that they "can't give up on them," even if this runs counter to the elder's wishes.

Despite the family's grief and pain, they must give the patient permission to die; let the loved one know that it is all right to let go and leave them. This gesture is the last act of love and dignity that the family can offer. Occasionally, no family is available to say, "It's okay to let go." The task then falls to the nurse who has developed a meaningful relationship with the person through caring.

❖ IMPLICATIONS FOR GERONTOLOGICAL NURSING AND HEALTHY AGING

The needs of the dying are like threads in a piece of cloth. Each thread is individual but necessary to the integrity and completeness of the fabric. If one thread is pulled, it affects the other threads, and the material's appearance, the thread placement, and the stability of the cloth. When one need is unmet it will affect all others because they are interdependent and interwoven.

A good and appropriate death is one that a person would choose if choosing were possible. It is one in which one's needs are met to the extent possible. The responsibility of the nurse is to provide safe conduct as the dying and their families navigate through unknown waters to a good and appropriate death (Boxes 28.5 and 28.6). There are several ways the nurse can intervene to promote healthy aging even while one is dying; one of these is to apply Weisman's six C's approach (1984).

The Six C's Approach

Weisman (1984) identified six needs of many persons who are dying: care, control, composure, communication, continuity, and closure. Although they are most applicable to those of northern European descent, they can provide a place to begin to think about caring for persons from all cultures.

BOX 28.5 Safe Conduct

The responsibility of the nurse is to provide what is referred to as "safe conduct," helping the dying and their families navigate through unknown waters to a good and appropriate death—that is, a death that the person would choose if choosing were possible. A good and appropriate death is one in which the person's needs are met for as long as possible, and life is never without meaning.

BOX 28.6 A Good and Appropriate Death

- Care needed is received, and it is timely and expert.
- One is able to control one's life and environment to the extent that is desired and possible and in a way that is culturally consistent with one's life.
- One is able to maintain composure when necessary and to the extent desired.
- One is able to initiate and maintain communication with significant others for as long as possible.
- Life continues as normal as possible while dying with the added tasks that may be needed to deal with and adjust to the inevitable death.
- One can maintain desirable hope at all times.
- One is able to reach a sense of closure in a way that is culturally consistent with one's practices and life patterns.

Care

As an advocate, the gerontological nurse makes sure that the best care is received; this includes expert management of pain (see Chapter 18), other symptoms, and support at all times. Care also goes beyond the physical to psychological pain, induced by depression, anxiety, fear, and unresolved emotional conflicts. When these needs are not met, the total pain experience is intensified and should be addressed in a manner that is acceptable to the person.

Dying calls for great amounts of energy for persons to cope with the emotional and physical assault of illness on the body. Two almost universal problems are a sense of breathlessness and fatigue. Caring means helping the person conserve energy (Glare et al., 2011). How much can the individual do without becoming physically and emotionally taxed? Is there something in particular that causes more or less shortness of breath? Would having oxygen available provide comfort? What everyday activities are most important for the person to do independently? How much energy is needed for the patient to be able to talk with visitors or staff without becoming exhausted? Only the person can answer these questions, and the nurse can advocate for the person to be given the opportunity to do so; and in doing so, the patient is able to remain in better control and maintain composure.

A detailed discussion of common symptoms addressed in palliative care can be found at http://consultgerirn.org, a service of the Hartford Institute for Geriatric Nursing.

Control

As people move toward physiological death and, in the case of dementia, loss of memories, they are in the process of losing everything they have ever known or will ever know. The potential loss of identity, independence, and control over bodily functions can lead to a sense of having lost self-esteem as well. The person may begin to feel ashamed, humiliated, and like a "burden." Control is the need to remain in a collaborative role relating to one's own living and dying and as an active participant in one's care to the extent desired. Once nurses know the elder's preferences, including cultural expectations, they can help the person meet these needs by taking every opportunity to return this level of control and in doing so bolster the person's self-esteem. Whenever possible the nurse can have the person decide when to groom, eat, wake, sleep, and so forth. The nurse never has the right to determine the activities of the individual, especially in relation to visitors and how time is spent.

Composure

Composure is the modulation of emotional extremes. Although Weisman describes this as a need for those who are dying, it is highly variable by culture; in some (e.g., Italian) it is a time of great emotional expression; in others (e.g., German) a time of stoicism. If the goal is one of composure, it is not to avoid the sadness but to have moments of relief.

Communication

The need for communication is broad, from the need for information as family members search for meaning, make decisions, or inform others of the actual or pending loss. Although the type and content of communication that are acceptable to the person vary by culture, the nurse has a responsibility to make sure that the dying have an opportunity to communicate how and what they choose.

In a study of terminal illness among the patient, family, and hospital staff, Glaser and Strauss (1963) identified four types of communication: *closed awareness, suspected awareness, mutual pretense,* and *open awareness*. Each of these influenced the work on the nursing home or hospital unit and the care of the patient.

- ***Closed awareness*** is described as "keeping the secret." Hospital staff and the family and friends know that the patient is dying, but the patient does not know it or knows and keeps the secret as well. Generally, caregivers invent a fictitious future for the patient to believe in, in hopes that it will boost the patient's morale. Although this happens less today because of legislation related to patients' rights, it still occurs. In some cultures, such as in many Latino families, it is expected.
- In ***suspected awareness,*** the person suspects he or she is dying, but because it is not discussed it cannot be confirmed. Inquiries on the part of the person are indirect or avoided by others. Hints are bandied back and forth, and a contest ensues for control of the information.
- ***Mutual pretense*** is a situation of "let's pretend." Everyone knows the patient has a terminal illness, but no one talks about it—real feelings are kept hidden.
- ***Open awareness*** occurs when the patient, family, friends, nurses, and physicians openly acknowledge the eventual death of the patient. The patient may ask, "Will I die?" and "How and when will I die?" The family grieves with the patient rather than for the patient. The nurse can encourage open awareness whenever possible while at the

same time respecting the patient's culture (Steinberg, 2011). In some cultures, talking about an anticipated death is deemed helpful. In others, one can be aware of the dying but talking about it openly may be taboo, such as in the traditional Haitian culture.

Continuity

The need for continuity equates to preserving as normal a life as possible; to maintaining at least some level of equilibrium while dying. Too often a dying person can feel shut off from the rest of the world at a time when he or she is still capable of being involved and active in some way. Loneliness is the result of a loss of continuity with one's life. The nurse may ask about the person's life and those things most valued and work with the family and the patient or resident on a plan to remain engaged in as many of the activities and past roles as possible. A father who watches a certain ballgame with his son every Sunday can continue to do this regardless of the need to be in a hospital, in a nursing home, or an inpatient hospice unit. If the person is at home and is bedridden, it may make more sense to have the bed in a central area rather than in a distant room. Treating the person who is dying as an intelligent and competent adult at all times is a powerful expression of caring.

One approach people have taken to obtain continuity of their lives after death is in the establishment of legacies. Legacies can take many different forms and may range from memories that will live on in the minds of others to bequeathed fortunes. A grandmother who is likely to die before a favorite grandchild's wedding can create a legacy when she participates with planning, regardless of the age of the grandchild if this is important to them, thereby leaving an enduring and special legacy.

Closure

Finding closure is an opportunity for reconciliation and transcendence. Reminiscence is one way of putting one's life in order, in other words, to evaluate the pluses and minuses of one's life and find that it had some value (Box 28.7). It is a means of resolving conflicts, giving up possessions, and making final good-byes. Learning to say "good-bye" today leaves open the possibility of many more "hellos." Pain and other symptoms that are not well controlled may interfere with this reconciliation, making appropriate interventions by the nurse especially important.

When the person feels that physiological death is approaching the nurse can look for signs when the person begins using "coded communication," such as saying good-bye instead of the usual goodnight, giving away cherished possessions as gifts, urgently contacting friends and relatives with whom the person has not communicated with for a long time, and having direct or symbolic premonitions that death is near.

For some, closure means coming to terms with their spiritual selves, with Jesus, God, Allah, or Buddha, for example. Pastoral support may be offered but should never be facilitated without the person's express permission. The nurse can foster transcendence by providing patients with the time and privacy for self-reflection as well as an opportunity to talk about whatever they need to talk about, especially about the meanings of their lives and the meanings of their deaths.

Care, control, composure, communication, continuity, and closure create the borders necessary to complete the fabric of needs of the dying. Their influence is omnipresent in the other needs. Without them, the cloth can fray, and attempts to meet the needs will be limited.

BOX 28.7 The Inherent Value of Every Life

The director of a long-term care facility asked me to do a presentation on death and dying. I brought my usual materials for staff training. However, when I entered the room I was shocked to see 20 or so residents of the facility sitting in wheelchairs. Most were leaning over and appeared to be asleep. I realized that they probably knew much more than I did. Instead I asked them, "As you get closer to the end of your natural lives, what is one thing you want to be remembered for?" Holding a microphone I went around the room to even those who from all appearances could not participate. The answers were amazing from "I grew wonderful roses" to "I designed a bridge." It was a life-changing experience for me.

Kathleen Jett

DYING AND THE NURSE

Nurses are professional grievers experiencing the death of their patients and residents over and over again. Nursing assistants are often "invisible grievers" as they watch the slow death or decline of someone they have intimately cared for over the years (Anderson & Gaugler, 2006–2007). Some consider the death of a patient as a failure, that they have "lost" the person they cared for; yet, when they are good deaths, they can be viewed as professional successes each time we share the special and very personal experience of providing safe conduct for elders while dying and gentle caring for their survivors. We can use the reminders of our own mortality as motivation to live the best we can with what we have. Nurses can seek support and give it to one another. As grievers, we too may need to tell the story of the dying, or the person, to those professionals around us, either in formal or in informal support groups; and we must listen to those stories of our colleagues over and over again until they become part of the fabric of our colleagues' lives as well.

Caring for older adults requires knowledge of the grieving and dying processes as well as skills in providing relief of symptoms or palliative care (Table 28.1). However, it is also acknowledged that constantly working with the grieving or dying is an art. The development of the art calls for inner strength and personal coping skills (Box 28.8). The most important coping skills for nurses may be meaning-making of the person's life and the ability to disengage after the death (Desbiens & Fillion, 2007). The effective gerontological nurse has developed a personal philosophy of life and of death. Although this can and does change over time, it will help when times are difficult. Emotional maturity allows the nurse to deal with disappointment and postponement of immediate needs or desires. Maturity means that the nurse can reach out for help when needed. Finally, in order to provide comfort to grieving persons, nurses must be comfortable with their own lives or at least be able to set aside their own sadness and grief while working with the sadness and grief of others.

TABLE 28.1 Best Nursing Practice: Signs and Symptoms of Approaching Death

Physical	Rationale	Intervention
Coolness	Diminished peripheral circulation to increase circulation to vital organs	Socks, light cotton blankets or warm blankets if needed; do not use electric blanket
Increased sleeping	Conservation of energy	Respect need for increased rest; inquire as to patient's wishes regarding timing of companionship
Disorientation	Metabolic changes	Identify self by name before speaking to patient; speak softly, clearly, and truthfully
Fecal and/or urinary incontinence	Increased muscle relaxation	Change bedding as needed; use bed pads; avoid indwelling catheters
Noisy respirations	Poor circulation of body fluids, immobilization, and the inability to expectorate	Elevate the head with pillows, or raise the head of the bed, or both; gently turn the head to the side to drain
Restlessness	Metabolic changes and relative cerebral anoxia	Calm the patient by speech and action; reduce light; gently rub back, stroke arms, or read aloud; play soothing music; do not use restraints
Decreased intake of food and fluids	Body conservation of energy for function	Provide nutrition within limits expressed by patient or in advance directive; semisolid liquids easiest to swallow; protect mouth and lips from discomfort of dryness
Decreased urine output	Decreased fluid intake and decreased circulation to kidney	None
Altered breathing pattern	Metabolic and oxygen changes	Elevate the head of bed; speak gently to patient
Emotional or Spiritual	**Presumed Rationale**	**Intervention**
Withdrawal	Prepares the patient for release and detachment and letting go	Continue communicating in a normal manner using a normal voice tone; identify self by name; give permission to die
Vision-like experiences of dead friends or family; religious vision	Preparation for transition	Accept the reality of the experience for the person; reassure the person that the feeling is normal
Restlessness	Tension, fear, unfinished business	Listen to patient express his or her fears, sadness, and anger; facilitate completion of business if possible
Unusual communication	Signals readiness to let go	Say what needs to be said to the dying patient; kiss, hug, cry with him or her as appropriate

BOX 28.8 Nursing Skills Needed for Palliative Care

- Have ability to talk to patients and families about dying.
- Be knowledgeable about symptom control and pain-control techniques.
- Have ability to provide comfort-oriented nursing interventions.
- Recognize physical changes that precede imminent death.
- Deal with own feelings.
- Deal with angry patients and families.
- Be knowledgeable and deal with the ethical issues in administering end-of-life palliative therapies.
- Be knowledgeable, and inform patients about advance directives.
- Be knowledgeable of the legal issues in administering end-of-life palliative care.

Modified from White KR, Coyne PJ, Patel UB: Are nurses adequately prepared for end-of-life care? *J Nurs Scholarsh* 33:147–151, 2001, Sigma Theta Tau International.

Palliative Care

Gerontological nurses routinely care for elders who have irreversible and progressive conditions, such as Alzheimer's disease and Parkinson's disease. Other elders have exhausted all treatment options for conditions such as cancer or end-stage heart or renal disease. A nursing home resident may elect to remain at a care facility rather than return (ever) to a hospital, even if faced with an acute event such as a stroke or the more protracted end-stage heart disease. These elders are receiving a type of care called *palliative care*—with the goal of comfort rather than cure, the treatment of symptoms rather than disease, and the *quality* of life left rather than the *quantity* of life remaining (Goldstein & Morrison, 2014). Nurses function in a variety of roles in the provision of palliative care: as a staff nurse giving direct care, as a coordinator implementing the plan of the interdisciplinary team, as an executive officer responsible for clinical care, or as an advocate for humane care for persons who are dying and their families.

Nurses have also been involved in the establishment of programs such as the POLST (Physician Orders for Life-Sustaining Treatment) program. Originating in Oregon in the 1990s, the POLST program supports effective communication of patient desires and respect for these wishes in end-of-life care (http://www.ohsu.edu/polst). Both master's degrees and national certifications in this program are now available (http://www.nhpco.org; http://www.hpna.org).

Some type of palliative care can be provided anywhere by anyone sharing these goals and skills. It can even be provided at the same time a person is receiving curative care for something else, such as receiving treatment for a bladder infection while terminally ill with heart disease (Batchelor, 2010). Palliative care affirms life, regards dying as a normal process, and neither hastens nor postpones death (World Health Organization [WHO], 2016). Good end-of-life care should focus more on what we as nurses provide than what we forgo (ANA Center for Ethics and Human Rights, 2012).

The scope and specialty of palliative care has grown considerably over the years; research has been conducted, professional organizations have been formed, and standardized curricula have been developed. With the support of the American Association of Colleges of Nursing and City of Hope Medical Center, a broad initiative (ANA-ELNEC) was organized in 1999, "Dedicated to Educating Nurses in Excellent Palliative Care" (http://www.aacn.nche.edu/ELNEC; http://www.cityofhope.org/education/health-professional-education/nursing-research-and-education-programs-for-health-professionals). It is hoped that by training nurses and faculty, nursing as a profession can provide the highest level of palliative care. Whereas initially palliative care was the specialty of community-based organizations referred to as hospices, specialized units and staff are now seen in many long-term care and acute care facilities.

Hospice

The term *hospice* refers to a formalized structure from which a significant amount of the palliative care is delivered. It derives its meaning from the medieval concept of hospitality in which a community assisted a traveler at dangerous points along his or her journey. The dying are indeed travelers along the continuum of life within a community consisting of friends, family, and specially prepared people to care, that is, the hospice/palliative care team.

The concept of the contemporary hospice was made famous by Dr. Cicely Saunders, founder of Saint Christopher's Hospice in London in 1967. In 1974 Dr. Florence Wald (Dean of the College of Nursing at Yale), two pediatricians, and a chaplain brought the hospice concept to the United States when they established the Connecticut Hospice in Branford, Connecticut.

Both for-profit and not-for-profit hospice organizations are now in many locations in the United States and provide comprehensive and interdisciplinary care to persons assessed to be in the last 6 months of life. A hospice organization is expected to provide medical, nursing, nursing assistant, chaplain, social work, and volunteer support 24 hours per day if needed. Other services may include massage, music, art, and pet therapy. Hospices provide care not only to the dying but also to the dying person's families and friends through support before and after the death of loved ones.

The majority of hospice care occurs at home. The home becomes the primary center of care, provided by family members or friends who are taught basic nursing care and how to administer the medications needed to ensure their loved one remains comfortable. A growing number of inpatient hospice facilities exist as well for those with symptoms that could not be managed at home or those without caregivers, or to provide short periods of rest from caring (respite) for the caregivers. These may be associated with a community hospice program—free-standing or small units within other types of care facilities. Hospice nurses and others may also see patients who are residents in assisted living facilities and work with the staff to supplement care and provide expertise in symptom management. Special units in acute care hospitals and some long-term care facilities may also provide palliative care services guided by traditional hospice principles. Pain control and the opportunity to die at home are the key principles that people associate with hospice services. In actuality, hospice represents much more. It supports and guides the family in patient care and ensures that the patient will not die alone and that the family will not be abandoned. Bereavement services for the family extend for a period of time on an emergency and regular basis after the death of the patient. In contrast to palliative care, hospice services are limited to the time when one's life expectancy is anticipated to be 6 months or less.

DECISION-MAKING AT THE END OF LIFE

Decision-making at the end of life has become a legal, ethical, medical, and personal concern. The lines between living and dying are blurred as a direct result of technological advances. This results in ambivalence concerning whether death is to be delayed and for how long and under what circumstances. Decisions need to be made if a death is acceptable only when aggressive medical procedures are no longer effective or what is referred to a "natural death" can occur without the use of death-delaying actions.

The issue of who has the authority to make end-of-life decisions and for whom has been the subject of research, debate, and, in the United States, federal legislation. An adult who has not been adjudicated to lack capacity (see Chapter 7) is recognized as the final decision-maker; however, this assumption is based on a very Euro-American or Western perspective. Persons who are from non-Western traditions place less emphasis on the individual and more on the needs of the family or community (see Chapter 2) (Mazanec & Tyler, 2003). Nurses have an obligation to know the legal requirements in their jurisdictions and then work with the elder and the family to determine how these will fit with their cultural patterns and needs related to end-of-life decisions.

Advance Directives

Whereas people have always had opinions about their wishes, their right to refuse medical treatment was not established in the United States until 1990 by the Patient Self-Determination Act (PSDA) and implemented in all states in 1991. Under the PSDA, the adult was recognized as the ultimate authority to accept or reject medical care, including death-delaying treatment. Through the legislation related to the PSDA, adults were granted the legal authority to complete what are known as advance health care directives (AHCDs)—or statements about their wishes and directions to others before the need for a decision arises. These directives may be as vague as "no treatment if I am terminally ill" to as detailed with a breakdown of decisions about dialysis, antibiotics, tube feedings, cardiopulmonary resuscitation (CPR), and so on. The AHCD provides a mechanism for an adult to appoint another adult of his or her choosing to make decisions if he or she is unable to do so (see Chapter 7).

The common forms of advance directives are known as living wills, durable powers of attorney for health care (DPAHC), and medical powers of attorney (see Chapter 7) (Gittler, 2011). In each of these the person creating it appoints a proxy or surrogate to act on his or her behalf should a time come when the person is unable to do so. A living will is usually restricted to represent a person's wishes specific to a terminal illness. In contrast, a person appointed in a DPAHC can speak for the other in most or all matters of health care. In many states, advance directives are legally binding documents that nurses, physicians, and health care institutions are required to respect. Both the proxy and the health care surrogate are expected to use what is known as *substituted judgment*, that is, a decision the person would make if able to do so. This may include turning off a ventilator, turning off tube feedings, or stopping intravenous fluids.

All agencies in the United States that receive Medicare and Medicaid funds are required to disseminate PSDA information to their patients and inquire as to the existence of advance directives. Hospitals and long-term care facilities are responsible for providing written information at the time of admission about the individual's rights under law both to refuse medical and surgical care and to provide this decision in writing and in advance. Health maintenance organizations (HMOs) are required to do the same at the time of member enrollment as are home health agencies before the patient comes under the care of the agency. Hospices are obliged to inform patients of their rights on the initial visit. Providers (physicians and nurse practitioners) are encouraged but are not under obligation to provide this same information to their patients, although a health care visit for the sole purpose of a discussion of advance planning is now covered (paid for) by Medicare.

Although the exact format and signature (e.g., notarization) requirements vary from state to state, the PSDA is a federal mandate and applies to persons in all jurisdictions. There are multiple sources of related information available on the Internet.

Although the nurse cannot provide legal information, she or he does have a responsibility to serve as a resource person ready to answer basic questions people have about end-of-life decision-making. The nurse may be called upon to determine the cultural barriers to completing advance directives (Box 28.9). The nurse is often the person who asks about the presence of an existing advance directive such as a living will, ensures that it still reflects the person's wishes, advocates that the wishes are followed, and makes sure that existing or newly created advance directives are available in the appropriate locations in the medical record.

Euthanasia, Assisted Suicide, and Aid-in-Dying

The recognition of the right to refuse life-sustaining medical treatment renewed age-old questions over persons' rights to make their own decisions regarding the continuation of their natural lives as well. Some people, especially those who are suffering from a terminal illness, have ended their lives. Others have asked for assistance in accomplishing this in the most painless way. Among those asked have been many gerontological nurses (Box 28.10).

BOX 28.9 Cultural Barriers to the Use of Advance Directives and Hospice

- Distrust of the health care system (especially in groups who have experienced violence or discrimination in the United States or their country of origin)
- Collectivism: Family rather than individual is "decision-maker"
- Preference for physician, as expert, to make the decision
- Taboo to talk about death or dying
- Influence of faith and spirituality: Illness as a test of faith
- Belief that life is a gift from God that must be protected
- Death as a part of the cycle of life and must not be disturbed
- Dying away from home may lead to a disturbance of the spirits
- Cannot die at home because the spirit will linger

From Coolen PR: Cultural relevance in end-of-life care, *EthnoMed,* May 1, 2012. Available at https://ethnomed.org/clinical/end-of-life/cultural-relevance-in-end-of-life-care. Accessed June 2016.

Euthanasia, physician-assisted suicide, and *physician aid-in-dying* are the phrases most commonly heard in discussions around this topic today. "Euthanasia means that someone other than the patient commits an action with the intent to end the patient's life, for example injecting a patient with a lethal dose of medication" (ANA Center for Ethics and Human Rights, 2013). In both physician-assisted suicide and physician aid-in-dying, the patient is given the means to end his or her life (usually in the form of access to a lethal dose of medications) and instructions on the safe way to do this on his or her own, if he or she chooses. If the dose is administered by the physician or nurse, even at the request of the patient, this is considered euthanasia and always illegal and considered professionally unethical in the United States.

Rules allowing and regulating physician aid-in-dying began in the United States in 1994 in the state of Oregon. Since that time it has become legal in four additional states (Montana, California, Washington State, and Vermont). As of September 2016, 19 additional states are considering what is referred to as "death with dignity" legislation (Death with Dignity, 2016). In the remaining states, it remains illegal. Physician-assisted suicide is legal in several European countries and Columbia. Euthanasia is permitted only in Switzerland. It is important to note that the numbers of persons who have chosen to take their lives in this way remain relatively few, and the majority have end-stage cancer, are highly educated, and are elderly (The Economist, 2015).

As the ethical questions surrounding end-of-life issues become increasingly complex, so do the questions regarding nurses' roles relative to these. Over the years the American Nursing Association has developed a number of Position Statements that provide nurses with the professional expectations and guidance related to the care they provide (ANA, 2012, 2013). Individual statements now include *Forgoing Nutrition and Hydration* (2011), *Nursing Care and Do Not Resuscitate (DNR) and Allow Natural Death (AND) Decisions* (2012), and *Euthanasia, Assisted Suicide, and Aid in Dying* (2013). In

BOX 28.10 Can I Help You?

One day when checking on a woman with end-stage pulmonary disease, I asked, "Is there anything I can do for you?" She responded quickly asking if I knew how she could reach Dr. Kevorkian, a physician who had been known for assisting people commit suicide. I knew that I had to be much more proactive in finding ways to make her more comfortable while she waited to die.

Kathleen Jett at 40

all cases the nurse is expected to strive to completely understand the desires of the patient, explain the options available to the patient, and provide the highest level of care needed to achieve comfort. It is recommended that the term "allow a natural death" instead of "do not resuscitate" be used because of vagueness of the latter term and the negative connotations that have been attributed to it (i.e., "doing nothing").

While the purpose of palliative care is always to promote comfort and alleviate suffering, there are times when this seems impossible. For some, refractory and unendurable symptoms cannot be controlled as death draws near. This may be the time (with the patient's or surrogate's permission) when palliative sedation is used. This is the controlled and carefully monitored use of nonopioid medications to lower the patient's level of consciousness to the extent necessary to achieve comfort. In some cases this will indeed hasten the timing of the death, but the purpose of palliative sedation is only for comfort care and is not considered physician-assisted (or nurse-assisted) suicide (ANA, 2013). "… The ethical justification that supports palliative sedation is based in precepts of dignity, respect for autonomy, beneficence, fidelity, nonmaleficence, and the principle of double effect, which evaluates an action based on intended outcome and the proportionality of benefit and harm" (ANA, 2013, p. 1). This type of symptom management was formerly referred to as terminal sedation but is more accurately described by the term palliative sedation (Box 28.11).

BOX 28.11 Providing Comfort in the Final Moments of a Natural Life: Palliative Sedation

A patient of mine had been admitted to a long-term care facility. She told me that she had been in and out of the hospital for congestive heart failure eight times in the last 2 months, and while she had just been discharged she could tell the failure was returning since she was having increased sense of breathlessness and anxiety even with supplemental oxygen. She begged not to be sent back to the hospital because she knew death was close. She asked only that she remain as comfortable as possible. I had the amount of Ativan available to achieve this and reassured her I would not let her suffer. When she began to have more shortness of breath and associated distress, we were able to give her very small doses of the Ativan until she could relax and not struggle with fear. The restlessness began again when she started to feel "air hunger," like many persons do as they die. We did not wait the usual "4 hours" but continued to administer the Ativan so that she was consistently comfortable. After a few hours she was sleeping in apparent comfort. No further Ativan was needed and in a couple of hours she died.

Nurses have had strong opinions related to all aspects of end-of-life care, yet the profession's opposition to nurse participation in euthanasia does not negate the obligation of the nurse to provide compassionate, ethically justified end-of-life care that includes the promotion of comfort and the alleviation of suffering, the provision of adequate pain control, and (at all times) the support of the patient's decision to forego life-sustaining treatments.

KEY CONCEPTS

- Loss occurs within a system consisting of the individual who has experienced the loss and his or her significant others. Loss includes the death of a member of the system.
- Grief is an emotional reaction and strongly influenced by the type of loss, the individual's ability to cope, and the system's ability to address chaos.
- Helping persons who are dealing with loss is part of the daily work of the gerontological nurse.
- The dying older adult is a living person with all the same needs as others for good and natural relationships with people.
- The goal of palliative care is to promote comfort at all times.
- Advance directives allow an individual control over life and death decisions by written communication and the appointment of a person (a proxy) to be an advocate when he or she is no longer able to dictate his or her wishes.
- Physician aid-in-dying and euthanasia are very different concepts as defined by both the World Health Organization and the American Nurses Association and any number of other organizations.
- The purpose of palliative sedation is only to reduce the person's level of awareness, to the point of symptom relief. It is never for the purpose of hastening death, even if in doing so this occurs.

ACTIVITIES AND DISCUSSION QUESTIONS

1. Explore your response to being given a terminal diagnosis. What coping mechanisms work for you? With which awareness approach would you be comfortable?
2. Describe how you would deal with a dying person and his or her family when they are especially protective of one another.
3. Describe and strategize how you would bring up the topic of advance directives.

4. What advance directive is legally recognized in your state?
5. Describe how you would introduce the topic of dying with a patient who is critically ill and not expected to live.

REFERENCES

Alward PD: Betty Newman's system model. In Parker ME, Smith MC, editors: *Nursing theories and nursing practice*, ed 3, Philadelphia, 2010, FA Davis, pp 182–201.

ANA Center for Ethics and Human Rights: *Nursing care and do not resuscitate (DNR) and allow natural death (AND) decisions,* 2012. Available at http://www.nursingworld.org/MainMenuCategories/EthicsStandards/Ethics-Position-Statements.

ANA Center for Ethics and Human Rights: *Euthanasia, assisted suicide, and aid in dying,* 2013. Available at http://www.nursingworld.org/MainMenuCategories/EthicsStandards/Ethics-Position-Statements.

Anderson KA, Gaugler JE: The grief experiences of certified nursing assistants: Personal growth and complicated grief, *Omega (Westport)* 54(4):301–318, 2006–2007.

Batchelor NH: Palliative or hospice care? Understanding the similarities and differences, *Rehabil Nurs* 35(2):60–64, 2010.

Carr D, Sonnega J, Nesse RM, et al: Do special occasions trigger psychological distress among older bereaved spouses? An empirical assessment of clinical wisdom, *J Gerontol B Psychol Sci Soc Sci* 69(1):113–122, 2014.

Chow A, Chan C, Ho S: Social sharing of bereavement experience by Chinese bereaved persons in Hong Kong, *Death Stud* 31(7):601–618, 2007.

Corr CA, Nabe CM, Corr DM: *Death and dying, life and living*, ed 3, Stamford City, CT, 2000, Wadsworth.

Death With Dignity: *Death with dignity around the U.S.,* September 7, 2016. Available at https://www.deathwithdignity.org/take-action. Accessed September 2016.

Desbiens J, Fillion L: Coping strategies, emotional outcomes and spiritual quality of life in palliative care nurses, *Int J Palliat Nurs* 13(6):291–300, 2007.

Doka KJ: *Disenfranchised grief: New direction, challenges, and strategies for practice*, Champaign, IL, 2002, Research Press.

The Economist: *Doctor-assisted suicide: The right to die,* June 27, 2015. Available at http://www.economist.com/news/leaders/21656182-doctors-should-be-allowed-help-suffering-and-terminally-ill-die-when-they-choose. Accessed February 2016.

Gerdner LA, Yang D, Cha D, et al: The circle of life, *J Gerontol Nurs* 33(5):20–31, 2007.

Giacquinta B: Helping families face the crisis of cancer, *Am J Nurs* 77(10):1585–1588, 1977.

Gittler J: Advance care planning and surrogate health care decision making for older adults, *J Geriatr Nurs* 37(5):15–19, 2011.

Glare P, Miller J, Nikolova T, et al: Treating nausea and vomiting in palliative care: A review, *Clin Interv Aging* 6:243–259, 2011.

Glaser BG, Strauss AL: *Awareness of dying*, Chicago, 1963, Aldine.

Glaser BG, Strauss AL: *Time for dying*, Chicago, 1968, Aldine.

Goldstein C, Anapolsky E, Park J, et al: Research guiding practice related to cultural issues at end of life care, *Geriatr Nurs* 25:58–59, 2004.

Goldstein NB, Morrison BS, et al: Palliative care. In Ham RJ, Sloane PD, Warshaw GA, editors: *Primary care geriatrics: A case-based approach*, ed 6, Philadelphia, 2014, Elsevier, pp 164–174.

Hall C: Beyond Kübler-Ross: Recent developments in our understanding of grief and bereavement, *InPsych* 2011. Available at http://www.psychology.org.au/publications/inpsych/2011.

Horacek BJ: Toward a more viable model of grieving and consequences for older persons, *Death Stud* 15:459–472, 1991.

Kübler-Ross E: *On death and dying*, New York, 1969, Macmillan.

Lewis ID, McBride M: Anticipatory grief and chronicity: Elders and families in racial/ethnic minority groups, *Geriatr Nurs* 25(1):44–47, 2004.

Maccallum F, Bryant RA: Imagining the future in complicated grief, *Depress Anxiety* 28(8):658–665, 2011.

Mazanec P, Tyler MK: Cultural considerations in end-of-life care: How ethnicity, age and spirituality affect decisions when death is imminent, *Am J Nurs* 103(3):50–59, 2003.

Metzger PL, Gray MJ: End-of-life communication and adjustment: Pre-loss communication as a predictor of bereavement-related outcomes, *Death Stud* 32(4):301–325, 2008.

National Cancer Institute: *Grief, bereavement and coping with loss,* 2013. Available at http://www.cancer.gov/about-cancer/advanced-cancer/caregivers/planning/bereavement-pdq#section/all.

Neimeyer RA, Sands DC: Meaning reconstruction in bereavement: From principles to practice. In Neimeyer RA, Harris DL, Winokuer HR, et al, editors: *Grief and bereavement in contemporary society: Bridging research and practice*, New York, 2011, Routledge.

Pattison EM, editor: *The experience of dying*, Englewood Cliffs, NJ, 1977, Prentice-Hall.

Paun O, Farran CJ: Chronic grief management for dementia caregivers in transition, *JGN* 37(12):28–35, 2011.

Rando TA: Grief and mourning: Accommodating to loss. In Wass H, Neimyer RA, editors: *Dying—Facing the facts*, Philadelphia, 1995, Taylor & Francis, pp 211–241.

Richardson VE, Bennett KM, Carr D, et al: How does bereavement get under the skin? The effects of late-life spousal loss on cortisol levels, *J Gerontol B Psychol Sci Soc Sci* 70(3):341–347, 2013.

Steinberg SM: Cultural and religious aspects of end-of-life care, *Int J Crit Illn Inj Sci* 1(2):154–156, 2011.

Sveen CA, Walby FA: Suicide survivors' mental health and grief reactions: A systematic review of controlled studies, *Suicide Life Threat Behav* 38(1):13–29, 2008.

Taylor DH Jr, Kuchibhatla M, Ostbye T, et al: The effect of spousal caregiving and bereavement on depressive symptoms, *Aging Ment Health* 12(1):100–107, 2008.

Utz RL, Caserta M, Lund D: Grief, depressive symptoms, and physical health among recently bereaved spouses, *Gerontologist* 52(4):460–471, 2012.

Ward L, Mathias JL, Hitchings SE: Relationships between bereavement and cognitive functioning in older adults, *Gerontology* 53(6):362–372, 2007.

Weisman A: *Coping with cancer*, New York, 1979, McGraw-Hill.

Weisman A: *The coping capacity: On the nature of being mortal*, New York, 1984, Human Sciences Press.

World Health Organization (WHO): *WHO definition of palliative care,* 2016. Available at http://www.who.int/cancer/palliative/definition/en.

INDEX

A

AACN. *see* American Association of Colleges of Nursing (AACN)
AAMI. *see* Age associated memory impairment (AAMI)
Absorbent products, for urinary incontinence, 161
Absorption, in pharmacokinetics, 112
Abuse, of elder, 393, 393*b*
Accessory organs, of digestive system, 33–34
Accidental bowel leakage, 167
  assessment for, 168
  implications of, for gerontological nursing and healthy aging, 168
  interventions for, 168
Acetaminophen, 112, 243–244, 243*b*
Acquired immunodeficiency syndrome (AIDS), 379–381, 380*f*
Actinic keratosis, 187–188, 188*f*
Activities of daily living (ADLs)
  assessment of, 103, 103*b*
  living with chronic illness and, 229*b*
  providing care for, 351–352, 351*f*
Activity
  in FANCAPES, 98, 98*f*
  respiratory disorders and, 294
Activity theory of aging, 41
Acupressure, 245
Acupuncture, 245
Acute care settings
  documentation of, 106
  generalist gerontological nurses' roles, 61–62
Acute dystonia, 123
Acute grief, 400
Acute illness, 229, 229*b*
Acute myocardial infarction, 288
Acute pain, 237–238
Acute rehabilitation care setting, documentation of, 106
Adjuvant drugs, 244–245
ADLs. *see* Activities of daily living (ADLs)
Administration, in safe medication use, 125–126, 126*b*
ADRs. *see* Adverse drug reactions (ADRs)

Figure numbers followed by *b*, *f*, and *t* indicate boxes, figures, and tables, respectively.

ADS. *see* Adult day services (ADS)
Adult children, elders and, 367–368
Adult day services (ADS), 67
Adults
  information technology and, 52
  later life, 51–52, 51*b*
  learning opportunities, 51–52
Advance directives, 410–412, 411*b*
Advanced practice nurses, 60
  working in LTC settings, 61*b*
Advanced practice registered nurses (APRNs), 60
Adverse drug reactions (ADRs), 118–119, 119*b*
Aeration, in FANCAPES, 98
Affordable Care Act, 312
  components of, 83*t*
African-American
  diabetes in, 269
  glaucoma and, 251–253
  health disparity and, 13*b*
  osteoporosis and, 277
Age, sexuality and, 373, 374*t*, 375–376
Age associated memory impairment (AAMI), 50
Ageism, 14, 15*b*
Agency for Healthcare Research and Quality (AHRQ), 196
Age-related macular degeneration, 252*f*, 254–255, 255*f*
Age-related physical changes, 22–39
Age-stratification theory of aging, 42
Aging
  activity and, 178–179, 179*b*
  biological theories of, 22–26
  brain and, 49*b*
  cardiovascular changes with, 29–30, 29*t*
  cellular functioning and, 23
  chronological, 3–6
  cognition and, 48–50, 49*b*
  contemporary theories of, building blocks of, 23*b*
  cross-cultural caring and, 11–21
    culture, 12
    diversity, 12–13
    health disparities and inequities, 13
    implications for gerontological nursing and, 17–20
    integrating concepts of, 20, 20*b*
Aging *(Continued)*
  cross-link theory, 23*b*
  definition of, 1
  DNA and, 25–26
  endocrine system changes with, 31–32
  free radical theory of, 24–25, 25*b*
  gastrointestinal system changes with, 32–34, 33*t*
  global, 3
  health and wellness, 7
  healthy, 1–10, 55
  immune system changes with, 37–38, 37*t*
  immunological theory of, 25
  implications for gerontological nursing and, 8
  life expectancy at birth, 4*f*
  moving toward healthy, 6–8
  musculoskeletal changes with, 28–29, 28*t*
  neurological changes with, 34–35, 34*t*
  pharmacokinetics and, 111, 111*f*
  phenotype, 4*b*
  physical changes that accompany, 26–38
  psychosocial theories of, 41–45
  recognize as "old", 3
  renal system changes with, 31
  reproductive system changes with, 32
  research on, 59–60
  respiratory changes with, 30–31, 30*f*, 31*b*
  sensory changes with, 35–37, 35*t*, 36*b*
  sleep and, 171–172, 172*b*
    changes in, 171*b*
  society, 56
  spirituality and, 46–47, 46*f*
  telomeres and, 25–26, 25*b*
  wear-and-tear theory, 23*b*
  years ahead, 2–3, 2*f*–3*f*
AHRQ. *see* Agency for Healthcare Research and Quality (AHRQ)
AIDS. *see* Acquired immunodeficiency syndrome (AIDS)
Akathisia, 123
Alarms, in fall risk reduction, 211
Alaskan Natives, diabetes in, 268, 268*t*

Albuterol, 116*t*–117*t*
in herb-medication and herb-disease interactions, 116*t*–117*t*
Alcohol
medications interacting with, 329*b*
withdrawal, acute, 331–332
Alcohol use disorder, 328–329
assessment of, 329–330, 330*t*, 331*b*
consequences of, 329
gender issues in, 328–329
interventions for, 330–332
physiology of, 329
prevalence and characteristics of, 328
ALFs. *see* Assisted living facilities (ALFs)
Allergic rhinitis, rhythmical influences on, 114*t*
Alprazolam, in herb-medication and herb-disease interactions, 116*t*–117*t*
Alzheimer's Association, 68–69
Alzheimer's disease, 303–304, 303*b*
depression and, 323
insomnia and, 172
American Association of Colleges of Nursing (AACN), 58
American Indian, diabetes in, 268, 268*t*
American Medical Association, 82
American Society on Aging (ASA), 58–59
Amiodarone, for hyperthyroidism, 266, 266*b*
Amlodipine, in herb-medication and herb-disease interactions, 116*t*–117*t*
Amsler grid, 255, 255*f*
Analgesics
aging and, 113*t*
nonopioid, 243–244
opioid, 244
Anomia, 305
Anomic aphasia, 306
Anthropomorphic measurements, 140
Antianxiety agents, 121–122
Antibiotics, aging and, 113*t*
Anticipatory grief, 400
Anticoagulant, in herb-medication and herb-disease interactions, 116*t*–117*t*
Antidepressants, 121
for bipolar disorder, 321
in herb-medication and herb-disease interactions, 116*t*–117*t*
Antidiabetic drugs, in herb-medication and herb-disease interactions, 116*t*–117*t*
Antihypertensives, in herb-medication and herb-disease interactions, 116*t*–117*t*
Antimetabolites, in herb-medication and herb-disease interactions, 116*t*–117*t*
Antiplatelet drug, in herb-medication and herb-disease interactions, 116*t*–117*t*
Antipsychotics, 122–124
for delirium, 342
Antiseizure drugs, in herb-medication and herb-disease interactions, 116*t*–117*t*
Anti-vascular endothelial growth factor (anti-VEGF) therapy, 255
Anxiety disorders, 313
assessment of, 313–314, 314*b*
interventions for, 314–315
nonpharmacological approaches for, 315, 315*b*
pharmacological approaches for, 314–315
prevalence and characteristics of, 313
Aphasia, 305–306
Apnea, sleep, 176
assessment for, 176
interventions for, 176–178
APRNs. *see* Advanced practice registered nurses (APRNs)
Aromatherapy, for sleep disorders, 174
Arterial blood pressure, rhythmical influences on, 114*t*
Arthritides, 279–282, 279*t*
assessment of, 282–284, 283*f*
giant cell arteritis, 280–281
gout, 281–282, 282*b*
interventions for, 282–284, 283*t*
intimacy and, 376*t*–378*t*
osteoarthritis, 277*f*, 279–280, 279*t*, 280*f*
polymyalgia rheumatica, 280–281
by race/ethnicity, prevalence of, 279, 280*t*
rheumatoid, 281, 281*b*
rhythmical influences on, 114*t*
Arthritis. *see* Arthritides
ASA. *see* American Society on Aging (ASA)
Asian Americans, diabetes among, 268, 268*t*
Aspiration, prevention of, in patients with dysphagia, 137, 137*b*
Aspirin, 243*b*
in herb-medication and herb-disease interactions, 116*t*–117*t*
Assessment
for accidental bowel leakage/fecal incontinence, 168
activities of daily living in, 103, 103*b*
of activity, 98, 98*f*, 179
of aeration, 98
arthritides, 282–284, 283*f*
for bowel incontinence, 165
of cardiovascular disease, 290
caregiver, 390–391, 391*b*
cognitive measures in, 99–100
of communication, 98
comprehensive geriatric, 103–105
data, collecting, 93
of dehydration, 146–147
diabetes mellitus, 270–271
of elimination, 99
FANCAPES in, 96
of fluids, 96–98
of frail and medically complex elder, 96–99
functional, 102–103
grief, 362–363, 402
health history in, 94–96, 95*b*
instrumental activities of daily living in, 103, 103*b*
of mental status, 99–102, 99*b*
mood measures in, 100–102
nutritional, 98, 135–136
of oral health, 150
of pain, 99
physical, 96–99, 97*t*
process, 93–94, 93*b*
of respiratory disorders, 292–293, 293*b*
in safe medication use, 124, 125*b*
of sexuality, 381–382, 382*b*
for sleep disordered breathing and sleep apnea, 176
for sleep disorders, 173, 173*b*
of socialization and social skills, 99, 99*b*
spirituality, 47–48, 47*b*
for urinary incontinence, 156–157, 160*f*
resources for, 159*b*
tips for best practice in, 158*b*
Assisted living facilities (ALFs), 68–69, 68*b*–69*b*
Assistive devices
in fall risk reduction, 210–211
low-vision, 257–258
personal listening, 260
Association for Gerontology in Higher Education, 58–59
Asthma, rhythmical influences on, 114*t*

Ataque de nervios (attack of nerves), 311*b*
Atrial fibrillation, 288–289
Attitudes, mental health care and, 310–311
Avastin, for age-related macular degeneration, 255
Awareness
  closed, 406
  cultural, 15, 15*b*
  open, 406–407
  suspected, 406

B
"Baby Boomers", 6
Balance exams, 8*t*
Barthel Index (BI), 103
Basal cell carcinoma, 190, 190*f*
Bathing, dementia and, 351–352, 352*b*, 352*f*
"Beers criteria", 120, 120*b*
Behavioral interventions, for urinary incontinence, 157–161, 159*b*
Beliefs, mental health care and, 310–311
Benign prostatic hyperplasia (BPH), 32
Benzodiazepine receptor agonists, 176
Benzodiazepines, 113, 122, 127*t*
  for anxiety, 314
Bereavement overload, 398
Bergstrom, Nancy, 197
Beta blockers, in herb-medication and herb-disease interactions, 116*t*–117*t*
BI. *see* Barthel Index (BI)
Bill of rights, for residents, 73, 73*b*
Biochemical analysis, for nutrition, 140–141
Biofeedback, 168
  for pain, 245
"Biological clock" theory, 23*b*
Biomedical model, 17
Biorhythm, and sleep, 171
Bipolar disorder, 320, 321*b*
Birth, life expectancy at, 4*f*
Bisphosphonates, 279
Bladder
  diary, 160*f*
  function of, 154–155
  healthy, promotion of, 155*b*
  overactive, 161
  training, 159
Blindness, cultural, 14
Blood glucose, self-monitoring, 272–273, 272*b*
Blood plasma volume, rhythmical influences on, 114*t*
Blood pressure
  home measurement of, 287*b*
  reducing, evidence-based practice on benefits of, 287*b*
Blood urea nitrogen (BUN), 147
Blood vessels, 30
BMI. *see* Body mass index (BMI)
Body composition, 28–29
Body mass index (BMI), 133, 140
Body water distribution, changes in, 29*f*
Bone, and joint problems, 276–285
Bowel elimination, 163–165
Bowel function, 154–155
BPH. *see* Benign prostatic hyperplasia (BPH)
Braden, Barbara, 197
Braden Scale, 197
Brain, 34
  aging and, 49*b*, 50
Breast cancer
  intimacy and, 376*t*–378*t*
  screening, 8*t*
Breathing, sleep disordered, 176
  assessment for, 176
  interventions for, 176–178
Bulk laxatives, 166–167
Bulk-forming agents, 166–167
BUN. *see* Blood urea nitrogen (BUN)
BuSpar, 122
Buspirone, 122

C
Calcitonin, 279
Calcium, 133
  sources of, 278, 278*b*
Caloric restriction theory, 23*b*
Canadian Gerontological Nursing Association (CGNA), 59
Cancer
  breast, 376*t*–378*t*
  intimacy and, 376*t*–378*t*
  rhythmical influences on, 114*t*
Candidiasis *(Candida albicans)*, 189–190
Capacity, 88
Cardiac disease, rhythmical influences on, 114*t*
Cardiovascular disease (CVD), 286–289, 290*b*
  atrial fibrillation, 288–289
  heart disease, 288
  heart failure, 289
  hypertension, 287–288, 288*b*
  intimacy and, 376*t*–378*t*
  promoting healthy aging in persons with, 291*b*
Cardiovascular system, aging-related changes with, 29–30, 29*t*
Care
  for dying patients, 406
  gerontological nursing across the continuum of, 66–78
  managers, 62
  palliative, 397–413
    dying, death and, 404–405
  quality of, in skilled nursing facilities, 71–72, 72*b*, 73*f*
  transitional
    improving, 75–76, 76*b*–77*b*
    outcomes, factors contributing to poor, 75, 75*b*
Caregiving, 386–396
  assessment of, 390–391, 391*b*
  description of, 386–390, 387*b*
  of developmentally disabled children, 389
  elder mistreatment and, 392–394, 392*b*, 394*b*
    definition of, 392
    prevention of, 395, 395*b*
  of grandparents raising grandchildren, 389–390, 390*b*
  impact of, 387–388
  for individuals with dementia, 388–389, 391–392
  interventions for, 391–392
  long-distance, 390
  needs of, 387*b*, 388
  neglect in, 393, 394*b*
  spousal, 388
  stress and, 387–388, 388*b*
Case and care management roles, generalist gerontological nurses' roles, 62, 62*b*
Cataracts, 250–251, 252*f*
Catecholamines, rhythmical influences on, 114*t*
Catheter-associated urinary tract infections (CAUTIs), 163, 163*b*
Catheterization, intermittent, 162
CAUTIs. *see* Catheter-associated urinary tract infections (CAUTIs)
CCRCs. *see* Continuing care retirement communities (CCRCs)
CDC. *see* Centers for Disease Control and Prevention (CDC)
Centenarians, 5, 6*f*
Centers for Disease Control and Prevention (CDC), 201
Centers for Medicare and Medicaid Services (CMS), 69, 82, 193, 201–202
  on feeding assistants, 141
Central nervous system (CNS), 34

Cerebrovascular diseases, 298–300, 298*f*
  hemorrhagic events, 299–300
  ischemic events, 298–299
Certification in gerontological nursing, 60
Certified nursing facilities, generalist gerontological nurses' roles, 62–63
Cerumen, 259, 259*f*
Cervical cancer screening, 8*t*
Cessation, driving, 222–223
CGNA. *see* Canadian Gerontological Nursing Association (CGNA)
CGNO. *see* Coalition of Geriatric Nursing Organizations (CGNO)
CHF. *see* Congestive heart failure (CHF)
Chromosomes, with telomere caps, 25*f*
Chronic care, 70
Chronic diseases, nutrition and, 135, 135*f*
Chronic illness
  intimacy and, 376, 376*f*, 376*t*–378*t*
  living with, 228–235, 229*b*–230*b*, 230*f*
    acute illness and, 229, 229*b*
    challenges, for person with, 234*b*
    chronic illness trajectory and, 231–232, 232*b*, 232*t*
    elder with, assessment of, 233
    implications for gerontological nursing and healthy aging and, 233–234
    interventions in, 233–234
    management models, characteristics of, 234*b*
    nursing roles, in caring for persons with, 234*b*
    prevention of, 231, 231*b*
    Shifting Perspectives Model, 232–233
    theoretical frameworks for, 231–233
Chronic illness trajectory, 231–232, 232*b*, 232*t*
Chronic obstructive pulmonary disease (COPD), 291–292, 294*b*–295*b*, 376*t*–378*t*
Chronic pain, 237–238
Chronological aging, 3–6
Chronopharmacology, 114–115, 114*t*
Cimetidine, 127*t*
Circadian rhythm, 171
  sleep disorders, 178
Clinical Institute Withdrawal Assessment (CIWA) scale, 332
Clock Drawing Test, 99–100, 100*b*, 101*f*
Clonazepam, 177–178
Closed awareness, 406
Closure, death and, 407*b*
CMS. *see* Centers for Medicare and Medicaid Services (CMS)
CNS. *see* Central nervous system (CNS)
Coalition of Geriatric Nursing Organizations (CGNO), 59
Cochlear implants, 260, 260*f*
Cockcroft-Gault equation, 113–114
Cognition
  definition of, 48
  promotion of cognitive health, 50–51, 51*b*
Cognitive behavioral therapy, for insomnia, 173
Cognitive health, 50
  practice for, 51*b*
Cognitive impairment, 44
  in fall risk reduction, 207
  pain and, 238–239, 239*b*, 241*b*
Cognitive measures, for mental status, 99–100
Cognitive reserve, 49
Cognitive-behavioral therapy (CBT)
  for anxiety, 314
  for posttraumatic stress disorder, 317
Cohort, 5, 372–373
Cold discomfort, preventing, 220*b*
Colorectal screening, 8*t*
Colposuspension, 162
Comfort, Alex, 49*f*
Comfort, pain and, 236–248
Communication
  dying and, 406–407
  dysarthria and, 306*b*
  in FANCAPES, 98
  hearing impairment and, 262*b*
  for neurocognitive disorders, 344–345, 344*b*, 346*b*
  neurological disorders and, 306–307
  pain and, 238–239, 239*b*
  visual impairment and, 257*b*
Community- and home-based setting, generalist gerontological nurses' roles, 62
Community care, 67–69
  adult day services, 67
  assisted living facilities, 68–69, 68*b*–69*b*
  continuing care retirement communities, 67–68
Community care *(Continued)*
  Program of All-Inclusive Care for the Elderly, 67
  residential care/assisted living, 67*t*, 68–69
Community-acquired disease (CAD), pneumonia, 292
Complementary and alternative interventions, 284
Complicated grief, 400–401
Composure, 406
Comprehensive fall assessment, 207
Comprehensive geriatric assessments, 103–105
Condom catheters, 163
Conductive hearing loss, 259
Congestive heart failure (CHF), 289
Conservators, 89–90
Constipation, 164–165
  assessment for, 165, 165*b*
  criteria for, 164*b*
  fecal impaction and, 164–165
  implications of, for gerontological nursing and healthy aging, 165–167
  interventions for, 165–167
    alternative treatments as, 167
    bowel training program for, 166*b*
    enema for, 167, 167*b*
    nonpharmacological treatment as, 165–166
    pharmacological treatment for, 166–167
    physical activity as, 165–166
    positioning as, 166
    toileting regimen as, 166
Continuing care retirement communities (CCRCs), 67–68
Continuity, death and, 407
Continuity theory of aging, 42
Continuous positive airway pressure (CPAP), for sleep apnea, 176–177
Control, dying and, 406
COPD. *see* Chronic obstructive pulmonary disease (COPD)
Cornea, 35
Cornell Scale for Depression in Dementia (CSD-D), 324–325
Coronary artery disease (CAD). *see* Heart disease
Coronary heart disease (CHD). *see* Heart disease
Costs, of long-term care, 67*t*, 71
Coumadin, 118
Countercoping, 403–404
Couples
  nontraditional, 367
  traditional, 366–367

Crepitus, definition of, 280
Cross-cultural caring
  aging and, 11–21
    culture, 12
    diversity, 12–13
    health disparities and inequities, 13
    implications for gerontological nursing and, 17–20
    integrating concepts of, 20, 20*b*
  model for, 14*f*
Cross-link theory, 23*b*
Cryopexy, 255
Crystallized intelligence, 50
CSD-D. *see* Cornell Scale for Depression in Dementia (CSD-D)
Cultural awareness, 15, 15*b*
Cultural blindness, 14
Cultural competence, 15
Cultural destructiveness, 13–14
Cultural diversity, 12
Cultural influences, sexuality and, 372–373
Cultural knowledge, 15–17
Cultural precompetence, 14–15
Cultural proficiency, 15
Culturally sensitive assessment, explanatory model for, 19*b*
Culture, 12
  on expressions of pain, 237*b*
  mental health and, 311–312, 311*b*
Culture change movement, 74, 74*b*–75*b*
Cutaneous stimulation, 245
CVD. *see* Cardiovascular disease (CVD)
Cyclooxygenase-2 (COX-2) inhibitors, 243–244
Cytochrome P450 (CYP450), 113, 113*b*

D

DASH. *see* Dietary Approaches to Stop Hypertension (DASH)
Data, collecting assessment, 93
Death, 397–413
  advance directives prior to, 410–411, 411*b*
  care for persons facing, and dying, 406
  closure and, 407, 407*b*
  communication and, 406–407
  composure and, 406
  continuity and, 407
  control and, 406
  decision-making about, 410–412
  and dignity, 411
  dying, and palliative care, 404–405
Death *(Continued)*
  euthanasia and, 411–412, 411*b*–412*b*
  hospice and, 409–410
  nurse and, dying and, 407–410, 408*t*, 409*b*
  palliative care for, 409
  of spouse/life partner, 362, 362*b*
Debridement methods, 198
Decision-making at end of life, 410–412, 411*b*–412*b*
Deep tissue pressure injury (DTPI), 193, 193*f*
Dehydration, 145–146
  assessment of, 146–147
  interventions for, 147
  risk factors for, 146, 146*b*
  signs and symptoms of, 146–147
  simple screen for, 146*b*
Delirium, 336–340
  assessment of, 340–341, 340*b*
  causes of, 339*b*
  clinical subtypes of, 339, 339*b*
  cognitive assessment of, 340
  consequences of, 339–340, 340*b*
  dementia, depression and, 337, 338*t*
  diagnosis of, 337*b*
  etiology of, 337
  incidence and prevalence of, 337
  recognition of, 338
  risk factors for, 338–339, 339*b*
  superimposed on mild and major neurocognitive disorders, 337–338
Delirium tremens, 332
Delusions, 319, 319*b*
Dementia, 337–338, 340*b*
  assessment of, 348–349, 348*b*, 349*t*
  bathing and, 351–352, 352*b*, 352*f*
  caregiving of individuals with, 388–389, 391–392
  delirium, depression and, 337, 338*t*
  driving and, 222
  interventions for, 341–342, 349–351
  intimacy, sexuality and, 379
  nonpharmacological approaches for, 341–342, 341*b*–342*b*, 350–351, 350*f*, 351*b*
  nursing roles for, 354–355, 356*f*
  nutrition and, 136–138, 137*b*, 353–354, 354*f*, 355*b*
  pharmacological approaches for, 342, 343*b*, 343*f*, 349–350, 349*b*–350*b*
  wandering and, 353, 353*b*–354*b*
Dentures, care of, 150–152, 151*b*
Depression, 321–323
  assessment of, 323–325, 324*b*, 324*f*
  collaborative care for, 325
Depression *(Continued)*
  consequences of, 322
  etiology of, 322–323, 323*b*
  family and professional support for, 327*b*
  interventions for, 325–326
  medications and, 323*b*
  nonpharmacological approaches for, 325, 325*f*
  pharmacological approaches for, 325–326
  prevalence of, 321–322
  racial, ethnic and cultural considerations for, 322
  risk factors for, 323*b*
  treatment of, 326
Dermis, 27
Destructiveness, cultural, 13–14
Detached retina, 255
Developmental theory of aging, 42
Developmentally disabled children, 389
Dextranomer, 168
Diabetes mellitus (DM), 267–270
  aging process and, 272*b*
  assessment of, 270–271
  cardiovascular risk in persons with, 270, 270*b*
  complications of, 269–270, 269*b*
  distribution of age, at diagnosis of, 269*f*
  evidence-based practice and, 270, 271*b*
  exercise and, 273
  Healthy People 2020 and, 270, 271*b*
  intimacy and, 376*t*–378*t*
  long-term care and, 274
  management of, 271–273
  medications and, 273–274
  nutrition and, 273
  prevalence of, 267–268
  by race/ethnicity, 268, 268*t*
  risk factors for, 267, 268*b*
  self-management (DSM), 272–273, 272*b*
  signs and symptoms of, 268–269, 269*b*
Diabetes screening, 8*t*
Diabetes self-management (DSM), 272–273, 272*b*
  training, 8*t*
Diabetic macular edema (DME), 254
Diabetic retinopathy, 252*f*, 253–254
Diazepam, 113
Dietary Approaches to Stop Hypertension (DASH), 131
Dietary education, respiratory disorders and, 294

Digestive system, 32
Digoxin, 127*t*
in herb-medication and herb-disease interactions, 116*t*–117*t*
Diphenhydramine, 175
Disease-modifying antirheumatic drugs (DMARDs), 281
Disenfranchised grief, 401
Disengagement theory of aging, 41–42
Disparity, health, 13
examples of, 13*b*
Distraction, in pain management, 245
Distribution, in pharmacokinetics, 112
Diuretics, aging and, 113*t*
Diversity, 12–13, 12*f*
Divorce, 366–367
DM. *see* Diabetes mellitus (DM)
DMARDs. *see* Disease-modifying antirheumatic drugs (DMARDs)
DME. *see* Diabetic macular edema (DME)
Domestic medicine, 16–17
Driving, 218*b*, 221–223
cessation, 222–223
dementia and, 222
safety, 221–222, 222*b*–224*b*
skills, 223*b*
Drug-drug interactions, 118, 118*b*
Dry eye, 256
DSM. *see* Diabetes self-management (DSM)
DTPI. *see* Deep tissue pressure injury (DTPI)
Dual-energy x-ray absorptiometry (DEXA), for osteoporosis, 277
Dysarthria, 306, 306*b*
Dysfunction, sexual, 373–375
Dysphagia, 135, 136*b*
risk factors for, 136*b*
symptoms for, 136*b*
Dyspnea, 289
Dysthymia, 322

E
Early-onset schizophrenia, 318
Ears, aging-related changes to, 36–37, 36*f*
EASY. *see* Exercise and Screening for You (EASY)
Eating habits, lifelong, 135
Economic issues, 79–91
Medicaid, 86–87
Medicare, 82–86, 82*b*, 83*t*
Social Security and, 80–81, 80*t*
Supplemental Security Income and, 81
Veterans Health Administration (VA), 87
Ectropion, 35
ED. *see* Erectile dysfunction (ED)
Eden Alternative, 74
Education
gerontological nursing, 58
respiratory disorders and, 294
in safe medication use, 124–125, 125*b*
Elder mistreatment, 392–394, 392*b*, 394*b*
definition of, 392
neglect and, 393–394
prevention of, 395, 395*b*
self-neglect and, 393–394
Elder-friendly communities, 225, 226*f*
Electroconvulsive therapy (ECT), for depression, 326
Elimination, 154–169
in FANCAPES, 99
implications of, for gerontological and healthy aging, 156–163
Endocrine system, 31–32
Endogenous nocturnal melatonin, 175
Enemas, 167, 167*b*
Enteral feeding, 137–138
Entropion, 35
Environmental assessment, in postfall assessment suggestions, 209
Environmental modifications, in fall risk reduction, 210
Environmental temperatures, 217–220
hyperthermia and, 218–219, 219*b*
hypothermia and, 219–220, 220*b*
thermoregulation and, 218, 218*b*
Epidermis, 26–27
EPUAP. *see* European Pressure Ulcer Advisory Panel (EPUAP)
Epworth Sleepiness Scale, 173, 176
Erectile dysfunction (ED), 373
Esophagus, 33
Essentials of Baccalaureate Education for Professional Nursing Practice (AACN), 58
Established incontinence, 156
Estrogen, in herb-medication and herb-disease interactions, 116*t*–117*t*
Eszopiclone, 176
Ethnocentrism, 15*b*
European Pressure Ulcer Advisory Panel (EPUAP), 192
Euthanasia, death and, 411–412, 411*b*–412*b*
Evidence-based practice
blood pressure and, 287*b*
Parkinson's disease and, 304*b*
pneumonia and, 292*b*
screening for hypertension, 288*b*
Evista, 279
Excretion, in pharmacokinetics, 113–114
Exercise
guidelines for, 180*b*
tolerance, respiratory disorders and, 294
Exercise and Screening for You (EASY), 179
Exposure therapy, for posttraumatic stress disorder, 317
External urinary catheters, 163
Extraocular changes, aging-related, 35
Extrapyramidal reactions, 123–124
Extrapyramidal symptoms, in schizophrenia, 318
Extrinsic risk factors, in fall, 204
Eye contact, in LEARN model, 18
Eyelids, 35
Eyes
aging-related, 35–36
diseases and disorders of, 250–256

F
Fainting, 289
Fall risk reduction, 201–216
falls, 201–206, 202*b*
consequences of, 202–204
interventions of, 209–211, 210*b*
postfall assessment, 208–209, 209*b*
prevention, 202*b*
restraint alternatives, 203*b*
risk assessment instruments, 207–208
risk factors, 204–206
screening and assessment of, 207
programs, 209–210
Fallophobia, in fall risk reduction, 203–204, 204*b*
Falls, 201–206, 202*b*
consequences of, 202–204
fallophobia, 203–204, 204*b*
hip fractures, 202–204
traumatic brain injury, 202–203
multifactorial nature of, 204*f*
postfall assessment, 208–209, 209*b*
prevention, 202*b*
restraint alternatives, 203*b*
risk assessment instruments, 207–208
risk factors, 204–206
foot deformities, 205–206
gait disturbances, 204–205
screening and assessment of, 207

Families, 364–369
- death and, 404–405
- elders and adult children in, 367–368
- fictive kin in, 369
- grandparents in, 368–369, 368*f*–369*f*, 369*b*
- multigenerational, 364–365, 365*b*
- nontraditional couples in, 367
- orientation to, 16
- relationships, 365–366, 366*f*
- siblings in, 369
- traditional couples in, 366–367
- types of, 366–369

FANCAPES, 96
Fats, 131–132
Fecal impaction, 164–165
Fecal incontinence, 167
- assessment for, 168
- implications of, for gerontological nursing and healthy aging, 168
- interventions for, 168

Feeding tubes, 136–138
Female reproductive system, age-changes with, 32
Fiber, 132
Fibrate drugs, in herb-medication and herb-disease interactions, 116*t*–117*t*
Fibrinolytic activity, rhythmical influences on, 114*t*
Fictive kin, 369
FIM. *see* Functional Independence Measure (FIM)
First generation psychosocial theories, of aging, 41
Fleming, Alexander, 5–6
Flower model, 7*f*
Fluent (Wernicke's) aphasia, 305
Fluid intelligence, 50
Fluids
- in FANCAPES, 96–98
- hydration management and, 145

Folk healing, 16–17
Folk medicine, 16–17
Food/nutrient intake, 139–140
Foot assessment, in fall risk reduction, 206*b*
Foot deformities, in fall risk reduction, 205–206
Frail and medically complex elder, comprehensive physical assessment of, 96–99
Frailty, assessing, 230*b*
Free radical theory, of aging, 24–25, 25*b*
Friendships, 363–364, 364*f*
Full-thickness skin
- loss, 194, 194*f*
- and tissue loss, 194, 194*f*

Fulmer, Terry, 57*b*
Fulmer SPICES, 104
Functional assessment, in postfall assessment suggestions, 209
Functional disruption, 398, 402*b*–403*b*, 403
Functional incontinence, 157*t*
Functional Independence Measure (FIM), 103
Furosemide, 127*t*

G

Gait disturbances, in fall risk reduction, 204–205
Garlic, in herb-medication and herb-disease interactions, 116*t*–117*t*
Gastric system, rhythmical influences on, 114*t*
Gastroesophageal reflux disease (GERD), 33
Gastrointestinal system, aging-related changes to, 32–34
GCA. *see* Giant cell arteritis (GCA)
GCNS. *see* Gerontological clinical nurse specialist (GCNS)
GDS. *see* Geriatric Depression Scale (GDS)
Generalist roles in gerontological nursing, 61–63
Geragogy, 51
GERD. *see* Gastroesophageal reflux disease (GERD)
Geriatric anxiety, 313
Geriatric Depression Scale (GDS), 102, 102*t*, 324–325
Geriatric nursing, 56
Geriatric Nursing Leadership Academy, 57–58
"Geriatric syndromes", 230*b*
Geriatricians, shortage of, 56
Gerontological clinical nurse specialist (GCNS), 60–61
Gerontological nurse practitioners (GNPs), 60–61
Gerontological nurses, 186
Gerontological nursing, 56, 60*f*
- across the continuum of care, 66–78
- in acute care settings, 61–62
- care for older adults, 55–56
- in case and care management roles, 62, 62*b*
- certification and, 60
- in certified nursing facilities, 62–63

Gerontological nursing *(Continued)*
- in community- and home-based setting, 62
- current initiatives in, 57–58
- current leaders in the field of, 56–57, 57*b*
- education, 58
- gerontological clinical nurse specialist (GCNS), 60–61
- gerontological nurse practitioners (GNPs), 60–61
- gerontology organizations and, 58–59
- healthy aging and, 55–65
  - implications for, 73–74, 76–77, 90, 90*b*
- history of, 56–58
- legal issues in, 88–90
  - advance care planning, 88–90
  - decision-making in, 88
- pioneers, 56–57, 57*b*
- reflections on, 57*b*
- research, 59–60
- roles, 60–63

Gerontological Nursing: Scope and Standards of Practice (ANA), 57
Gerontological Society of America, 58
Gerontology organizations, 58–59
Geropsychiatric nursing, 311
Gerotranscendence theory of aging, 43
Giacquinta, Barbara, 398
Giant cell arteritis (GCA), 280–281
Ginkgo, in herb-medication and herb-disease interactions, 116*t*–117*t*
Ginseng, in herb-medication and herb-disease interactions, 116*t*–117*t*
Glaucoma, 251–253, 252*f*, 253*b*
Global aphasia, 305–306
Global Deterioration Scale, 100, 101*t*
Global flu pandemics, 5*t*
Glomerular filtration rate (GFR), 31
Glucose self-monitoring, 272
GNPs. *see* Gerontological nurse practitioners (GNPs)
Gout, 281–282, 282*b*
Grandparents, 368–369, 368*f*–369*f*, 369*b*, 389–390, 390*b*
Graves' disease, 266
Green tea, in herb-medication and herb-disease interactions, 116*t*–117*t*
Grief, 398–401. *see also* Loss
- acute, 400
- anticipatory, 400
- assessment, 362–363, 402
- complicated, 400–401

Grief *(Continued)*
coping with loss, factors affecting, 401, 401*b*
countercoping, 403–404
definition of, 412
disenfranchised, 401
interventions, 363, 363*b*, 402–404, 403*b*
shadow, 400, 400*b*
for a spouse/life partner, 362, 362*b*
types of, 399–401
Grieving, definition of, 398
Guardians, 89–90

H

HACs. *see* Health care-acquired conditions (HACs)
Hair, 27–28
Hallucinations, 319, 319*b*
Hand weights, 180
Hartford Institute for Geriatric Nursing, 57
Hawthorn, in herb-medication and herb-disease interactions, 116*t*–117*t*
HDL. *see* High-density lipoprotein (HDL)
Health
sexual, 370*b*, 371–373
sleep as barometer of, 171
Health aging, moving toward cultural proficiency and, 14*b*
Health beliefs, 16–17
comparison of, 17*t*
Health care insurance plans, in later life, 81–88. *see also* Insurance plans, health care; Medicaid; Medicare
long-term care insurance, 87–88
TRICARE for Life, 87
Health care proxy, 89, 89*b*
Health care-acquired conditions (HACs), 193
Health disparity, 13
examples of, 13*b*
Health inequities, 13
Health information, technology and, 52
Health maintenance organizations (HMOs), 85, 410–411
Healthy aging, moving toward, 6–8
Healthy People 2020, 250*b*
activity and, 179*b*
COPD goals and, 295*b*
diabetes and, 270, 271*b*
goals
for geriatric health care, 56
to reduce potentially preventable infections, 37*b*
Healthy People 2020 (Continued)
heart failure goals of, 290*b*
nutrition goals of, 131, 131*b*
Office of Disease Prevention and Health Promotion [ODPHP], 2015, 231
of older adults, 8*b*
on oral health, 149*b*
sleep health in, 171*b*
stroke and, 300*b*
Healthy People 2000 (CDC, 2009), 231
Hearing
diseases affecting, 249–264
in fall risk reduction, 207
Hearing aids, 259–260, 260*b*
Hearing exams, 8*t*
Hearing impairment, 258–259, 258*b*
aging-related, 36–37
assessment of, 261–262, 261*b*
assistive listening and adaptive devices for, 260–261
cochlear implants for, 260, 260*f*
communication and, 262*b*
consequences of, 258
hearing aids for, 259–260, 260*b*
interventions of, 262, 262*b*
tinnitus, 262–263
types of, 258–259, 259*f*
Heart, 29–30
Heart disease, 288
older adult with, exacerbation of illness in, 288*b*
risk factors for, 287*b*
Heart failure, 289, 290*b*
HELP. *see* Hospital Elder Life Program (HELP)
Hemoglobin A_{1c} test, 267, 268*t*
Hendrich II fall risk model, 205, 205*f*
Herb-medication and herb-disease interactions, 116, 116*t*–117*t*
Herpes zoster, 188–189
High-density lipoprotein (HDL), 131–132
Hip fractures, in fall risk reduction, 202
Hip protectors, in fall risk reduction, 211
Hispanics, diabetes among, 268, 268*t*
History
health, in optimal care, 94–96, 95*b*
in postfall assessment suggestions, 209
HIV. *see* Human immunodeficiency virus (HIV)
HMOs. *see* Health maintenance organizations (HMOs)
Home care, documentation of, 106
Home safety, 217, 218*b*
Hospice, 409–410
Hospital Elder Life Program (HELP), 342
Hospital-acquired condition (HAC), pneumonia, 292
Hospitals
oral hygiene in, 152
sleep in, 174–175, 175*b*
Human immunodeficiency virus (HIV), 379–381, 380*b*, 380*f*
screening, 8*t*
Hydration
management of, 145
and oral care, 145–153, 148*b*
Hyperactive delirium, 339*b*
Hyperemia, 196–197
Hypertension, 287–288, 288*b*
nutrition and, 130
Hyperthermia, 218–219, 219*b*
Hyperthyroidism, 266
Hypoactive delirium, 339*b*
Hypodermis, 27
Hypodermoclysis, 147
Hypoglycemia, 270
Hypothermia, 219–220, 220*b*
Hypothyroidism, 266, 266*b*

I

IADLs. *see* Instrumental activities of daily living (IADLs)
IES-R. *see* Impact of Event Scale-Revised (IES-R)
IHS. *see* Indian Health Service (IHS)
Imagery, in pain management, 245–246
Immune system
aging-related changes in, 37–38, 37*t*
Healthy People 2020 goals related to, 37*b*
Immunosuppressants, in herb-medication and herb-disease interactions, 116*t*–117*t*
Impact of Event Scale-Revised (IES-R), 317, 317*b*
Impaction, fecal, 164–165
Improve health outcomes, moving toward cultural proficiency to, 13
Indian Health Service (IHS), 87
Influenza immunizations, promoting, 8*t*
Information technology, adults and, 52
Informed consent, 88, 88*b*
Insomnia, 172, 172*b*
Alzheimer's disease and, 172
interventions for, 174*b*
Institution-centered culture, 74

Instrumental activities of daily living (IADLs)
assessment of, 103, 103*b*
driving as, 221
living with chronic illness and, 229*b*
Insulin, 267
in herb-medication and herb-disease interactions, 116*t*–117*t*
Insurance plans, health care, 81–88. *see also* Medicaid; Medicare
long-term care insurance, 87–88
TRICARE for Life, 87
Integument, 27
Intelligence, in older people, 50
Interactions, drug, 115–118
Intermittent catheterization, 162
International Institute for Reminiscence and Life Review, 43
Internet, adults and, 52
Interventions
for accidental bowel leakage/fecal incontinence, 168
for activity, 179–182
for arthritides, 282–284, 283*t*
for bowel elimination, 165–167
for cardiovascular disease, 290–291, 291*b*
for caregiving, 391–392
for dysphagia, 136–138
for grief, 363, 363*b*, 402–404, 403*b*
for hydration management, 147, 148*b*
for insomnia, 174*b*
nutritional, 141–142, 141*b*
for oral health, 150–152, 151*b*
for osteoarthritis (OA), 283
for respiratory disorders, 293
in sexuality, 382
for sleep disordered breathing and sleep apnea, 176–178
for sleep disorders, 173–176
for urinary incontinence, 157–163, 159*b*
Interview, in assessment, of nutrition, 139–141
Intestines, 33
Intimacy, 369–370, 370*f*. *see also* Sexuality
chronic illness and, 376, 376*f*, 376*t*–378*t*
dementia and, 379
in long-term care facilities, 376–379
Intraocular changes, aging-related, 36
Intrinsic risk factors, in fall, 204

J
Johnson, Lyndon B., 82
Joint problems, bone and, 276–285

K
Kayser-Jones Brief Oral Health Status Examination (BOHSE), 148, 150
Kennedy Terminal Ulcer, 195
Keratoconjunctivitis sicca, 256
Keratoses, 187–188
Ketoprofen, in herb-medication and herb-disease interactions, 116*t*–117*t*
Khyâl cap (wind attacks), 311*b*
Knee brace, 283–284
Knowledge, cultural, 15–17
Kübler-Ross, Elisabeth, 398

L
Late life income, 79–81, 81*b*
Late-life anxiety, 313
Late-onset schizophrenia, 318
Later life
learning in, 51–52
relationships in, 363–364
transitions, 360–361
death of a spouse/life partner, 362, 362*b*
retirement, 360–361, 362*b*
Laxatives
bulk, 166–167
natural, recipe for, 167*b*
stimulant, 167
LDL. *see* Low-density lipoprotein (LDL)
LEARN model, 18–20, 18*b*
Learning opportunities for adults, 51–52
Legal issues, 88–90
capacity, 88
guardians and conservators, 89–90
health care proxy, 89, 89*b*
power of attorney, 89
Lemon glycerin swabs, 152*b*
Lesbian, gay, bisexual, and transgender (LGBT), older, 367, 367*b*, 375
Levodopa, 127*t*
Levodopa-carbidopa, 303*b*
Levothyroxine
appropriate administration of, 267*b*
for hyperthyroidism, 266
for hypothyroidism, 266
Life expectancy, at birth, 4*f*
Life review, 45, 45*f*
Life story, 43
Lifelong eating habits, 135
Lifestyle modifications, for urinary incontinence, 160–161
Lingler, Jennifer, 57*b*
Lithium, for bipolar disorder, 321
Long stay quality measures, 72
Long term care (LTC) setting, 60–61
outcomes of APNs, 61*b*
Long-distance caregiving, 390
Long-term care, 70–71, 70*f*, 71*b*
costs of, 71
culture change movement, 74, 74*b*–75*b*
elder with diabetes and, 274
facilities
documentation of, 106
intimacy and sexuality in, 376–379
nutrition in, 136, 137*b*
oral hygiene in, 152
resident bill of rights, 73, 73*b*
Long-term care insurance (LTCI), 87–88
Loss, 397–413. *see also* Grief
factors affecting coping with, 401, 401*b*
Loss Response Model, 398–399, 399*f*
Loss Response Model (LRM), 398–399, 399*f*
Low-density lipoprotein (LDL), 131–132
Low-vision optical devices, 257–258
LRM. *see* Loss Response Model (LRM)
LTCI. *see* Long-term care insurance (LTCI)
Lucentis, for age-related macular degeneration, 255
Lungs, aging-related changes in, 30*f*, 31*b*

M
Macular degeneration, age-related, 252*f*, 254–255, 255*f*
Macular edema, diabetic, 254
Male reproductive system, age-changes with, 32
Malnutrition (undernutrition), 133–134. *see also* Nutrition
characteristics of, 134
consequences of, 133
incidence of, 133
interventions for, 141–142, 141*b*
interview and, 139–141
patient education on, 142
pharmacological therapy for, 142
risk factors of, 133, 134*f*
Managed care plan (MCP), 85
Mandatory reporting, of abuse, 394–395
MCP. *see* Managed care plan (MCP)
Meaning, searching for, 402*b*, 403
Medicaid, 86–87
costs of LTC and, 71

Medical device-related pressure injury, 193–195
Medicare, 82–86, 82*b*, 83*t*
costs of LTC and, 71
parts
A, 83–84, 83*b*
B, 84–85, 84*b*
C, 85
D, 85, 86*b*
Medication review, 176
Medication-food interactions, 116–118, 117*t*, 118*b*
Medication-herb/supplement interactions, 116, 116*t*–117*t*
Medication-related problems, and older adults, 115–120
adverse drug reactions in, 118–119, 119*b*
drug interactions in, 115–118
misuse of drugs in, 119–120, 119*b*
polypharmacy in, 115, 115*f*
Medications
affecting sleep, 172*b*
diabetes and, 273–274
in fall risk reduction, 207
osteoporosis and, 279
respiratory disorders and, 294
Meditation, 245–246
Melanoma, 191, 192*b*, 197*b*
Melatonin, endogenous nocturnal, 175
Memories, reframing, 402*b*, 403
Memory, 50
Mental disorders, mental health and, 310*b*
Mental health, 309–335
factors influencing, 310–313
mental disorders and, 310*b*
settings of, 312–313
Mental health disorders, 313
alcohol use disorder as, 328–329
assessment of, 329–330, 330*t*, 331*b*
consequences of, 329
gender issues in, 328–329
interventions for, 330–332
physiology of, 329
prevalence and characteristics of, 328
anxiety disorders as, 313
assessment of, 313–314, 314*b*
interventions for, 314–315
nonpharmacological approaches for, 315, 315*b*
pharmacological approaches for, 314–315
prevalence and characteristics of, 313
bipolar disorder as, 320, 321*b*
Mental health disorders *(Continued)*
depression as, 321–323
assessment of, 323–325, 324*b*, 324*f*
collaborative care for, 325
consequences of, 322
etiology of, 322–323, 323*b*
family and professional support for, 327*b*
interventions for, 325–326
medications and, 323*b*
nonpharmacological approaches for, 325, 325*f*
pharmacological approaches for, 325–326
prevalence of, 321–322
racial, ethnic and cultural considerations for, 322
risk factors for, 323*b*
treatment of, 326
posttraumatic stress disorder as, 315–316, 316*b*
psychotic symptoms of, 318–319
assessment of, 319–320
delusions as, 319, 319*b*
hallucinations as, 319, 319*b*
interventions for, 320, 320*f*
schizophrenia as, 317–318, 317*b*
substance use disorders as, 328–329
suicide and, 326–327
Mental status, assessment of, 99–102, 99*b*
Metabolic disorders, 265–275
diabetes, 267–270
thyroid disease, 265–267, 266*b*
Metabolism, in pharmacokinetics, 112–113, 113*b*, 113*t*
Minerals, 132–133
Mini Nutritional Assessment (MNA), 139, 354
Mini-Cog, 100, 100*b*
Mini-Mental State Exam-2 (MMSE-2), for delirium, 341
Mini-Mental State Examination (MMSE), 99
Minimum Data Set 3.0 (MDS 3.0), 104–105, 105*b*, 139
for assessment of urinary incontinence, 157
Mistreatment, elder, 392–394, 392*b*, 394*b*
definition of, 392
neglect and, 393–394
prevention of, 395, 395*b*
self-neglect and, 393–394
Mitochondria, in young and old cells, 24*f*
Mixed incontinence, 157*t*
Mixed pain, 237*b*
MNA. *see* Mini Nutritional Assessment (MNA)
Modernization theory of aging, 42
Monitoring, in safe medication use, 126–128, 127*b*, 127*t*
Mood measures, for mental status, 100–102
Mood stabilizers, 122
Morse Falls Scale, 208
Motion sensors, in fall risk reduction, 211
Mourning, 398
Mouth, age-related changes to, 32–33
Mouth care, respiratory disorders and, 295
Mouth dryness, 149
Mucosal membrane pressure injury, 195
Multidisciplinary care, for respiratory disorders, 294–295
Multigenerational families, 364–365, 365*b*
Musculoskeletal system, 276
aging-related changes in, 28–29, 28*t*
arthritides, 279–282, 279*t*
assessment of, 282–284, 283*f*
gout, 281–282, 282*b*
interventions for, 282–284, 283*t*
osteoarthritis, 277*f*, 279–280, 279*t*, 280*f*
polymyalgia rheumatica and giant cell arteritis, 280–281
by race/ethnicity, prevalence of, 279, 280*t*
rheumatoid, 281, 281*b*
Healthy People 2020 and, 282, 282*b*
osteoporosis, 277–278, 277*f*
pharmacological interventions for, 278–279, 278*b*–279*b*
reducing risk and injury related to, 278
risk factors for, 277, 277*b*
Mutual pretense, 406
MyPlate, 131, 132*f*
Myxedema coma, 266–267

N

Nails, age-related changes in, 27–28
National Council on Aging (NCOA), 58–59
National Elder Law Foundation (NELF), 90
National Eye Health Education Program (NEHEP), 250
National Family Caregiver Support Program (NFCSP), 390

National Institute of Nursing Research (NINR), 59
National Pressure Ulcer Advisory Panel (NPUAP), 192
Native intelligence, 50
Natural disasters, vulnerability to, 218*b*, 221
Naturalistic model, 17*t*
Naylor, Mary, 76
NCOA. *see* National Council on Aging (NCOA)
Need-driven dementia-compromised behavior model, 347–348
Neglect, of elder, 393–394
NEHEP. *see* National Eye Health Education Program (NEHEP)
NELF. *see* National Elder Law Foundation (NELF)
Neurocognitive disorders, 336–359
  activities of daily living and, 351–352, 351*f*
  behavior concerns and nursing models of care for, 346–348
  communication for, 344–345, 344*b*, 346*b*
  delirium as, 336–340
    assessment of, 340–341, 340*b*
    causes of, 339*b*
    clinical subtypes of, 339, 339*b*
    cognitive assessment of, 340
    consequences of, 339–340, 340*b*
    dementia, depression and, 337, 338*t*
    diagnosis of, 337*b*
    etiology of, 337
    incidence and prevalence of, 337
    recognition of, 338
    risk factors for, 338–339, 339*b*
    superimposed on mild and major neurocognitive disorders, 337–338
  dementia as, 337–338, 340*b*
    assessment of, 348–349, 348*b*, 349*t*
    delirium, depression and, 337, 338*t*
    interventions for, 341–342, 349–351
    nonpharmacological approaches for, 341–342, 341*b*–342*b*, 350–351, 350*f*, 351*b*
    nursing roles for, 354–355
    pharmacological approaches for, 342, 343*b*, 343*f*, 349–350, 349*b*–350*b*
  wandering and, 353, 353*b*–354*b*
  mild and major, 342–344
Neurocognitive disorders *(Continued)*
  need-driven dementia-compromised behavior model for, 347–348
  person-centered care for, 343–344, 344*b*
  progressively lowered stress threshold model for, 347, 347*b*
  reality orientation for, 345
Neurodegenerative disorders, 301–304
  Alzheimer's disease, 303–304, 303*b*
  aphasia, 305–306
  communication and persons with, 305–307
  dysarthria, 306
  nursing care for, 304
  Parkinson's disease, 301–303
Neuroleptic malignant syndrome (NMS), 123
Neuroleptics, 122–124
Neurological disorders, 297–308
  cerebrovascular diseases, 298–300, 298*f*
    hemorrhagic events, 299–300
    ischemic events, 298–299
  enhancing communication and, 306–307
  neurodegenerative disorders, 301–304
    Alzheimer's disease, 303–304, 303*b*
    aphasia, 305–306
    communication and persons with, 305–307
    dysarthria, 306
    nursing care for, 304
    Parkinson's disease, 301–303
Neurological system, aging-related changes to, 34–35, 34*t*
Neuropathic pain, 237*b*
Neuroplasticity, 49–50
Never-married older adults, 368
NFCSP. *see* National Family Caregiver Support Program (NFCSP)
NICHE. *see* Nurses Improving Care for Health system Elders (NICHE)
NIHL. *see* Noise-induced hearing loss (NIHL)
NINR. *see* National Institute of Nursing Research (NINR)
NMS. *see* Neuroleptic malignant syndrome (NMS)
Nociceptive pain, 237*b*
Nocturia, 289
Noise-induced hearing loss (NIHL), 258
Nonblanchable erythema, of intact skin, 193, 193*f*
Nonfluent (Broca's) aphasia, 305
Non-Hispanic blacks, diabetes among, 268, 268*t*
Non-Hispanic whites, diabetes among, 268, 268*t*
Nonopioid analgesics, 243–244
Non-rapid eye movement (NREM) sleep, 171
Nonsteroidal anti-inflammatory medications (NSAIDs), 127*t*
  in herb-medication and herb-disease interactions, 116*t*–117*t*
  pain and, 243
Nontraditional couples, 367
Nosocomial, pneumonia, 292
NPUAP. *see* National Pressure Ulcer Advisory Panel (NPUAP)
NSAIDs. *see* Nonsteroidal anti-inflammatory medications (NSAIDs)
Nurse
  dying and, 407–410, 408*t*, 409*b*
  goal of, 197–198
Nurse Competence in Aging, 57
Nurses Improving Care for Health system Elders (NICHE), 61–62
Nursing, spirituality and, 47–48, 47*b*
Nursing assessment, in fall risk reduction, 208*t*
Nursing homes, 69–70
  sleep in, 174–175, 175*b*
Nursing roles, in caring for persons with chronic illness, 234*b*
Nutrition, 130–144
  aging and, 135–138, 150–152
  assessment of, 135–136
  chronic diseases and conditions and, 135
  COPD and, 294*b*
  dehydration and, 145–146, 146*b*
  dementia and, 136–138, 137*b*, 353–354, 354*f*, 355*b*
  diabetes and, 273
  dysphagia and, 131
  in FANCAPES, 98
  food/ nutrient intake and, 139–140
  Healthy People 2020 on, 131, 131*b*
  hydration management and, 145
  hypertension and, 130
  lifelong eating habits and, 135
  MyPlate on, 131, 132*f*
  obesity and, 133
  for older adults, 131, 132*b*, 132*f*
  patient education on, 142
  screening for, 139, 139*f*
  socialization and, 135
  socioeconomic deprivation and, 138

Nutrition *(Continued)*
transportation and, 138
weight/ height considerations and, 140

O
OA. *see* Osteoarthritis (OA)
OAA. *see* Older Americans Act (OAA)
OARS. *see* Older Americans Resources and Services (OARS)
OARS Multidimensional Functional Assessment Questionnaire (OMFAQ), 104
Obesity (overnutrition), 133
OBRA. *see* Omnibus Budget Reconciliation Act (OBRA)
Obscured full-thickness skin, tissue loss and, 194, 194*f*
Obstructive sleep apnea (OSA), 176
risk factors for, 176*b*
Ocular changes, aging-related, 35–36
Olanzapine, in herb-medication and herb-disease interactions, 116*t*–117*t*
"Old," recognize as, 3
OLD CART acronym, 239–240, 240*b*
Older adults
adult children and, 367–368
alcohol guidelines for, 329
alcohol problems in, 331*b*
care of, 55–56, 56*b*
dental health goals for, 149*b*
emerging issues in health of, 8*b*
gerontological nurses and, 63, 63*f*
gerontological nursing and healthy aging, 8
HIV/AIDS and, 379–381
medication-related problems and, 115–120
never-married, 368
nutrition for, 131, 132*b*, 132*f*
psychotic disorders in, 318–319
Older Americans Act (OAA), 135
Older Americans Resources and Services (OARS), 104
"Older generation", 6
OMFAQ. *see* OARS Multidimensional Functional Assessment Questionnaire (OMFAQ)
Omnibus Budget Reconciliation Act (OBRA), 71–72
Open awareness, 406–407
Opioid analgesics, 244
Optimal care, 92–109
assessment process of, 93–94, 93*b*
comprehensive geriatric assessments of, 103–105
Fulmer SPICES in, 104
Optimal care *(Continued)*
OARS Multidimensional Functional Assessment Questionnaire in, 104
Outcome and Assessment Information Set (OASIS-C1) in, 105
Resident Assessment Instrument (RAI)/Minimum Data Set (MDS 3.0), 104–105, 105*b*
functional assessment of, 102–103
health history of, 94–96, 95*b*
implications of, for gerontological nursing and healthy aging, 107
mental status in, assessment of, 99–102
cognitive measures in, 99–100
mood measures in, 100–102
physical assessment in, 96–99, 97*t*
frail and medically complex elder, 96–99
quality care and, documentation for, 105–106
Oral cancer, 149, 150*b*
Oral care, 149–150
in hospitals and long-term care, 152
hydration and, 148*b*
provision of, 151*b*
Oral health, 148–150
assessment of, 150
Healthy People 2020 on, 149*b*
interventions for, 150–152, 151*b*
promoting, 149*b*
Oral problems, 149
Organizations, gerontology, 58–59
Orthopnea, 289
Orthostatic, in fall risk reduction, 206
OSA. *see* Obstructive sleep apnea (OSA)
Osteoarthritis (OA), 277*f*, 279–280, 279*t*, 280*f*
interventions for, 283
rhythmical influences on, 114*t*
Osteopenia, 277
Osteophytes, 280
Osteoporosis, 277–278, 277*f*
pharmacological interventions for, 278–279, 278*b*–279*b*
reducing risk and injury related to, 278
risk factors for, 277, 277*b*
Osteoporosis treatment, in fall risk reduction, 211
Outcome and Assessment Information Set (OASIS-C1), 105, 105*b*
Overactive bladder, 161
Overnutrition, 133
Over-the-counter (OTC) sleep aids, 175
Oxidative stress theories, 23–25

P
PACE. *see* Program of All-Inclusive Care for the Elderly (PACE)
PACSLAC. *see Pain Assessment Checklist for Seniors with Limited Ability to Communicate* (PACSLAC)
Pain, comfort and, 236–248
acute, 237–238
assessment of, 239–241, 240*b*, 241*f*
chronic, 237–238
cognitive impairment and, 238–239, 239*b*, 241*b*
communication and, 238–239, 239*b*
culture on expressions of, 237*b*
evaluation of, 246–247, 246*b*
fact and fiction about, 239*b*
interventions of, 241–246, 242*b*
management of, 238*b*
nonpharmacological, 245–246
pain clinics, 246
pharmacological, 243–245
mixed or unspecified, 237*b*
neuropathic, 237*b*
nociceptive, 237*b*
persistent, 237, 237*b*
visual analog scales for, 240, 241*f*
Pain Assessment Checklist for Seniors with Limited Ability to Communicate (PACSLAC), 241
Pain Assessment in Advanced Dementia Scale (PAINAD), 241, 242*t*
Pain clinics, 246
PAINAD. *see Pain Assessment in Advanced Dementia Scale* (PAINAD)
Palliative care, 397–413
dying, death and, 404–405
Pancreas, age-related changes in, 31
Paranoia, in schizophrenia, 318
Paranoid ideation, 319–320
Parkinsonian symptoms, 123
Parkinson's disease, 301–303
annual medical exam for, 304*b*
genetics and, 302*b*
management of, 302–303
signs and symptoms of, 302, 302*b*
Paroxetine, in herb-medication and herb-disease interactions, 116*t*–117*t*
Partial-thickness skin loss, with exposed dermis, 194, 194*f*

Patient education
  on diabetes self-management, 272–273, 272*b*
  on nutrition, 142
  on osteoporosis, 278
Patient Self-Determination Act (PSDA), 410
Payne-Martin classification, in skin tears, 187
Pelvic floor muscle exercises (PFMEs), 159
Penicillin, 5–6
Percutaneous endoscopic gastrotomy (PEG) tubes, 137, 137*b*
Peripheral nervous system, 34–35
Persistent depressive disorder, 322
Persistent pain, 237, 237*b*
Personalistic model (magicoreligious), 17*t*
Person-centered culture, 74
PFMEs. *see* Pelvic floor muscle exercises (PFMEs)
Pharmacodynamics, 114
Pharmacokinetics, 111–114
  absorption in, 112
  aging and, 111, 111*f*
  definition of, 111
  distribution in, 112
  excretion in, 113–114
  metabolism in, 112–113, 113*b*, 113*t*
Pharmacological therapy, for malnutrition, 142
Phenotype, of aging, 4*b*
Physical activity, 170–184
  aging and, 178–179, 179*b*
  assessment of, 179
  for constipation, 165–166
  guidelines for, 180, 180*b*
  health benefits of, 178*b*
  Healthy People 2020 and, 179*b*
  incorporation of, into lifestyle, 180
  interventions for, 179–182
  osteoporosis and, 278
  screening for, 179
  special considerations for, 180–182, 181*f*–182*f*
Physical assessment, 96–99, 97*t*
Physical contact, in LEARN model, 18
Physical examination, in postfall assessment suggestions, 209
Physician Orders for Life-Sustaining Treatment (POLST) program, 409
Physician-assisted suicide, 411
Pioneer Network, 74
Pittsburgh Sleep Quality Index (PSQI), 173
Planning, retirement, 361
Platelet activation, rhythmical influences on, 114*t*
PLISSIT model, 382, 382*b*
PMR. *see* Polymyalgia rheumatica (PMR)
Pneumococcal immunizations, promoting, 8*t*
Pneumococcal vaccine, 295
Pneumonia, 292, 292*b*
POA. *see* Power of attorney (POA)
Pocket-sized amplifier, 261, 261*f*
Polio infection, 5–6
Polymyalgia rheumatica (PMR), 280–281
Polypharmacy, 115, 115*f*
Polysomnogram, 176
Porous bone. *see* Osteoporosis
Positioning, for constipation, 166
Postherpetic neuralgia, 238
Postprandial hypotension, in fall risk reduction, 206
Posttraumatic stress disorder, 315–316
  assessment of, 316–317, 317*b*
  interventions for, 317
  prevalence of, 315–316, 316*b*
  symptoms of, 316
Posture, 28–29
Potassium excretion, rhythmical influences on, 114*t*
Power of attorney (POA), 89
PPOs. *see* Preferred provider organizations (PPOs)
Precompetence, cultural, 14–15
Preferred provider organizations (PPOs), 85
Presbycusis, 36, 258
Presbyopia, 35
Prescription bottle magnifier, 257*f*
Pressure injuries, 192–196, 193*b*
  characteristics of, 193
  classification of, 193–195, 195*b*
  consequences of, 196
  cost and regulatory requirements of, 193
  definition of, 192
  factors to consider in, 198*b*
  mnemonic for, 198*b*
  prevention of, 196
    and treatment, 188*b*
  risk factors, 195–196
  scope of the problem, 192–193
  stages of, 193*b*–194*b*
Pressure Ulcer Scale for Healing (PUSH) tool, 198
Prevention, of respiratory disorders, 295
Proficiency, cultural, 15
Progesterone, in herb-medication and herb-disease interactions, 116*t*–117*t*
Program of All-Inclusive Care for the Elderly (PACE), 67
Progressively lowered stress threshold model, 347, 347*b*
Promoting safety, 217–227
  elder-friendly communities and, 225, 226*f*
  emerging technologies for, in older adults, 223–225
  environmental temperatures and, vulnerability to, 217–220
  gerontological nursing and healthy aging and, implications for, 220, 223
  home safety and, 217
  natural disasters and, vulnerability to, 218*b*, 221
  transportation safety and, 221–223, 222*b*–224*b*
Prompted voiding, 160, 161*b*
Proprioception, 34–35
Prostate screening (PSA and DRE), 8*t*
Protease inhibitors, in herb-medication and herb-disease interactions, 116*t*–117*t*
Protein, 132
Pruritus, 186
PSDA. *see* Patient Self-Determination Act (PSDA)
PSQI. *see* Pittsburgh Sleep Quality Index (PSQI)
Psychoactive medications, 120–124
  aging and, 113*t*
  antianxiety agents as, 121–122
  antidepressants as, 121
  antipsychotics as, 122–124
  mood stabilizers as, 122
Psychoeducation, bipolar disorder and, 321
Psychosis, 122
Psychosocial theories, of aging, 41–45
  first generation, 41
  second generation, 41–43
  third generation, 43–45
Psychotic symptoms, 318–319
  assessment of, 319–320
  delusions as, 319, 319*b*
  hallucinations as, 319, 319*b*
  interventions for, 320, 320*f*
Purines, foods high in, 282, 282*b*

Q
Quality care, documentation for, 105–106
Quality of care, in skilled nursing facilities, 71–72, 72*b*, 73*f*

R
RA. *see* Rheumatoid arthritis (RA)
Race and ethnicity, chest pain, 288*b*
Racism, 14*b*
RAI. *see* Resident Assessment Instrument (RAI)
Ranitidine, 127*t*
Rapid eye movement (REM) sleep, 171
 behavior disorder, 177–178
Rapid transcranial magnetic stimulation (rTMS), for depression, 326
RDA. *see* Recommended Dietary Allowance (RDA)
Readmissions, 75
Reality orientation, for neurocognitive disorders, 345
Recommended Dietary Allowance (RDA), 132
Red yeast rice, in herb-medication and herb-disease interactions, 116*t*–117*t*
Reframing memories, 402*b*, 403
Rehabilitation
 after stroke, 300
 respiratory disorders and, 295
Rehydration methods, 147
Reimbursement, documentation and, 106, 107*b*
Relationships. *see also* Sexuality
 families and, 364–369
  elders and adult children in, 367–368
  fictive kin in, 369
  grandparents in, 368–369, 368*f*–369*f*, 369*b*
  nontraditional couples in, 367
  siblings in, 369
  traditional couples in, 366–367
  types of, 366–369
 intimacy and, 369–370, 370*f*
  chronic illness and, 376, 376*f*, 376*t*–378*t*
  dementia and, 379
  in long-term care facilities, 376–379
 roles, and transitions, 360–385
Relaxation, in pain management, 245–246
Religion, spirituality and, 46
Remeron, 121
Reminiscence, 43–45
 encouraging, 44*b*
Renal system, 31
Reperfusion therapy, 299, 300*b*
Reproductive system, age-changes with, 32
Research, gerontological nursing, 59–60
Resident Assessment Instrument (RAI), 104–105, 105*b*
Residential care/assisted living (RC/AL), 67*t*, 68–69
Resilience, 309
Respiratory disorders, 291–292
 assessment of, 292–293, 293*b*
 chronic obstructive pulmonary disease, 291–292
 interventions for, 293
 multidisciplinary care for, 294–295
 pneumonia, 292
Respiratory system, 30–31, 30*f*, 31*b*
Rest, 170–184
 sleep and, 170–172
Restless legs syndrome/Willis-Ekbom disease (RLS/WED), 177
Restraints, 212–214
 consequences of, 212
 definition and history of, 212
 prevention interventions in, 214*b*
 side rails and, 212
Restraints-free care, 212–214, 213*f*
Retina, detached, 255
Retinopathy, diabetic, 252*f*, 253–254
Retirement, 360–361, 362*b*
 planning, 361
 special considerations in, 361
Rheumatoid arthritis (RA), 281, 281*b*
 rhythmical influences on, 114*t*
Risk reduction
 falls, 201–216, 202*b*
  consequences of, 202–204
  interventions of, 209–211
  postfall assessment, 208–209, 209*b*
  prevention, 202*b*
  restraint alternatives, 203*b*
  risk assessment instruments, 207–208
  risk factors, 204–206
  screening and assessment of, 207
 programs, 209–210
RLS/WED. *see* Restless legs syndrome/Willis-Ekbom disease (RLS/WED)
Road Scholar program, 51–52
Robots, 225
Role theory of aging, 41
Rome III criteria, for constipation, 164*b*
Roosevelt, Franklin D., 82

S
SAFE DRIVE, 223, 223*b*
Safe medication use, 110–129
 chronopharmacology, 114–115, 114*t*
 for gerontological nursing and healthy aging, 124–128
Safe medication use *(Continued)*
 medication-related problems, and older adults, 115–120
 pharmacodynamics, 114
 pharmacokinetics, 111–114, 111*f*
 psychoactive medications, 120–124
Safe patient handling, in fall risk reduction, 211, 211*b*
Safety, promoting, 217–227
 elder-friendly communities and, 225, 226*f*
 emerging technologies for, in older adults, 223–225
 environmental temperatures and, vulnerability to, 217–220
 gerontological nursing and healthy aging and, implications for, 220, 223
 home safety and, 217
 natural disasters and, vulnerability to, 218*b*, 221
 transportation safety and, 221–223, 222*b*–224*b*
Sarcopenia, 28
Sarcoptes scabiei, 186–187
Satir, Virginia, 369
Saunders, Cicely, 409
Scabies, 186–187
 treatment of, 187
Scheduled (timed) voiding, 158–159
Schizophrenia, 317–318, 317*b*
Searching for meaning, 402*b*, 403
Sebaceous glands, 27
Seborrheic keratosis, 187, 188*f*
Second generation psychosocial theories, of aging, 41–43
Selective serotonin reuptake inhibitors (SSRIs), 121
 for depression, 326
Self-monitoring blood glucose (SMBG), 272–273, 272*b*
Self-neglect, elder, 393–394
Sensorineural hearing loss, 258
Sexuality, 370–371
 activity levels and, 372, 372*f*
 alternative sexual lifestyles and, 375
 assessment of, 381–382, 382*b*
 biological changes with age and, 373, 374*t*
 cohort and cultural influences in, 372–373
 dementia and, 379
 expectations about, 372
 female dysfunction and, 374–375
 interrelationship of dimensions of, 371*f*
 interventions in, 382
 in long-term care facilities, 376–379
 male dysfunction and, 373–374

Sexuality *(Continued)*
  sexual dysfunction and, 373–375
  sexual health and, 370*b*, 371–373, 371*f*
Shadow grief, 400, 400*b*
Shifting Perspectives Model of chronic illness, 232–233
Shingles vaccination, 8*t*
Short Michigan Alcoholism Screening Test-Geriatric Version, 330, 330*t*
Short stay quality measures, 72
Siblings, 369
Sigma Theta Tau's Center for Nursing Excellence in Long-Term Care, 57–58
Six C's approach, to dying, 405–407, 405*b*
Skilled nursing facilities, 69–70
  quality of care in, 71–72, 72*b*, 73*f*
Skin, 186
  aging-related changes in, 26–28, 26*t*
  cancers, 190–191
    basal cell carcinoma, 190
    facts and figures, 190
    melanoma, 191, 192*b*, 197*b*
    squamous cell carcinoma, 190–191
  common skin problems, 186–190
    candidiasis *(Candida albicans)*, 189–190
    herpes zoster, 188–189
    keratoses, 187–188
    photo damage of, 190
    pruritus, 186
    purpura, 187
    scabies, 186–187
    skin tears, 187
    xerosis, 186
  pressure injuries, 192–196, 193*b*
    characteristics of, 193
    classification of, 193–195, 195*b*
    consequences of, 196
    cost and regulatory requirements of, 193
    definition of, 192
    factors to consider in, 198*b*
    mnemonic for, 198*b*
    prevention, and treatment, 188*b*, 196
    risk factors, 195–196
    scope of the problem, 192–193
    stages of, 193*b*–194*b*
  promoting healthy, 185–200, 192*b*
Skin failure, 195
Skin flaps, 187
Skin tears, 187
  management of, 187
Sleep, 170–184
  aging and, 171–172, 172*b*
    changes with, 171*b*
  biorhythm and, 171
Sleep *(Continued)*
  disorders in, 172
    assessment of, 173, 173*b*
    circadian rhythm, 178
    insomnia, 172, 172*b*
    interventions for, 173–176
    nonpharmacological treatment for, 173–175
    pharmacological treatment for, 175–176, 175*b*–176*b*
    rapid eye movement sleep behavior, 177–178
    restless legs syndrome/Willis-Ekbom disease (RLS/WED), 177
    sleep apnea, 176
  Healthy People 2020 and, 171*b*
  in hospitals and nursing homes, 174–175, 175*b*
  insufficient, 171
  non-rapid eye movement (NREM), 171
  rapid eye movement (REM), 171
  rest and, 170
Sleep aids, over-the-counter, 175
Sleep diary, 173, 173*b*
Sleep study, 176
Sliding scale insulin, 273–274
Smart homes, 224–225
SMBG. *see* Self-monitoring blood glucose (SMBG)
Social aging, 3
Social exchange theory of aging, 42
Social networks, adults and, 52
Social Security, 80–82, 80*t*
Social Security Act, 80
Social skills, in FANCAPES, 99, 99*b*
Socialization
  in FANCAPES, 99, 99*b*
  nutrition and, 135
Specialist roles in gerontological nursing, 60–61
Speech, apraxia of, 305
Spiritual distress, 46–47
  identifying elders at risk for, 47*b*
Spiritual well-being, 46
Spirituality
  aging and, 46–47, 46*f*
  assessment of, 47–48, 47*b*
  definition of, 46
  interventions, 48, 48*b*
  of nurses, 48
  nursing and, 47–48, 47*b*
  religion and, 46
Spousal caregiving, 388
Squamous cell carcinoma, 190–191
SSI. *see* Supplemental Security Income (SSI)
Steri-Strips, 187
Stimulant laxatives, 167
St.John's wort, in herb-medication and herb-disease interactions, 116*t*–117*t*
Stomach, 33
Stool softeners, 167
Storytelling, 43, 45*f*
Streptococcal immunizations, promoting, 8*t*
Stress, factors influencing, 310*b*
Stress incontinence, 157*t*
Stroke
  assessment of, 300*b*
  complications of, 299
  intimacy and, 376*t*–378*t*
  management of, 299–300
  rate of, 298
Sub-acute care, 69–70, 69*b*
Substance use disorders, 328–329, 328*b*
Substituted judgment, 410
Suicide, 326–327
  assessment of, 327, 327*b*
  depression and, 326–327
  interventions for, 328
Sulfonylureas, 127*t*
Super-centenarians, 4–5, 5*b*
Supplemental Security Income (SSI), 81
Surgical treatment, for urinary incontinence, 162
Suspected awareness, 406
Susto (fright), 311*b*
Systemic insulin level, rhythmical influences on, 114*t*

T
Tai chi, for sleep disorders, 174
Tardive dyskinesia, 123–124
T-cell function, 37
TCM. *see* Transitional Care Model (TCM)
Telehealth, 224
Telomere caps, chromosomes with, 25*f*
Telomeres, 25–26, 25*b*
Temperature
  environmental, 217–220
    hyperthermia and, 218–219, 219*b*
    hypothermia and, 219–220, 220*b*
    thermoregulation and, 218, 218*b*
  monitoring, in older adults, 218
Temporal arteritis. *see* Giant cell arteritis (GCA)
TENS. *see* Transcutaneous electrical nerve stimulation (TENS)
Tetracyclic antidepressant mirtazapine, 121
TFL. *see* TRICARE for Life (TFL)

Theophylline, in herb-medication and herb-disease interactions, 116*t*–117*t*
Thermoregulation, 218, 218*b*
Third generation psychosocial theories, of aging, 43–45
Throat cancer, 150*b*
Thyroid, age-related changes in, 31–32
Thyroid disease, 265–267, 266*b*
  complications of, 266–267
TIA. *see* Transient ischemic attack (TIA)
Time, orientation to, 16
TimeSlips program, 45
Tinnitus, 262–263
Toileting regimen, for constipation, 166
Tonometry, 253
Touch therapies, 245
Traditional couples, 366–367
Tramadol, in herb-medication and herb-disease interactions, 116*t*–117*t*
Transcutaneous electrical nerve stimulation (TENS), 245
Transient incontinence, 156
Transient ischemic attack (TIA), 299
  assessment after, 300*b*
  complications of, 299
  management of, 299–300
  signs and symptoms of, 299
  stroke risk after, 299*b*
Transitional care
  improving, 75–76, 76*b*–77*b*
  outcomes, factors contributing to poor, 75, 75*b*
Transitional Care Model (TCM), 76
Transitions
  across the continuum, 74–76
  later life, 360–361
    death of a spouse/life partner, 362, 362*b*
    retirement, 360–361, 362*b*
Transportation, nutrition and, 138
Transportation safety, 221–223
  driving and, 221–223
Traumatic brain injury, in fall risk reduction, 202–203
  signs and symptoms of, 203*b*
Trazodone, 121
TRICARE for Life (TFL), 87
Triptans, in herb-medication and herb-disease interactions, 116*t*–117*t*
Tube feeding, oral hygiene and, 152
Tylenol (acetaminophen), 243–244, 243*b*

U
Unspecified pain, 237*b*
Urge incontinence, 157*t*
Urinary catheters, 162–163
  external, 163
  indwelling, indications for use of, 162, 162*b*
Urinary incontinence, 155–156
  alcohol use disorder and, 329
  assessment for, 156–157, 160*f*
    resources for, 159*b*
    tips for best practice in, 158*b*
  consequences of, 156
  definition of, 155
  facts and figures, 155–156
  interventions for, 157–163, 163*b*
    behavioral, 157–161, 159*b*
    lifestyle modifications as, 160–161
    nonsurgical devices as, 162–163
    pharmacological treatment in, 161–162
    promotion of continence friendly environment as, 161
    surgical treatment as, 162
  prevalence of, 155
  risk factors for, 156, 156*b*
  symptoms of, 157*t*
  types, 156, 157*t*
Urinary tract infections, 156, 163
  catheter-associated, 163, 163*b*
Urine
  color of, hydration and, 147
  creatinine, 31

V
VA. *see* Veterans Health Administration (VA)
Vaginal screening, 8*t*
Validation therapy, for delirium, 345
Verbal apraxia, 305
Verbal communication, in LEARN model, 18
Veterans Health Administration (VA), 87
Vision
  diseases affecting, 249–264
  in fall risk reduction, 207
Visual analog scales, 240, 241*f*
Visual impairment, 249–250
  aging-related, 35–36
  assessment of, 256
  communication and, 257*b*
  consequences of, 250
  disease-related, 250–256
    age-related macular degeneration, 252*f*, 254–255
    cataracts, 250–251, 252*f*
    detached retina, 255
Visual impairment *(Continued)*
    diabetic macular edema, 254
    diabetic retinopathy, 252*f*, 253–254
    dry eye, 256
    glaucoma, 251–253, 252*f*, 253*b*
  interventions to enhance vision, 256–258, 256*f*
  low-vision optical devices for, 257–258
  prevention of, 250, 250*b*–251*b*
Vitamin D supplementation, in fall risk reduction, 211
Vitamin K, warfarin and, 289
Vitamins, 132–133
Voice-clarifying headset system, 261*f*
Voiding
  prompted, 160, 161*b*
  scheduled (timed), 158–159
Voiding diary, 158*b*, 160*f*

W
Wandering, dementia and, 353, 353*b*–354*b*
Warfarin
  in atrial fibrillation, 289
  in medication-herb/supplement interactions, 116, 116*t*–117*t*
Wear-and-tear theory, 23*b*
Weight history, 140
Weisman, Avery, 403
Wellbutrin, for depression, 326
Wellness
  definition of, 7
  example of interventions to promote, 8*t*
Wellspring Model, 74
Western model, 17, 17*t*
Wheelchairs, in fall risk reduction, 211
Wolanin, Mary Opal, 57*b*
Women, sexuality and, 372–373, 375
Working with interpreters, in LEARN model, 18–19, 19*b*
World Health Organization, 371–372

X
Xerosis, 186
Xerostomia, 32–33, 149

Y
Years ahead, of older adults, 2–3, 2*f*–3*f*
"YouTube" reminiscence therapy, 44

Z
Zaleplon, 176
Zolpidem, 176